FASCIA in the OSTEOPATHIC FIELD

FASCIA in the OSTEOPATHIC FIELD

Edited by
Torsten LIEM
Paolo TOZZI
Anthony CHILA

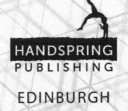

HANDSPRING
PUBLISHING

EDINBURGH

HANDSPRING PUBLISHING LIMITED
The Old Manse, Fountainhall,
Pencaitland, East Lothian
EH34 5EY, United Kingdom
Tel: +44 1875 341 859
Website: www.handspringpublishing.com

First published 2017 in the United Kingdom by Handspring Publishing

Reprinted 2019

ISBN 978-1-909141-27-8

British Library Cataloguing in Publication Data
A catalogue record for this book is available from the British Library

Important notice
Neither the publishers nor the authors will be liable for any loss or damage of any nature occasioned to or suffered by any person or property in regard to product liability, negligence or otherwise, or through acting or refraining from acting as a result of adherence to the material contained in this book.

Commissioning Editor Mary Law
Design direction Bruce Hogarth
Cover design Bruce Hogarth
Copy editing Sally Davies
Typesetter DSMSoft
Printer Severn, UK

The
Publisher's
policy is to use
paper manufactured
from sustainable forests

Contents

Contents

4 CLINICAL ASPECTS OF FASCIA

4.1 Therapeutic considerations

4.2 Manual techniques

Torsten Liem MSc(Ost), MSc(PaedOst), DO, DPO, GOsC (GB)

Torsten Liem is Joint Principal of the German School of Osteopathy, a practicing osteopath, international lecturer in osteopathy and head of several osteopathic MSc programs in Germany and Europe. He has developed an osteopathic approach to the treatment of trauma and emotional integration. He is the author and editor of 14 books and has written more than 50 articles. Torsten Liem is co-organizer of the international osteopathy symposia in Berlin and founder of an osteopathic teaching clinic and of the charitably financed centre for paediatric osteopathy in Hamburg.

A board member of the German and European Societies of Pediatric Osteopathy, Torsten Liem is also co-founder and co-editor of the journal *Osteopathische Medizin* (Elsevier), member of the Advisory Board of the *International Journal of Osteopathic Medicine,* and co-founder of Breathe Yoga. He is the author and co-editor of *Foundations of Morphodynamics in Osteopathy,* also published by Handspring Publishing.

His core vision is the implementation of osteopathic principles in practice, and connecting them with the principles of classical Chinese medicine and yoga, and with psychological and energetic aspects.

Paolo Tozzi MSc(Ost), DO, PT

Paolo Tozzi is former Treasurer of the Osteopathic European Academic Network (OsEAN), and former Vice Principal of the school of osteopathy CROMON in Rome.

He lectures widely on osteopathy and he is a member of the Fascia Science and Clinical Applications Advisory Board of the *Journal of Bodywork and Movement Therapies.* He is the co-editor of *Teaching Osteopathic Research – Proceedings of the OsEAN Open Forum 2012,* and of *The Five Osteopathic Models,* also to be published by Handspring Publishing.

Anthony G. Chila DO, FAAO DIST, FCA

Anthony Chila received his degree as Doctor of Osteopathy (USA) in 1965. After 11 years in general practice he embarked on an academic career, teaching first at Michigan State University College of Osteopathic Medicine, and latterly at Ohio University College of Osteopathic Medicine/Heritage College of Osteopathic Medicine. At Ohio University he was Chairman of the Department of Family Medicine for 10 years, and is now Professor Emeritus, Department of Family Medicine. He is dually board-certified by the American Osteopathic Association in Family Practice and Neuromusculoskeletal Medicine.

Anthony Chila has been active as office holder in the American Osteopathic Association and other national groups, and was recognized as Educator of the Year by the American Osteopathic Foundation in 2013. His many writing and editorial activities include the executive editorship of the third edition of the standard textbook *Foundations of Osteopathic Medicine.* He also served as Editor-in-Chief of *The AAO Journal.* For many years, he has been a peer reviewer for *The Journal of the American Osteopathic Association* and *The Journal of Craniomandibular & Sleep Practice.*

Contributors

Phillip Beach DO, DAc
Osteopath in private practice, Wellington, New Zealand; lecturer in the USA, Europe, and Australasia on the subjects of whole-organism movement patterns and biomechanical assessment via archetypal postures

Jean-Marie A. T. Beuckels DO (GB/B/G), Phd (Ost. Dep.), MSc Ost. (GB), BSc (Hons) Ost. Med. (GB), DF (F), PGCF (F), PT(B), Lic. Mot. Rehab. (B), PGCE (D)
Private osteopathic practitioner, Belgium; Lecturer in Osteosophy™ and Clinical Osteopathy at institutes, colleges, and universities in Europe, the USA, and Russia; Head of the Department of Osteopathic Medicine and Research, Faculty of Health at the Witten/Herdecke University, Germany; former Clinical Associate Professor, Philadelphia College of Osteopathic Medicine, Philadelphia, Pennsylvania, USA

Julia Bierbaum MSc, PT
Research Assistant in Physiotherapy, Adullam Foundation, Basel, Switzerland

**Davide Bongiorno
MD, General Surgery Postgraduate Degree, DO**
Private practitioner; lecturer, and teacher in echographic dynamic anatomy (Fascial-motion Ultrasonographic Anatomic Evaluation – FUSAE), Italy and Europe; lecturer, SIUMB. Courses, Milan and Pavia University, Italy; Member of Italian Register of Osteopaths (ROI), Italy

**Peter J. Brechtenbreiter
BSc (Ost), MSc (OPT), DO, OSD, OMT**
Private practitioner in osteopathy, Stuttgart, Germany; teacher in osteopathy

Maurice César DO, MRO (B)
Private practitioner, teacher, and lecturer, Huy, Belgium

Susan L. Chapelle RMT
Visiting Researcher, University of New England Center for Excellence in Neuroscience; Practitioner, Squamish Integrated Health, Squamish, British Columbia, Canada; Board of Directors, Howe Sound Women's Centre, Squamish, British Columbia, Canada; teacher and international lecturer in science communication in manual therapy; National Institute of General Medical Science investigator in postsurgical abdominal adhesions

Bruno Chikly MD, DO
President/CEO, Chikly Health Institute (CHI), Scottsdale, Arizona, USA; Curriculum Director, Lymph Drainage Therapy and the Brain Therapy curriculi; former Adjunct Professor, Union Institute and University Graduate College, University of Ohio, Athens, Ohio, USA; former member, Advisory Board, *International Journal of Therapeutic Massage & Bodywork*, Churchill Livingstone; former Consultant, Riekes Center for Human Enhancement, Health and Athletic Department, California, USA

Cristian Ciranna-Raab BSc, MSc, DO, DPO
Director, German School of Osteopathy (OSD), Hamburg, Germany; Board Member, Bundesarbeitsgemeinschaft Osteopathie (BAO) [Federal Association of Osteopathy], Wiesbaden, Germany; Board Member, Scandinavian School of Osteopathy (SKOSH), Gothenburg, Sweden; former Vice President, Osteopathic European Network (OsEAN), Vienna, Austria

Bradley S. Davidson PhD
Assistant Professor, Mechanical and Materials Engineering, University of Denver, Denver, Colorado, USA

Julie A. Day PT
Physiotherapist, Centro Socio Sanitario dei Colli, Padua, Italy

Michael J. Decker PhD
Senior Research Consultant, Daniel Felix Ritchie School of Engineering and Computer Science, Department of Mechanical and Materials Engineering, University of Denver, Denver, Colorado, USA

William H. Devine DO, BS C-NMM, OMM, C-FM, OMT
Clinical Professor Midwestern University, Arizona College of Osteopathic Medicine, Glendale, Arizona, USA; Fellow, Osteopathic Research; former Midwestern University OPTI Program Director, Osteopathic Principles and Practice for Postgraduate Education; former Director of Medical Education and Program Director, Midwestern University Osteopathic Specialty Clinic, Neuromusculoskeletal Medicine and Osteopathic Manipulative Medicine Residency, Arizona Campus, Glendale, Arizona, USA

Darrell J. R. Evans BSc, PhD
Vice-Provost, Learning and Teaching; Professor of Developmental Tissue Biology, Monash University, Melbourne, Australia

Christian Fossum DO

Associate Professor, Norwegian School of Health Sciences, Kristiania University College, Oslo, Norway; former Vice Principal, European School of Osteopathy, Maidstone, UK; former Assistant Professor, Department of Osteopathic Manipulative Medicine, Kirksville College of Osteopathic Medicine, Kirksville, Missouri, USA; former Associate Director, A. T. Still Research Institute, A. T. Still University of Health Sciences, Kirksville, Missouri, USA

Cristina Gioja DO

Classical Osteopathy and Body Adjustment specialist, Rome, Italy; international postgraduate and undergraduate lecturer

John C. Glover MS, DO, FAAO, C-FP, C-OMM

Professor of Osteopathic Manipulative Medicine, Touro University, Vallejo, California, USA

Rüdiger C. Goldenstein MD, MSc (PaedOst) DO, DAAO, DPO

Private practitioner; national and international teacher of osteopathy; Chairman, German Association of Paediatric Osteopathy (DGKO); Member, Principal Team, German School of Osteopathy (OSD), Hamburg, Germany

Serge Gracovetsky PhD

Professor Emeritus, Concordia University, Montréal, Québec, Canada

Jean-Claude Guimberteau MD, Surgeon

Former President, French Plastic Surgery Society; Member, French Academy of Surgery; previously surgeon, Institut Aquitain de la Main et Membre Supérieur [Aquitaine Hand and Upper Limb Institute], Pessac, France

Michael Hamm LMP, CCST

Practitioner and presenter based in Seattle, WA, USA; Former Trustee, Massage Therapy Foundation; Former faculty at Cortiva Institute-Seattle, and the Brian Utting School of Massage

Georg Harrer MD

Consultant in anesthesiology, intensive care, resuscitation, and pain therapy; Osteopath; FDM Instructor; Founder and first President of the European FDM Association (EFDMA); International Lecturer, Vienna School of Osteopathy (WSO) and Osteopathieschule Deutschland (OSD)

Laurie S. Hartmann DO

Former Head, Department of Technique, British School of Osteopathy, London, UK

Lisa M. Hodge PhD

Associate Professor, Department of Cell Biology and Immunology, Osteopathic Heritage Basic Science Research Chair, The Osteopathic Research Center, University of North Texas Health Science Center, Fort Worth, Texas, USA

David J. Hohenschurz-Schmidt MOst(Hons)

Private practitioner in osteopathy, Berlin, Germany; clinic tutor and lecturer, German School of Osteopathy (OSD)

Peter A. Huijing PhD

Professor Emeritus, Vrije Universiteit, Amsterdam, The Netherlands; Assistant, University of Minnesota, Minneapolis, Minnesota, USA; Visiting Professor, København Universitetet and Arbejdsmiljøinstituttet [University of Copenhagen and Institute of Occupational Health], Copenhagen, Denmark; Professor, University of Twente, Enschede, The Netherlands; Visiting Professor, Waseda University, Tokyo, Japan

Wilfrid Jänig MD

Professor Emeritus, Department of Physiology, University of Kiel, Germany; former Visiting Scientist, Department of Neurobiology & Behavior, Public Health Research Institute, New York University, New York, USA; former Visiting Professor: Neurobiology Unit, Life Sciences Institute, Hebrew University, Jerusalem, Israel; Department of Physiology, Monash University; Baker Institute and Florey Institute, Melbourne; Melbourne University; University of Queensland, Brisbane (John Mayne Professorship); Prince of Wales Medical Research Institute, University of New South Wales Sydney, Australia; Department of Physiology, University of Bristol, Bristol, UK; (Regent's Professor), University of California, San Francisco Campus, Department of Medicine, University of California, San Francisco, California, USA; Nagoya University, Japan

Kenzo Kase

Chairman and Founder, Kinesio Taping Association International; Honorary Chairman and past President, Natural Chiropractic College; Board of Executive Council of Japan Olympic Committee; Vice President, Japan Sepaktakraw Federation; Director, Japan Chiropractic Society; author of more than two dozen books on Kinesio Taping and other manual therapies; visiting lecturer at Tohoku University, Chiba University, Portland State University, University of New Mexico, University of Southern California, University of Hawaii, National Chiropractic College, Parker Chiropractic College, Hong Kong Techno University; presenter at clinical symposiums in Japan, the USA, the UK, Germany, Italy, Singapore, South Africa, Australia, Brazil, Argentina, Spain, and other countries

Werner Klingler MD, PhD

Lecturer, Ulm University, Germany; Director, Neurophysiological Laboratory, Ulm University at Bezirkskrankenhaus Günzburg, Günzburg, Germany; Adjunct Associate Professor, Faculty of Health, Clinical Sciences, Queensland University of Technology, Brisbane, Australia

Christian Lunghi DO, ND

Private practitioner in osteopathy and naturopathy in Italy; undergraduate and postgraduate professor and lecturer in osteopathy at various institutes and colleges in Italy; Board Member, Italian National Centre COME Collaboration Onlus; Member of Research Committee and National Examination Board of Italian Register of Osteopaths (ROI); author of and contributor to national and international books in the osteopathic field and articles published in indexed journals

Carol J. Manheim PT, LPC, MS, MEd

Visiting international instructor, Myofascial Release; private practitioner (retired), physical therapy and mental health counseling, Charleston, South Carolina, USA

Thomas W. Myers LMT

Advanced Structural Integration Practitioner; Director, Anatomy Trains, Maine, USA

Winfried L. Neuhuber MD

Professor of Anatomy and Chairman, Institute of Anatomy, Friedrich-Alexander University Erlangen-Nürnberg, Erlangen, Germany

Judith A. O'Connell DO MHA FAAO

Former President, American Academy of Osteopathy, Indianapolis, Indiana, USA; Clinical Professor, Osteopathic Manipulative Medicine, Pikeville University College of Osteopathic Medicine, Pikeville, Kentucky, USA; Clinical Professor, Osteopathic Manipulative Medicine, Ohio University Heritage College of Osteopathic Medicine, Athens, Ohio, USA

Serge Paoletti DO, MROF

International lecturer; Member, Scientific Community of the Russian Osteopathic Journal; Founding Member, French Osteopathic Academy, Chambéry, Savoy, France

Andrea Pasini PT, FMID

Instructor, Fascial Manipulation® for Internal Dysfunctions (FMID)

Andrzej Pilat PT

Director, Myofascial Therapy School 'Tupimek,' Madrid, Spain; Lecturer, Masters Degree Program, Physiotherapy School ONCE, Autonomous University, Madrid, Spain

Michel Puylaert MSc, DO, HP

Practitioner, private practice; national and international, teacher and lecturer in osteopathy, Munich, Germany

Robert Schleip PhD, MA

Director, Fascia Research Group, Ulm University, Germany; Research Director, European Rolfing Association, Munich, Germany

Fabio Schröter DO, DPT, ND

Private practitioner; teacher and lecturer; founder and Director, Collegio di Perfezionamento in Osteopatia R. Fulford DO (CPO Fulford DO) [R. Fulford DO College of Osteopathy], Rivanazzano Terme, Italy

Jay P. Shah MD

Senior Staff Physiatrist and Clinical Investigator, Rehabilitation Medicine Department, Clinical Center, National Institutes of Health, Bethesda, Maryland, USA

Jane E. Stark MS, DOMP

Director of Research, Canadian College of Osteopathy, Toronto, Canada; former Board Member, World Osteopathic Health Organization

Antonio Stecco MD, PhD

Clinical Instructor, New York University, Langone Medical Center, New York City, USA

Carla Stecco MD

Professor of Human Anatomy and Movement Science, University of Padua, Italy

Luigi Stecco PT

Former Honorary President, Fascial Manipulation Association, Vicenza, Italy

Nikki Thaker BS

Research Assistant, Rehabilitation Medicine Department, Clinical Center, National Institutes of Health, Bethesda, Maryland, USA

Francisco Toscano-Jimenez, BSc (Hons, OstMed), MRO (UK), MROE (Spain), MFEO

Director, Marbella Osteopathy Clinic, Marbella, Spain; former Director of Studies, John Wernham College of Osteopathy, Maidstone, UK

Frans van den Berg BSc, PT, MT, OMT

Senior instructor in orthopaedic manual therapy, Germany, Austria, and Turkey; founder and teacher, International Academy of Osteopathic and Manual Therapy (IAOMT), Germany, Austria and Turkey; lecturer, sports physiotherapy, Germany and Austria; former teacher, Master of Science Program, Department of Sport Sciences, University of Salzburg, Salzburg, Austria

Patrick Van Den Heede DO, MSc Physiotherapy

Practitioner in osteopathy; teacher at several European colleges; co-founder, Integrative Institute of Morphology, Orroir, Belgium

Jaap C. van der Wal MD, PhD

Associate Professor (retired), Anatomy and Embryology, University of Maastricht, Maastricht, The Netherlands

Ralf Vogt MSc, DO

Engineer, aircraft and spacecraft technologies; Member, Fascia Research Group, Ulm University guided by Robert Schleip PhD, Ulm, Germany; former Head, Visceral Osteopathic Division, German Osteopathic School (OSD), Germany; teacher of osteopathy in the cranial field at several schools

Maurizio Zanardi MSc Ost, DO, MRO (I), FT

Director General, European Institute for Osteopathic Medicine Padua, Italy

Paolo Zavarella MD, Surgeon, Specialist in Dentistry, DO

Former lecturer, Master of Posturology and Osteopathy, University of Rome Tor Vergata, Rome, Italy; former Principal, School of Osteopathy, CROMON–EDUCAM SOI; former Principal, School of Posturology, CROMON–EDUCAM SPI; former Principal, School of Osteopathy applied to Animals, CROMON–EDUCAM IFOA, Rome, Italy

Fascia is one of the most intriguing body tissues, and in the last decade it has been attracting the interest of both researchers and clinicians from different fields throughout the world. Although the definition of fascia itself is still under debate, this tissue undoubtedly displays different levels of structural and functional complexity, ranging from the intracellular to the body-wide organization. In health as well as in disease, it appears to respond to various physical and chemical forces, as a single structural continuum interacting with a multitude of regulatory functional properties. Therefore, such a multi-potential system provides the anatomical and physiological basis for several 'vital and deadly processes' as the old doctor, A. T. Still, founder of osteopathy, used to state.

Nowadays, our knowledge of fascia is still far from comprehensive, and it continues to draw experts from different fields to gather and share their data and experience in the attempt to achieve a deeper understanding of it. The first International Fascia Congress was held in 2007. Three further Fascia Research Congresses have been held in 2009, 2012 and 2015 and the Fascia World Congress of the Osteopathie Schule Deutschland in 2013. All these evolved without the benefit of guidance from Dr Still, but remarkably covered most of the concepts he proposed in his writings. Penetration, support and innervation were all presented at the first and second congresses but it was not until the third congress that fluid flow was addressed. Respiration and cancer have still to be covered.

In *Fascia in the Osteopathic Field* we have aimed to offer a multidimensional foundation of fascia from an osteopathic perspective by selectively collecting, thoroughly organizing and carefully discussing the main information currently available on this tissue from both research and clinical fields. The book firstly explores the fascial structural properties – such as anatomical arrangement, embryological development, and biomechanical qualities – from the most superficial to the deeper layers. Secondly, it examines the functional properties of fascia, such as fluidic, immune, hormonal and neural responses. Finally, it widens its perspective to address the most common manual approaches to treating this tissue, from the more traditional to the most recent ones, touching on their principles, methods of application, indications and mechanisms.

This book represents a unique piece of work. It brings together contributions from international experts on fascia, integrated with osteopathic principles and application. It offers the reader a solid osteopathic foundation to understand, assess and approach the fascial tissue. As Editors we hope it will provide a stimulus to further study and research as well as providing a valuable clinical reference.

Fascial concepts | 1

INTRODUCTION

Torsten Liem

The role of the fascia and how it relates to the musculoskeletal system as well as the entire structural integrity of the human body has become of raised interest in recent years, accompanied by an increase in research into various aspects of the human fascia. This section provides an overview of the foundations and basic terminology surrounding the term 'fascia'. The most recent scientific evidence is used to explore fascial anatomy and physiology, with the aim of creating a specific terminology that can be used for both clinical and scientific applications. The historical aspects of fascial approaches, described in this section, are of particular importance for the osteopathic understanding of fascia and may be of interest to many practitioners of manual therapy. With regard to embryological development, osteopathic strategies and fascial functions in relation to tissue development are explored and discussed. Finally, important aspects of the histology and cell biology of the fascia and connective tissue are reviewed, aiding the reader to fully understand the clinical importance of fascial structure and its implications in the genesis of dysfunctional patterns.

INTRODUCTION

Anthony G. Chila

The modern era of research involving the connective tissue system of the human body can be said to have begun in 2007. During that year, in Boston, MA (USA) a conference was held which had far-reaching ramifications. The title of the conference, Fascia Research, carried an explanatory subtitle: Basic Science and Implications for Conventional and Complementary Health Care. The proceedings of the conference, edited by Thomas Findley and Robert Schleip, were published in 2007.[1]*

In the Foreword to the proceedings, the editors discussed the two perspectives embraced in the book: a survey of what was then known about the basic science of fascia, and an exploration of the clinical implications of this knowledge for conventional medicine and complementary health care.

One of the key issues in this field was and remains the definition of fascia, and in the Introduction to the proceedings, Findley and Schleip offered a definition which has held through subsequent conferences on this subject:

'Fascia is the soft tissue component of the connective tissue system that permeates the human body forming a whole-body continuous three-dimensional matrix of structural support. It interpenetrates and surrounds all organs, muscles, bones and nerve fibers, creating a unique environment for body systems functioning. The scope of our definition and interest in fascia extends to all fibrous connective tissues, including aponeuroses, ligaments, tendons, retinacula, joint capsules, organ and vessel tunics, the epineurium, the meninges, the periostea, and all the endomysial and intermuscular fibers of the myofasciae. There is a substantial body of research on connective tissue generally focused on specialized genetic and molecular aspects of extracellular matrix. However, the study of fascia and its function as an organ of support has been largely neglected and overlooked for several decades. Since fascia serves both global, generalized functions and local, specialized functions, it is a substrate that crosses several scientific, medical, and therapeutic disciplines, both in conventional and complementary/alternative modalities.'

The conclusion to the Introduction contains the following remarks:

'This book ends with a discussion of new directions for research and new hypotheses coming very appropriately from the perspective provided by several osteopathic physicians. It is this group of physicians who more than 100 years ago championed both manual body work and the conceptual connection between bodywork and overall medical health.'†

Given the interest and momentum for the study of fascia just described, what is the place of the present text *Fascia in the Osteopathic Field?* The groundwork and original extensive preparation of content was carried out by Torsten Liem and Paolo Tozzi, who together mapped out four major areas of focus which form the book's main sections:

- Fascial Concepts

- Physiology and Functions of Fascia

- Anatomy and Structure of Fascia

---

*Further such conferences have been held in Amsterdam (2009); Vancouver (2012); and Washington (2015).

†In 2013, Findley and Shalwala published a paper which related Fascia Research Congress evidence to the perspective of Andrew Taylor Still.[2]

- Clinical Aspects of Fascia
  - Therapeutic Considerations
  - Manual Techniques

Under these headings, a wide range of presenters reflects various levels of interest and study. Liem and Tozzi have expended great effort in portraying the potential breadth and depth of the topic of fascia. Each has made his own contribution to the text as well as seeking broad representation in each area by numerous additional authors, recruited from across the world. All these come together to present a comprehensive account of the role of fascia in osteopathic practice, showing its significance as the substrate mentioned in the definition above, and its importance as a mediator in many forms of osteopathic intervention.

On this subject, readers should note the international differences in usage of terms such as *osteopathy, osteopath, osteopathic medicine, osteopathic physician*. This can best be focused by noting the standard for definition in the USA. There, the preparation for and study of osteopathic medicine culminates in degree recognition of a fully licensed osteopathic physician. While this may or may not be altogether true in other countries of the world, practitioners globally must meet the statutory regulations of their various governments. But whatever the reader's background and form of training and certification, he or she is following a path laid down by Andrew Taylor Still.

From the very beginnings of osteopathy in the 1870s, an assessment of the connective tissue has been considered fundamental to the treatment of a wide variety of conditions.[3] The role of fascia in osteopathic practice was seen as crucial: '... this philosophy [of Osteopathy] has chosen the fascia as a foundation on which to stand ...'[4] The vital function of fascia was so important that 'by its action we live and by its failure we shrink, or swell and die',[5] and it is probably due to this ambivalent potential as source of life and death that fascia was referred to by A.T. Still as the dwelling place of our spiritual being.[6] Still's concept of fascia continued to be developed by the early osteopaths and created the basis for much of our clinical understanding of this tissue, which is increasingly recognized as the unifying structural element of the body and key to understanding the reciprocal interrelation between structure and function, and the body's innate ability to heal itself.

References

1. Findley T. W., Schleip R. (eds) 2007. *Fascia Research: Basic Science and Implications for Conventional and Complementary Health Care.* Elsevier, Munich.

2. Findley T. W., Shalwala M. 2013. Fascia Research Congress. Evidence from the 100 Year Perspective of Andrew Taylor Still. *Journal of Bodywork and Movement Therapies* 17(3):356–364.

3. Lee P. R. 2006. Still's concept of connective tissue: lost in "translation"? *The Journal of the American Osteopathic Association* 106(4):176–177; author reply 213–214.

4. Still A. T. 1899. *Philosophy of Osteopathy.* A. T. Still, Kirksville, MO, p. 162.

5. Still A. T. 1899. *Philosophy of Osteopathy.* A. T. Still, Kirksville, MO, p. 164.

6. Still A. T. 1899. *Philosophy of Osteopathy.* A. T. Still, Kirksville, MO, p. 165.

FASCIAL CONCEPTS IN OSTEOPATHIC HISTORY

Jane E. Stark

Osteopathic physicians and nonphysician osteopaths* have given fascia a prominent position in their clinical reasoning and treatment approaches since 1897, when osteopathy's founder Andrew Taylor Still first used the term in his writing.[1] However, the word 'fascia', as well as the concept of fascia, did not originate with osteopathy; nor does the concept reside solely within the practice of osteopathy or osteopathic medicine. In fact, the term predates osteopathy by many centuries, and tissue known as fascia remains an integral consideration in a variety of manual therapy approaches.

The word fascia has its origin in Latin, in which it has been used for at least 1000 years to mean a band or a fillet.[2] Beyond fascia's Latin roots, a 1587 English translation of a fourth-century Greek work[3] used the term in conjunction with tying one's loose hair to one's head. However, fascia's original appearance as an English term can be traced a bit earlier – to 1573, in the first book on architecture known to be published in English.[4] In his chapter 'The first and chief groundes [grounds] of architecture vsed [used] in all the auncient [ancient] and famous monyments [monuments]', John Shute[5] used the term in reference to the lowest of the three layers that comprise the upper part of a temple or classical building. This upper part, known as the entablature, consists of the architrave (the lower layer of the entablature), the frieze (the middle layer), and the cornice (the uppermost layer).[6] Using a magnifying glass to read the words at the level of the architrave in Shute's engraved plate of a 'composite order' column, the word fascia can be seen three times.[5] These uses correspond to the *Oxford English Dictionary*'s entry for the first known architectural reference to fascia: 'the lowest Fascia ... the second Fascia ... the

third Fascia'.[2] According to classical architecture terminology, the architrave consists of one or more horizontal bands. Shute's use of the term fascia remains a popular architectural expression for a bandlike structural detail today – thus preserving the original Latin meaning. The *Oxford English Dictionary* further defines fascia as 'any object, or collection of objects, that gives the appearance of a band or stripe'.[2]

Besides noting its literary and architectural applications to a band or layer, the *Oxford English Dictionary* defines fascia in an anatomical sense, as a 'thin sheath of fibrous tissue investing a muscle or some special tissue or organ; an aponeurosis'.[2] The first English use of fascia as an anatomical term occurred in 1788, when it appeared in a serial publication known as *Medical Communications*, in an article under the title of *History of a contracture of forearm and fingers, with some remarks and reflections on bleeding of the arm*. This article was read aloud to the Society for Promoting Medical Knowledge[7] by a British surgeon named Henry Watson.[8] In his talk to society members, Watson described fascia not as a bandlike piece of tissue, but rather as a more encompassing tissue forming a compartment that created enough tension to prevent blood from escaping under it. According to Watson, the blood was retained by the fascia as a result of a medical intervention intended to cause bleeding from the cephalic median vein. Watson described this fascia as a 'tendonous expansion'.[8,p.256] He elaborated on this idea as follows:

'The use of the expansions is very great. They support
muscles, strengthen and increase the muscular
power when in action, confine and protect the blood
vessels in their proper situations, supply the place of
bone where a plate of bone could not so conveniently
answer the purpose, give firmness with flexibility to
the joints, preserve the symmetry of the limbs'.[8,p.268]

---

*For the remainder of the chapter, and for convenience's sake, osteopathic physicians and nonphysician osteopaths will be collectively referred to as osteopaths.

Early conceptions of fascia were mostly visual rather than textual. Dissected fascialike tissue, usually not labeled as such, can be seen depicted in fine art as well as medical engravings and illustrations dating back to the dawn of the Renaissance. At that time, anatomists performed dissections for physicians and surgeons to study and for artists to capture on canvas. Physicians and artists alike intended that the knowledge gained from dissecting human bodies would ultimately lead to preservation of human life. Men of medicine focused on the status of one's physical body, while artists concentrated on humankind's spiritual makeup. From an artistic perspective, anatomical renderings showed 'the dead as living embodiments of our form and fate'.[9,p.1] Therefore, in the latter centuries of the second millennium, the study of medicine was influenced by artistic renditions of the body depicting humans as both physical and spiritual.

One of the more famous portrayals of fascialike tissue is found in a 1559–1560 anatomical work titled *Anatomia del corpo humano* by the Spanish anatomist Juan Valverde de Amusco (c.1525–c.1587).[10] Although Valverde performed the dissections for his book, Gaspar Becerra is credited with making the illustrations and Nicolas Beatrizet with the engravings.[10] Some of Valverde's plates have been criticized for being little more than close copies of the work of Andreas Vesalius (1514–1564), one of Leonardo da Vinci's (1452–1519) contemporaries. Nevertheless, the plate on page 64 of *Historia de la composicion del cuerpo humano* 1551 is sufficiently different from the majority of Vesalius' anatomical illustrations to make it noteworthy. Here, the cadaver reveals the separation of his body and soul through the depiction of the knife in his hand.[11]

There are several other significant antique illustrative anatomy books that have brought fascia to life. These include *Anatomia Humani Corporis*[12] by Govard Bidloo (1649–1713), *The Anatomy of Humane Bodies*[13] by William Cowper (1666–1709), and *Traité Complet de l'Anatomie de l'Homme*[14] by Jean-Baptiste Bourgery (1797–1849). *Anatomy, Descriptive and Surgical*,[15] by Henry Gray (1825–1861), is considered to be the last of the great antique illustrative anatomy books. A. T. Still is known to have owned the 1893 13th edition of *Gray's Anatomy*.[16]

The ways in which fascia was depicted in the writings of A. T. Still and in the osteopathic literature up to the year 2000 constituted the subject of a lengthy thesis titled *Still's Fascia: A Qualitative Investigation to Enrich the Meaning Behind Andrew Taylor Still's Concepts of Fascia (Still's Fascia)*. The research for this thesis was conducted by the present author between 2001 and 2003,[17] with the thesis published in its entirety first in German[18] and then in English.[19] *Still's Fascia* reveals that A. T. Still had access to a substantial amount of previously recorded material on fascia and membranes, as well as fresh tissue samples of fascia and membranes. Still regularly interchanged his use of the terms fascia and membranes,[19,p.284] and his habit of substituting one word for the other created much difficulty in clearly defining his concept of fascia in isolation from his concept of membranes. The thesis research led to the conclusion that Still did not seek to distinguish fascia from membranes, as indicated by his phrase, '... this membrane we call the mesentery, the peritoneum, the fascia, muscular attachment or any other name we may select ...'.[20,p.124] Unfortunately, it is problematic for today's reader that the modern histologic classification of tissues typically reserves the term 'membrane' for epithelial tissue, whereas fascial tissues are classified in the connective tissue category.

Still thought intensely about fascia. In 1899, he stated that fascia 'stands before the world today, the greatest problem, the most pleasing thought'.[21,p.163] 'The fascia', he wrote, 'gives one of, if not the greatest problems to solve as to the part it takes in life and death'[21,p.164] and 'This life is surely too short to solve the uses of the fascia in animal forms'.[21,p.165] Perhaps Still's fascination was so pronounced because – unlike most of us today who view fascia only in photographic images, illustrative renditions, or preserved cadavers – Still observed 'fascia' and 'membranes' and 'this connecting substance'[21,p.166] in freshly killed animals, especially the deer that provided his family with food and clothing. Although Still is known to have owned dissection books, including Robert Harrison's *The Dublin Dissector*, published in 1859,[16,22] and Sir William Fergusson's *A System of Practical Surgery*, published in 1843,[23] those books were published several decades after he began to hunt. The advantage to Still of not having access to detailed dissection instructions was that, when field dressing the animals, he was not biased to disregard the fascia. Dissection instructions usually implied that fascia was merely an insignificant tissue to be cut away, because its presence obscured the underlying important structures of muscles, bones, vessels, and viscera.

In keeping with the ideas emanating from the Renaissance period – and unlike the majority of osteopathic authors who were to follow him – Still conceptualized the fascia as having both physical and spiritual features. He admitted that, anatomically, the fascia 'permeates, divides and sub-divides every portion of all animal bodies; surrounding and penetrating every muscle and all its fibers—every artery, and every fiber ... venous system ... lymphatics'.[21,p.164] He placed a great deal of emphasis on the relationship between the lymphatics and fascia.

Still also stated that fascia was the 'dwelling place of his [mankind's] spiritual being ...'[21,p.163] and 'the house of God'.[21,p.163] He wrote that 'the soul of man with all the streams of pure living water seems to dwell in the fascia of his body'.[21,p.165] *Still's Fascia* presented supporting evidence that Still's foregoing statement demonstrated his view of the human being as constituting the union of body, motion (or spirit, which was physiological, not spiritual), and mind (not a thinking mind, but a managing mind of divine origin). All three of these were united in the fascia.[24] This triple union concept was referred to elsewhere in Still's writing as the 'triune' nature of the man.[20,p.16]

The osteopaths and other individuals who wrote about fascia in the twentieth century can have their contributions regarding fascia classified into four broad categories. One category consists of those writers who simply quote A. T. Still, noting how profound his statements are but not trying to explain his intended meanings. Examples include Beryl E. Arbuckle's 1947 article *Reflexes*,[25] a section of Arbuckle's 1953 article *The Craniocervical Area*,[26] Mary A. Hoover's 1951 article *On Importance of Fascia*,[27] and Harold Magoun Sr's *Fascia in the Writings of A. T. Still.* Magoun's contribution was originally presented in 1953 as a lecture at a conference of the Osteopathic Cranial Association in Kirksville, Missouri.[28] The text of the lecture was initially published in 1954[28] and reissued in 1970.[29]

The other three categories of twentieth-century fascia contributions provide anatomical and/or physiological descriptions of the properties of fascia or connective tissue, expound upon fascia's mechanical properties, or describe features of fascia related to fluids, especially the lymphatics. The writings that fall into these three categories do not seem to demonstrate any progression of ideas or other obvious patterns of thought. However, with a few exceptions, there is a consistent theme that emerges from this diverse set of articles. As McConnell wrote in 1939, the ultimate effect of fascial disturbances and disruptions is on 'the cellular mechanism or processes'.[30]

The present review of contributions selected from the osteopathic literature, which were deemed either important or unique by this author, fall into the preciously noted four categories, which can be reworded as follows: 1) reiterations of Still's works, 2) anatomical or physiological descriptions, 3) mechanical properties, and 4) fascia related to fluid. The contributions are presented chronologically by publication date.

This review of fascial concepts in osteopathy is mostly limited to an American viewpoint, derived from the osteopathic literature written by osteopathic physicians and published in the United States. This limitation is the result of the sample of reviewed articles being based on the outcome of two literature searches – one conducted in June 2001 by Robert Sanders DO of the A. T. Still University of Health Sciences and the other in 2014 by Debra Loguda-Summers, the curator and special projects manager of the Museum of Osteopathic Medicine[SM] and International Center for Osteopathic History in Kirksville, Missouri. Literature searches, using the subject terms of 'fascia' or 'connective tissue', were conducted using the osteopathic databases OSTMED®[31] and OSTMED. Dr®. The 2001 search yielded 16 records with the subject term fascia and 10 records with the subject term connective tissue. The 2014 search produced approximately 40 titles (some being duplicates); only five titles were dated from 2001 or later, one a letter and another a review of a foreign-based study.[32]

Because OSTMED indexes only osteopathic medical literature, the majority of search results are US-based osteopathic medicine articles that were published in journals, primarily *JAOA – The Journal of the American Osteopathic Association*, and a collection of American Academy of Osteopathy (AAO) yearbooks. The retrieved articles did not include any clinical trial studies on fascia or connective tissue. Instead, each article was a review, an opinion piece, or anecdotal information.

Readers should be aware that foreign-based studies do exist, but they are likely not indexed in either OSTMED®[31] or OSTMED.Dr®. For example, in 2009, a predominately German group of researchers – J. Vagedes, C. M. Gordon, D. Beutinger, et al. – published a review titled *Myofascial Release in Combination with Trigger Point Therapy and Deep Breathing Training Improves Low Back Pain* in the conference proceedings of the Second International Fascia Research Congress.[33] In 2013, Italian-based researchers – P. Tozzi, D. Bongiorno, and C. Vitturini – published their work, *Low Back Pain and Kidney Mobility: Local Osteopathic Fascial Manipulation Decreases Pain Perception and Improves Renal Mobility*, in the *Journal of Bodywork and Movement Therapies*.[34] The American osteopathic literature provided a summary abstract of the study by Tozzi et al.[32]

There are fascia-related articles in the peer-reviewed osteopathic literature that are written by authors other than osteopathic physicians, such as *Mathematical analysis of the flow of hyaluronic acid around fascia during manual therapy motions*, by M. Roman, H. Chaudhry, B. Bukiet, A. Stecco, and T. W. Findley,[35] published in the *JAOA*. However, those articles are not discussed here, because they fall outside the focus of the present review. The *Journal of Bodywork and Movement Therapies* (*JBMT*), which, as the journal's title implies, caters to many forms of manual and movement therapies, is a richer source of peer-reviewed articles on fascia than are any of the peer-reviewed osteopathic journals. Yet, because this chapter is about the history of fascia in the osteopathic literature, a huge wealth of information published in the *JBMT* must be excluded, including such recent articles as: *The fourth phase of water: a role in fascia?* by G. Pollack;[36] *The anatomical and functional relation between gluteus maximus and fascia lata* by S. Antonio, G. Wolfgang, H. Robert, B. Fullerton, and S. Carla;[37] *Does fascia hold memories?* by P. Tozzi;[38] and a case

study titled *Could ultrasound and elastography visualize densified areas inside the deep fascia?* by T. Luomala, M. Pihlman, J. Heiskanen, and C. Stecco.[39]

The following contributions are briefly summarized, describing the focus of each article along with the significance of its author(s).

1923 – *Fascia—tension—light*[40] by Frank P. Millard DO.

This is a fascinating article, still relevant today, about how the lymphatic system and the fascia work in conjunction to maintain the body's 'life force'. Millard was a graduate of the American School of Osteopathy (ASO), class of 1900.[41] Therefore, he had the advantage of being exposed to the teachings of both A. T. Still and John Martin Littlejohn.[42]

1928 – *Studies in osteopathic pathology*[43] subtitled *Connective tissue and fascia* by Carl Philip McConnell DO.

Although not highly organized in its presentation, this article discusses how pathological conditions are reflected in the connective tissue and/or fascia in the form of fibrosis or edema. McConnell studied at ASO in one of the earliest classes (1896)[41] with a small cohort of 25 graduates.[44] He taught at ASO between 1897 and 1900,[42,45–47] before leaving to join the faculty with John Martin Littlejohn at the American College of Osteopathic Medicine and Surgery in Chicago.[48]

1936 – *Fascial reflexes: a new aid in diagnosis*[49] by Addison O'Neill DO.

This a short article that puts forth a novel idea by the author regarding palpable reflexes, differing from those of Chapman in the region of the spine covered. There is no biographical information available on the O'Neill article, other than it is estimated from his writing that he graduated (unlikely from ASO) in approximately 1902.[49]

1936 – *The role of fascia in osteopathic problems*[50] by Harold E. Kerr DO.

Rather than viewing fascia as an isolated tissue, this article recommends viewing the fascia in relation to the immediate anatomic structures in its vicinity. The physiological impacts of the anatomical disturbances are emphasized. Kerr graduated in 1934 from Midwestern University's Chicago College of Osteopathic Medicine.[51] Thus, this article is written by a relatively inexperienced DO.

1942 – *Old age and connective tissue*[52] by Charles H. Kauffman DO.

This article remains very relevant today, because it relates the importance of lymphatics to the connective tissue's viability – a theme reminiscent of A. T. Still's writing.

1944 – Connective tissue and osteopathy[53] by Alan R. Becker DO.

This article presents a summary of the writing of Charles Kauffman, specifically intended to emphasize connective tissue. Although the majority of Kauffman's work was published decades after Still's death, Kauffman's writing is interesting because he attended ASO[41] while Still was alive, though not actively teaching.

1947 – Soft tissues in areas of osteopathic lesions[54] by J. Stedman Denslow DO.

Although Denslow did not attempt to distinguish muscle from fascia, he described the changes in tissue quality and palpation in regions of spinal dysfunction. According to William A. Kuchera and his son Michael L. Kuchera, Denslow was the first osteopathic physician 'educated to use the modern scientific method in a clinical setting to investigate what was then called the osteopathic lesion'.[55,p.32]

1947 – The fascias: manipulative treatment removes lesion and normalizes reflex arc[56] by Alan R. Becker DO.

This article draws on the writings of Still and Kauffman, as well as Becker's own experience that facial treatment should focus on lymphatic drainage and be indirect. Alan Becker was the son of Arthur Becker, a faculty member of ASO from 1910 to 1912, during Still's involvement with the school.[57,58] Alan Becker was also a devoted student of William Garner Sutherland, and he later served on ASO's faculty along with his more famous brother, Rollin E. Becker.[59] Becker was a professor of anatomy at Kirksville College of Osteopathic Medicine (KCOM).

1952 – Fascia of the head and neck as it applies to dental lesions[60] by Angus G. Cathie DO.

This article describes, without the use of illustrations, the continuity of the fascia in the oral, head, and cervical regions. Cathie was a highly respected osteopathic anatomist. Soon after graduating from the Philadelphia College of Osteopathy in 1931, Cathie became a professor of osteopathy at that college and later the chair of the anatomy department, a position that he held from 1944 until his death in 1970.[61] Other articles on fascia by Cathie are also significant, including The fascia of the body in relation to function and manipulative therapy[62] and Considerations of fascia and its relation to disease of the musculoskeletal system.[63]

1952 – The role of the fasciae in the maintenance of structural integrity[64] by Leon E. Page DO.

This article focuses intently on the physical support provided to the body by connective tissue. Yet it concludes by emphasizing the role of connective tissue in maintenance of life through fluids and the lymphatics. Page graduated from ASO in 1917, the year of Still's death.[41]

1953 – A Clinical Conference on Osteopathy[65] held in Kirksville, and organized by the Osteopathic Cranial Association.

This five-day conference held at the Kirksville College of Osteopathy and Surgery (KCOS) included lectures from elite members of Sutherland's cranial faculty, as well as two prominent scientists on the faculty of KCOS – George Snyder PhD, and Irvin M. Korr PhD. Some of the cranial members giving oral presentations on fascia-related topics included Kenneth E. Little DO; Della B. Caldwell DO; Rollin R. Becker DO; Harold I. Magoun; Thomas Schooley DO; Anna Slocum DO; Rebecca C. Lippincott DO; and, of course, William Garner Sutherland.[66]

Although some of the lectures have been recorded in various journals, not all of them can be traced. However, both of Sutherland's lectures can be found in a book of his collected works called *Contributions of Thought*.[67,pp.278–289]

1954 – Embryology and physiology of fascia[68,69] by George E. Snyder PhD.

This article provided osteopathic clinicians with a comprehensive review of the physiological properties and importance of fascia. Although not an osteopath, Snyder describes fascia's embryologic origin from the mesoderm and its differentiation into the various forms of connective tissue, including the cells of the immune system, such as macrophages and mast cells. The article remains a worthwhile read today. Biographical information on Snyder is not available.

1956 – Fasciae – applied anatomy and physiology[70] by George E. Snyder PhD.

This article represents the second of Snyder's important articles on the physiological role and importance of connective tissue in 'all phases of body economy in both health and disease'.[70,p.75]

1959 – The circulation of the cerebrospinal fluid through the connective tissue system[71] by Ralph F. Erlingheuser DO.

This work was made famous by Harold Magoun Sr, in his book *Osteopathy in the Cranial Field*.[72,p.36,p.350] It was used as a reference for Sutherland's theory that the cerebral spinal fluid was continuous with every cell of the body through the lymphatic system and collagen fiber tubules. Considered a specialist in the connective tissue system, Erlingheuser was a 1940s graduate of the College of Osteopathic Physicians and Surgeons in Los Angeles.[73]

1969 – *The clinical importance of fascia*[74] written by the 1969 class at the Philadelphia College of Osteopathic Medicine (PCOM).

This 15-page article, edited by Angus G. Cathie DO and Robert W. England DO of the department of anatomy, represents the combined effort of the PCOM anatomy students to provide a published synopsis of the clinical importance of fascia. They divided the article into four sections: 1) fascia's role in support and protection, 2) its role in the musculoskeletal system, 3) its relationship to metabolism, and 4) consideration of fascia's chemical and pathologic aspects. This article would probably be more useful to osteopathic students than to experienced DOs.

1975 – *Fascial considerations in treatment of the head and neck*[75] by Philip Greenman DO.

This article, like so many before it, relates the importance of fascia to circulation and lymphatic drainage. However, unlike previous articles, this one provides a step-by-step approach to examining the face, head, and neck. Philip E. Greenman DO graduated from PCOM in 1952, while Angus G. Cathie was on the faculty. After 20 years in private practice, Greenman became professor and associate dean of the College of Osteopathic Medicine at Michigan State University, where he stayed until his retirement in 2004.[76]

1975 – *The meaning of fascia and fascial continuity*[77] by R. Frederick Becker PhD.

This article provides a useful synopsis of the types of connective tissues that should not be classified as fascia. It also offers an historical overview of how the naming of fascia caused fascia to be conceptualized as discrete pieces of tissue instead of seeing its continuity. This article is nicely illustrated. In 1940, Roland Frederick Becker obtained a PhD in anatomy from Northwestern University, and he spent his early career at Duke University. Between 1969 and 1975 he was at Michigan State University,[78] where he served in the department of biomechanics.[77]

1979 – *Some clinical considerations on fascia in diagnosis and treatment*[79] by Gerald J. Cooper DO.

This article describes some of the reactions of fascia to physical and chemical environmental stressors and fascia's consequent impact on the body's functioning. It also provides a list of treatment options, for which Cooper credits Angus Cathie with describing to him in personal communications. A past president of the Cranial Academy, Cooper was a 1956 graduate of the Des Moines College of Osteopathic Medicine, where he later served on the faulty.[80]

1994 – *Introducing the fascial distortion model*[81] by Stephen P. Typaldos DO.

This article introduces the idea of distinct and classifiable distortions in the fabric of the fibrous fascia. This type of distortion had its own accompanying 'body language' and 'signature presentation'.[82] Over the course of 15 years in practice, Typaldos noticed a poor response to conventional forms of therapy. In his introductory article, he outlined four distortion types, though the Fascial Distortion Model (FDM) training seminar website now lists six types of distortions.[83] According to his family, Typaldos hoped that his FDM would one day 'revitalize medicine by providing new insight into cardiology, internal medicine and neurology'.[84] His sudden death in 2006, at the age of 49, left his students to continue to teach his method. Typaldos was a 1986 graduate of the University of Health Sciences College of Osteopathic Medicine in Kansas City, Missouri.[84]

1995 – *The nature of fascia and the role of lower extremity fascia in low back pain*[85] by Dallas D. Hessler DO.

This article emphasizes the importance of examining and treating the fascia of the lower extremity in patients with low back pain. A 1975 graduate of the A. T. Still University of Health Sciences,[86] Hessler had the benefit of being in general family practice for 20 years when he wrote this article.

2006 – *The effects of manipulation on ligaments and fascia from a fluids model perspective*[87] by William T. Crow DO.

This twenty-first-century article ties together the words of A. T. Still and several other prominent American osteopathic physicians, including Cathie and Magoun Sr. Ultimately the article emphasizes the role of fascia in the fluid dynamics of the body. Crow is a 1987 graduate of the Texas College of Osteopathic Medicine, where he is listed as serving on its faculty in the osteopathic manipulative medicine department.[88]

There have been two books written on fascia, one by an osteopathic physician and the other by a non-physician osteopath. The first book, *Bioelectric Fascial Activation and Release: The Physician's Guide to Hunting with Dr. Still*, is a treatment manual based on what the author, Judith A. O'Connell DO calls a bioelectrical activation model.[89] It was originally published in 1998. The second book, *Les fascias: rôle des tissus dans la mécanique humaine*, is written by Serge Paoletti DO, a graduate of the European School of Osteopathy in Maidstone, England. The book was originally published in French in 1998.[90] In 2001, it was translated into German.[91]

The English translation was initially published in 2006 as *The Fascia: Anatomy, Dysfunction and Treatment*.[92] The book serves as a good overview of fascia.

Although the term fascia originated as a structural feature of architecture, artists whose work served the medical profession in the latter parts of the first millennium depicted fascia as having both physical and spiritual qualities. A. T. Still developed his concepts of osteopathy and fascia by means of his exposure to fresh fascia through necessary dressing, skinning, and dissection of prey. Thus, it seems that he experienced the properties of life found in *living* fascia. His exposure to fresh fascia, shortly after the animal was killed, likely contributed to the formation of such statements as 'the soul of man with all the streams of pure living water seems to dwell in the fascia of his body'.[21,p.165] and the belief that fascia was a 'dwelling place of his [mankind's] spiritual being'.[21,p.163] However, of those published osteopaths writing on fascia in the American literature, A. T. Still was the only one to discuss fascia in terms other than physical. While the physical properties of fascia are certainly important, it seems imperative to give further consideration to such statements as fascia being the 'dwelling place of his [human's] spiritual being'.[21,p.163]

In the first of the American Osteopathic Association's four tenets of osteopathic medicine[93] – or '4 key principles of osteopathic philosophy'[94] – the body is a unit, and the person is a unit of body, mind, and spirit. It then follows that one's spirit is a valued and essential element of the human makeup. Still may not have been correct, but at least he considered the union of body, mind, and spirit as the triune nature of a person, displayed in the fascia. Perhaps the profession would benefit from some open dialogue about the nonphysical properties of fascia.

The final take-home message is that although the osteopathic literature houses some germane articles on fascia, dating back 100 years, it sorely lacks published data on bench or clinical trial research on fascia, its properties, or its treatment. That information is now beginning to percolate into the scientific literature. If osteopathic medicine intends to continue to consider fascia as an important tissue requiring the attention of osteopaths in assessment and treatment

regimens, then research into fascia assessment and treatment should be a future 'must' in the peer-reviewed osteopathic literature.

References

1. Still A. T. Preparatory studies essential. *Journal of Osteopathy*. 1897;August:4(4):182–184.

2. *Oxford English Dictionary*. Oxford University Press; 2013.

3. Underdowne T. W. C. *An Æthiopian History written in Greek … Englished by Thomas Underdowne Anno 1587. With an introduction by Charles Whibley*; 1895.

4. Columbia University Libraries. Treasures of Columbia University Libraries Special Collections: Art & Architecture, #58: John Shute (d. 1563). Available at: http://www.columbia.edu/cu/lweb/eresources/exhibitions/treasures/html/58.html [accessed January 11, 2016].

5. Shute J. The first and chief groundes of architecture vsed in all the auncient and famous monymentes. *In Fletestrete nere to Sainct Dunstans churche by Thomas Marshe*. Was available at: http://gateway.proquest.com/openurl?ctx_ver=Z39.88-2003&res_id=xri:eebo&rft_val_fmt=&rft_id=xri:eebo:image:1835 [accessed December 20, 2013].

6. Small J. *The Five Orders of Classical Architecture: The Architecture of Robert Adam (1728–1792)* 2002. Available at: http://sites.scran.ac.uk/ada/documents/general/orders/classical_orders.htm [accessed July 14, 2014].

7. Gray, Ford. Preface. *Medical Communications*. Vol. 1. London: Joseph Johnson, St. Paul's Church-Yard; 1784.

8. Watson H. History of a contracture of forearm and fingers, with some remarks and reflections on bleeding of the arm. Read February 19, 1788. *Medical Communications*. Vol. 2. London: Joseph Johnson, St. Paul's Church-Yard; 1790:251–276.

9. Rifkin B. A., Ackerman M. J. *Human anatomy: from the Renaissance to the Digital Age*. New York: Abrams; 2006.

10. Valverde de Amusco J. *Historia de la composición del cuerpo humano*. Roma: Per Ant. Salamanca, et Antonio Lafreri; 1559 or 1560.

11. U.S. National Library of Medicine. History of Medicine: Anatomica del corpo humano. Available at: http://www.nlm.nih.gov/dreamanatomy/da_g_I-B-2-01.html [accessed January 11, 2016].

12. Bidloo G., de Lairesse G. *Anatomia Humani Corporis/Centum & Quinque Tabulis, per Artificiosiss. G. de Lairesse ad Vivum Delineatis, Demonstrata*: Henrici & Viduae Theodori Boom; 1685.

13. Cowper W. *The Anatomy of Humane Bodies, with Figures Drawn After the Life*. Walford, London: Oxford: Printed at the Theater, for Sam. Smith and Benj.; 1698.

14. Bourgery J-B. M. *Traité Complet de l'anatomie de l'homme comprenant la médecine opératoire avec planches lithographiées*. Paris: C. A. Delaunay; 1831–1854.

15. Gray H. *Anatomy, Descriptive and Surgical*. London: J. W. Parker; 1858.

16. Onsager L. W. The Personal Library of A. T. Still. Revised. 2001. Unpublished paper. Still National Osteopathic Museum. Kirksville, Missouri; 1992.

17. Stark J. E. *Still's Fascia: A Qualitative Investigation to Enrich the Meaning Behind Andrew Taylor Still's Concepts of Fascia*. Toronto, Canada, Canadian College of Osteopathy; 2003.

18. Stark J. *Stills Faszienkonzepte: Eine Biografie üder den Entdecker der Osteopathie*. Pähl, Germany: Jolandos; 2006.

19. Stark J. *Still's Fascia: A Qualitative Investigation to Enrich the Meaning Behind Andrew Taylor Still's Concepts of Fascia*. Pähl, Germany: Jolandos; 2007.

20. Still A. T. *The Philosophy and Mechanical Principles of Osteopathy*. Kansas City, Missouri: Hudson-Kimberly Publishing Company; 1902.

21. Still A. T. *Philosophy of Osteopathy*. Kirksville, Missouri: A. T. Still; 1899.

22. Harrison R. *The Dublin Dissector, or System of Practical Anatomy*. London: Hodges and Smith; 1859.

23. Fergusson W., Sir. *A System of Practical Surgery*. Philadelphia: Lea and Blanchard; 1843.

24. Stark J. E. *Still's Fascia*. Pahl Germany: Jolandos; 2007.

25. Arbuckle B. E. Reflexes. *Journal of the American Osteopathic Association*. 1947;46(7):405–407.

26. Arbuckle B. E. The craniocervical area. *Journal of the American Osteopathic Association*. 1953(52):415–422.

27. Hoover M. A. Importance of fascia. *AAO Yearbook*. 1951:55–72.

28. Magoun HI. Fascia in the writings of A. T. Still. *Journal of the Osteopathic Cranial Association*. 1954;1954:16–25.

29. Magoun H. I. Fascia in the writings of A. T. Still. *AOA Yearbook*. 1970:159–168.

30. McConnell CP. Fundamental fragments. IV Fascia. *Journal of the American Osteopathic Association*. 1939;December, 39(4):204.

31. Ostmed® – Osteopathic Literature Database. University of North Texas Health Science Center at Fort Worth, Gibson D. Lewis Health Science Library. Sponsored by the American Osteopathic Association and American Academy of Osteopathic Medicine. Was available at: http://library.hsc.unt.edu/ostmed/ [accessed June, 2002].

32. Seffinger M. A. Osteopathic fascial manipulation reduces low back pain and increases kidney mobility [Abstract]. *Journal of the American Osteopathic Association*. 2013;113(1):102–102.

33. Vagedes J., Gordon C. M., Beutinger D. et al. Myofascial release in combination with trigger point therapy and deep breathing training improves low back pain. *Fascia Research II, Basic Science and Implications for Conventional and Complementary Health Care, Elsevier*. 2009;249.

34. Tozzi P., Bongiorno D., Vitturini C. Low back pain and kidney mobility: local osteopathic fascial manipulation decreases pain perception and improves renal mobility. *Journal of Bodywork and Movement Therapies*. 2012;16(3):381–391.

35. Roman M., Chaudhry H., Bukiet B., Stecco A., Findley T. W. Mathematical analysis of the flow of hyaluronic acid around fascia during manual therapy motions. *Journal of the American Osteopathic Association*. 2013;113(8): 600–610.

36. Pollack G. The Fourth Phase of Water: A role in fascia? *Journal of Bodywork and Movement Therapies*. 2013;17(4):510–511.

37. Antonio S., Wolfgang G., Robert H., Fullerton B., Carla S. The anatomical and functional relation between gluteus maximus and fascia lata. *Journal of Bodywork and Movement Therapies*. 2013;17(4):512–517.

38. Tozzi P. Does fascia hold memories? *Journal of Bodywork and Movement Therapies*. 2014;18(2):259–265.

39. Luomala T., Pihlman M., Heiskanen J., Stecco C. Case study: Could ultrasound and elastography visualized [sic] densified areas inside the deep fascia? *Journal of Bodywork and Movement Therapies*. 2014;18(3):462–468.

40. Millard F. P., DO Fascia–Tension–Light. *Journal of the American Osteopathic Association*. 1923;March.

41. Gracey C., Loguda-Summers D. American School of Osteopathy Alumni. 1894–1924, revised 2003. Kirksville, Missouri: Kirksville College of Osteopathic Medicine; 1999.

42. American School of Osteopathy. American School of Osteopathy. Session of 1899–1900. Kirksville, Missouri; 1899.

43. McConnell C. P. Studies in Osteopathic Pathology. *The Journal of the American Osteopathic Association*. 1928;28(3):167–170.

44. Graduates of the American School of Osteopathy. *Journal of Osteopathy*. 1900;October VII(5):244–248.

45. American School of Osteopathy. *Journal of Osteopathy*. 1897;IV(5):217–224, 254–258.

46. American School of Osteopathy. Catalogue of the American School of Osteopathy. Session of 1897–1898. Kirksville, Missouri: Journal Printing Co.; 1897.

47. American School of Osteopathy. Catalogue of the American School of Osteopathy. Session of 1898–1899.

48. Berchtold T. A. *To Teach, To Heal, To Serve! The Story of the Chicago College of Osteopathic Medicine. The First 75 Years (1900–1975)*. Chicago: The University of Chicago Printing Department; 1975.

49. O'Neill A. Fascial reflexes: a new aid in diagnosis. *Osteopathic Profession*. 1936;3(11):16–17.

50. Kerr H. E. The role of fascia in osteopathic problems. *Journal of the American Osteopathic Association*. 1936;May:418–419.

51. Editorial Staff. In Memoriam: Harold E. Kerr DO. *The DO*. Vol. August; 2007:58.

52. Kauffman C. H. Old age and connective tissue. *The Osteopathic Profession*. 1942;5(2):77–84.

53. Becker A. R. Connective Tissue and Osteopathy: Resumé of Lectures given by Charles H. Kauffman, DO MSC. *AAO Yearbook*; 1945:57–62.

54. Denslow J. S. Soft tissues in areas of osteopathic lesion. *Journal of the American Osteopathic Association*. 1947;February:46(6):334–337.

55. Kuchera W. A., Kuchera M. L. *Osteopathic Principles in Practice*. Kirksville, Missouri: Kirksville College of Osteopathic Medicine; 1993.

56. Becker A. R. The fascias. *Osteopathic Profession*. 1947;February:XIV(5):13–17, 36,38.

57. American School of Osteopathy. Nineteenth Annual Catalogue of the American School of Osteopathy and Sixth Annual Announcement of the Nurses Training School: Kirksville, Missouri; 1911.

58. American School of Osteopathy. Eighteenth Annual Catalogue of the American School of Osteopathy and Fifth Annual Announcement of the Nurses Training School. Session of 1910–1911. Kirksville, Missouri; 1910.

59. American School of Osteopathy. Fifteenth Annual Catalogue of the American School of Osteopathy: Kirksville, Missouri; 1907.

60. Cathie A. Fascia of the head and neck as it applies to dental lesions: a preliminary consideration. *Journal of the American Osteopathic Association*. 1952;Jan 51:260–261.

61. Philadelphia College of Osteopathic Medicine. Cathie, Angus G., D.O. - 1902–1970, Professor and Chairman, Department of Anatomy 1944–1970. Available at: http://digitalcommons.pcom.edu/portraits/26/ [accessed January 11, 2016].

62. Cathie A. Fascia of the body in relation to function and manipulative therapy. Originally recorded in 1960 – in Dr Cathie's PCOM Notebook – #C-17. *AAO Yearbook*. 1974;81–84.

63. Cathie A. Consideration of fascia and its relation to disease of the musculoskeletal system. Originally published in 1962. *AAO Yearbook*. 1974:85–88.

64. Page L. E. The role of the fasciae in the maintenance of structural integrity. *AAO Yearbook*. 1952;1952:70–73.

65. Association O. C. Program for A Clinical Conference on Osteopathy, January, 5–9, 1953, Offered by the Kirksville College of Osteopathy and Surgery and sponsored by the Osteopathic Cranial Association. 1953.

66. First clinical conference sponsored by the osteopathic cranial association a success. *Journal of Osteopathy*. 1953;February:11–13.

67. Sutherland A. S., Wales A. L, Sutherland Cranial Teaching Foundation Inc., eds. *Contributions of Thought: The Collected Writings of William Garner Sutherland, D.O., Pertaining to the Art and Science of Osteopathy Including the Cranial Concept in Osteopathy Covering the Years 1914–1954*. Fort Worth, Texas: Sutherland Cranial Teaching Foundation, Inc.; 1998.

68. Snyder G. E. Embryology and physiology of fascia. *Journal of the Canadian Chiropractic Association*. 1954;1954:4–15.

69. Snyder G. E. Embryology and physiology of fascia [reprint from 1954]. *AAO yearbook*. 1970:147–158.

70. Snyder G. E. Fasciae – Applied anatomy and physiology. *AAO Yearbook*. 1956:65–75.

71. Erlingheuser R. F. The circulation of the cerebrospinal fluid through the connective tissue system. *AAO Yearbook*. 1959:77–87.

72. Magoun H. I. *Osteopathy in the Cranial Field*. 3rd ed. Kirksville Missouri: The Journal Printing Co. 1976.

73. Golden Nugget's Los Angeles Biographies. Los Angeles County biographies: Ralph F. Erlingheuser D.O. Available at: http://freepages. genealogy.rootsweb.ancestry.com/~npmelton/laerli.htm [accessed January 12, 2016].

74. PCOM Class of 1969. *The Clinical Importance of Fascia*; 1968.

75. Greenman P. E. Fascial considerations in treatment of the head and neck. *Osteopathic Annals*. 1975;February, 3(2):34–42.

76. Legacy.com. Obituary: Philip E. Greenman Available at: http://www.legacy.com/obituaries/tucson/obituary.aspx?n=philip-e-greenman&pid=162974024#sthash.DCO3pZVx.dpuf [accessed January 12, 2016].

77. Becker F. The meaning of fascial and fascial continuity. *Osteopathic Annals*. 1975;February:8–32.

78. Duke University Medical Center Archives. Becker, R. Frederick, Papers, 1942–1969. Available at: https://archives.mc.duke.edu/mcabeckerr.html [accessed January 12, 2016].

79. Cooper G. J. Some clinical considerations on fascia in diagnosis and treatment. *Journal of the American Osteopathic Association*. 1979; 78:363–347.

80. Register TDM. Dr Gerald J. Cooper Sr. Obituary Available at: http://www.legacy.com/obituaries/desmoinesregister/obituary.aspx?pid=171714789 [accessed January 12, 2016].

81. Typaldos S. Introducing the fascial distortion model. *AAO Journal*. 1994;4:14–18, 30–36.

82. American Fascial Distortion Model Association. The Fascial Distortion Model (FDM). Available at: http://www.afdma.com/ [accessed January 12, 2016].

83. Select Seminar Services, LLC. The Fascial Distortion Model TM, find it and fix it fast. Available at: http://www.fascialdistortion.com/ [accessed January 12, 2016].

84. Typaldos Family. Stephen P. Typaldos tribute. Available at: www.typaldos.org [accessed January 12, 2016].

85. Hessler D. D. The nature of fascia and the role of lower extremity fascia in low back pain. *Journal of the AAO*. 1995;5:15–19.

86. Vitals. Dallas D. Hessler, DO Available at: http://www.vitals.com/doctors/Dr_Dallas_Hessler/credentials#education [accessed January 12, 2016].

87. Crow T. The effects of manipulation on ligaments and fascia from a fluids model perspective. *The American Academy of Osteopathy*. 2006;September:13–19.

88. University of Texas Health Sciences Center. William Crow: Professor – Osteopathic Manipulative Med. Available at: https://profile.hsc.unt.edu/profilesystem/viewprofile.php?pid=100783&onlyview=1 [accessed January 12, 2016].

89. O'Connell J. A. *Bioelectric Fascial Activation and Release: The Physician's Guide to Hunting with Dr. Still*. Indianapolis: American Academy of Osteopathy; 1998.

90. Paoletti S. *Les fascias: rôle des tissus dans la mécanique humaine*. Vannes: Éditions Sully; 2009.

91. Paoletti S. *Faszien: Anatomie, Strukturen, Techniken, spezielle Osteopathie*. München; Jena: Urban und Fischer; 2001.

92. Paoletti S. *The Fasciae: Anatomy, Dysfunction and Treatment*. Seattle: Eastland Press; 2006.

93. American Osteopathic Association. Tenets of Osteopathic Medicine Available at: http://www.osteopathic.org/inside-aoa/about/leadership/Pages/tenets-of-osteopathic-medicine.aspx [accessed January 12, 2016].

94. Seffinger M. A., King H. H., Ward R. C., Jones III J. M., Rogers F. J., Patterson M. M. Osteopathic Philosophy. In: Chila A. G., American Osteopathic Association, eds. *Foundations of Osteopathic Medicine*. Philadelphia: Wolters Kluwer Health/Lippincott Williams & Wilkins. 2011;3–22.

NOMENCLATURE OF FASCIA

Werner Klingler, Julia Bierbaum, Robert Schleip

Introduction

At the end of the nineteenth century, Andrew Taylor Still documented his knowledge about fascia based on many years of experience and clinical experiments, but it took more then a century for his work to receive particular attention in modern science. This trend is demonstrated by the increasing number of movement therapies, manual therapies, massage techniques, and types of training equipment aimed at improving fascial tissue function, which have a positive impact on health and sports performance. On the basis of the immense plasticity of the tissue, it can be assumed that short-term as well as long-term changes in functional capability can be achieved if loading stimulations are applied regularly.[1-3]

In the last two decades the significance of experiences and empirical data has been analyzed scientifically, using laboratory investigations and imaging techniques, for example, high-resolution ultrasound. Objective views of anatomy and histology verify possible connections between form, function, intervention, and patients' symptoms.[4,5]

Notably, the presentation of scientific research and the interdisciplinary exchange of therapists and scientists in four fascia research congresses so far (2007, 2009, 2012, 2015)[6] demonstrate an increasing interest in the fascinating tissue of fascia, but also highlight the lack of a uniform language to define fascia. Previous definitions of fascia are diverse and depend on the perspective of the author. The two most commonly cited terminologies are the nomenclature proposed by the Federative Committee on Anatomical Terminology in 1998 and by *Gray's Anatomy* in 2008.[7,8] The first defines fascia as 'sheaths, sheets or other dissectible connective tissue aggregations' and distinguishes structures dependent on their histology. Therefore, this terminology includes connective tissue with high density and excludes loose tissue layers. *Gray's Anatomy* specifies fascia depending on fiber arrangement. It gives priority to connective tissue with interwoven structure and thus excludes one-directional orientated tissue such as ligaments, tendons, and aponeuroses. Since *Gray's Anatomy*'s definition is widely accepted, it is commonly used in communication with medical professionals.

Boston terminology

The Boston terminology is proposed by the Fascia Research Society and presents a function associated definition. Meeting the scientific findings about fascia, multidisciplinary experts came to the following conclusion regarding a standardized nomenclature:[9]

Fascia is the soft tissue component of the connective tissue. It interpenetrates and surrounds muscles, bones, organs, nerves, and blood vessels. Fascia is an uninterrupted, three-dimensional web of tissue that appears as well-defined membranes with an undulating structure permeating the whole body.[6] The tissue varies in fiber-orientation and density dependent on specific tensional demands (Figure 3.1).

The fundamental layers of fascial tissue are 1) superficial fascia, 2) deep fascia, and 3) organ-specific layers.[9]

1. The superficial fascia surrounds the body as a subcutaneous layer of non-dense, organized collagen and elastin fibers. The presence of mechanoreceptors, nociceptors, and proprioceptors as well as a network of free nerve endings, nerve fibers staining positive for calcitonin-related peptide and substance P, and sympathetic nerves, indicates the great impact of fascial tissue on proprioception and pain and demonstrates the connection between fascia and the sympathetic

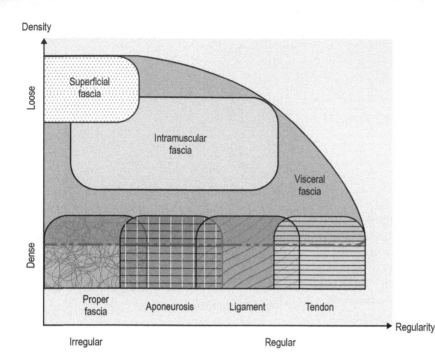

Density

Loose

Superficial fascia

Intramuscular fascia

Visceral fascia

Dense

Proper fascia   Aponeurosis   Ligament   Tendon

Regularity

Irregular   Regular

Figure 3.1
Differentiation of fascial tissue depending on density and fiber alignment. The structure adapts specifically to local tensional demands. Reproduced with permission from Schleip et al.[3]

nervous system. A high water content enables adjacent layers to move freely against one another.

2. The deep fascia is distributed throughout the whole body as a continuous sheet of mostly dense, irregular connective tissue. Due its stiffness it maintains the shape of the muscular body and provides structural support. Myofibroblasts, located in deep fascia, are important for the extent of tissue crimp and elastic recoil after elongation.

3. The organ-specific fascia merges with the deep layer and in some areas is not clearly assigned to one or the other. The term includes internal organ and joint capsules, ligaments and tendons, neurovascular sheaths, and muscle-related fascia. The latter consists of the epimysium, perimysium, and endomysium, which form fibrous compartments for the muscle, and which interconnect muscle fibers with connective tissue and the muscle with tendons. Thus, it increases strength, transmits muscle tension, and serves structural integrity.

Boston terminology highlights the fascial network as a body-wide force transmission system based on its tensegrity structure. Tensegrity originally describes a construction principle in architecture, where interconnected solid and elastic elements keep their stability

through a state of equilibrium between tension and compression. The term can be applied to fascia (biotensegrity) in humans, whose tissues extend in longitudinal and transverse direction throughout the entire body, transmitting tension from bottom to top, from outside to inside, and vice versa. With regard to the tension modulatory function of fascia, important for an upright posture and efficient body movements, biotensegrity also explains that symptom and cause location may differ. It is interesting clinically to look for interrupted mobility of fascia, for example, fascial scars, ruptures, or immobility-dependent adhesions, and for gaps in force transmission leading to impaired function along the fascial connections.[10,11]

Figures 3.2A and B show an example of how different nomenclatures of fascia affect anatomical dissections, and demonstrate their functional consequences.

Boston nomenclature – importance for manual therapists

Interest in manually applied interventions aimed at improving fascial function, such as osteopathic manipulative therapies, manual therapy/physiotherapy, connective tissue manipulation, trigger point therapy, Rolfing structural integration, and fascial manipulation has grown now that more evidence-based information about the structure and function of fascia is available.

In the manual treatment of soft tissue it is important to know about its structure, tension, and fiber arrangement; to understand its location, function, and mobility; and to be familiar with its connections and integration in different structural and functional networks. The nomenclature presented in this chapter will help in the assessment of physiological

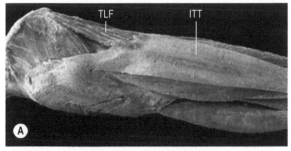

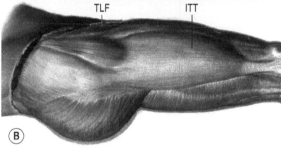

Figure 3.2

(A) An example of fascia dissection of the ITT based on the classification of *Gray's Anatomy*, in which the terms fascia and aponeurosis are treated as different structures. Therefore, the tissue connecting the ITT with the lateral iliac crest has been removed, as it does not fit to the remaining portions of the ITT as an aponeurotic structure. (B) ITT shown as a fascial structure according to Boston Terminology, which classifies fascia mainly as a tensional transmission system and therefore also includes aponeurotic structures. In the case of the ITT, the important portion of the lateral functional chain between pelvis and knee, the direct attachment of ITT with the iliac crest above glutei medius and minimus, is shown. TLF = thoracolumbar fascia; ITT = iliotibial tract

and pathological conditions of fascia and enable the therapist to choose the appropriate intervention.[12,13,1]

The terms used to refer to types of of applied fascia-related techniques differ depending on the authors and their treatment concepts. The results of recent histological and biomechanical research have led to some basic practical applications.

The following examples of recent fascia-related insights support the advantages of our proposed terminology, in which intramuscular connective tissues as well as tendinous tissues are seen as contributing elements of a body-wide fascial network. After application of mechanical load via stretching or local compression, where a significant amount of water is pushed out, fascia refills with new fluid. Increased interstitial fluid flow allows adjacent tissue layers to move one against the other, and is likely to improve mobility in that area. It might also induce myofibroblast differentiation and collagen alignment, contributing to an increase in elasticity. In tissue conditions associated with pathological water content, such as inflammatory processes, edema, or the increased accumulation of free radicals, squeezing the tissue can result in adequate rehydration.

Long-term fascial adaptation, in the form of length, strength, and the ability to shear, happens as a slow but constant reaction of fibroblasts to everyday strain as well as to specific training. Due to the plasticity of collagenous fibers, fascia steadily remodels its fibrous network arrangement. For expected treatment effects it needs to be considered that the turnover of connective tissue is more than 18 months, thus loading stimuli should continuously be applied throughout the entire period.

An increased density of myofibroblasts found in thoracolumbar fascia is associated with the amplitude of crimp in collagen fibers as well as with resting muscle tone. Tendinous and aponeurotic tissues have been shown to be the basis for the 'catapult effect' in jumping kangaroos as well as running antelopes, horses, and humans. Muscle-related connective tissue stores energy while being prestretched, and can generate high acceleration of movements by releasing the tension. Soft elastic bounces in the end ranges of available motion are recommended to increase elastic recoil, contributing to elasticity and effectiveness in daily activity.

Fascial layers and main contents	Main function	Fascial adaptation due to manually applied stimuli and training
Superficial fascia • Subcutaneous layer • Continuous sheath of loose connective tissue • Mechanoreceptors, nociceptors, and proprioceptors • Pain-related nerves • Sympathetic nerves	'Communication' Posture and movement awareness Pain generation Interaction with autonomous nervous system Shaping of muscular body	Adequate hydration ↑ Pain ↓ Tension release and increase Proprioception ↑ Length ↑ Elasticity ↑
Deep fascia • Continuous sheath of mostly dense, irregular connective tissue • Collagen and elastin fibers • Myofibroblasts	Shaping of muscular body Structural support Tension transmission Elastic recoil Wound healing	
Organ-specific fascia • Sheaths of muscles, nerves, vessels, and bones • Capsules of internal organs and joints	Organ protection Muscle strength Muscle tension transmission Structural integrity	
Intermuscular septa • Closely packed bundles of collagen fibers	Separation of different muscle groups	
Intramuscular and extramuscular aponeuroses • Multiple layers of collagen bundles with various directions • Muscle fiber attachment	Force transmission between muscle groups	
Interosseal membrane • Thin collagen membrane	Connection of two bones	
Neurovascular tract • Dense, irregular connective tissue sheaths for vessels and nerves	Protection	
Periosteum • Bilayered collagen membrane for the bone	Blood supply	

Table 3.1
Fascial nomenclature: key points

If excessively active, myofibroblasts are involved in pathological fascial contractures such as fibromyalgia, scleroderma, and frozen shoulder, and some cases of low back pain (LBP) may also be associated with a similar stiffening of the thoracolumbar fascia (TLF), which could be described as 'frozen lumbars'. Moreover, these structural changes could constrict nerve and vessel pathways through the layers. Reduction in blood supply or venous return is one reason for various symptoms like compartment syndrome, while nerve compression could lead to inappropriate muscle innervation and increased tensile stress distally and proximally.[1,14,15,5]

Recent research into thoracolumbar fascia demonstrates that a tissue-specific pain pattern appears when a pain-inducing stimulus is applied. Compared to the sensory reactions of back muscles, fascial pain is higher in intensity, longer in duration, wider in spread, and is of a more affective quality (agonizing, heavy ...). A high density of sympathetic nerves were found in fascia and this suggests that fascia is a source of at least some cases of LBP and, more than that, potentially explains why some patients with LBP report increased intensity of pain when they are under psychological stress. It seems useful to integrate these findings into clinical reasoning processes in order to differentiate structures in the origin of pain. Slowly applied stretching forces are likely to reduce mechanical sensitivity and functional limitations, and may lead to improved body awareness.[5,16,17,4]

Stiffening of fascia seems to be important in the stabilization of underlying joints. Willard et al. summarized current evidence about the biomechanical properties of the TLF due to its multiple muscle attachments. Contraction of the latissimus dorsi, gluteus maximus, and transversus abdominis muscles, for example, transmits tension through the TLF, thus stiffening the lumbar spine and increasing force-closure of the sacroiliac joint. Both tensioning fascial chains during functional movements and increasing trunk stability essentially contribute to force transmission between the upper and lower body.[5]

Conclusion

It can be concluded that the nomenclature presented in this chapter explains facts about the anatomy and physiology of the fascia according to scientific research. It highlights the important findings and thus is useful for therapists treating fascia since it will enable them to understand the form, structure, and function of fascia and it could complement the patient's previous assessment and therapy. The terminology provides a common language for manual therapists and other experts, both in practical use and in science.

References

1. **Schleip, R. & Muller, D. G. 2013.** Training principles for fascial connective tissues: scientific foundation and suggested practical applications. *J Bodyw Mov Ther*, 17, 103–115.

2. **Still, A. T. 1899.** *Philosophy of Osteopathy*, Kirksville, Missouri, A. T.Still.

3. **Schleip, R., Jager, H. & Klingler, W. 2012.** What is 'fascia'? A review of different nomenclatures. *J Bodyw Mov Ther*, 16, 496–502.

4. **Findley, T., Chaudhry, H., Stecco, A. & Roman, M. 2012.** Fascia research—a narrative review. *J Bodyw Mov Ther*, 16, 67–75.

5. **Willard, F. H., Vleeming, A., Schuenke, M. D., Danneels, L. & Schleip, R. 2012.** The thoracolumbar fascia: anatomy, function and clinical considerations. *J Anat*, 221, 507–536.

6. **Fascia Research Congress. Recordings and Proceedings Books.** http://www.fasciacongress. org/2015/conference/dvd-recordings-and-books/ [accessed January 18, 2016].

7. **Federative Committee on Anatomical Terminology (FCAT). 1998.** *Terminologia Anatomica: International Anatomical Terminology*. Stuttgart: Georg Thieme Verlag.

8. **Standring, S. (ed) 2008.** *Gray's Anatomy: The Anatomical Basis of Clinical Practice*, 40th edn. Churchill Livingstone Elsevier.

9. **Langevin, H. M. & Huijing, P. A. 2009.** Communicating about fascia: history, pitfalls, and recommendations. *Int J Ther Massage Bodywork*, 2, 3–8.

10. **Bordoni, B. & Zanier, E. 2013.** Skin, fascias, and scars: symptoms and systemic connections. *J Multidiscip Healthc*, 7, 11–24.

11. **Swanson, R. L., 2nd. 2013.** Biotensegrity: a unifying theory of biological architecture with applications to osteopathic practice, education, and research—a review and analysis. *J Am Osteopath Assoc*, 113, 34–52.

12. **Findley, T. W. & Shalwala, M. 2013.** Fascia Research Congress evidence from the 100 year perspective of Andrew Taylor Still. *J Bodyw Mov Ther*, 17, 356–364.

13. **Schleip, R. F., Findley, T.W.; Chaitow, L.; Huijing, P. A. 2012.** *Fascia The Tensional Network of the Human Body*, Churchill Livingstone Elsevier.

14. **Schleip, R., Duerselen, L., Vleeming, A., Naylor, I. L., Lehmann-Horn, F., Zorn, A., Jaeger, H. & Klingler, W. 2012.** Strain hardening of fascia: static stretching of dense fibrous connective tissues can induce a temporary stiffness increase accompanied by enhanced matrix hydration. *J Bodyw Mov Ther*, 16, 94–100.

15. **Ng, C. P., Hinz, B. & Swartz, M. A. 2005.** Interstitial fluid flow induces myofibroblast differentiation and collagen alignment in vitro. *J Cell Sci*, 118, 4731–4739.

16. **Schilder, A., Hoheisel, U., Magerl, W., Benrath, J., Klein, T. & Treede, R. D. 2014.** Sensory findings after stimulation of the thoracolumbar fascia with hypertonic saline suggest its contribution to low back pain. *Pain*, 155, 222–231.

17. **Corey, S. M., Vizzard, M. A., Bouffard, N. A., Badger, G. J. & Langevin, H. M. 2012.** Stretching of the back improves gait, mechanical sensitivity and connective tissue inflammation in a rodent model. *PLOS One*, 7, e29831.

THE EMBRYOLOGY OF FASCIA: PROVIDING THE CAPACITY FOR MOVEMENT AND INTEGRITY

Darrell J. R. Evans

Introduction

The developmental journey of the human embryo is a fascinating one filled with explosions of cell division and growth, complex sets of interactions between cells and their surroundings, a continuous series of movements and positioning, and incremental patterns of structural intricacies. Developing the 'masterplan' of the embryo is the result of a defined interconnection between mechanical, genetic, chemical, and morphological factors and relies on the necessary populations of cells being in the right place at the right time and ready for action. The developmental journey is not just confined to the embryonic period (up until the end of the eighth week of gestation) and is instead a continuous and ever-changing process until the end of puberty. Birth simply acts as a change in environment for the developing human, without an interruption in tissue development, growth and maturity. The continuous nature of change during development has been likened to the art of origami where the folding to form an elaborate structure relies on a precise and sequential set of steps and if one fold is missing or incorrectly made there are consequential effects on the final structure.[1]

The study of embryology has often been demonstrated as a static set of events or been explained by concentrating on the development of a specific structure without reference to the surrounding players, other cell populations, their movements, and the forces acting on them. The importance of biokinetics and biodynamics during development has been demonstrated through the work of Erich Blechschmidt and latterly Raymond Gasser.[2,3] Their work shows that developmental processes are 'kinetically related', with physical forces evoking changes in the differentiation and interrelations of cell populations and the shape and size configurations that occur as development proceeds. An appreciation of these interrelationships allows us to better understand the basis of the functional and dynamic architecture of the adult anatomy.

While the importance of biodynamics during the development journey is often underplayed, the formation and functional role of the fascia during development is largely overlooked. In anatomy, fascia is often seen as the nuisance tissue that needs to be cleaned away to see the real constituent tissues of the particular structure. However, as we know, it is the fascia that really provides the balanced functional ability of tissues and structures in the body. In the case of the musculoskeletal system, the fascia is responsible for the transmission of contractile or tensional forces within the musculoskeletal unit, resulting in movement. The essential intimate and integrated association of the fascial connective tissues with other players such as the muscle arises during development and is the result of a precise spatial and temporal sequence of events.[4] The establishment of a detailed pattern of integration is achieved even though the precursors of the component elements have different embryological origins and exhibit independent differentiation sequences. Unlike the other tissues of the body, there is a continuous and singular fascial network: the fascial web or net.[5] This network interconnects all fascia within the body and becomes apparent quite early in development. However, it is unclear exactly what role the fascia might play in determining the movement, positioning, and integration of other embryonic cell populations, although it is likely to be key.

This short chapter is therefore designed to outline some of the main stages of embryogenesis, with a focus on establishing the origins and early formation of tissues including fascia, and also to highlight the importance of demonstrating some of the dynamics underlying the developmental journey. Using the developing limb as an example, a demonstration will be made of how the connective tissues play a specific and dynamic role in determining the arrangement, formation, and functionality of an integrated structural unit. The processes outlined in this chapter are influenced by an array of signaling interactions (which articulate with and respond to kinetic factors), but these will not be covered in any detail. The understanding of the embryology leading to and providing the basis for the adult anatomy should enhance the ability of osteopathic practitioners to diagnose and apply their therapies.

Early embryology – from fertilized egg to the trilaminar embryo

Following fertilization the resulting zygote undergoes a division process called cleavage, which produces a cluster of cells in a solid mass called a morula, resembling the morphology of a mulberry. Over the next day or so the cells become stretched and a cavity forms within the morula, with cells becoming defined either within an outer layer of cells called the trophoblast (which will form the embryonic part of the placenta) or within an inner cell mass (which will form the embryo itself) located against part of the trophoblast wall. This is known as a blastocyst.

Once within the uterine body, the blastocyst attaches to and implants into the endometrial wall. The trophoblast differentiates into an inner layer of cells, the cytotrophoblast, which both surrounds the inner cell mass and continually forms new trophoblastic cells that are pushed outwards into the endometrium. These fuse to form a syncytiotrophoblast layer, which expands as a multinucleated mass and continues to invade the endometrium, gradually contributing to the formation of the placenta. Meanwhile the cells within the inner cell mass start to alter shape in response to changes around them and form a disc-like structure that eventually arranges as two layers of cells: a thick, overlying epiblast layer of columnar cells and a thin, underlying hypoblast layer of cuboidal cells. This is known as the bilaminar embryonic disc (Fig. 4.1).

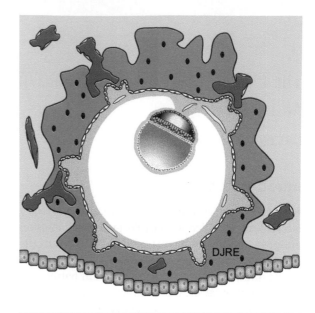

Figure 4.1

Implanted blastocyst with formation of the bilaminar embryonic disc and associated structures

Two cavities form around the embryonic disc. The amniotic cavity first develops as a cavitation within the epiblast layer as the outer cytotrophoblast expands and pulls away from the embryonic disc. The cells separating from the epiblast are called aminoblasts and form the roof of the cavity. The aminoblasts gradually transform into the amniotic membrane that surrounds the amnion and the growing embryo. Another cavity forms below the hypoblast called the primary umbilical vesicle (formerly called the yolk sac, but which in humans contains no yolk). The embryonic disc therefore becomes situated between the amniotic cavity and the primary umbilical vesicle.

Whilst the trophoblast layers provide the network of supporting tissues for the embryo, the embryonic disc is the focus for embryo formation. The most significant process during this period is gastrulation, which produces the three germ layers, arranged as a trilaminar embryonic disc. The highly dynamic process of gastrulation begins with the appearance of the primitive streak in the epiblast surface of the disc and

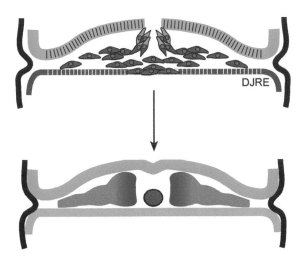

DJRE

Figure 4.2

The process of gastrulation: formation of the trilaminar embryonic disc (ectoderm = blue; mesoderm = red; endoderm = green)

The developing mesoderm – an array of different roles

The mesoderm layer of the embryo, while initially a homogeneous and mesenchymal population of cells, gives rise to various cell types in response to location, cell-to-cell interactions and movements, and response to kinetic and genetic patterning signals. The mesodermal mesenchyme forms all the supporting tissues of the body, including the connective tissues. These mesoderm-derived connective tissue cells migrate and inhabit much of the developing embryo, except in the head region where connective tissues are mainly derived from another population of embryonic cells called neural crest cells. Despite their different origins, all the connective tissue cells seamlessly interact to form a continuous connective tissue framework extending throughout the embryo. This framework is essentially the prelude to the fascial net and provides a flexibility and consistency that allows cells to move and interact to become appropriately positioned and integrated as development proceeds.

results from rapidly dividing epiblast cells migrating to the midline and forming a narrow groove with a small pit at one end. This defines the main cranio–caudal axis and thus the head and tail, left and right sides, and dorsal and ventral aspects of the embryo. Epiblast cells around the pit and along the streak change shape because of their location, gradually become detached, and move between the epiblast and hypoblast layers forming a mesenchyme (loose aggregation of intermingling cells). Because of their close apposition to the hypoblast the first cells invade and displace hypoblast cells laterally and form a definitive embryonic endoderm layer. The space between the epiblast and newly formed endoderm layers gradually expands as more cells move beneath the epiblast, and these cells are pushed laterally and cranially to form an internal layer of mesoderm called the intraembryonic mesoderm. As the definitive endoderm and mesoderm layers are formed, the epiblast becomes known as the ectoderm. A trilaminar disc is now evident, with all three germ layers derived from the epiblast. Gastrulation continues as the embryo elongates, forming new mesoderm until about week four of gestation, with the primitive streak regressing thereafter (Fig. 4.2).

The mesoderm cells that derive from those cells entering the sub-epiblast space through the primitive pit move forward in the midline to form a rod-like organization of cells that becomes a very important signaling structure known as the notochord. The notochord will initiate the development of a range of other surrounding structures and provides some structural integrity to the early developing embryo. In humans the remains of the notochord form the nucleus pulposus of the intervertebral disc. An example of the importance of the notochord as a signaling center is demonstrated with the formation of the neural tube, which will become the brain and spinal cord. However, it is the combination of genetic and kinetic signaling that enables the neural tube to form. In response to signals from the notochord the overlying ectoderm cells are induced to become neuroectoderm and form a neural plate. Cell shape changes within the plate and the apposition and subsequent anchoring of the midline cells to the notochord causes an invagination in the plate and the creation of the neural groove surrounded by lateral neural folds. Continued cell proliferation in the adjacent ectoderm forces the neural folds to push towards one another, eventually fusing in the midline and forming the

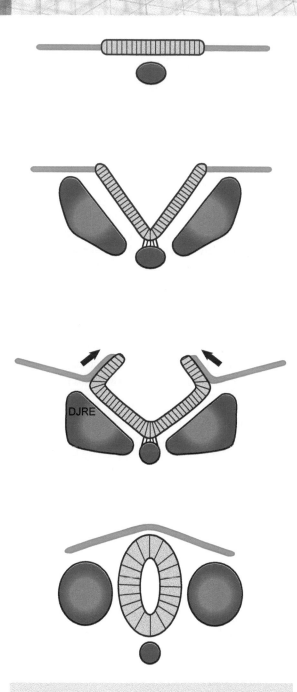

Figure 4.3

The process of neurulation: formation of the neural tube

and become a continuous layer that later contributes to the epidermis. The neural tube gradually becomes displaced into the mesodermal mesenchyme. The dorsal aspect of the neural tube is where the neural crest cells originate and migrate within the embryo (Fig. 4.3).

Cells that enter the sub-epiblast space though the primitive streak become displaced laterally, with mesoderm becoming regionalized and segregated and thereby destined for differing fates. The cells located closest to the midline and immediately adjacent to the developing neural tube are known as the paraxial mesoderm, while the cells pushed to the lateral edges of the trilaminar disc form a sheet-like layer and are known as the lateral plate mesoderm. Those cells in between are called the intermediate mesoderm. The paraxial mesoderm, which appears as longitudinal bands of cells, is one of the key players in the development of the musculoskeletal system, forming an array of tissues including some of the connective tissues. Initially a mesenchyme, the paraxial mesoderm becomes divided into discrete blocks of tissue called somites. Somites form in a cranial to caudal sequence, although the paraxial mesoderm in the head region remains unsegmented. Somites give rise to the axial skeleton; epaxial, hypaxial and limb skeletal muscle; axial tendons; and also the dermis of neck and trunk.[6] As such the somites are critical transient structures that establish the segmented body plan of vertebrates, the organization of which allows our integrated movements (Fig. 4.4).

Each somite is initially an epithelialized rosette of cells surrounding a core of mesenchymal cells. Signals from surrounding structures induce the ventral cells of the somite to lose their epithelial organization and develop into the sclerotome, while the remaining dorsal epithelial cap becomes the dermomyotome.[6] As proliferation increases, ventral cells of each sclerotome move and surround the notochord forming the rudiment of the vertebral body, while the dorsal sclerotome cells come to surround the neural tube and form the rudiment of the vertebral arch. The dermomyotome of each somite gives rise to skeletal muscle and dermis. Proliferating and elongating cells at the lips of the dermomyotome generate the myotomes, which in turn gives rise to epaxial and

neural tube. This zippering process continues along the length of the embryo. The neural tube disassociates from the ectoderm as the ectoderm cells reseal

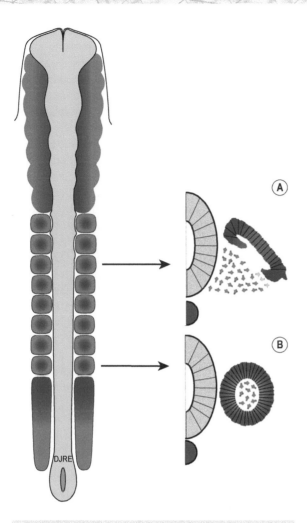

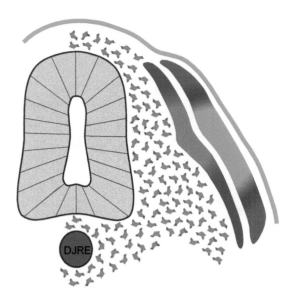

Figure 4.5
Late somite differentiation: sclerotome envelops neural tube; and dermatome and myotome become distinct

Figure 4.4
The formation and early differentiation of somites. (A) Differentiating somite with sclerotome and dermomyotome evident. (B) Newly formed somite: an epithelialized ball of mesoderm

hypaxial skeletal muscle. Cells at the lateral margin of the dermomyotome give rise to limb muscle precursors in the regions of developing limbs. As the neighboring ectoderm expands outwards, the dermatome becomes separated from the myotomes and goes on to contribute to the dermis of the neck and back. Interaction between the myotome and the ventral sclerotome produces the syndetome, which is the origin of the tendons of the vertebral region (Fig. 4.5).

This elaborate series of continuous events provides the foundations of much of the musculoskeletal system. However, it is the lateral plate mesoderm that plays a significant role in shaping the placement and integration of structures, due in part to it being the main connective tissue production centre of the body. Whilst starting out as two sheets of cells on the two lateral edges of the embryo, small gaps start to appear within the mesoderm due to the growth and expansion of the embryo pulling the layers of cells apart. These gaps gradually merge to create a large cavity known as the intraembryonic coelom. This leaves a somatic mesoderm layer associated with the outer ectoderm, which subsequently gives rise to the body wall lining tissues and the mesenchyme of the developing limbs, and the splanchnic mesoderm that associates with the endoderm and gives rise to the coverings of the viscera. The elaborate process of embryonic folding that now ensues uses all these layers and the intraembryonic coelom, which expand and change shape to help form the body cavities in the thorax and abdomen (Fig. 4.6).

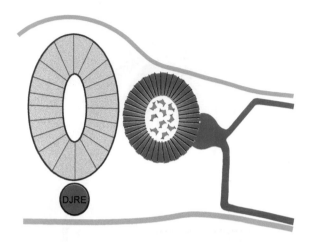

Figure 4.6
Separation of lateral plate mesoderm into somatic and splanchnic mesoderm

Embryonic folding – a result of differential growth

The process of embryonic folding is essential as it transforms the flat trilaminar disc formed during gastrulation into the start of a recognizable human embryo. Folding results mainly from the differential growth of various embryonic structures and involves a range of mesenchymal populations of cells, including those of the mesoderm. The developing notochord, neural tube and somites stiffen the dorsal axis of the embryo, thereby restricting folding mainly to the flexible outer rim of the disc. The most distinctive period of folding involves the cranial, caudal, and lateral margins of the disc folding underneath the dorsal axial structures to give rise to the ventral surface of the embryo. Initially the pericardial tissues of the embryo lie at the most cranial end of the embryo, however, as the body axis lengthens between relatively fixed attachments, the disc buckles and the pericardium rotates through 180 degrees. The head fold is further enhanced by a flexure of the neural tube. A small portion of the primary umbilical vesicle becomes trapped and incorporated into the embryo as the *foregut* (primitive pharynx). It is surrounded by the layer of splanchnic mesoderm and ends blindly at the membrane covering the future mouth. The tail fold occurs later than the head fold and results from the growth of the neural tube, caudally. Growth causes another buckling, with the tail region rotating ventrally and a small part of the primary umbilical vesicle becoming incorporated into the embryo as the *hindgut* (primitive colon), ending blindly at the membrane covering the future anus and again surrounded by splanchnic mesoderm. Folding of the lateral sides of the embryo first ventrally and then towards the midline is due to the inability to expand further laterally and results in the creation of a cylindrical embryo. As the abdominal wall forms, part of the primary umbilical vesicle becomes trapped and incorporated into the embryo as the *midgut* (primordium of small intestines) and the beginnings of the peritoneal cavity. As a consequence of this embryonic folding, the ectoderm, lined by somatic mesoderm, covers the entire embryo except in the region of the body stalk. The lateral edges of the embryo fuse ventrally to create the gut tube and are surrounded by splanchnic mesoderm, which provides the smooth muscle and connective tissue of the viscera. The heart becomes a centralized structure in the future thoracic region. Further folding and reshaping occurs within the embryo and is essentially a continuous process throughout the developmental journey, one that uses the interconnecting net of connective tissue and the differential growth of intermingling cells and tissues (Fig. 4.7).

The developing limb – a pattern of integration for musculoskeletal development

The first sign of the limbs are small out-pocketings from the upper (cervical) and lower (lumbar/sacral) body wall areas, which gradually develop into the limb buds. These buds are formed from the rapid proliferation of lateral plate mesoderm cells, resulting in a limb mesenchyme covered by ectoderm. The limb mesenchyme produces all the connective tissues of the limb including tendons, ligaments, and fascia as well as the cartilages and bones.[7,8,9] At the distal end of the limb bud there is a thickened area of external ectoderm called the apical ectodermal ridge (AER). The AER is important as it produces factors that keep cells at the distal region in a state of proliferation and stops them differentiating. As the limb grows out from the body wall, due to the rapid proliferation of cells, the cells that are more proximal lose the influ-

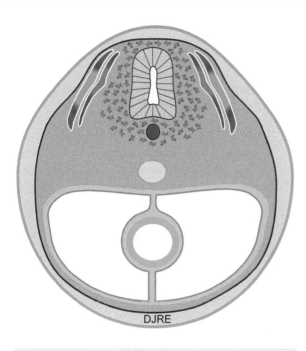

DJRE

Figure 4.7
Section of developing embryo postembryonic folding with gut tube internalized and ectoderm covering the embryo

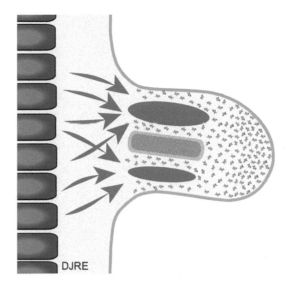

DJRE

Figure 4.8
Developing limb bud demonstrating early formation of musculoskeletal components

ence of these factors and are able to stop dividing and start to differentiate (Fig. 4.8).

The development of the limb skeleton

Some cells condense within the core region of the limb bud to form cartilaginous elements that act as the templates for the subsequent skeletal components of the limb.[10] The spatial patterning of the limb is under the control of various genes, which are responsible for the laying down of the skeletal elements in a particular sequence. Such a pattern is fascinatingly repeated in almost all mammals, although modifications to the pattern allow for the required functional adaptations in each animal. As the limb extends further a hand or footplate is formed, appearing initially as a flattened paddle-shaped feature. Some cells within the plates condense to form cartilaginous digital rays in a sequence so that formation is from the fifth to the first digit. The tissue between each ray gradually undergoes programmed cell death, revealing the

fingers and toes. Once formed, the limb cartilages undergo endochondral ossification to form bone, a process that doesn't stop in long bones until adulthood (Fig. 4.9).

The formation of the joints is a characteristic feature during the differentiation of the limb skeleton, and synovial joints form once the mesenchymal condensations have taken shape.[11] The formation of the joint is first apparent as an area of higher cell density within the cartilaginous mesenchymal rods, which is known as the interzone. This region gradually undergoes cavitation, which produces two opposing and separate elements. Joint morphogenesis can now take place with the mesenchyme at the ends of the developing skeletal primordia becoming a dense, fibrous tissue that gradually forms articular cartilage, covering the ends of the bones. The cartilage allows the smooth articulation between opposing skeletal elements in the adult. The capsule of the joint forms from connective tissue cells that surround the interzone and gradually form a protective fibrous tissue layer. The movement of the embryo and muscle contractility in particular appear to be necessary requirements for appropriate joint formation.[12]

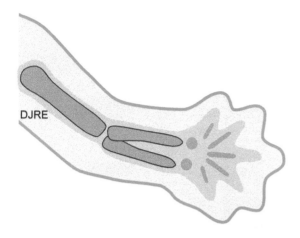

Figure 4.9
Developing limb demonstrating laying down of skeletal elements and formation of the hand plate

Developing muscles, tendons, and connective tissues – an intimate association

The muscular components of the limbs originate in the somites, with limb muscle precursor cells delaminating from the lateral edge of the dermomyotome region of somites adjacent to the limb bud.[13] These cells actively migrate into the limb in response to specific signals from surrounding tissues and keep pace with the distal outgrowth of the limb bud.[14] Muscle precursors become aggregated and form a large muscle mass close to the first forming skeletal elements. In response to growth and invading connective tissues, the masses separate to form a dorsal (extensor) and ventral (flexor) mass, continuing to differentiate. Precursor cells within the masses differentiate into myoblasts, which begin to line up against a scaffold of connective tissue and extracellular matrix molecules and fuse together to form multinucleated myotubes. The myotubes gradually differentiate as the characteristic organelles of skeletal muscles such as myobibrils develop and the myotubes mature to become muscle fibers, a process that continues during the fetal period up until around birth. No new fibers form after birth and instead growth results from hypertrophy of the fibers as more myofilaments are formed and more myoblasts are added. The initial connective scaffold enables an intimacy with developing muscle fibers to be formed. As the connective tissues extend and invest further they become the epimysium, perimysium, and endomysium of the muscle. Initial functionality of the limb muscles occurs during the embryonic period as motor axons (ventral primary rami) from the developing spinal cord enter the limb, and divide into dorsal and ventral divisions in order to innervate the dorsal and ventral muscle masses respectively. Cues within the limb mesenchyme are responsible for guiding the early direction of the growing axons into and within the limb (Fig. 4.10). The developing perimysium surrounds a bundle of muscle fibers to form a fascicle (the linkages of the words fascia and fascicle demonstrate the functionality that is the fascia binding together the fibers as a bundle that creates the fascicle) and provides a conduit for the nerve fibers to travel as well as the growing network of the blood vessels.

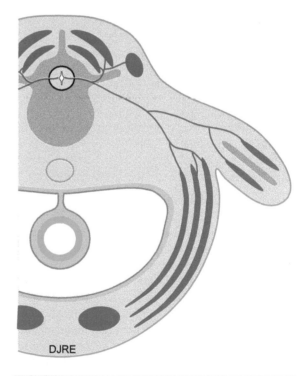

Figure 4.10
Section of developing embryo demonstrating axons invading muscular components

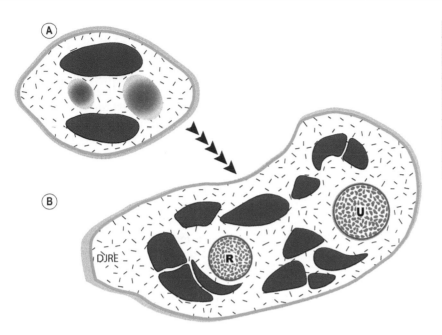

Figure 4.11
Sections of developing limb. (A) Formation of dorsal and ventral muscle masses. (B) Individuation of muscles around the developing ulna (U) and radius (R)

Early contact between the nerve and muscle cells is a prerequisite for functional differentiation to become complete. The muscle masses themselves gradually undergo cleavage, the pattern of which is determined by the intervening connective tissue and results in the formation of the individual muscles of the limb, which grow in length in response to the expansion and elongation of the skeleton. Muscles are capable of contracting by the early fetal period, although maturation of the muscle architecture continues until after birth (Fig. 4.11).

The tendons in the limb are derived from connective tissue cells within the limb mesenchyme aggregating to form blastemas, which subsequently develop into the tendinous bands of dense, fibrous connective tissue. Developing tendons become associated with their respective muscles at the myotendinous junction, a structural interface formed through an intricate association of muscle, tendon, and muscle connective tissue cells. These come together to produce a functional zone that permits appropriate force transmission. The blastemas that give rise to the limb tendons form in the absence of developing muscles, but failure to establish muscle connections results in the nascent tendons gradually breaking down into disorganized connective tissue.[15] The exact nature of the interaction between muscle and

tendon and connective tissue cells once the early connective tissue pattern is established is unknown. Full differentiation and maturation of the tendon body, myotendinous junction, and enthesis can only occur once muscle contractility is possible.

The influence of the developing limb connective tissues

It must be remembered, as highlighted above, that the process of skeletal and muscle formation takes place within a dynamic mesenchymal environment, dominated by cells that will contribute to the fascia of the limb and embedded in a collagen fiber-rich matrix. These populations of cells will need to become closely associated with skeletal and muscular tissues in a controlled and organized manner to ensure appropriate functionality of the resulting musculoskeletal unit and ability to maintain its integrity under differing loads. In the case of muscle morphogenesis this connectivity is achieved despite the precursors having different origins and demonstrating, at least initially, independent differentiating steps.[4] Whilst these tissues will have an intimate relationship within the adult anatomy, the role that the connective tissue plays in determining the movement and specification of muscle primordia within the embryo is not clear. We are aware that connective tissue has a profound influencing effect on the spatial pattern of muscle morphogenesis, with the defined spatial organization being initially established within the connective tissues, an arrangement that appears to be imposed on the later-forming muscle by providing specific differentiation 'addresses'. Studies in the limb demonstrate that, prior to the arrival of the myogenic primordia, connective tissues become positionally specified,[9,16] a pattern that is maintained whether myogenic cells eventually localize to this destination or not.[17] It appears that within the limb mesenchyme specific populations of cells are responsible for establishing a prepattern within the environment of the limb. This subsequently dictates the basic pattern of individuated muscles and enables the intimate musculofascial organization to develop. It is unclear whether this prepattern is purely a structural patterning cue that guides the spacialization of the muscle progenitors, or whether additional mechanisms come into play including the action of the invading blood vessels.[4]

In the head where neural crest cells generate the connective tissues and tendons of the muscles, the sequence of interaction is different, with neural crest cells interacting with their muscle precursor counterparts at different stages of morphogenesis.[18] Individual muscle and connective tissue precursors arise in close registration and maintain contiguity during the migration to their destination, however, integration of the precursors doesn't occur until they have reached the destination. The relationship formed at that point is maintained and matured. The investing connective tissues and distal attachment regions of the muscle are formed at an even later stage, although it is unclear whether the neural crest cells determine these attachment sites.[19,20,18]

Conclusion

The developmental journey in humans is characterized by interactions of cell populations; waves and flows of cell movement; differential expansion and growth of tissues; and the developing maturation of structural integrity. All this relies on an exquisite intercommunication of dynamic mechanical, genetic, chemical, and morphological factors. Such an articulation of factors also governs the

functionality and biodynamics of the adult anatomy and demonstrates a deep relationship with our embryonic past. An understanding of the dynamic cooperation of the component elements during development and the major role played by the fascia in providing a spatial architecture will provide osteopathic practitioners with a more holistic view of the interplays at work and will hopefully enhance their ability to diagnose and apply appropriate therapy.

References

1. **Avison J. S. (2015).** *Yoga: Fascia Anatomy and Movement.* Handspring Publishing: Edinburgh.

2. **Blechschmidt E. (2004).** *The Ontogenetic Basis of Human Anatomy: A Biodynamic Approach to Development from Conception to Birth,* trans. B. Freeman. North Atlantic Books, Berkeley: CA.

3. **Blechschmidt E., Gasser R. F. (2012)** *Biokinetics and Biodynamics of Human Differentiation: Principles and Applications.* North Atlantic Books, Berkeley: CA.

4. **Evans D. J. R., Valasek P., Schmidt C., Patel K. (2006)** Skeletal muscle translocation in vertebrates. *Anat Embryol (Berl)* 211:43–50.

5. **Myers T. W. (2014)** *Anatomy Trains: Myofascial Meridians for Manual and Movement Therapists.* Churchill Livingstone Elsevier.

6. **Christ B., Huang R., Scaal M. (2007)** Amniote somite derivatives. *Develop Dyn* 236:2382–2396.

7. **Christ B., Jacob H. J., Jacob M. (1977)** Experimental analysis of the origin of the wing musculature in avian embryos. *Anat Embryol (Berl)* 150:171–186.

8. **Ordahl C. P., Le Douarin N. M. (1992)** Two myogenic lineages within the developing somite. *Development* 114:339–353.

9. **Kardon G. (1998)** Muscle and tendon morphogenesis in the avian hind limb. *Development* 125:4019–4032.

10. **Egawa S., Miura S., Yokoyama H., Endo T., Tamura K. (2014)** Growth and differentiation of a long bone in limb development, repair and regeneration. *Develop Growth Differ* 56:410–424.

11. **Decker R. S., Koyama E., Pacifici M. (2014)** Genesis and morphogenesis of limb synovial joints and articular cartilage. *Matrix Biol* 39:5–10.

12. **Yasuda H., de Crombrugghe B. (2009)** Joint formation requires muscle formation and contraction. *Developmental Cell* 16:625–626.

13. **Christ B., Ordahl C. (1995)** Early stages of chick somite development. *Anat Embryol (Berl)* 191:381–396.

14. **Musumeci G., Castrogiovanni P., Coleman R, Szychlinska MA, Salvatorelli L, Parenti R, Magro G., Imbesi R. (2015)** Somitogenesis: from somite to skeletal muscle. *Acta Histochem* 117:313–328.

15. **Schweitzer R., Zelzer E., Volk T. (2010)** Connecting muscles to tendons: tendons and musculoskeletal development in flies and vertebrates. *Development* 137:2807–2817.

16. **Kardon G., Campbell J. K., Tabin C. J. (2002)** Local extrinsic signals determine muscle and endothelial cell fate and patterning in the vertebrate limb. *Dev Cell* 3:533–545.

17. **Kardon G., Harfe B. D., Tabin C. J. (2003)** A Tcf4-positive mesodermal population provides a prepattern for vertebrate limb muscle patterning. *Dev Cell* 5:937–944.

18. **Evans D. J., Noden D. M. (2006)** Spatial relations between avian craniofacial neural crest and paraxial mesoderm cells. *Dev Dyn* 235:1310–1325.

19. **Trainor P. A., Tam P. P. (1995)** Cranial paraxial mesoderm and neural crest cells of the mouse embryo: co-distribution in the craniofacial mesenchyme but distinct segregation in branchial arches. *Development* 121:2569–2582.

20. **Matsuoka T., Ahlberg P. E., Kessaris N., Iannarelli P., Dennehy U., Richardson W. D., McMahon A. P., Koentges G. (2005)** Neural crest origins of the neck and shoulder. *Nature* 436:347–355.

HISTOLOGY OF FASCIA
Frans van den Berg

Introduction

Before we describe the histology of the fascia in more detail, we first have to understand the basic principles of connective tissue. The most basic question to consider is: why do we have connective tissue, and what are its functions in the human body?

One reason that we have connective tissue is because it protects the cells, the tissues, and the organ systems of the body. Another reason is that it allows the different tissues to move friction-free against each other. This friction-free movement is extremely important, because permanent friction would adversely affect health. Unrelieved friction would mean that the body would never be able to stabilize its core temperature at a constant level of approximately 37° C.

In addition, the connective tissue enables, by the specific structure of the extracellular matrix, the diffusion processes to occur and the cells to receive their nutrients. Moreover, the connective tissue is an important information and coordinating system. It communicates with the central nervous system and the autonomic nervous system, and it controls their coordination (see also Chapter 6).

Protection

The primary purpose of connective tissue is protection of the cells. When we study the origin of life on this planet, we suspect that it started with the development of single-celled organisms that lived in water. The border between the inside of the cell and the external water was formed by the cell membrane, which was built of a double layer of phospholipids (Fig. 5.1).

Single-celled microorganisms essentially possess all the major functional abilities that our multicellular bodies possess. They can absorb and remove chemical substances. They have organs, or organelles, that can absorb, convert, reduce, and utilize nutrients as energy. They have sensory and controlling systems – the integrated membrane proteins (channel proteins) that transport substances into and out of the cell. But there are also receptor proteins that transfer information from the outside to the inside of the cell, controlling the activity of the cell nucleus and, thus, the genetic material.[1,2,3] The single cell possesses contractility and, in this way, it can change its form, and it is mobile.

The only major multicellular-type functional characteristic that the single cell does not possess is protection against mechanical loading. The thin cell membrane, with its phospholipid components, does not lend the cell a significant amount of mechanical protection. This was not a problem when cells first evolved billions of years ago, because the first microbes were presumably filled with water and were living in water, thus the cell membrane was not exposed to higher mechanical loadings.[4]

The next step in evolution was the development of multicellular organisms. This evolutionary milestone was enabled by the development of intercellular connections, such as tight junctions. These structures formed the basis for the later development of the Metazoan animals (e.g., fish, amphibians, reptiles, birds, mammals), the body plans of which can be traced to the 'Cambrian explosion' between approximately 570 million and 530 million years ago.[5,6]

Due to these developments, there was a necessity for the cells of the multicellular organism to be protected against mechanical loading. To achieve this protection, the cells produce an extracellular matrix. This extracellular matrix is connected to the cell membrane by integrins.[1,2] If the cell is mainly loaded with

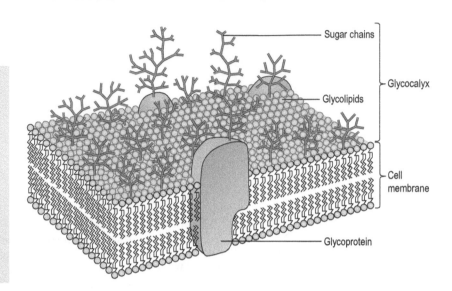

Figure 5.1
Cell membrane.
Reproduced with
permission from van
den Berg *Angewandte
Physiologie Band 1*,
Georg Thieme Verlag.
3. Auflage, Stuttgart.
[*Applied Physiology
Volume 1*, Georg
Thieme publishers, 3rd
edition, Stuttgart]. 2011.
Fig. 1.36, page 49

tensile loading, then it primarily produces collagen fibers – mostly collagen type I. Collagen type I is the main collagen in the human body (making up 95% of the body's collagen). It is also the thickest and the strongest of all collagens.

When the loading also includes dynamics, then it is important to produce a certain amount of elastic fibers. The elastic fibers have the task of reducing the speed at which the tissue and collagen fibers are loaded. Recall the physical formula $F = M \times a$ (loading = mass × acceleration).

For the collagen fibers to move friction-free against each other during loading, the cell produces a small amount of ground substance that is able to bind water, resulting in a lubricating film. The ground substance and the bound water are vital for the cells, because all of our cells must 'feed' themselves through the process of diffusion – just like the original single-cell microbes did on Earth. Diffusion requires water.

Cells that mainly produce fibers are understandably called fibroblasts, or fibrocytes. By contrast, cells that are primarily loaded by compression forces produce large amounts of ground substance, which enables the binding of water in tissue. The ground substance is kept together and stabilized by a small amount of collagen type II. Such cells are called chondroblasts, or chondrocytes. Figure 5.2 is a diagram of the components of connective tissue.

One might compare the articular cartilage with a plastic bottle filled with water. The more water there is in the bottle, the less deformation and the more stability there is. The same phenomenon is seen with the tire of a car, only that stability is not achieved by the storage of water but of air.[4]

Crucial for the development of the Metazoa was the construction of the basal membranes, which allow histologically different tissues to be separated from each other. In this way, the development of different tissues and organs was enabled. An extremely important basal membrane is the basal membrane that lies between the epidermis and the dermis, which ensures that body fluids cannot leak out of the body, preventing the body from drying out.

The terms 'blasts' and 'cytes' refer to the amount of synthesizing activity of the cells. When a cell is very active, it requires a lot of energy, which is generated by mitochondria. Furthermore, the synthesis takes place at the endoplasmic reticulum. Thus, the cell has to be rich in such organelles. When referring to such cells, we speak of 'blasts'. By contrast, 'cytes' refers to cells that have only a few mitochondria and endoplasmic reticula.

The extracellular matrix provides a framework of fibers and ground substance that is attached with connecting proteins to the cell membrane. When a mechanical load works on the matrix, it is transferred through the connecting proteins to the inside of the

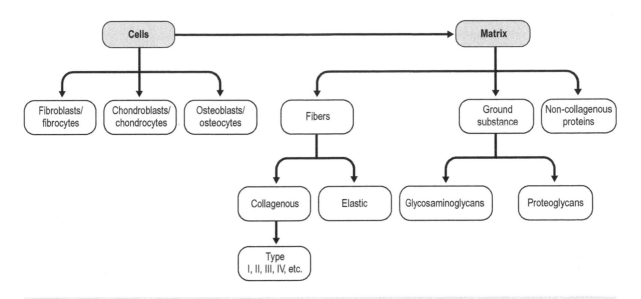

Figure 5.2
Components of connective tissue

cell. In this way, the cell receives information about the kind and intensity of the loading. In the cell nucleus, this information leads to transcription and duplication of part of the DNA into mRNA, which is important for synthesis of the necessary matrix components. Thus, it is clear that stimuli external to the cell steer the activity of the DNA. This phenomenon is a major aspect of epigenetics.[4,7,2,1]

The connective tissue in the body is constantly adapting to the momentary loading. This loading capacity is based on the fact that connective tissue is in a perpetual process of reconstruction. Because the different components of the extracellular matrix have certain defined lifespans, matrix components are continuously being degraded and replaced. Complete turnover of the ground substance happens every 2 to 10 days. By contrast, turnover of collagen fibers requires approximately between 300 and 500 days, though collagen turnover in some tissues can take much longer.[4]

In order for the cell to produce new matrix components, it needs a stimulus that informs it about the amount and intensity of the loading. As previously mentioned, this information tells the cell which parts of DNA must be duplicated and what substances must be produced by the cell.[2,8]

In our society, most people hardly load their locomotor system in daily living, meaning that matrix components are removed but they are not replaced by new ones. In this way, the connective tissue loses stability, elasticity, and mobility. These losses lead to atrophy of the tissues, which, in muscles, can be seen with the naked eye. Although hidden from view, atrophy also occurs in the bones (as osteoporosis), the intervertebral discs (as sintering), the tendons, the ligaments, the menisci, and other tissues.

If the connective tissue is increasingly loaded, the synthesis activity of the cell will rise, and more matrix components will be produced. In muscle and connective tissue, these events can lead to hypertrophy. For example, at birth, the tibial and fibular joint capsules of the ankle joint are equally thick. When a child starts to stand and walk, the continuous valgus movement of the foot increasingly stimulates the cells in the tibial capsule. In this way, that part of the capsule grows thicker and more stable. Similar tissue development occurs in the lumbar spine, where, over the course of many years, the anterior ligament grows thicker, broader, and more stable.

Depending on the type of loading that is working on the tissue, the connective tissue becomes differently organized and constructed. Where the loading is working with much repetition in the same direction, the collagen fibers are more likely to orient themselves parallel to the direction of the loading forces. In this way, tightly formed fibrous connective tissue is developed, such as the tendons and ligaments. These structures are primarily constructed for stability and possess an enormous loading capacity ($500-1,000 \, kg/cm^2$).[4] That is why, regardless of how much and how often the quadriceps muscle is contracted (or trained), the patellar tendon will never grow longer – but it will become thicker to better absorb the steadily increasing loading.

Where the loading direction is always changing, a framework of criss-crossing collagen fibers emerges. In these cases, unformed, tight fibrous connective tissue is developed, such as the joint capsules and intramuscular connective tissue. These structures must allow mobility while assuring stability at the end of the movement.[4]

The mobility and unfolding capacity of the collagen network – including in the joint capsule, fascia, and intramuscular connective tissue – can be disturbed under pathologic circumstances (e.g., immobilization) by the formation of biochemical connections between crossing collagen fibers. This pathologic cross-linking can be recognized in the form of decreased mobility.[4]

In the clinical setting, the effect of the treatment of this decreased mobility used to be explained by mechanical 'stretching' of the capsule. Fundamentally, of course, connective tissue cannot be stretched due to its enormous loading capacity. When we try to stretch the capsule, we are actually trying to remove the pathologic cross-links. As we apply a rhythmic, mild stretch to the connective tissue, the cells increase the liberation of the enzyme collagenase, which is capable of biochemically breaking down the pathologic cross-links.[9] But if we apply stretching impulses at a high intensity, the cells may act to limit the threat posed by these impulses by increasing the production of collagen. In such a case, an increase of mobility is unlikely. Furthermore, there is a danger with high-intensity stretching of causing injuries to the connective tissue – in which case the patient would likely experience pain some hours after the treatment.

We may occasionally see signs that certain parts of the joint capsule become increasingly loaded in the same direction. These signs include a thickening of the capsule and a parallel orientation of the collagen fibers. Thickenings of the capsule (e.g., fibrous membrane) are called ligaments by anatomists. Histologically, we use the term intracapsular ligaments.[4]

Besides mechanical loading, another important issue for the development of tissue is the tissue's supply of oxygen. The oxygen supply determines in what way the cells will produce energy. In tissues that are not well supplied with vessels and where the oxygen level is low, the cells produce energy primarily in an anaerobic manner. As a consequence, much lactate is produced in the tissue, lowering the tissue's pH value. Examples of such tissues include the joint cartilage and nucleus pulposus. By contrast, in tissues that are well supplied with vessels, the cells produce their energy in an aerobic manner. In those tissues, the pH value is normally neutral.

When the pH value becomes lower than 6.5 (a condition called acidosis), the cells cannot perform synthesis, and normal remodeling processes cannot take place. This condition usually leads to tissue degeneration. Furthermore, wound healing cannot take place under such conditions, and training impulses will not lead to an increase of functions.[4]

The cause for acidosis is typically related to nutrition. Strong acid-forming food substances include animal proteins, refined sugar, coffee, black tea, alcohol, milk products, and many cereal products. Acid-base-forming food products include many fruits and vegetables. The nutrition of many of our patients consists mostly of acid-forming food.

Research by Vormann and colleagues showed that allocations of the Basica® mineral supplement caused a statistically significant reduction of symptoms in 76 of 82 patients with chronic low back pain.[10] Birklein and colleagues demonstrated a direct correlation between a local acidosis and pain in patients with complex regional pain syndrome.[11]

Lubrication and protection against friction

Due to the ground substance and the water bound to it within the extracellular matrix, tissue movement can take place without friction. During movement, the deformation of the matrix forces the ground substance to release water, which will be absorbed again when the tissue is relaxed again. This water moves through the tissue but also leaks into neighbouring tissues. An example is the intervertebral disc, where leaking water will pass through the endplate into the vertebral body. The same phenomenon occurs in the articular cartilage, the bursae, and tendon sheets. In the paratenon, the outer sheet of the tendon constantly produces a fluid similar to synovial fluid. In fact, all tissues permanently form a fluid film to ensure lubrication during movement.

Fascia also has this lubrication effect. Fascia incorporates a water-dense vascular system, which enables different fasciae to slide friction-free against each other.[12,13,14] The fluid production in the fascia can be disturbed under pathologic circumstances, such as decreased circulation caused by increased sympathetic reflex activity. An example would be the development of subcutaneous connective tissue zones, in which we find reduced mobility as well as a decrease in the possibility of lifting the skin from the bottom layer. The tension and mobility changes found in osteopathic listening tests are additional examples of these changes.

Due to the different forms of loading and circulation of the tissue, various kinds of connective tissue have developed. The names of these tissues depend on several factors, including their location, function, form, and thickness (Fig. 5.3).

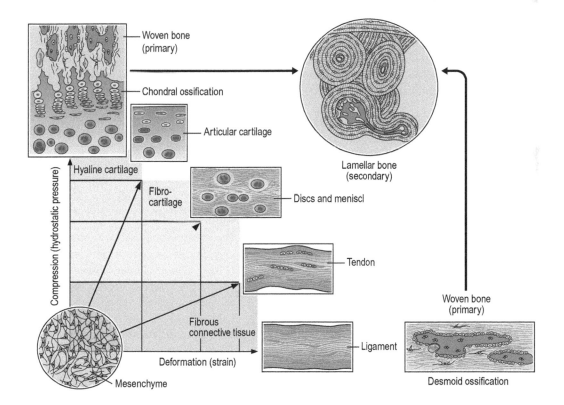

Figure 5.3

Pauwel's Theory: cells subjected to stress and strain differentiate into fibroblasts and chondroblasts. Reproduced with permission from van den Berg, *Angewandte Physiologie Band 1*, Georg Thieme Verlag. 3. Auflage, Stuttgart. [*Applied Physiology Volume 1*, Georg Thieme publishers, 3rd edition, Stuttgart]. 2011. Fig. 1.56, page 5

Anatomically, fascia is described as connective tissue sheets that surround the whole body inside the skin and each and every body structure internally. Fascia also separates, and sometimes connects, body structures with each other. Some fasciae are thin, fragile, and transparent, but others are thick, strong, and opaque. The stronger fasciae are typically subjected to greater daily mechanical loading, which affects their architecture and structure.

Paoletti is of the opinion that all connective tissues in the body should be called fascia.[15] I am of the opinion that we should generally speak about connective tissue – which has acquired from anatomists different, descriptive names, such as joint capsule, ligament, tendon, aponeurosis, retinaculum, periosteum, and endosteum – but also fascia.

Histology of fascia

So what exactly is fascia? As indicated in the previous paragraph, there are different opinions regarding what we can call or should call fascia. According to one definition, which was proposed at the First International Fascia Research Congress in 2007, fascia is the soft tissue component of the connective tissue system. This definition emphasizes fascia's uninterrupted three-dimensional weblike extensions and its functional attributes. According to this definition, joint and organ capsules, muscular septa, tendons, ligaments, aponeuroses, retinacula, myofasciae, and neurofasciae are all specialized fasciae.

The Federative International Committee on Anatomical Terminology (FICAT) writes in its *Terminologia Anatomica* (1998) that fascia is sheaths, sheets, or other dissectible connective tissue aggregations. FICAT describes fascia according to the following characteristics:

1. Its location: fascia of the head and neck, fascia of the trunk, and fascia of the limbs.

2. Its relation to surrounding structures: subcutaneous fascia, visceral fascia, parietal fascia, fascia of the muscles, and fascia extraserosalis.[16]

FICAT considers the terms 'superficial' and 'deep fascia' to be incorrect.[17]

Kumka and Bonar suggest the following four categories of fascia:

1. Linking fascia (connecting)

2. Fascicular fascia

3. Compression fascia

4. Separating fascia (disconnecting)[17]

   a. The linking fascia is built of connective tissues ordered in a parallel manner, with collagen type I dominating. Linking fascia can be categorized into dynamic and passive divisions. Dynamic divisions are the fascia of the trunk and the limbs. They are rich in myofibroblasts, giving them the ability to actively contract the tissue. Their innervation is primarily by free nerve endings and Pacini corpuscles. The passive divisions are the fascia of the muscles, head, neck, and limbs. They create muscular insertion points and have the task of absorbing mechanical stretch and loading. They are innervated by free nerve endings, Ruffini receptors, and Golgi receptors.

   b. The fascicular fascia forms tunnels for the vessels in the bones, muscles, nerves, and tendons. This fascia consist of irregular, dense connective tissues, as well as loose connective tissues. Its collagen fibers are mainly types I and III, but also types V, VI, XII, and XIV. Fascicular fascia is innervated primarily by Golgi receptors.

   c. The compression fascia is built of regular and irregular dense connective tissue and loose connective tissue. As an ensheathment of whole limbs, the fascia enables and/or improves the venous drainage from the limbs. In the limbs, we see the thickest fascia, such as the crural fascia (924 µm thick) and the fascia lata (944 µm thick).[18] These tissues consist of two or three layers, in which the collagen fibers run parallel to each other. But between the different layers, the fibers cross at angles of approximately 70° to 80°.[19,18] Also between the layers there is a small amount of loose connective tissue, enabling the layers to slide against each other. The fascia of the upper limbs is thinner (e.g., brachial fascia = 700 µm) than the fascia of the lower limbs. The fascia on the anterior side of the body is thinner than the fascia on the posterior side. And the fascia of males is thinner than that of females.[20]

d. The separating fascia is built of irregular, dense connective tissue and loose connective tissue. The predominant collagen type is type III, with smaller amounts of types V and VII. This fascia contains many elastic fibers. The separating fascia divides the body into sheets and layers, allowing for friction-free movement between these layers. Pacini and Ruffini receptors innervate the fascia.

Cells

The main cells in the fascia are fibroblasts and myofibroblasts. Besides these cells, we see adipocytes and many migrating leucocytes (white blood cells).

It has long been observed that the cells in the fascia are contractile. Paoletti describes a rhythmic contraction of the cells and fascia, with a rhythm of 8 to 12 cycles per second (Hz).[15] Randoll and colleagues, in research in Erlangen, Germany, displayed this so-called coherent vibration, or rhythm, in the cells by means of a video microscope. They too found that the cells in humans are moving at a rhythm of 8 to 12 Hz.[21]

Randoll and colleagues also showed that the 8–12 Hz rhythm is of central importance for the human body, because this frequency correlates with the frequency of the alpha waves in the brain.

Findings from space medicine have revealed that this frequency is important for generating gravitation-dependent resting periods of the body. In 2009, Randoll reported that brainwave entrainment, or synchronization, is a basic mechanism of life.[22] In 2005, Randoll and colleagues described cancer cells as distinctly showing more chaotic rhythms and cell dynamics than normal cells.[23]

The rhythms that are most often addressed in medicine, namely the artery pulse and the heart rhythm, are caused by rhythmic contractions of cells in the heart and vessel walls. The peristaltic waves of the intestines are based on the same mechanism.

The transport of cerebrospinal fluid could be caused by rhythmic contractions of the cells of the cerebral membranes. These same contractions could form the basis of the explanation of the so-called craniosacral rhythm, which is often spoken about in osteopathy. Strogatz and colleagues have shown that cells that lie close enough to each other synchronize their rhythms – as can be seen in the area of the heart's sinus node.[24] Synchronization can also emerge in the brain cellular rhythm. Nakagaki and colleagues have demonstrated that cellular rhythms can be influenced by external stimuli, such as light impulses.[25]

An important principle to keep in mind is that all connective tissue cells have the capacity to contract. Spector demonstrated this contractility in fibroblasts as well as chondroblasts and osteoblasts.[26] The contractile characteristics of these connective tissue cells can increase significantly during wound-healing processes and fibrosis processes. In such cases, we are speaking about myofibroblasts.

During an injury of a connective tissue, there is typically also an injury of the vessels. This causes an emission of leukocytes from the vessel system into the connective tissue, leading to changes in the activation of the extracellular matrix. This activation, in turn, stimulates the leukocytes to liberate cytokines, chemokines, and degrading enzymes. The memory T lymphocytes have, through the beta-1 integrins, a major influence on the cell–cell connections and on the cell–matrix connections. The result is that the extracellular matrix can bind to growth factors, such as tumor necrosis factor alpha (TNF-α), interleukins 7 and 2 (IL-7, IL-2), macrophage inflammatory protein-1 beta (MIP-1β), transforming growth factor beta (TGF-β), and basic fibroblast growth factor beta (BFGF-β).[3]

Within the cell, TGF-β1 causes an increase in the development of actin chains, which leads to a doubling of their contractility.[27] Later, there is also the development of actin chains outside of the cells – within the extracellular matrix and between the cells. These chains provide the basis for the contractility of the tissue.[28,29,30,31,32,27] TGF-β1 protects myofibroblasts against apoptosis.[33] This action explains why we find myofibroblasts in the tissue after an injury, resulting in wound contraction during the first phase of the wound-healing process.[28]

In order for the myofibroblasts to move through the tissue, the cell–cell connections must be unfastened. Prompted by the extracellular stimuli, small GTPases (Rac, Rho, and Cdc-42) are produced within the cell. Rac stimulates the production of actin chains along the edges of the cell, as well as the development of pseudopodia, and it loosens the cell–cell connections. Rho stimulates the development of actomyosin chains, but it increases the amount of cell–cell connections. Cdc-42 enables the development of filopodia by the cell.[34]

Reasons and factors that lead to the development of myofibroblasts and fibrosis of the tissue under pathologic situations (e.g., Dupuytren's contracture) are discussed in detail in Chapter 9.

Depending on the loading of the tissue, cells can change from fibroblasts to chondroblasts. For example, when tendons or ligaments are confronted with increasing compression, the fibroblasts change into chondroblasts and start to produce fibrocartilage tissue.[35,36,37]

Fibers – collagen and elastic: The collagen fibers of the fascia are, as we would expect, in tissues that are under tensile loading. These are mainly collagens of the types I, III, IV, V, VI, XII, XIV, and XXI. Beside these collagen fibers, we also find many elastic fibers, which are relatively short and lie between the collagen fibers.

Ground substance: The ground substance consists mainly of dermatan sulfate and chondroitin sulfate, some heparan sulfate and hyaluronic acid, and small amounts of keratan sulfate.

The amount of water in the fascia is relatively high for tissues that are under tensile loading. This relatively high amount of water is probably responsible for the smooth mobility of the fascia against other anatomical structures and of the different fascial sheets against each other.

Non-collagenous proteins: The non-collagenous proteins consist primarily of the connecting proteins fibronectin, tenascin, and laminin. In addition, there are so-called link-proteins that bind, within the ground substance, the different proteoglycans to the hyaluronic acid chain.

Circulation and innervation: Fascia has its own rich vessel system, which strongly anastomizes with vessels in surrounding tissues. The nerves run through the fascia much like the vessels; the fascia is richly innervated. According to Schleip, there are 10 times more receptors in the fascia than in the muscles.[38]

Within the fascia, there are many Ruffini corpuscles, Pacini corpuscles, nociceptors, and interstitial myofascial receptors (which consist mainly of free nerve endings).[39,40,41] The interstitial myofascial system responds to temperature, mechanical pressure, and vibration.

Stecco and colleagues and Schleip have found that in the knee, between the superficial and deep fascia, there are numerous proprioceptive nerve endings. Because of this tissue's strong vascular supply, it also possesses many sympathetic nerve endings, which control the lumen of the vessels and are closely connected to the myofibroblasts.[42,38]

The presence of many Ruffini and Pacini receptors suggests that the fascia probably also fulfils proprioceptive tasks. In the fascia, we often see that collagen fibers are in close contact with nerves. The capsules of the Ruffini and Pacini receptors are often connected to collagen fibers. The significance of these facts for the organism is still unclear.[43] The possible significance of the strong neural supply of the fascia and the interaction between cells, receptors, and vessel systems will be more extensively discussed in Chapter 6.

References

1. Hynes R. O. Extracellular matrix: not just pretty fibrils. *Science.* 2009;326(5957):1216–1219.

2. Ramage L. Integrins and extracellualr matrix in mechanotransduction. *Cell Health and Cytoskeleton.* 2012;4:1–9.

3. Vaday G. G., Lider O. Extracellular matrix moieties, cytokines, and enzymes: dynamic effects on immune cell behavior and inflammation. *J Leuk Biol.* 2000;67:149–159.

4. van den Berg F. *Angewandte Physiologie: Das Bindegewebe des Bewegungsapparates verstehen und beeinflussen (Band 1)*. 3. Auflage. [*Applied Physiology Volume 1*, 3rd edition] Thieme Verlag: Stuttgart, 2011.

5. Geiger B., Yamada K. M. Molecular architecture and function of matrix adhesions. *Cold Spring Harbor Perspectives in Biology*. 2011;3:a005033.

6. Abedin M., King N. Diverse evolutionary paths to cell adhesion. *Trends Cell. Biol*. 2010;20(12): 734–742.

7. Özbek S., Balasubramanian P. G, Chiquet-Ehrismann R. et al. The evolution of extracellular matrix. *Mol Biol Cell*. 2010;21:4300–4305.

8. Kim S.-H., Turnbull J., Guilmond S. Extracellular matrix and cell signalling: the dynamic cooperation of integrin, proteoglycan and growth factor receptor. *Journal of Endocrinology*. 2011;209:139–151.

9. Carano A., Siciliani G. Effect of continuous and intermittent forces on human fibroblasts in vitro. *Journal of Orthodontics*. 1996;18:19–26.

10. Vormann J., Worlitschek M., Goedecke T., Silver B. Supplementation with alkaline minerals reduces symptoms in patients with chronic low back pain. *J Trace Elem Med Biol*. 2001;15:179–183.

11. Birklein F., Weber M., Ernst M. et al. Experimental tissue acidosis leads to increase *pain* in complex regional pain syndrome (CRPS). Pain. 2000;87(2):227–234.

12. Guimberteau J., Delage J., McGrouther D., Wong J. The microvascular system: how connective tissue sliding works. *J Hand Surg Eur*. 2010;35(8):614–622.

13. Guimberteau J., Sentucq-Rigall J., Panconi B.. Introduction to the knowledge of subcutaneous sliding system in humans. *Ann Chir Plast Esth*. 2005;50(1):19–34.

14. Langevin H., Stevens-Tuttle D., Fox J. et al. Ultrasound evidence of altered lumbar connective tissue structure in human subjects with chronic low back pain. *BMC Musculoskelet Disord*. 2009;10(1):151–161.

15. Paoletti S., Faszien. München-Jena. Urban & Fischer Verlag. 2001.

16. Federative Committee of Anatomical Terminology (FCAT). *Terminologia Anatomica: International Anatomical Terminology*. Thieme: Stuttgart. 1998: pp. 1–292.

17. Kumka M., Bonar J. Fascia: a morphological description and classification system based on a literature review. *J Can Chiropr Assoc*. 2012;56(3):179–191.

18. Stecco C., Pavan P., Porzionato A. et al. Mechanics of crural fascia: from anatomy to constitutive modelling. *Surg Radiol Anat*. 2009;31(7):523–529.

19. Benetazzo L., Bizzego A., De Caro R. et al. 3D reconstruction of the crural and thoracolumbar fasciae. *Surg Radiol Anat*. Published online January 4, 2011. Doi: 10.1007/s00276-010-0757-7.

20. Stecco C., Macchi V., Porzionato A. et al. The fascia: the forgotten structure. *It J Anat Embryol*. 2011;116(3):127–138.

21. Randoll U. G., McCutcheon R., Hennig F. F. Matrix-Rhythmus-Therapie und der osteopatische Ansatz. *Osteopatische Medizin*. 2006;7J(1)28–34.

22. Randoll U. G., Hennig F. F. Matrix-Rhythmus-Therapie, Zellbiologische Grundlagen, Theorie und Praxis. *Zeitschrift für Physiotherapeuten*. 2009;61(6):545–549.

23. Randoll U. G., Hennig F. F. Matrix-Rhythmus-Therapie für Zeitstrukturen und Prozesse. *GZM Netzwerkjournal – Praxis und Wissenschaft*. 2005;10J(1).20–25.

24. Strogatz S. H., Stewart I. Coupled oscillators and biological synchronization. *Scientific American*. December 1993;68–74.

25. Nakagaki T, Yamada H, Ueda T. Modulation of cellular rhythm and photoavoidance by oscillatory irradiation in the Physarum plasmodium. *Biophysl Chem*. 1999;82(1):23–28.

26. Spector M. Musculoskeletal connective tissue cells with muscle: expression of muscle actin in and contraction of fibroblasts, chondrocyles, and osteoblasts. *Wound Repair Regen*. 2001; 9:11–18.

27. Hinz B., Phan S. H., Thannickal V. J., Galli A., Bochaton-Piallat M.-L., Gabbiani G. The Myofibroblast; One function, Multiple Origins. *Am J Pathol*. 2007;170 (6):1807–1816.

28. Gabbiani G. The evolution of the myofibroblast concept: a key cell for wound healing and fibrotic diseases. *G Gerontol*. 2004;52:280–282.

29. Meek R. M. D., McLellan S., Crossan J. F. Dupuytren's disease: a model for the mechanism of fibrosis and its modulation by steroids. *J Bone Joint Surg*. 1999;81–B(4):732–738.

30. Kozma E. M., Glowacki A., Olcyk K., Ciecierska M. Dermatan sulfate remodelling associated with advanced Dupuytren´s contracture. *Acta Biochemica Polonica*. 2007;54 (4):821–830.

31. Singer I. I., Kawka D. W., Kazakis D. M., Clark R. A. F. In vivo co-distribution of fibronectin and actin fibers in granulation tissue: immunofluorescence and electron microscope study of the fibronexus at the myofibroblast surface. *J Cell Biol.* 1984;98:2091–2106.

32. Wipff P.-J., Rifkin D. B., Meister J.-J., Hinz B. Myofibroblast contraction activates latent TGF-beta1 from the extracellular matrix. *J Cell Biol.* 2007;179 (6):1311–1323.

33. Lee S., Baytion M., Reinke D. L. et al. Dupuytren contracture. E-Medicine Orthopaedics. 2010. http://emedicine.medscape.com/article/1238712-overview [accessed January 31, 2016].

34. Alexandrova A. Y. Evolution of cell interactions with extracellular matrix during carcinogenesis. *Biochemistry* (Moscow). 2008;73(7):733–741.

35. Benjamin M., Ralphs J. R. Fibrocartilage in tendons and ligaments – an adaptation to compressive load. *J Anat.* 1998;193(4):481–494.

36. Milz S., Benjamin M., Putz R. Molecular parameters indicating adaptation to mechanical stress in fibrous connective tissue. *Adv Anat Embryol Cell Biol.* 2005;178:1–71.

37. Bank R., TeKoppele J., Oostingh G., Hazleman B., Riley G. Lysylhydroxylation and non-reducible crosslinking of human supraspinatus tendon collagen: changes with age and in chronic rotator cuff tendinitis. *Ann Rheum Dis.* 1999; 58:35–41.

38. Schleip R., Findley T. W., Chaitow L., Huijing P. A. (eds).*Fascia: The Tensional Network of the Human Body.* 2012. Churchill Livingstone Elsevier.

39. Yahia L. H., Rhalmi S., Newman N., Isler M. Sensory innervation of human thoracolumbar fascia. *Acta Orthop Scand.* 1992;63(2):195–197.

40. Schleip R. Fascial plasticity – a new neurobiological explanation: Part 1. *J Bodyw Mov Ther.* 2003;7 (1):11–19.

41. Schleip R. Fascial plasticity – a new neurobiological explanation: Part 2. *J Bodyw Mov Ther.* 2003;7 (2):104–110.

42. Stecco C., Porzionato A., Lancerotto L. et al. Histological study of the deep fasciae of the limbs. *J Bodyw Mov Ther.* 2008;12(3):225–230.

43. Stecco C., Porzionato A., Macchi V. et al. A histological study of the deep fascia of the upper limb. It *J Anat Embryol.* 2006;111(2):105–110.

Physiology and functions of fascia | 2

2

INTRODUCTION

Torsten Liem

This section explores various clinical aspects of fascia, which may be important in the application of manual therapeutic approaches, for example, the role of the connective tissue in acting against tensile forces and tissue repair, and the physiological mechanisms of tissue response after the application of manual therapy. Furthermore, the interaction of fascia with the lymphatic system will be explored together with its role in the inflammatory process. This section contains several noteworthy concepts that have direct clinical implications. Existing biomechanical models are challenged and presented in light of available evidence with a view to incorporating fascia as a component into these models, which has not been considered in conventional teaching and/or practice of manual therapy to date. This section will provide the reader with a basic knowledge of how various manual treatment approaches may be able to help with the recovery process of the human body.

PHYSIOLOGY OF FASCIA

Frans van den Berg

Introduction

As previously mentioned in Chapter 5 on histology, it is the task of the fascia and all of the connective tissue to protect the cells, the tissues, and the entire body against mechanical loading – including tensile loading, compression, and friction – as well as to enable the repair process after injury.

How can the fascia be capable of continually performing these tasks? It is important that the connective tissue cells of the fascia perform their synthesizing activity so that normal physiological remodeling processes can take place. But how can the cells ensure that no permanent injuries to the tissue occur, that they constantly have enough nutrients for their synthesizing activity, and that the tissue can be repaired after repeated injuries?

For these tasks to occur, there must be an intense interaction and exchange between the cells and each other and between the cells and the extracellular matrix, as well as between the fascia and other protective structures, such as the muscles. By the activation of receptors in the fascia, the muscles can be activated through reflexes that can protect the tissue. In order for the cells to continually obtain sufficient nutrients (e.g., vitamins, enzymes), the tissue must constantly receive sufficient circulation. For that reason, there is close contact and exchange between receptors of the fascia and the autonomic nervous system.

Communication

Communication among cells and between cells and the extracellular matrix

As described in Chapter 5, cell activity is directed by mechanical impulses that are transferred from the matrix to the cells. Depending on the intensity, direction, and other characteristics of the loading, the cells are informed about the specific matrix components that are needed at any moment. The mechanical loading also influences the way the matrix is build up – that is, the matrix architecture.

Through intercellular connections (i.e., tight junctions), not only single cells but also complete cell groups are activated by the mechanical deformation of the matrix.

Communication between fasciae and the central nervous system

During the course of human evolution, the nervous system developed and became increasingly optimized. The development of receptors and reflexes gave the cells, the tissues, and the whole body increasingly optimal protection against the rapid changes of loading and overloading. The changes in the tissue initiated by the nervous system are a lot faster than the changes taking place in the tissue themselves initiated by cell activity.

Receptors in the joint capsules, ligaments, tendons, muscles, intervertebral discs, and menisci – and also in the fascia – send their afferent impulses (i.e., information) to the spinal cord and brain. These afferent impulses lead to stimulations in the spinal cord, including the motor neurons of the anterior horn.

It is common knowledge that a stimulus of a muscle spindle results in activation and contraction of the muscle. But exactly how is the muscle spindle activated? A quick stretch of the muscle could be responsible for the activation – for example, a sudden inversion movement of the foot. At the same time, receptors of the joint capsule are stimulated. In this way, an arthrokinetic reflex or arthrokinematic reflex is provoked.[1-6] This means that, due to a rapid movement, receptors in the joint capsule, muscle, skin, and fascia are activated, leading to a contraction of the muscle. In this way, the joint is stabilized and protected against injury.

When the joint capsule is injured, the joint receptors are facilitated by means of a decrease of the stimulus threshold, which is elicited by the release of inflammatory and pain mediators caused by the injury.[7] This leads to an increased reaction of the arthrokinetic reflex, resulting in earlier activation of the protective and stabilizing muscles and protection of the joint against excessive stretch. This phenomenon is referred to in physiotherapy as a capsular pattern.

Stecco and colleagues[8,9] have found that between the superficial and deep fascia of the knee there are many proprioceptive nerve endings. These receptors could be responsible for the activation of the muscles. It is also possible that after an injury or threat of an injury the muscles are inhibited in their activity.

Yerys and colleagues were able to find that inflammation and swelling of the knee joint lead to an inhibition of the quadriceps muscle.[4] The type I receptors have a controlling function on muscle tone in the more tonic-orientated muscles, which are responsible for upright posture and activity against gravity. The type II receptors primarily control motion sequence and coordination between the muscles that are active during movement. These receptors are probably also important for balance and balance reactions, with a greater influence on the more fascicle-oriented muscles.

Similar to the research performed by Yerys and colleagues,[4] Makofsky and colleagues have shown that, as a result of stretching treatment on the joint capsule of the hip, the force of the gluteal muscles increased. They proposed that the inhibition of the hip muscles was reduced by this treatment.[6]

Another protective reflex is elicited by the activation of the so-called Golgi tendon receptor. The Golgi receptor is a stretch receptor that has a high conduction velocity, meaning that the impulse from this receptor progresses at a very high speed to the spinal cord. The afferent activity of the Golgi receptor leads to an inhibition of the alpha motor neuron in the spinal cord and, in this way, to an inhibition (or relaxation) of the muscles.

Because this receptor has such a high stimulation threshold, only a very high loading can activate it. Apparently, the main function of this receptor is to relax the muscles and reduce the loading of the structure at the point where the loading becomes so great that an injury is threatened. In the clinical situation, we know this as 'giving way', where the patient loses control over his or her muscles.

The fasciae are richly innervated. According to Schleip, there are 10 times more receptors in the fasciae than in the muscles.[9] The receptors that are found here are mechanoreceptors, such as Ruffini receptors, Pacini receptors, and Golgi receptors. In particular, there are a large amount of free nerve endings. This system, according to Schleip, makes up the largest sensory organ in the body. Most of the sensory nerves are connected with the myofascial system.[9] These receptors mainly serve thermoregulation and chemoregulation purposes, but they can also be stimulated mechanically. A distinction is made between receptors with a high stimulation threshold (HTP = high threshold pressure) and those with a low stimulation threshold (LTP = low threshold pressure). The Achilles tendon, for example, consists of approximately 50% LTP receptors. The stimulation of these receptors leads to reduced activity of the gamma motor neurons.[10,11] During conditions of pain, there is a large release of neuropeptides, which causes a decrease of the stimulation threshold of all receptors.

Communication between fascia and the autonomic nervous system

Mechanical stimulation of the receptors in fascia can produce effects in the autonomic nervous system. A stimulation of type IV receptors (free nerve endings) can raise the arterial blood pressure. By contrast, a stimulation of type III receptors can either raise or lower the arterial blood pressure. When constant pressure is applied to a muscle, blood pressure, muscle tone, and EMG activity decrease.[10,11]

A stimulation of the Ruffini receptors leads to a decrease of sympathetic reflex activity. It has also been shown that the application of pressure in the area of the belly and pelvis can influence parasympathetic activity, causing a reduction of EMG activity, a synchronization of EEG activity, and an increase of vagus nerve activity. This effect is called hypothalamic (or trophotropic) tuning. Further effects of hypothalamic tuning include reduction of muscle tone, especially in the lower extremities, and synchronization of cortical activity, as well as a reduction of emotional activity.[10,11]

The stimulation of the type III and type IV receptors in the interstitial myofascial system achieve a local vasodilatation of the vessels, as well as a reduction of muscle tone. The vasodilatation is probably caused by a reduction of sympathetic reflex activity and an increase in the release of histamine. Besides the vasodilatation of the vessels, there is also a local increase in the permeability of the vessel wall, which leads to increased leakage of fluid from the vessel system. The leakage further alters the viscosity of the connective tissue, causing a transformation from a gelatinous (gel) condition to a more soluble (sol) condition. In this thixotropic change, tissue deformation becomes easier.

The complete intestinal system is rich in fasciae and receptors. This enteric nervous system, which contains more then 100 million receptors, is the so-called brain of the gut, working independently from the cortical nervous system. Activation of the extremely mechanosensitive enteric nervous system causes many neuroendocrine changes, such as increased production and release of serotonin and histamine (Fig. 6.1).[10,11]

Energetic communication (fascia and acupuncture)

The main principle of traditional Chinese medicine (TCM) is to transport energy through the body. It is claimed that an acupuncture point is the place where the triad of a vein, an artery, and a nerve (non-myelinated) pass through a superficial body fascia. Heine confirms that this is exactly the case in more then 82% of the 361 acupuncture points that are described in TCM.[12] When the pathways of the fascia in the human body are examined, we find great similarity with the pathways of the meridians on which acupuncture points are localized.

Langevin et al. describe that the majority of the fibroblasts are connected with each other by connexin 43 and, in this way, build a large network within the fascia and throughout the body.[13] Information is exchanged via these cell–cell connections.[14] In addition, information is distributed throughout the whole body over/via the collagen network and over/via the ground substance. Langevin also found that

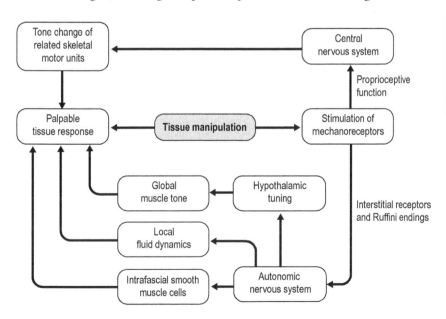

Figure 6.1

The fascia and the autonomic nervous system. After Schleip (2003a, 2003b)

the insertion and twisting of an acupuncture needle cause a mechanical stress in the tissue that is transferred to the cells.[15,16]

Wound healing

After an injury, the body attempts to repair the damaged tissue. This wound-healing process passes through the following phases: the inflammatory phase (days 0–5), the proliferation phase (days 5–21), the consolidation phase (days 21–60), and the remodeling phase (days 60–360). These phase lengths are only average approximations. The actual lengths in any particular case depend on the size of the injury, the tissue that is injured, and the circulation to the tissue.[7]

Inflammatory phase

The inflammatory phase is divided into a vascular subphase (days 0–2) and a cellular subphase (days 3–5). In the vascular phase, coagulation and the stabilization of the vessels are the major priorities. In the cellular phase, myofibroblasts migrate from surrounding tissue to the borders of the wound.

A typical injury, in addition to damaged connective tissue, consists of damage to the vascular system, resulting in leakage of leucocytes from the vascular system into the connective tissue. This causes an activation of the extracellular matrix, leading, in turn, to an activation of the leukocytes, which then release cytokines, chemokines, and degrading enzymes. The T-memory lymphocytes, via beta-1 integrins, have a major influence on the cell–cell and cell–matrix connections. The extracellular matrix now binds to growth factors, such as tumor necrosis factor alpha (TNF-α), interleukins 7 and 2 (IL-7 and -2), macrophage inflammatory protein-1 beta (MIP-1β), transforming growth factor beta (TGF-β), and basic fibroblast growth factor beta (BFGF-β).[17]

TGF-β1 causes an increased production of actin chains within the cells, which double their contractility.[18] Later, extracellular matrix actin chains are built outside the cells, including between the cells and between the cells and the matrix. This forms the basis for the contraction of the tissue.[19–21,18]

In this way, myofibroblasts emerge in the tissue after an injury, resulting in wound contraction during the first phase of the wound-healing process.[19] For the myofibroblasts to be able to move through the tissue during the cellular phase, the cell–cell connections must be released. For this purpose, the cells produce small GTPases (Rac, Rho, Cdc 42). Rac stimulates the production of actin chains along the edges of the cell, as well as the development of pseudopodia and the release of cell–cell connections. Rho stimulates the production of actomyosin bundles and an increase in the amount of cell–cell connections. Cdc 42 enables the development of filopodia in the cells.[22]

The myofibroblasts move in the direction of the borders of the wound. Once there, they produce thin collagen fibers of collagen type III. Besides producing collagen type III to close the wound, the myofibroblasts also function to draw the tissue around the wound back together. In this way, the wound is made smaller (through wound contraction), and it can be fully closed and healed faster. Furthermore, the wound becomes stabilized in this way.

Proliferation phase

In the proliferation phase, the production of collagen, primarily type III, is increased, leading to wound closure on approximately day 21. In this phase, the production of ground substance is low. The wound becomes stabilized through the activity of the myofibroblasts. As the provisional network of collagen type III progresses, the myofibroblasts move over this network from the border deeper into the wound.

Consolidation phase

When the wound is closed with collagen type III after approximately 21 days, the turnover from collagen type III to the more stable collagen type I begins. At the same time, the production of ground substance increases. In this way, the tissue becomes more stable, and the necessity of a wound contraction by myofibroblasts diminishes.

Remodeling phase

In the remodeling or maturation phase, which is essentially a flowing transition from the consolidation phase, the tissue becomes increasingly stable. The synthesizing activity of the cells remains high until day 120, after which it is gradually reduced.

At 150 days, 85% of the collagen type III has been transformed into collagen type I. After that point, the amount of collagen type III cells continues to be slowly reduced until approximately only 3% to 5% of the cells remain.

Mechanical loading during wound healing (Fig. 6.2)

During the inflammatory phase, one should be reluctant regarding application of mechanical loading to the tissue, because the tissue is still very unstable and can easily be injured again. Loading should be performed in an absolutely pain-free and resistance-free area of motion. It is also physiologically acceptable in this phase to immobilize the tissue.

During the proliferation phase, mechanical loading is an absolute necessity, because the cells need to receive a stimulus and information in order to build a functional collagen network. However, one should be careful with the intensity of the loading in this phase.

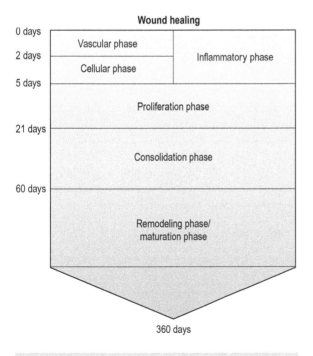

Figure 6.2
Wound healing

In the consolidation and remodeling phases, the loading of the tissue must be slowly increased in order to properly promote the transformation of collagen type III to collagen type I. The cells need to be confronted with gradually heavier loading so that more and more collagen type I continues to be produced. How far loading should be increased in any individual patient is dependent on the kind of loading that he or she is confronted with during daily living. If the individual works all day in an office and does not participate in athletic activities, then it is not necessary to raise the loading very much during therapy. By contrast, if the individual performs hard labor during the day and also regularly participates in intense athletic activities, then the loading must be increased accordingly.[7]

Therapeutic effects during mobilization treatments

One problem with which therapists are confronted on a regular basis is reduced mobility, or hypomobility. In attempting to treat this problem, all manner of mobilization techniques are used at various intensities. Interestingly, there are also multiple explanation models associated with these different techniques. Despite the many therapists using many different techniques, they may achieve the same outcome: increased mobility of their patients during treatment.

Another problem is that, in most cases, therapists have no idea as to what is causing the limitation of movement. Possible causes could include the development of pathologic cross-links within the collagen network, protective changes in the muscles, and protective changes in the connective tissue cells and matrix.

For this reason, I divide the movement limitations into reflectory and structural hypomobilities. Reflectory hypomobilities are caused by mechanisms trying to protect the injured tissue against excessive loading. Such hypomobilities can be recognized by the pain associated with the borders of movement. Structural hypomobilities are pain free and are caused by the building of pathologic cross-links and adhesions.[7]

In the following section, some commonly used explanation models for the effects of mobilizing therapies are discussed.

Changes in the matrix and cell activity

Creep and stress-relaxation

Creep and stress-relaxation are phenomena that are often used as a possible explanation for the mobilizing effect. This is one of the oldest explanation models in manual therapy. A fact that is often overlooked, however, is that in order to achieve these effects, one has to keep the tissue under constant loading (creep) or under constant length (stress-relaxation) over a period of several hours.[23]

Loading in the linear area of the stress–strain curve can lead to trauma or microtrauma in the tissue.[24] For example, when the iliotibial tract is loaded for one hour with a tensile load of 60 kg, causing an elongation of 1% to 1.5% microtrauma already occurs. At an elongation of 3% to 8%, tears arise, followed by inflammation (representing wound healing).[10,11] This means that higher loads are more likely to cause injury, rather than simple elongation of the tissue. If we keep the physical formula $F = M \times a$ in mind, the risks of manipulative thrust become clear as the stretch is applied on the tissue with extreme speed.

Thus, one must conclude that creep and stress-relaxation cannot be explanations for the mobilizing effects observed during treatment. For those explanations to be plausible, we would have to stretch the tissue over several hours, and it would very likely cause injury and pain (Fig. 6.3).

Thixotropy

As previously mentioned, the warmth and mechanical deformation of the tissue caused by therapy results in the ground substance transforming from a gelatinous (gel) condition into a more soluble (sol) condition. This means that the tissue gets more watery as the viscosity is reduced. Schleip compares this change with the transformation of butter into a gel (or jelly) form.[10,11] During this transformation, the tissue can be deformed more easily. This effect, called thixotropy, occurs only as long as the warmth and/or mechanical loading is applied. Furthermore, the stimuli must be applied for more then two minutes.

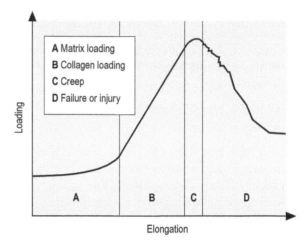

Figure 6.3

Collagen stress-strain curve. Reproduced with permission from van den Berg *Angewandte Physiologie Band 1*, Georg Thieme Verlag. 3. Auflage. Stuttgart. [*Applied Physiology Volume 1*, Georg Thieme publishers, 3rd edition, Stuttgart] 2011. Fig. 1.59, page 53

Piezoelectric activity

Due to repetitive loading and unloading of the tissue, the fluid transport through the tissue is increased. In this way, the electrical loading of the tissue also changes in a phenomenon known as the piezoelectric effect, which stimulates cell synthesis and remodeling processes in the tissue.[7] However, because remodeling of the ground substance requires anywhere from 2 to 10 days, the question remains whether the fast changes of mobility observed during treatment can be explained with this effect.

Collagenase production

Because it is assumed that one of the reasons for hypomobility is the development of pathologic cross-links within the collagen networks, one of the goals of therapy is to remove these cross-links. Carano & Siciliani have found that intermittent stretch can cause the cells to boost release of the enzyme collagenase by more than 200%. This enzyme is capable of removing the pathologic cross-links (see Fig. 9.1).[25]

Adhesions

A further cause of limited movement is the formation of adhesions, such as adhesions between capsular folds. These adhesions are initially caused by fatty deposits between parts of the capsule. In therapy, it is our goal to release these adhesions mechanically – meaning that this is one of the rare situations in which more force is needed during therapy. Our mobilization force must be larger than the adhesion force. That is why manipulative thrusts can be very useful in these cases.[7]

Neurophysiologic explanation models

Additional explanation models for the mobilizing effects can be found within neurophysiology. It is known that, in an activated situation, the Golgi tendon receptors inhibit the alpha motor neurons and relax the muscles. This means that when we stretch the tissue, we activate the Golgi receptors and relax the muscles. Golgi tendon receptors can be activated only when the muscle simultaneously contracts, thereby stabilizing the contractile elements and bringing mechanical loading on the tendon. A passive stretch of the muscle cannot stimulate the Golgi tendon receptors, because now there is no loading of the tendon.

Only about 10% of the Golgi receptors are located in the tendon, while 90% are in the area of the muscle–tendon junction, in the connective tissue of the muscle belly, in the ligaments, in the fascia, in the joint capsule, and in other locations.[10,11] Thus, a passive stretch of these noncontractile tissues is able to activate Golgi receptors. However, the Golgi receptors have a very high stimulation threshold, meaning that we have to apply a relatively strong stretch to the tissue. The stimulation of the mechanoreceptors of the ligaments of the knee generates only a small change in alpha motor activity, but a large change in gamma motor activity and muscle tone.

In the fascia, there are also numerous Pacini and Ruffini receptors. These are mechanoreceptors that react during stretch of the tissue. The main difference between these two receptors is their adaptation speed. The Pacini receptors adapt very quickly and, therefore, they can be activated only by intermittent stretches (vibrations). By contrast, the Ruffini receptors adapt very slowly and can be activated by static stretching.[10,11,26]

Furthermore, there are many so-called interstitial myofascial receptors. These are primarily free nerve endings that serve as thermoreceptors, though they can also be activated mechanically. As previously noted, a distinction is made between receptors with a high stimulation threshold and those with a low stimulation threshold.[10,11]

Changes in the autonomic nervous system

It was mentioned earlier that the mechanical stimulation of these receptors can also produce effects on the autonomic nervous system – a phenomenon called hypothalamic tuning. For example, hypothalamic tuning can influence the muscle tone and the circulation within the tissue.[10,11] In addition, due to the mechanical impulses on the tissue, mast cells are stimulated to increase the release of histamine, which enhances circulation within the tissue.

Influence on myofibroblasts

The contraction of myofibroblasts has long been discussed as one of the causes for limited movement (see Chapter 5). It was formerly assumed that myofibroblasts could be found only in the areas of the ovaries, uterus, testicles, heart, spleen, vessels, periodontal ligaments, pulmonary fascia, and other fascia. We now know that myofibroblasts can be found in all connective tissues.[27] Carbon dioxide, interstitial pH value, sympathetic reflex activity, and vasoactive substances all influence the tone of the myofibroblasts. Serotonin probably also has an influence on the activity of the myofibroblasts. Serotonin reduces the stimulation threshold of the type IV receptors (i.e., free nerve endings), which are especially nociceptive active. For example, patients with fibromyalgia have very high serotonin levels.[7]

Summary and explanation of possible mobilization effects

This chapter makes it clear that mobilization effects can and must be ascribed to multiple factors, including the following:

• relaxation of muscles

- hypothalamic tuning → increased circulation of the tissue:
  - increased cell activity and increased remodeling of the tissue
  - thixotropy (transformation from 'gel' to 'sol')
  - relaxation of myofibroblasts

- increased piezoelectric activity → increased cell activity and remodeling

- increased release of collagenase

- release of adhesions.

It is important that the stimuli are not applied with a high intensity, because this would increase the risk of injuring the tissue, causing such problems as pain, increased myofibroblast activity, and reduced tissue circulation. Mobilization is, in most cases, a gentle play with cells and receptors – the only exception being in regard to adhesions of capsular folds and other forms of adhesions.

References

1. Cohen L. A., Cohen M. L. Arthrokinetic reflex of the knee. *Am J Physiol.* 1956;184:433–437.

2. Clark R. K., Wyke B. D. Temporomandibular arthrokinetic reflex control of the mandibular musculature. *Br J Oral Surg.* 1975;13(2):196–202.

3. Serola R. A theory on the role of counternutation in self-bracing of the sacroiliac joint after injury. Poster Presentation. At: 3rd Interdisciplinary World Congress On Low Back Pain and Pelvic Pain. Vienna, Austria. November 19–21, 1998.

4. Yerys S., Makofsky H., Byrd C., Pennachio J., Cinkay J. Effect of mobilization of the anterior hip capsule on gluteus maximus strength. *J Man Manip Ther.* 2002;10(4):218–224.

5. Gordon R. C. *Manipulation Under Anesthesia: Concepts in Theory and Application.* Taylor & Francis Group (CRC). 2005.

6. Makofsky H., Panicker S., Abbruzzese J., Aridas C., Camp M., Derakes J., Franco C., Sileo R. Immediate effect of grade IV inferior hip joint mobilization on hip abductor torque: a pilot study. *J Man Manip Ther.* 2007;15(2):103–110.

7. van den Berg F. *Angewandte Physiologie: Das Bindegewebe des Bewegungsapparates verstehen und beeinflussen Band 1.* 3. Auflage, Georg Thieme Verlag, Stuttgart. [*Applied Physiology Volume 1.* 3rd Edition. Stuttgart: Georg Thieme publishers. Stuttgart]. 2011.

8. Stecco C., Porzionato A., Lancerotto L. et al. Histological study of the deep fasciae of the limbs. *J Bodyw Mov Ther.* 2008;12(3):225–230.

9. Schleip R. Chapter 2.2 Fascia as an organ of communication. In: *Fascia: the Tensional Network of the Human Body.* Schleip R., Findley T. W, Chaitow L., Huijing P. A. (eds). 2012. Churchill Livingstone Elsevier.

10. Schleip R. Fascial plasticity – a new neurobiological explanation: Part 1. *J Bodyw Mov Ther.* 2003a;7(1):11–19.

11. Schleip R. Fascial plasticity – a new neurobiological explanation: Part 2. *J Bodyw Mov Ther.* 2003b;7(2):104–110.

12. Heine H. Functional anatomy of traditional Chinese acupuncture points. *Acta Anatomica.* 1995;152:293–296.

13. Langevin H. M., Cornbrook C. J., Taatjes D. J. Fibroblasts form a body-wide cellular network. *Histochem Cell Biol.* 2004;122(1):7–15.

14. Langevin HM, Bouffard NA, Badger GJ, Iatridis JC, Howe AK. Dynamic fibroblast cytoskeletal response to subcutaneous tissue stretch ex vivo and in vivo. Am J Physiol Cell Physiol. 2005;288:747–756.

15. Langevin H. M. Connective tissue: a body-wide signalling network? *Med Hypotheses.* 2006;66(6):1074–1077.

16. Langevin H. M., Bouffard N. A., Badger G. J., Churchill D. L., Howe A. K.. Subcutaneous tissue fibroblast cytoskeletal remodelling induced by acupuncture: evidence for a mechanotransduction-based mechanism. *J Cell Physiol.* 2006;207:767–774.

17. Vaday G. G, Lider O. Extracellular matrix moieties, cytokines, and enzymes: dynamic effects on immune cell behaviour and inflammation. *J Leukoc Biol.* 2000;67:149–159.

18. Hinz B., Phan S. H., Thannickal V. J., Galli A., Bochaton-Piallat M.-L., Gabbiani G. The myofibroblast: one function, multiple origins. *Am J Pathol.* 2007;170(6):1807–1816.

19. Gabbiani G. The evolution of the myofibroblast concept: a key cell for wound healing and fibrotic diseases. *G Gerontol.* 2004;52:280–282.

20. Kozma E. M., Glowacki A., Olcyk K., Ciecierska M. Dermatan sulfate remodeling associated

with advanced Dupuytren's contracture. *Acta Biochemica Polonica*. 2007;54(4):821–830.

21. Wipff P.-J., Rifkin D. B., Meister J.-J., Hinz B. Myofibroblast contraction activates latent TGF-beta1 from the extrecellular matrix. *J Cell Biol*. 2007;179(6):1311–1323.

22. Alexandrova A. Y. Evolution of cell interactions with extracellular matrix during carcinogenesis. *Biochemistry* (Moscow). 2008;73(7):733–741.

23. Currier D., Nelson R. *Dynamics of Human Biologic Tissues*. 1st ed. Philadelphia:F. A. Davis Company. 1992.

24. Threlkeld A. J. The effects of manual therapy on connective tissue. *Phys Ther*. 1992;72 (12):893–902.

25. Carano A, Siciliani G. Effect of continuous and intermittent forces on human fibroblasts in vitro. *Journal of Orthodontics*. 1996;18:19–26.

26. van der Wal J. C. Chapter 2.2 Proprioception. In: *Fascia: the Tensional Network of the Human Body: the Science and Clinical Applications in Manual and Movement Therapy*. Schleip R., Findley T. W, Chaitow L., Huijing P. A. (eds). 2012. Churchill Livingstone Elsevier.

27. Spector M. Musculoskeletal connective tissue cells with muscle: expression of muscle actin in and contraction of fibroblasts, chondrocytes, and osteoblasts. *Wound Repair Regen*. 2001; 9:11–18.

FASCIA AS A SENSORY ORGAN
Robert Schleip

Treating a piece of fresh meat: what is missing?

A corpse is a body minus life. While it is easy to agree with that statement, a related set of more intriguing questions include:

- How exactly does 'life' affect the tissue response during manual therapy?

- Which physiological or other known mechanisms are involved in this?

- Could the answers to this also help in understanding the difference between tissue qualities in seemingly very 'alive' body parts and more neglected body parts that feel less 'alive' to the palpating hand?

Guided by these questions, the author and a group of colleagues conducted several exploratory experiments in which they gave manual mobilization techniques to freshly extracted animal fascia (lumbar fascia from pigs, cows, rats, and mice, taken a few minutes after their sacrifice – see Figure 7.1). While it was possible to loosen some of the tinier collagenous connections and adhesions, the practitioners involved left with the clear impression that many important tissue response aspects that are usually palpable when working with 'alive fascia' were missing in these artificial treatment sessions. In a similar set of exploratory experiments the author applied fascial mobilization techniques to patients under anesthesia in a hospital setting. Here, too, a lack of the normal tissue responsiveness was encountered. Whereas many previously tight muscular tissues (such as the upper trapezius or the hamstrings) appeared to be softer compared with their pre-anesthesia condition, none of the melting or release responses that are familiar to fascial therapists could be detected during application of deep tissue mobilization techniques (Schleip, 2012).

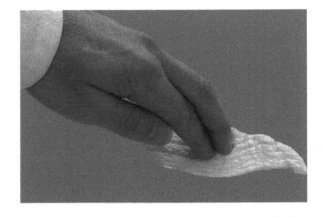

Figure 7.1
Experimenting with different myofascial techniques on a fresh piece of animal fascia. While most of the inherent fibroblastic cells are still alive (for several hours after sacrifice of the donor), several tissue responses could not be elicited that are familiar to fascial therapists when working with fascia in normal conditions. Could this lack of responsiveness be related to the disrupted neural connections with the central nervous system? (© fascialnet.com)

While these explorations did not include sufficient methodological rigor and therefore cannot be scientifically relied upon, they seem to be in agreement with the results of an extensive study conducted by Chaudhry et al. (2008). Here it was shown that the mechanical forces used in myofascial mobilization are capable of inducing an immediate and lasting tissue deformation in very loose connective tissues such as the nasal fascia. However, these forces are not sufficient to induce lasting effects in dense fascial tissues (such as the lumbar fascia, fascia lata, or plantar fascia). The study authors therefore suggested that fascial therapies with palpable results may involve stimulation of sensory nerve endings in fascia, which, via their link with the central nervous system, could elicit physiological or neuromuscular responses that indirectly influence the tissue responsiveness (beyond the original biomechanical tissue deformation effect explored in that study).

Fascial tissues are richly innervated

What is actually known about the sensory innervation of fascia? In fact, for most medical professionals fascia had long been considered to be an inert wrapping organ, giving mechanical support to other more important structures, such as muscles and organs. Whereas there existed some early histological reports about the presence of sensory nerves in fascia (Stillwell, 1957; Sakada, 1974), these were hardly noticed and did not affect the general understanding of musculoskeletal dynamics. While other manual therapy pioneers – such as Moshe Feldenkrais as well as Ida Rolf, founders of the related somatic therapies – were apparently not aware of the importance of fascia as a sensory organ, it was the founder of osteopathy, A. T. Still, who proclaimed that 'No doubt nerves exist in the fascia ...' and suggested that all fascial tissues should be treated with the same degree of respect as if dealing with 'the branch offices of the brain' (Still, 1902). However, his writings included hardly any detail about how he had arrived at that conclusion, what specific nerve types he meant, and how these respond to different kinds of mechanical stimulation.

A great contribution to this field was later made by van der Wal, who documented with painstaking detail the rich presence of sensory nerve endings in the fascia of rats (van der Wal, 1988; van der Wal, 2009). Unfortunately, this important finding was hardly noticed in the medical and therapeutic community for several decades. Concerning ligaments – as very specialized fascial tissues – their proprioceptive innervation was recognized during the 1990s, which subsequently influenced the guidelines for joint injury surgeries (Johansson et al., 1991). Similarly, the plantar fascia as a specialized tissue was found to contribute to the sensorimotor regulation of postural control in standing (Erdemir & Piazza,

2004). However, what really changed the general perspective in a more encompassing and powerful manner was the first international Fascia Research Congress, held at Harvard Medical School in Boston in 2007. During the Congress, three teams from different countries reported, independently, their findings of a rich presence of sensory nerves in fascial tissues (Findley & Schleip, 2007).

Figure 7.2 gives an example of the richness of nerve supply in a piece of human fascia. If one follows the terminology laid out in Chapter 3 and recognizes all dominantly fibrous connective tissues – such as ligaments, organ capsules, or intramuscular connective tissues – to be part of a body-wide tensional network referred to as 'fascia', then fascia contains at least several hundred thousand nerve endings, all of which link the peripheral fascial tissues with the central somatic or autonomous nervous system (Mitchell & Schmidt, 1977). In return, fascia is supplied by a rich

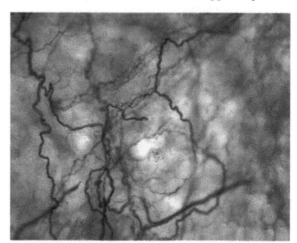

Figure 7.2

Demonstration of the rich presence of nerves in a piece of human lumbar fascia. The image length is approximately 0.5mm. Use of a pan-neuronal antibody permitted the visible marking of all neural tissues (here in dark brown). Reproduced from Tesarz J., Hoheisel U., Wiedenhöfer B., Mense S. (2011) Sensory innervation of the thoracolumbar fascia in rats and humans. *Neuroscience.* 194:302–308, with permission from Elsevier

supply of efferent sympathetic nerve endings, which influence the local vasomotor activity and could possibly have additional (yet to be understood) functions (Tesarz et al, 2011).

Based on this it seems not presumptuous to look at the body-wide fascial web as a sensory organ. With regard to the sheer quantity and richness of nerve endings, the facial web can 'stand up' to our senses of seeing, not to mention hearing, or any other of what are usually considered our sensory organs. When the intricate system of intramuscular sacs and septi of collagenous connective tissues is included as contributing an element of this tensional network, fascia can also be seen as our largest sensory organ in terms of overall surface area.

According to Tesarz et al. (2011), the innervation pattern of fascia – examined in rodent as well as human lumbodorsal fascia – follows a segmental pattern, comparable to the congruence of the well-known myotome and dermatome innervation maps. The term 'fasciatome' was suggested for fascial areas innervated from respective levels of the spinal cord.

Areas with a particularly rich innervation

Does it make a difference which locations of the fascial network are stimulated in a manual treatment in order to supply the spinal cord with new proprioceptive input? Two new insights regarding the density of sensory receptors in fascia provide valuable insight into this question. First, recent histological studies from the group around Mense at the University of Heidelberg have shown that in both human and rodent lumbar fascia the density of sensory neurons is significantly higher in the most superficial tissue layers, i.e., in those between the dermis and fascia profunda (Tesarz et al., 2011). In our own experiments at Ulm University we also observed an increased density of visible nerves in the transitional shearing zone between fascia profunda and fascia superficialis. In healthy body regions, this zone is where a lateral 'skin sliding' movement, in relation to the underlying tissues, can easily be induced. It is also the zone whose architecture determines whether a skin fold can be pulled away from the body or not. This may serve as background for the plausible assumption that

the lateral gliding movements provided by everyday movements provide an important source of fascial proprioception. In relation to this, it is also possible to speculate that the often profound anecdotal effects of various skin-taping techniques in sports medicine may partially be explained by their local amplification of respective skin movements in normal joint functioning. Further research is necessary to confirm these assumptions.

The second recent insight comes from the Stecco group at Padua University in Italy (Stecco et al., 2007). Their histological examinations of upper and lower limb fasciae in human cadavers revealed huge differences in the density of proprioceptive nerve endings, such as Golgi, Pacini, and Ruffini corpuscles. Their data indicates that fascial tissues, which clearly serve an important force-transmitting function (such as the lacertus fibrosus on the upper forearm as an extension of the biceps femoris), hardly contain any proprioceptive endings. On the other hand, the researchers observed that other fascial structures seem to have very little role in force transmission, as witnessed when cutting them away, as is the case of the retinacula around ankle and wrist region. Interestingly, these more obliquely running fascial bands seem to be located at specific narrow distances from major joints and they contain a very high density of proprioceptive nerve endings. It was even suggested that the prime function of these fascial bands may not be their biomechanical but their sensorial function in providing detailed proprioception to the central nervous system. If verified, this could suggest that proprioception-enhancing approaches in manual therapy could possibly be augmented in their respective therapeutic effectiveness by stimulating fascial tissues in regions with an increased proprioceptive innervation.

Different mechanosensory receptor types and their functions

Figure 7.3 illustrates the typical composition of a musculoskeletal nerve bundle, such as the sciatic nerve in the leg or the radial nerve in the arm. One of the many interesting aspects about this composition is that a vast number of nerves are devoted to the fine-tuning of nutrient delivery via the vascular supply, which is regulated by the sympathetic nervous system.

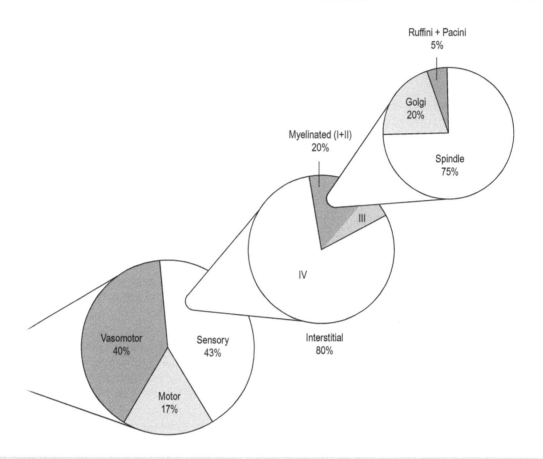

Figure 7.3
Neuronal composition of a peripheral nerve. The proportions illustrated were derived from quantitative analysis of the individual axons that make up a larger nerve bundle supplying a peripheral region (in this case the combined nerve supplying the lateral gastrocnemius and soleus muscle of a cat; data taken from Mitchell & Schmidt, 1977). While a small portion of the interstitial neurons may terminate inside bone, the remaining neurons can all be considered to terminate in fascial tissues. Even the sensory devices called muscle spindles are nestled within perimysial or endomysial fascial tissues. Interstitial neurons terminate in free nerve endings. Some of these clearly have a proprioceptive, interoceptive, or nociceptive function. Recent investigations, however, suggest that the majority of the interstitial neurons in fascia serve a polymodal function, which means that they are open for nociceptive as well as nonnociceptive stimulation (© fascialnet.com)

The remaining portion, dealing with sensorimotor regulation, is then not at all equally devoted to motor and sensory pathways. In contrast, the body architecture devotes more than twice as many neurons for the 'listening' or feeling aspect of communication as it does to 'talking' and giving instructions towards the periphery. Could this wise architectural principle be one of the explanations why sometimes the body's

innate intelligence by far surpasses the effectiveness of an old-fashioned bossy CEO who tries to direct his company by a multitude of demands and with only scarcely developed listening skills?

A quarter of the sensory axons are made up of relatively fast-conducting myelinated neurons that can clearly be regarded as proprioceptive pathways. Their termination includes the Pacini, Golgi, and Ruffini corpuscles. They usually terminate in fascial tissues, in either the epimysial or tendinous portions or in the intramuscular connective tissues.

Note that the muscle spindles – which are from an evolutionary perspective a fairly recent invention for the fine-tuning of movement of land animals – can be regarded as sensory devices that are also located within the perimysial or endomysial collagenous tissues of the intramuscular fascial network. It is plausible that if the surrounding collagenous tissues suffer from a loss of elasticity, then the functioning of these spindles may be corrupted. Possibly this could be a contributing factor in conditions such as chronic muscle stiffness or in fibromyalgia, as an increased endomysial thickness has been shown to be a characteristic of fibromyalgia patients (Liptan, 2010). Furthermore, it is also interesting to learn from meat scientists that an increased perimysial thickness has been found to account for the difference in stiffness between tough meat muscles versus tender meat muscles within the same animal (Schleip et al., 2006).

While much is known about the functioning of these different mechanosensitive neurons, the majority of sensory nerves in fascial tissue terminate in interstitial free nerve endings (see Figure 7.3), which are much less understood and are still considered as intriguingly mysterious by those who investigate. Classical neurology divides these further into the type III neurons, whose axons contain a very thin myelin sheet, and type IV neurons, with unmyelinated axons. For our purposes, however, they can largely be considered to behave in a similar manner, although the speed of the type IV neurons (also called C-fibers in another classification category) is even slower than the already slow type III axons (also called A-δ fibers).

For the regularly myelinated neurons – supplying muscle spindles, Golgi, Pacini, and Ruffini endings – it is clear that they function as proprioceptive devices. Among these the Ruffini endings have been reported to be highly sensitive to shear loading (i.e., a directional difference in tensional loading between one tissue layer and an adjacent one), whereas the Pacini endings respond to rapid changes only and they tend to be unreceptive to any nonchanging stimulations.

While the Golgi receptors were previously considered to exist only in tendinous tissues, their presence in other fascial tissues has been independently confirmed by different international studies (Yahia et al., 1992; Stecco et al., 2007; Stecco et al., 2008). Stimulation of Golgi receptors tends to trigger a relaxation response in those muscle fibers, which are serially connected with the stimulated collagen fiber bundles. However, if tendinous tissues are stretched with the serially connected myofibers in a relaxed condition, then most of the respective elongation will be 'swallowed' by the more compliant myofibers. Imagine a rope consisting of a dense string in line with a soft, compliant string. When pulling on both, all lengthening will first happen within the softer portion, while hardly any lengthening will be seen in the serially connected denser portion. This is congruent with Jami's article, which states that stretching impulses with simultaneously relaxed muscles may not provide sufficient stimulation for eliciting any muscular tonus change (Jami, 1992).

Stimulation of Ruffini endings has been reported to trigger a decrease in sympathetic activation. Ruffini endings seem particularly responsive to shear loading. It is an intriguing thought that slow, melting myofascial techniques – incorporating 'local listening' skills about the preferred release direction of tissue – may be particularly effective in stimulating these receptors. Such techniques are frequently utilized in the Rolfing method (Jones, 2004) as well as related deep tissue manipulation approaches.

Pacini corpuscles, on the other hand, prefer rapid changes, since they are fast-adapting receptors. They could be particularly involved in high-velocity manipulations, but also in more gentle rocking motions such as are used in the Trager approach or in Lederman's harmonic technique (Trager, 1987; Schleip, 2003; Lederman, 2005).

Stimulation of mechanosensory interstitial free nerve endings, particularly those with a high mechanical threshold, has been shown to induce an altered local fluid supply, via increased local vasodilation as well as plasma extrusion (Mitchell & Schmidt, 1977).

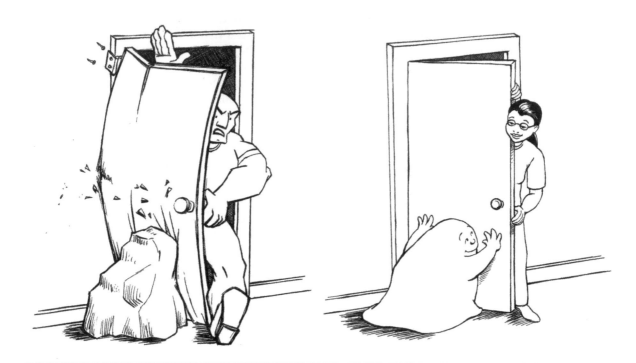

Figure 7.4
Two ways to open a blocked door or joint. A door blocked by a mechanical object requires a different approach compared with one that is blocked by an animated obstacle. Similarly, a blocked joint or immobile tissue can be approached in purely mechanical terms, as if dealing with dead tissues. Alternatively, these can be approached as an active self-regulatory mechanism. The choice of approach depends largely on whether the practitioner is aware of any neural dynamics involved in the specific situation on the patient's side (© fascialnet.com, with kind permission of Twyle Weixl)

See Table 7.1 for a review of different sensory receptors in fascia that can be targeted with manual therapy approaches. For a more clinically oriented extension of this overview, see Chapter 25, Table 25.1.

Fascia as a potent pain generator

That fascial nerve endings can be the origin of soft tissue pain has been convincingly shown by Tesarz et al. (2011). This study documented the rich presence of free nerve endings with a clear nociceptive function in both rodent and human lumbar fascia. This has also been confirmed by different provocation tests via injection of hypotonic saline into human lumbar fascia

(Schilder et al., 2014). Interestingly, it was found that the related interstitial neurons in fascia seem to be particularly responsive, in terms of a subsequently long-lasting hypersensitivity, to repeated mechanical or biochemical irritation.

Similar provocation tests with hypotonic saline revealed that much of the sensation known as delayed onset muscle soreness (DOMS) after strenuous eccentric exercise seems to originate from nociceptive interstitial neurons in the fascial layer of the muscular epimysium (Gibson et al., 2009).

The new perspective of fascia being a potential pain generator could offer important implications for the

Receptor	Preferred location	Particular responsiveness
Muscle spindle	• Perimysium • Endomysium • Around epimysial origin of muscular septi	• Rapid, unexpected elongation
Golgi receptor	• Myotendinous junctions • Epimysium • Joint capsules	• Slow elongation of related collagen fibers above a certain strain threshold (may require muscular resistance)
Pacini corpuscle	• Spinal ligaments • Inner layer of joint capsules	• Rapid changes in local tension and/or compression
Ruffini endings	• Outer layer of joint capsules • Dura mater • Fascia profunda in areas that are frequently exposed to extension	• Slow deformation along tangential vectors (shear loading)
Interstitial free nerve endings	• Periosteum • Subdermal connective tissue (tactile C-fibers) • Superficial layers of lumbar fascia • Visceral and intramuscular connective tissues	• Nociception • High threshold mechanoreception • Low threshold mechanoreception • Polymodal receptivity

Table 7.1
Review of different sensory receptors in fascia that can be targeted with manual therapy approaches

understanding and treatment of low back pain. While some cases of low back pain are definitely caused by deformations of spinal discs, several large MRI studies clearly revealed that for the majority of low back pain cases the origins may have to be looked for elsewhere in the body, as the discal alterations are frequently incidental (Jensen et al., 1994; Sheehan, 2010). Based on this background, a new hypothetical explanation model for low back pain was proposed by Panjabi (2006) and subsequently elaborated on by others (Langevin & Sherman, 2007; Schleip et al., 2007). According to these authors, microinjuries in lumbar connective tissues may lead to nociceptive signaling and further downstream effects associated with low back pain. Microinjuries in human lumbar fascia have indeed long been documented in low back pain patients (for a review see Willard et al., 2012). However their presence in comparable healthy people had not been quantified and therefore a causal relationship remained questionable. However, recently an extensive sonographic study by Langevin and Sherman compared the lumbar fascia in patients with

chronic low back pain with a group of comparable healthy persons. Here this fascial layer was shown to be more densely (or more adherently) connected with the underlying musculature in patients compared with their healthy controls. This finding, together with the previously reported innervations studies, suggests that the lumbar fascia should be recognized as an important factor in the understanding and treatment of at least some cases of low back pain (Langevin & Sherman, 2007).

Polymodal receptors in fascia

It is important to realize that not all free nerve endings can be classified as nociceptive. Some of them are sensory devices for thermoception. Others report changes of muscular activity to the sympathetic nervous system in order to allow for locally specific fine-tuning of the blood flow to respective muscle portions, which is known as ergoreception.

Interestingly, in fascial tissues the majority of the interstitial neurons are so-called 'wide dynamic range' receptors or polymodal receptors, meaning that they are responsive to more than one kind of stimulation (Sandkühler, 2009). While their respective synapses in the posterior horn of the spinal cord are hungry and eager for 'any' kind of stimulation, they seem to be easily satisfied if sufficient proprioceptive information is supplied to them via these polymodal receptors. However, in cases of insufficient supply with proprioceptive stimulation (e.g., because of alterations in the connective tissue matrix surrounding the respective nerve endings) these neurons tend to actively lower their threshold for nociceptive stimulation. In addition, they may actively extrude cytokines that sensitize polymodal neurons in their neighborhood and predispose them towards a nociceptive function. A seemingly miniscule mechanical stimulation, such as a leg length difference of 1 mm only, can then lead to a nociceptive response within the intricate network of these intrafascial polymodal receptors.

Based on the mutually inhibiting dynamics between proprioceptive and nociceptive intrafascial stimulation, many therapeutic approaches are exploring the use of movement and/or touch in order to supply the respective polymodal receptors with novel

SUMMARY

In a nutshell:

- Touching fascia on a living person requires a different approach to treating a piece of dead meat. In fact, fascia constitutes a body-wide fabric that serves as our largest sensory organ. It provides our most important orientation for sensing our physical self.

- Related sensory nerves include receptors that signal proprioceptive information. Different manual techniques may function well by providing new proprioceptive stimulation to these receptors, resulting in receptor-specific neuromuscular and physiological effects.

- Fascia can also be the origin of pain, including some cases of low back pain transmitted via nociceptive nerve endings.

- Other nerve endings in fascia serve an interoceptive function and tend to influence the insular cortex and its somatoemotional self-sensing function.

- The widespread existence of polymodal receptors in fascia provides a useful basis for understanding the beneficial analgesic effects of several fascia-related therapeutic approaches.

proprioceptive input. This can be done with many different methods, whether it be the guided exploration of new movement patterns (as in the Feldenkrais method), the use of active micromovements of the client at an amplitude of few millimetres only (as in continuum movement), or use of a caliper to improve two-point discrimination when touched at decreasing two-point distances on the skin, among many others (Buchanan & Ulrich, 2001).

Apparently induction of novel nociceptive input – from slightly different locations within the same fasciatome – can also lower a previous hypersensitivity of polymodal receptors. Doing so on the highly innervated periosteum (or at the tendon–periosteum transitions) seems to be particularly effective in this respect, which could be one of the explanatory mechanisms behind more vigorous treatments such as *Chua K'a* massage and behind several aspects of Typaldos' fascial distortion model (Typaldos, 1999).

Interoceptive innervation

Several free nerve endings in fascia are neither related to somatosensory nor nociceptive signaling. Instead they inform the insular cortex of the forebrain about physiological tissue conditions, such as warmth, pH changes, or visceral sensations (Craig, 2002). A particular richness of such interoceptive endings is located in visceral connective tissues and constitutes the so-called enteric brain. Interestingly, several dysfunctions common to osteopaths seem more related to a disturbed interoception, rather than to proprioception. The list of these conditions includes irritable bowel syndrome, eating disorders, anxiety, depression, alexithymia (emotional blindness), and possibly fibromyalgia. It can be speculated that treatment of those conditions could profit from a more interoceptive rather than proprioceptive mindful attention of the patient during treatment. On the other hand, treatment of conditions with a known proprioceptive impairment may work best with enhanced proprioceptive stimulation and attention, which would then include low back pain, scoliosis, phantom pain, whiplash injuries, and complex regional pain syndrome (CRPS) (Schleip et al., 2012).

The recent discovery of 'tactile C-fibers' in subcutaneous connective tissues of human skin has shed a new light on the powerful and complex dynamics of grooming behavior in primates. Stimulation of these nerve endings can provide important interoceptive signaling to the insular cortex, with resultant downstream effects on psychoendocrine function, immune system, and vegetative regulation (Schleip et al., 2012).

References

Buchanan P. A., Ulrich B. D. (2001) The Feldenkrais Method: a dynamic approach to changing motor behavior. *Res Q Exerc Sport* 72(4):315–323.

Chaudhry H. Schleip R., Ji Z. et al., (2008) Three-dimensional mathematical model for deformation of fascia in manual therapy. *J Am Osteop Assoc* 108:379–390.

Craig A. D. (2002) How do you feel? Interoception: the sense of the physiological condition of the body. *Nat Rev Neurosci* 3(8):655–666.

Erdemir A., Piazza S. J. (2004) Changes in foot loading following plantar fasciotomy: a computer modeling study. *J Biomech Eng* 126(2):237–43.

Findley W. T. & Schleip R. (eds) (2007) *Fascia Research: Basic Science and Implications for Conventional and Complementary Health Care.* Munich: Elsevier Urban & Fischer.

Gibson W., Arendt-Nielsen L., Taguchi T. et al., (2009) Increased pain from muscle fascia following eccentric exercise: animal and human findings. *Exp Brain Res* 194(2):299–308.

Jami A. (1992) Golgi tendon organs in mammalian skeletal muscles: functional properties and central actions. *Physiol Rev* 72(3):623–666.

Jensen M. C., Brant-Zawadzki M. N., Obuchowski N. et al., (1994) Magnetic resonance imaging of the lumbar spine in people without back pain. *NEJM* 331(2):69–73.

Johansson H., Sjölander P., Sojka P. (1991) A sensory role for the cruciate ligaments. *Clin Orthop Relat Res* 268:161–178.

Jones T. A. (2004) Rolfing. *Phys Med Rehabil Clin N Am* 15(4):799–809.

Langevin H. M., Sherman K. J. (2007) Pathophysiological model for chronic low back pain integrating connective tissue and nervous system mechanisms. *Med Hypotheses* 68(1):74–80.

Lederman E. (2005) *Harmonic Technique.* Churchill Livingstone, Edinburgh.

Liptan G. L. (2010) Fascia: a missing link in our understanding of the pathology of fibromyalgia. *J Bodyw Mov Ther* 14(1):3–12.

Mitchell J. H., Schmidt R. F. (1977) Cardiovascular reflex control by afferent fibers from skeletal muscle receptors. In: Shepherd J. T. Abboud F. M. (eds) Handbook of Physiology, Section 2, Vol. III, Part 2, pp. 623–658.

Panjabi M. M. (2006) A hypothesis of chronic back pain: ligament subfailure injuries lead to muscle control dysfunction. *Eur Spine J* 15(5):668–767.

Sakada S (1974) Mechanoreceptors in fascia, periosteum and periodontal ligament. *Bull Tokyo Med Dent Univ* 21 Suppl:11–13.

Sandkühler J. (2009) Models and mechanisms of hyperalgesia and allodynia. *Physiol Rev* 89(2):707–758.

Schilder A., Hoheisel U., Magerl W., et al., (2014) Sensory findings after stimulation of the thoracolumbar fascia with hypertonic saline suggest its contribution to low back pain. *Pain* 155(2):222–231.

Schleip R. (2003) Fascial plasticity—a new neurobiological explanation. Part 1. *J Bodyw Mov Ther* 7(1):11–19.

Schleip R. (2012) Chapter 2.1 Fascia as an organ of communication. In:Schleip R., Findley T. W., Chaitow L., Huijing P. A. (eds.) *Fascia: the Tensional Network of the Human Body.* Churchill Livingstone Elsevier, pp.77–79.

Schleip R., Naylor I. L., Ursu D., et al., (2006) Passive muscle stiffness may be influenced by active contractility of intramuscular connective tissue. *Med Hypotheses* 66(1):66–71.

Schleip R., Vleeming A., Lehmann-Horn F., Klingler W. (2007) Letter to the Editor concerning "A hypothesis of chronic back pain: ligament subfailure injuries lead to muscle control dysfunction" (M. Panjabi). *Eur Spine J* 16(10):1733–1735.

Stecco C., Gagey O., Belloni A. et al., (2007) Anatomy of the deep fascia of the upper limb. Second part:study of innervation. Morphologie 91(292):38–43.

Stecco C., Porzionato A., Lancerotto L. et al., (2008) Histological study of the deep fasciae of the limbs. *J Bodyw Mov Ther* 12(3):225–230.

Still A. T. (1902) *The Philosophy and Mechanical Principles of Osteopathy.* Hudson-Kimberly Publishing Company, Kansas City, p. 62.

Stillwell D. L. (1957) Regional variations in the innervation of deep fasciae and aponeuroses. *Anat Rec* 127:635–648.

Tesarz J., Hoheisel U., Wiedenhöfer B., Mense S. (2011) Sensory innervation of the thoracolumbar fascia in rats and humans. *Neuroscience* 194:302–308.

Trager M., Guadagno-Hammond C., Turnley Walker T. (1987) *Trager Mentastics: Movement as a Way to Agelessness.* Station Hill Press, Barrytown.

Typaldos S. (1999) Orthopathic Medicine: *The Unification of Orthopedics with Osteopathy through the Fascial Distortion Model.* Orthopathic Global Health Publications.

van der Wal J. C. (1988) The organization of the substrate of proprioception in the elbow region of the rat [PhD thesis]. Maastricht, Netherlands: Maastricht University, Faculty of Medicine.

van der Wal J. (2009) The architecture of the connective tissue in the musculoskeletal system: an often overlooked functional parameter as to proprioception in the locomotor apparatus. In: Huijing P. A. Hollander P., Findley T. W., Schleip R. (eds), *Fascia Research II: Basic Science and Implications for Conventional and Complementary Health Care.* Munich: Elsevier GmbH.

Willard F. H. , Vleeming A., Schuenke M. D. et al., (2012) The thoracolumbar fascia:anatomy, function and clinical considerations. *J Anat* 221(6):507–36.

Yahia L., Rhalmi S., Newman N., Isler M. (1992) Sensory innervation of human thoracolumbar fascia: an immunohistochemical study. *Acta Orthop Scand* 63(2):195–197.

THE ROLE OF THE FASCIA IN IMMUNITY AND INFLAMMATION

Lisa M. Hodge

Introduction

The lymphatic system maintains tissue fluid homeostasis by returning excessive interstitial fluid to the blood circulation.[1,2] Lymph formation in the soft tissue creates pressure gradients that drive the movement of lymph through lymphatic vessels.[3] However, other factors such as lymphatic vessel contraction, movement of the skeletal system, respiration, peristalsis, and arterial pulsation will alter this gradient.[4,2] Compression of tissue by external forces, exercise, massage, and body-based manipulative medicine techniques[5–10,11,12,13,14,15,16] have also been shown to increase lymph flow.

Fascia is a form of connective tissue that envelops muscles, nerves, bones, and organs.[17,18] It is a continuous structure and is thought to transmit mechanical forces generated by muscular activities throughout the body.[17,19] Inflammation may increase the thickness of the fascia, thereby reducing its flexibility and range of motion, which may predispose tissue to pain and further injury.[17,19,18] Therefore, body-based manipulative techniques may promote the healing of muscle and fascia by releasing tightness, relieving pressure, and restoring blood and lymph circulation.

The lymphatic system

The lymphatic system helps to maintain extravascular homeostasis by providing a unidirectional transport system between the interstitial space and blood circulation. As blood travels from the branching arteries to the capillary beds, excess plasma leaks into the interstitial space. This interstitial fluid is convected into the lymphatic capillaries. This transported tissue fluid is referred to as 'lymph', and can contain white blood cells, tumor cells, apoptotic cells, proteins, pathogens, and antigens that exist in the interstitial space.[1,2]

Interstitial fluid flow plays an important role in tissue function. For example, interstitial flow creates shear stress that controls myogenic tone;[20,21] enhances endothelial cell wound closure;[22] and stimulates blood and lymphatic endothelial cell morphogenesis.[23] The lymphatic capillaries are anchored to the extracellular matrix via anchoring filaments, which are highly sensitive to these interstitial fluid stresses.[24,2]

Initially, the lymphatic capillaries drain lymph from the interstitial space into the larger collecting lymph vessels. The collecting lymph vessels then deliver the lymph to the nodes and ducts. Segments of lymphatic vessels between valves, called lymphangions, cyclically contract and propel the lymph. The movement of lymph through the lymphatic vessels is also aided by the phasic contractions of smooth muscle cells within the lymph vessel walls.[3] A series of valves along the vessels also ensures the unidirectional flow of lymph toward blood circulation.[2]

In addition to transporting lymph, the lymphatic system also transports white blood cells, proteins, and lipids. During infection and inflammation, lymph vessels transport antigens and immune cells from infected tissues into regional lymph nodes, where specific immune responses are initiated.[1,2] Once these lymphocytes become activated, they are returned to venous circulation. These primed lymphocytes then traffic to the affected tissue where they perform their effector functions. Therapies that increase lymphatic flow, such as massage and osteopathic manipulative treatment (OMT), may drain inflammatory mediators from diseased tissue and redistribute them to lymph nodes where they can boost immunity.

Osteopathic manipulative techniques

Central to osteopathic practice is the belief that improving lymph flow will cleanse the interstitial space of blood cells, particulate matter, exudates, toxins, and bacteria that could predispose the fascia and surrounding tissue to disease.[25,18,26] Considering the importance of the lymphatic system in maintaining tissue homeostasis and immunity, manual medicine techniques that enhance lymph output may be the best approach when treating inflammatory and infectious diseases. In support, OMT has been reported to increase vaccine-specific antibodies,[27,28] reduce intravenous antibiotic use,[29] protect against lower respiratory tract disease,[30,31] and shorten the duration of hospital stay in elderly patients with pneumonia.[32,33]

While there are numerous manual therapies designed to enhance lymph flow, lymphatic pump techniques (LPT) have been experimentally proven to enhance lymphatic flow.[5–9,11,14] LPT are used clinically to treat patients with congestive heart failure, upper and lower gastrointestinal dysfunction, respiratory tract infection, and edema. They can be applied to the feet and legs (pedal pump), thoracic cage (thoracic pump), abdomen (abdominal pump), and the areas of the spleen and liver.[26] Considering the volume of lymphatic pools within the abdominal trunk,[34,35,36,37] repeated compression or stimulation of the mesenteric viscera may be a global approach to release large amounts of lymph into circulation. However, when addressing local edema of the peripheral tissues, such as lymphedema secondary to cancer or surgery, techniques such as pedal pump and manual lymph drainage may be more effective at relieving the tissue and fascia of edematous fluid.

Lymphatic pump techniques and immunity

While LPT has been applied clinically for more than 90 years to enhance immunological function, it is very surprising that the mechanisms of action have only been recently investigated. LPT may protect against infectious and inflammatory diseases by mobilizing leukocytes into lymphatic circulation. To test this hypothesis, the thoracic ducts of eight anesthetized mongrel dogs were catheterized and lymph flow was measured by timed collection and analyzed for the concentration of leukocytes.[5] Specifically, lymph was collected under 1) resting (baseline) conditions, and 2) during application of LPT. To apply LPT, the anesthetized animal was placed in a lateral recumbent position and the operator contacted the animal with the hands placed bilaterally at the costo-diaphragmatic junction. Pressure was exerted medially sufficient to compress the lower ribs until significant resistance was encountered, and then the pressure was released. Rib compressions were administered at a rate of approximately one per second for a total of eight minutes. For details pertaining to the experimental design see Hodge et al. (2007).[5]

LPT significantly ($P < 0.05$) increased thoracic duct lymph flow and the numbers of macrophages, neutrophils, T cells, and B cells in the lymph. Increased mobilization of immune cells is likely an important mechanism responsible for the enhanced immunity and recovery from infection of patients treated with LPT.

Early lymphatic studies found that the output of lymphocytes from the intestinal lymph duct was almost equal to the output of the thoracic lymph duct,[34,35,36,37] suggesting that thoracic duct lymphocytes are gathered from a pool drained by the intestinal duct. Rhythmic compressions on the abdomen during LPT compress the abdominal area, including the gastrointestinal lymphoid tissues, which may facilitate the release of leukocytes from these tissues into lymphatic circulation. To this hypothesis, a catheter was inserted into either the thoracic or the large intestinal lymph ducts of dogs.[6] In addition, to determine if LPT enhanced the release of leukocytes from the mesenteric lymph nodes (MLN) into thoracic duct lymph, the MLN were fluorescently labeled in situ. Lymph samples were collected during four minutes of baseline, four minutes of LPT, and ten minutes following cessation of LPT (recovery). The application of LPT significantly ($P < 0.05$) increased lymph flow and leukocytes in both intestinal and thoracic duct lymph. LPT had no preferential effect on any specific leukocyte population, since neutrophil, monocyte, T cell, and B cell numbers were similarly increased (Table 8.1). Thus, the hypothesis that

	Baseline	LPT	Recovery
Neutrophils	0.27 ± 0.12	3.67 ± 0.96[d]	0.75 ± 0.23
Monocytes	0.34 ± 0.14	4.24 ± 1.18[d]	0.91 ± 0.25
Lymphocytes	10.32 ± 4.53	81.1 ± 22.2[b]	18.3 ± 6.62
CD4[+] T cells	3.25 ± 0.62	43.7 ± 5.57[b]	12.4 ± 4.74
CD8[+] T cells	1.24 ± 0.37	16.3 ± 4.12[b]	5.31 ± 2.00
IgA[+] B cells	0.65 ± 0.18	9.02 ± 0.86[c]	1.48 ± 0.53
IgG[+] B cells	1.06 ± 0.21	13.4 ± 4.81[c]	1.95 ± 0.45

[a] Data are means × 10^6 leukocytes/min ± SE from 6 experiments. [b] Greater than baseline and recovery (P < 0.01). [c] Greater than baseline (P < 0.001) and recovery (P < 0.01). [d] Greater than baseline (P < 0.01) and recovery (P < 0.05). From Hodge et al.[6] Reprinted with permission from *Lymphatic Research & Biology*, 2010, Vol. 8, Issue 2, pp. 103–110, published by Mary Ann Liebert, Inc., New Rochelle, NY

Table 8.1

Abdominal LPT increases leukocyte flux in thoracic duct lymph[a]

LPT facilitates mobilization of leukocytes from the gastrointestinal tissues into the lymphatic circulation is supported.

Historically, large animal models have been used to study lymphatic function. However, this research is complex, expensive, and molecular tools are often limited in these species. Rodents have been used to study the lymphatic system[38,37] and provide a reasonable alternative to the use of large animals for research. To determine if LPT would also enhance the lymph flow of the rat, the cisterna chyli of 10 rats were cannulated and lymph was collected during 1) four minutes of pre-LPT baseline, 2) four minutes of LPT, and 3) ten minutes of post-LPT recovery.[9] LPT treatment was applied to the rat to simulate, as much as possible, how LPT is applied to the abdomen of humans. Figure 8.1 displays the application of LPT in a rat under light anesthesia.[6] To perform LPT, the operator contacted the abdomen of the rat with the thumb on one side and index finger and middle finger on the other side of the medial sagittal plane. The fingers were placed bilaterally caudal to the ribs (see Figure 8.1), and pressure was exerted medially and cranially to compress the abdomen until significant resistance was met against the diaphragm, then the pressure was released. Compressions were administered at approximately one per second for the duration of the four minutes of treatment.

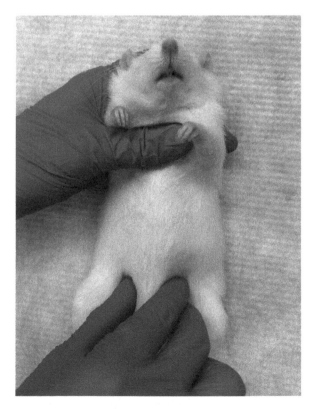

Figure 8.1

Application of lymphatic pump technique in a rat under light anesthesia

LPT increased (P < 0.05) lymph flow from a baseline of 24 ± 5 µl/minute to 89 ± 30 µl/minute. The baseline lymph flux was 0.65 ± 0.21 x 10⁶ lymphocytes/minute, and LPT increased lymph flux to 6.10 ± 0.99 x 10⁶ lymphocytes/minute (P < 0.01). Similar to studies in the dog,[5,6] LPT had no preferential effect on any lymphocyte population, since T cell and B cell numbers were similarly increased. To determine if LPT mobilized gut-associated lymphocytes into the lymph, gut-associated lymphocytes in lymph were identified by staining lymphocytes for the gut homing receptor integrin α4β7. LPT significantly increased (P < 0.01) the lymphatic flux of α4β7 positive lymphocytes from a baseline of 0.70 ± 0.03 x 10⁵ lymphocytes/minute to 6.50 ± 0.10 x 10⁵ lymphocytes/minute during LPT. Collectively, these results suggest that LPT may enhance immune surveillance by increasing the numbers of lymphocytes released into lymphatic circulation, especially from the gut-associated lymphoid tissue.

Inflammation

During infection and edema, inflammatory cytokines, chemokines, reactive oxygen species (ROS), and reactive nitrogen species (RNS) are generated in the tissue and released into blood and lymph.[1,2] Therefore, therapies that drain the fascia and surrounding tissue of these inflammatory mediators may reduce pain and facilitate tissue recovery. In support, OMT has been shown to alter serum cytokines in both healthy[39] and diseased subjects.[33]

To determine if LPT would mobilize inflammatory mediators into the lymphatic circulation, thoracic or intestinal lymph of dogs was collected at resting (pre-LPT), during four minutes of LPT, and for ten minutes following LPT (post-LPT). The lymphatic concentrations of interleukin-2 (IL-2), IL-4, IL-6, IL-10, interferon-γ (IFN-γ), tissue necrosis factor α (TNFα), monocyte chemotactic protein-1 (MCP-1), keratinocyte chemoattractant, superoxide dismutase (SOD), and nitrotyrosine (NT) were measured. LPT significantly (P < 0.05) increased the flux of thoracic and intestinal duct cytokines and chemokines compared to their respective pre-LPT flux.[15] Specifically, LPT increased the thoracic duct lymphatic flux of IL-6 (615%), IL-8 (944%), IL-10 (917%), MCP-1 (1505%), KC (788%), SOD (367%), and NT (373%) compared

with pre-LPT. In addition, LPT increased lymphatic flux of SOD and NT. Furthermore, LPT significantly increased the mesenteric duct lymphatic flux of IL-6 (394%), IL-8 (741%), IL-10 (556%), MCP-1 (651%), and KC (496%). The cytokines IL-2, IL-4, IFN-γ and TNFα were not detectable in thoracic or mesenteric duct lymph at any of the time points. Ten minutes following cessation of LPT, the thoracic and intestinal lymphatic flux of cytokines, chemokines, NT, and SOD were similar to pre-LPT, demonstrating that their flux was transient and a response to LPT. This redistribution of inflammatory mediators during LPT may provide scientific rationale for the clinical use of LPT to enhance immunity and treat infection.

Lymphedema

Inflammation, cancer, surgery, irradiation, and other factors can damage the lymphatic vessels and slow the transport of fluid away from the tissue. As protein-rich fluid accumulates in the tissue, edema forms in the dermis, subcutaneous tissue, muscular fascia, and muscles.[2,40] Lymphedema treatment is limited to manual medicine techniques designed to reduce the volume of edematous fluid and relieve pain. Complete decongestive therapy (CDT) is a treatment used to reduce lymphedema. CDT typically consists of manual lymph drainage, compression bandaging, exercise, compression garments, and skin care. Studies have demonstrated that CDT can reduce edematous limbs and improve quality of life,[12] though little is known about the mechanisms of action of these techniques.

Manual therapies such as massage, lymphatic pump/drainage techniques and intermittent compression may drain excess fluid from the edematous tissue and fascia into circulation. Therefore, understanding the pathways of lymph and tissue fluid flow may aid manual therapists during the treatment of edema. A recent study examined the pathways of lymph and tissue fluid flow during pneumatic massage of the limb using lymphoscintigraphy.[40] This study was carried out on 15 subjects with lymphedema (stage II–IV) of one of the lower limbs for 2–15 years. Lower limb lymphoscintigraphy was performed before treatment and seven days later, following a 45-minute limb pneumatic compression massage. Compression massage was achieved using a biocompression device[40] and strain gauge plethysmography was used to measure changes in limb circumference. Lymphscintigrams demonstrated that pneumatic compression mobilized the isotope in the lymph of the functioning lymphatics, the tissue fluid, and the interstitial space toward the inguinal region and femoral channel. There was no isotope crossing the inguinal crease or moving to the gluteal area. Isotope injected intradermally in the hypogastrium did not spread during manual massage to the upper and contralateral abdominal quadrants. These data suggest pneumatic compression can mobilize stagnant tissue fluid toward the groin in cases of lymphedema.

Animal studies have also provided insight into the mechanisms of lymphatic drainage/pumping techniques. In a study by Takeno et al. indocyanine green (ICG) lymphography was used to visualize lymph fluid accumulating in edematous limbs of rats.[41] To induce lymphedema, the ipsilateral popliteal fossa and lymph nodes with surrounding adipose tissue were excised from the inguinal region. Five weeks after lymphadenectomy, rats were randomly divided into two groups, no intervention or CDT. On day one, ICG was injected into the edematous limb, and either no intervention or CDT was applied for two weeks. CDT consisted of 15 minutes of massage, during which a compression bandage and exercise were used. ICG lymphography and circumferential measurements were done every two days during the two weeks. Nonedematous limbs served as negative controls. During edema, a high-intensity fluorescent signal concentrated around the ICG injection site, suggesting lymph stasis. As seen with edema, the circumferential lengths of the edematous limbs were longer than the nonedematous limbs. Of interest, two weeks of CDT reduced the high-intensity area at the injection site and the circumferential length of the edematous limb, suggesting CDT encourages lymph fluid to move from the periphery of edematous limbs.

The effect of LPT on lymph flow during edema has also been studied.[14] Edema was introduced by constriction of the inferior vena cava (IVC) of dogs. An ultrasonic flow transducer was placed on the thoracic lymph duct and catheters were placed in the

descending thoracic aorta and in IVC. Lymph flow and hemodynamic variables were measured in the presence and absence of edema during pre-LPT, four minutes of LPT, and post-LPT. Edema significantly ($P < 0.01$) increased thoracic duct lymph flow. LPT increased thoracic duct lymph flow in the presence and absence of edema. However, the incremental flow observed during LPT after edema was not significantly greater than the incremental flow observed during LPT before edema.

Collectively, these studies suggest that lymphatic draining/pumping therapies can enhance lymph flow and mobilize large pools of stagnant tissue fluid toward central circulation. Studies such as these support the use of manual therapies to treat lymphedema.

Infectious disease

While there are a few reports that support the use of OMT to treat infection,[30,42,31,43,32,29] very little is known about the mechanisms by which OMT may protect against infectious disease. By mobilizing lymph pools rich in inflammatory mediators, LPT may redistribute protective factors from the lymph to tissues, which could aid in the clearance of infection. Furthermore, by enhancing lymph flow, LPT might enhance the delivery of antibiotics to tissues.

LPT has been shown to reduce the bacterial load in the lungs of rats with acute pneumonia.[8] In this study, rats were nasally infected with 1×10^8 *Streptococcus pneumoniae* colony-forming units (CFU) and received either a daily sham treatment consisting of intravenous administration of anesthesia followed by four minutes of light touch, four minutes of LPT daily under anesthesia, or no treatment or anesthesia (control). The application of LPT to the rats was performed as previously described.[9] Eight days after infection, lungs were collected and measured for the number of *S. pneumoniae* bacteria. Both sham and LPT significantly ($P < 0.05$) reduced bacteria in the lungs compared to control; however, LPT cleared approximately 1.5×10^6 more *S. pneumoniae* CFU compared to sham treatment. These results suggest LPT may protect against pneumonia by inhibiting bacterial growth in the lung; however, the mechanism of protection is unclear.

Conclusion

The administration of OMT may facilitate the healing process by enhancing the lymphatic and immune systems, relieving restrictions to the fascia, and removing inflammatory mediators from the interstitial fluid space. However, we have only recently begun studying the mechanisms by which these therapies protect against disease. Once these mechanisms have been fully identified, OMT can be optimally applied to patients, which may substantially reduce morbidity, mortality, and the rate of hospitalization.

References

1. Olszewski W. L. The lymphatic system in body homeostasis: physiological conditions. *Lymphat Res Biol*. 2003, 1:11–21.

2. Swartz M. A. The physiology of the lymphatic system. *Adv Drug Deliv Rev*. 2001, 50:3–20.

3. Muthuchamy M., Zaweija D. Molecular regulation of lymphatic contractility. *Ann N Y Acad Sci*. 2008, 1131:89–99.

4. Bridenbaugh E. S., Gashev A. A., and Zaweija D. C. Lymphatic muscle: a review of contractile function. *Lymphat Res Biol*. 2003, 1:147–158.

5. *Hodge L. M., King H. H., Williams A. G., Reder S. .J., Belavadi T. J., Simecka J. W., Stoll S. T., and Downey H. F.* Abdominal lymphatic pump treatment increases leukocyte count and flux in thoracic duct lymph. *Lymphat Res Biol*. 2007, 5:127–132.

6. Hodge L. M., Bearden M. K., Schander A., Huff J. B., Williams A. Jr, King H. H., and Downey H. F. Abdominal lymphatic pump treatment mobilizes leukocytes from the gastrointestinal associated lymphoid tissue into lymph. *Lymphat Res Biol*. 2010, 8:103–110.

7. Hodge L. M., and Downey H. F. Lymphatic pump treatment enhances the lymphatic and immune systems. *Exp Biol Med*. 2011, 236:1109–1115.

8. Hodge L. M. Osteopathic lymphatic pump techniques to enhance immunity and treat pneumonia. *Int J Osteopath Med*. 2012, 15:13–21.

9. Huff J. B., Schander A., Downey H. F., and Hodge L. M. Lymphatic pump treatment augments lymphatic flux of lymphocytes in rats. *Lymphat Res Biol*. 2010, 8:183–187.

10. Ikomi F., and Ohhashi T. Effects of leg rotation on lymph flow and pressure in rabbit lumbar lymph circulation: in vivo experiments and graphical analysis. *Clin Hemorheol Microcirc*. 2000, 23:329–333.

11. Knott E. M., Tune J. D., Stoll S. T., and Downey H. F. Increased lymphatic flow in the thoracic duct during manipulative intervention. *J Am Osteopath Assoc*. 2005, 105:447–456.

12. Lasinski B. B., McKillip Thrift K., Squire D., Austin M. K., Smith K. M., Wanchai A., Green J. M., Stewart B. R., Cormier J. N., and Armer J. M. A systematic review of the evidence for complete decongestive therapy in the treatment of lymphedema from 2004 to 2011. *PMR*. 2012, 4:580–601.

13. McGeown J. G., McHale N. G. and Thornbury K. D. Effects of varying patterns of external compression on lymph flow in the hindlimb of the anaesthetized sheep. *J Physiol*. 1988, 397:449–457.

14. Prajapti P., Shah P., King H. H., Williams A. G. Jr, Desai, P., and Downey H. F. Lymphatic pump treatment increases thoracic duct lymph flow in conscious dogs with edema due to constriction of the inferior vena cava. *Lymphat Res Biol*. 2010, 8:149–154.

15. Schander A., Downey H. F., and Hodge L. M. Lymphatic pump manipulation mobilizes inflammatory mediators into lymphatic circulation. *Exp Biol Med*. 2012, 237:58–63.

16. Schander A., Padro D., Downey H. F., and Hodge L. M. Lymphatic pump treatment repeatedly enhances the lymphatic and immune systems. *Lymphat Res Biol*. 2013, 11:219–226.

17. Findley T., Chaudhry H., Stecco A., and Roman M. Fascia research—a narrative review. *J Bodyw Mov Ther*. 2012, 16:67–75.

18. Seffinger M. A., King H. H., Ward R. C., Jones J. M. III, and Rogers F. J. Osteopathic philosophy. In: R. C. Ward ed. *Foundations for Osteopathic Medicine, 2nd ed.* Philadelphia, PA: Lippincott Williams & Wilkins; 2003:3–12.

19. Langevin H. M., and Huijing P. A. Communicating about fascia: history, pitfalls, and recommendations. *Int J Ther Massage Bodywork* 2009, 2:3–8.

20. Kim, M. H. Harris N. R., Korzick D. H., and Tarbell J. M. Control of the arteriolar myogenic response by transvascular fluid filtration. *Microvasc Res*. 2004, 68:30–37.

21. Tada S., and Tarbell J. M. Interstitial flow through the internal elastic lamina affects shear stress on arterial smooth muscle cells. *Am J Physiol Heart Circ Physiol*. 2000, 278:H1589–H1597.

22. Albuquerque M. L., Waters C. M., Savla U., Schnaper H. W., and Flozak A. S. Shear stress enhances human endothelial cell wound

closure in vitro. *Am J Physiol Heart Circ Physiol.* 2000, 279:H293–H302.

23. Ng C. P. Helm C. L., and Swartz M. A. Interstitial flow differentially stimulates blood and lymphatic endothelial cell morphogenesis in vitro. *Microvasc Res.* 2004, 68, 258–264.

24. Swartz M. A., Kaipainen A., Nett P. A., Brekken C., Boucher Y., Grodzinsky A. J. and Jain R. Mechanics of interstitial-lymphatic fluid transport:theoretical foundation and experimental validation. *J Biomech.* 1999, 32:1297–1307.

25. Degenhardt B. F., and Kuchera M. L. Update on osteopathic medical concepts and the lymphatic system. *J Am Osteopath Assoc.* 1996, 96:97–100.

26. Wallace E., McPartland J. M., Jones J. M. III, Kuchera W. A., Buser B. R. Lymphatic system: lymphatic manipulative techniques. In: R. Ward ed. *Foundations for Osteopathic Medicine, 2nd ed.* Philadelphia, PA: Lippincott Williams & Wilkins, 2003:1056–1077.

27. Jackson K. M., Steele T. F., Dugan E. P., Kukulka G., Blue W., and Roberts A. Effect of lymphatic and splenic pump techniques on the antibody response to Hepatitis B vaccine: a pilot study. *J Am Osteopath Assoc.* 1998, 98:155–160.

28. Measel J. W. Jr. The effect of lymphatic pump on the immune response: preliminary studies on the antibody response to pneumococcal polysaccharide assayed by bacterial agglutination and passive hemagglutination. *J Am Osteopath Assoc.* 1982, 82:28–31.

29. Noll D. R., Degenhardt B. F., Morely T. F., Blais F. X., Hortos K. A., Hensel K., Johnson J. C., Pasta D. J., Stoll T. Efficacy of osteopathic manipulation as an adjunctive therapy for hospitalized patients with pneumonia: a randomized controlled trial. *Osteopath Med Prim Care.* 2010;4:2.

30. Allen T. W., and Pence T. K. The use of the thoracic pump in treatment of lower respiratory tract disease. *J Am Osteopath Assoc.* 1967, 67:408–411.

31. Kline, C. A. Osteopathic manipulative therapy, antibiotics, and supportive therapy in respiratory infections in children: comparative study. *J Am Osteopath Assoc.* 1965, 65:278–281.

32. Noll D. R., Shores J. H., Gamber R. G., Herron K. M., and Swift J. Jr. Benefits of osteopathic manipulative treatment for hospitalized elderly patients with pneumonia. *J Am Osteopath Assoc.* 2000, 100:776–782.

33. Licciardone J. C., Kearns C. M., Hodge L. M., and Bergamini M. V. Associations of cytokine concentrations with key osteopathic lesions and clinical outcomes in patients with nonspecific chronic low back pain: results from the OSTEOPATHIC Trial. *J Am Osteopath Assoc.* 2012, 112:596–605.

34. Mann J. D., and Higgins G. M. Lymphocytes in thoracic duct intestinal and hepatic lymph. *Blood.* 1950, 5:177–190.

35. Morris B. The hepatic and intestinal contributions to the thoracic duct lymph. *Q J Exp Physiol Cogn Med Sci.* 1956, 41:318–325.

36. Pabst R., and Binns R. M. *In vivo* labeling of the spleen and mesenteric lymph nodes with fluorescein isothiocyanate for lymphocyte migration studies. *Immunology* 1981, 44:321–329.

37. Smith M. E., and Ford W. L. The recirculating lymphocytes pool of the rat: a systematic description of the migratory behaviour of recirculating lymphocytes. *Immunology.* 1983, 49:83–94.

38. Gowans J. L. The recirculation of lymphocytes from blood to lymph in the rat. *J Physiol.* 1959, 146:54–69.

39. Walkowski S., Singh M., Puertas J., Pate M., Goodrum K., and Benencia F. Osteopathic manipulative therapy induces early plasma cytokine release and mobilization of a population of blood dendritic cells. *PLoS One.* 2014, 9:e90132.

40. Olszewski W. L., Cwikla J., Zaleska M., Domaszewska-Szostek A., Gradalski T., and Szopinska S. Pathways of lymph and tissue fluid flow during intermittent pneumatic massage of lower limbs with obstructive lymphedema. *Lymphology.* 2011, 44:54–64.

41. Takeno Y., Arita H., and Fujimoto E. Efficacy of complete decongestive therapy (CDT) on edematous rat limb after lymphadenectomy demonstrated by real time lymphatic fluid tracing. *Springerplus.* 2013, 2:225.

42. Degenhardt B. F., and Kuchera M. L. Osteopathic evaluation and manipulative treatment in reducing the morbidity of otitis media: a pilot study. *J Am Osteopath Assoc.* 2006, 106:327–334.

43. Mills M. V., Henley C. E., Barnes L. L. B., Carreiro J. E., and Degenhardt B. F. The use of osteopathic manipulative treatment as adjuvant therapy in children with recurrent acute otitis media. *J Am Osteopath Assoc.* 2003, 157:861–866.

PATHOPHYSIOLOGY OF FASCIA

Frans van den Berg

Introduction

In Chapter 6, the functions the fasciae have to fulfill and the ways in which they manage these tasks were described. The tasks of fascia are:

- to protect cells and also tissue against tension loading
- to enable repair of tissue after injury
- to allow resistance-free and friction-free movement.

It is pathologic when the fascia are unable to fulfill the tasks mentioned above. In the following text, the reasons for how and why the fascia are not able to perform their mechanical protective functions are discussed. These reasons are related to the changes that make the fascia cells unable to perform normal wound healing. The text further clarifies why and how friction-free movement can be disturbed. Finally, some typical diseases of the fascia are discussed.

Loss of stability

As mentioned in Chapters 5 and 6, connective tissue can retain its normal stability and mobility only when the cells are capable of performing their permanent physiological remodeling process. This means that any matrix components that are removed must be replaced by new matrix components. To allow this process, the cells need mechanical loading impulses, in order to produce matrix components that are capable of absorbing these mechanical loadings. Furthermore, the tissue needs this mechanical loading in order to integrate the matrix components into the normal tissue structure.

This process is disturbed because of the increasing lack of mobility and loading in our daily lives, but especially during immobilization after an injury. A lack of loading automatically leads to reduced loading capacity as well as a loss of mobility.

Due to reduced synthesizing activity of the cells, we see a loss of collagen, as well as a huge reduction in the amount of ground substance. This leads to a reduction of the distance between crossing collagen fibres within the collagen network – and finally to the formation of pathologic biochemical connections, called pathologic cross-links, between these crossing collagen fibres. The cross-links hinder the normal gliding capacity of collagen fibres against each other and, in this way, the mobility of the collagen network is adversely affected (Fig. 9.1).

Coinciding with the loss of collagen, we see a parallel loss of stability in the connective tissue structure. After 12 weeks of immobilization, we lose approximately 16% of the collagen (Currier & Nelson, 1992). Research on tendons and ligaments has indicated that stability is reduced by approximately 80% after an immobilization period of four weeks (Tabary et al., 1972).

Disturbances of wound healing

In order for the wound-healing process to take place after an injury, the cells require, as previously mentioned, mechanical loading. When the tissue is immobilized after an injury, a disturbance of normal wound healing occurs, at least in the proliferation phase (Fig. 9.2).

A further disturbance of wound healing could occur when the cells are not getting enough of the nutrients they need to build the matrix components. This could happen when the circulation in the tissue is not sufficient. For this reason, inflammatory mediators,

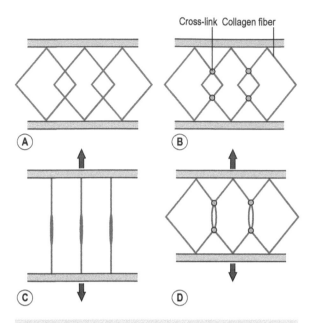

Cross-link Collagen fiber

Figure 9.1
Pathologic cross-links. Reproduced with permission from van den Berg *Angewandte Physiologie Band 1*, Georg Thieme Verlag. 3. Auflage, Stuttgart. [*Applied Physiology Volume 1*, Georg Thieme publishers, 3rd edition, Stuttgart], Fig. 2.131, page 245

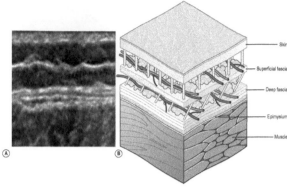

Figure 9.2
Normal tissue and tissue after wound healing with and without immobilization. Reproduced with permission from van den Berg *Angewandte Physiologie Band 1*, Georg Thieme Verlag. 3. Auflage, Stuttgart. [*Applied Physiology Volume 1*, Georg Thieme publishers, 3rd edition, Stuttgart], 2011, Fig. 2.131, page 245

such as prostaglandin-2, are produced in the injured tissue, as noted in the section on wound healing in Chapter 6. This, of course, implies that when the release of inflammatory mediators is inhibited or disturbed in wound healing, the healing of the wound will be delayed. This delay has already been proven in many scientific studies (Bergenstock et al., 2005; Kaftan & Hosemann, 2005; Marsolais et al., 2003; Murnaghan et al., 2006; Muscará et al., 2000; Sikiric et al., 2003; Tortland, 2007; Yugoshi et al., 2002).

The circulation within tissue can also be negatively influenced by the smoking of cigarettes (Battié et al., 1991; Zimmermann-Stenzel et al., 2008; Holm & Nachemson, 1988; Iwahashi et al., 2002; Oda et al., 2004; Pezeshki et al., 2007; Silcox et al., 1995; Hadley & Reddy, 1997); by atherosclerosis (Kurunlahti et al., 1999; Turgut et al., 2008; Tokuda et al., 2006; Kauppila et al., 2009; Dwivedi et al., 2003); and by increased sympathetic reflex activity (van den Berg, 2011).

Concerning increased sympathetic reflex activity, it is clear that pain, fear, anger, worry, and other strong feelings and emotions can trigger this increase (Soloweij, 2009, 2010a, 2010b; Soon & Acton, 2006; Gouin et al., 2008). That is why it is of extreme importance that the patient be informed about the processes that take place during normal wound healing, including the sense and purpose of pain during this process.

Relaxation techniques can be very helpful at this stage of the wound-healing process because they decrease sympathetic reflex activity and increase wound healing (Holden-Lund, 1988).

To prevent or decrease pain and to prevent an increase of sympathetic reflex activity, patients are usually given painkilling medications after trauma or surgery. The main danger of such medication is that it prevents the patient's brain from receiving sensory information about the momentary loading capacity of the healing tissue. As a result, the tissue could get injured over and over again, substantially delaying wound healing (Brower & Johnson, 2003; Dormus et al., 2003; Northcliffe & Buggy, 2003; Bislo & Tanelian, 1992; Scherb et al., 2009). To prevent this from taking place, the body releases the pain mediators.

For the cells to perform their synthesizing activity during the wound-healing process, it is extremely important that the internal environment in which the cells exist allows for optimal cell activity. One of the fundamental factors regulating this optimal activity is the pH level within the tissue. Fibroblasts can only produce matrix components when the interstitial pH level is 6.5 or higher. This means that when the pH level is below 6.5 the cells cannot produce matrix components, thus they cannot make a repair.

When we examine the conditions that can cause the pH level to drop below 6.5, we can see that this is often related to the nutritional habits of people in the industrialized world. Acid-producing compounds are especially common in animal proteins, sugar (including sugar-containing fluids and canned foods), alcohol, coffee, and black tea. Stress and smoking may also have an acidic influence on the pH level. By contrast, nutrients with an alkaline pH can be found in fruits and vegetables. When one examines the average nutritional habits of patients in the industrialized world, it is evident that acidic nutrients are consumed in far greater quantities then alkaline nutrients (van den Berg, 2011; Vormann et al., 2001; Birklein et al., 2000; Woo et al., 2004; Finlayson et al., 1964; Bibby et al., 2005; Bibby & Urban, 2004; Murphy & McPhee, 1965; Kellum et al., 2004).

When edema is present, the transport distance from the vessels to the cells is increased – meaning that the cells have more problems in getting their nutrients (van den Berg, 2011;). Therefore, the application of lymph drainage massage can be very helpful at this stage of wound healing.

As well as causing an increase in sympathetic reflex activity, stress can also cause an increase in the liberation of stress hormones, such as cortisol. Cortisol decreases the synthesizing activity of the cells, because it decreases the liberation of interleukin-6 and, in this way, the production of mRNA (Cole-King & Harding, 2001; Ebrecht et al., 2004; Marucha et al., 1998; Kiecolt-Glaser et al., 1995; Broadbent et al., 2003). Furthermore, cortisol weakens the immune system (Vileikyte, 2007; Weinman et al., 2008). A danger of a weakened immune system is the development of autoimmune diseases, such as rheumatoid arthritis (van den Berg, 2011).

In patients with diabetes mellitus, the inflammatory phase of wound healing is disturbed (or reduced), because fewer growth hormones (e.g., PDGF, FGF, TNFα) are produced. This disturbance leads, in turn, to a reduced production of matrix components (Ritzwoller et al., 2006; Ladhani et al., 2002; Greenhalgh et al., 1990; Seifter et al., 1981; Black et al., 2003; Darby et al., 1997; Peterson-Kim et al., 2001; Hoff et al., 2008; Mäntyselkä et al., 2008a, 2008b; Ekmektzoglou & Zografos, 2006).

Vitamins, minerals, and trace elements are essential for matrix synthesis and stability, because they enable stabilizing biochemical connections within the collagen structure (van den Berg, 2011; Geiersperger, 2009).

In order for inflammation to be minimized in the tissue (in the inflammatory phase), it is important that the body be capable of controlling the liberation of prostaglandin-2. For this reason, the body produces prostaglandin-1 and prostaglandin-3. Prostaglandin-2 is produced out of arachidonic acid (an omega-6 fatty acid), which can be found in meat (especially pork) and meat products. Prostaglandin-1 and prostaglandin-3 are produced from omega-3 fatty acids, which can be found in fish and other seafood, as well as in some cold-pressed oils (van den Berg, 2011).

It is clear that the above-mentioned factors not only negatively influence wound healing, but also the remodeling and regeneration processes.

Loss of mobility

As described in Chapters 5 and 6, fascia permanently produce fluid to allow for friction-free movement against other fascia and also against other anatomical structures (Guimberteau et al., 2010; Guimberteau et al., 2005; Langevin et al., 2009; van den Berg, 2011).

When the circulation within tissue is reduced – as the result of increased sympathetic reflex activity, atherosclerosis, or smoking – fascia cannot produce enough fluid and friction-free movement becomes impossible. One of the effects of manual therapy is that we decrease sympathetic reflex activity, which then leads again to increased mobility (van den Berg, 2011).

When fasciae are not moved sufficiently for long periods of time, morphologic changes in the tissue, such as fibrosis, can develop. This situation can be compared with the late phase in Dupuytren's contracture. The first changes occur in the matrix, especially in the ground substance. The dominant glycosaminoglycan (GAG) to be changed in this process is dermatan sulfate, as shown by Kozma and colleagues (Kozma et al., 2000, 2007). They demonstrated that the amounts of short and long chains increase. In this way, the networking (i.e., cross-linking) within the matrix is increased, and the fibrillogenesis of collagen is also influenced. Moreover, there is increased activity of growth hormones. This leads to a hypertrophy of the connective tissue, comparable to that which sometimes occurs with scars on the skin.

Dupuytren's contracture

Dupuytren's contracture or disease, also called morbus Dupuytren or palmar fasciitis, is a disease of the palmar fascia of the hand that manifests itself as increasing flexion contracture of the fingers (mainly the fourth and fifth fingers). The same disease can be found in the foot (morbus Ledderhose) and in the penis (Peyronie's disease). Changes in the liver (liver cirrhosis) can also be classified in this disease group. Recently, the cause of frozen shoulder has also been connected with these changes (Kumka & Bonar, 2012).

With Dupuytren's contracture, we can recognize two phases – first a contraction phase, and then a contracture phase.

Contraction phase

This phase is caused by increased activity of myofibroblasts. The question that needs to be answered is: why is the activity and contraction of the myofibroblasts increased?

The transformation of fibroblasts into myofibroblasts is prompted by the transforming growth factor beta-1 (TGF-β1). It causes the production of actin chains initially and primarily within – but later also outside – the cells. The latter chains connect the cell membrane with the extracellular matrix, forming the basis for contraction of the tissue (Gabbiani, 2004; Meek et al., 1999; Kozma et al., 2007; Singer et al., 1984; Wipff et al., 2007; Hinz et al., 2007). Furthermore, TGF-β1 protects the myofibroblasts against cell death (apoptosis) (Lee et al., 2010). This explains why myofibroblasts emerge in the palmar fascia, but not why more TGF-β1 is suddenly produced.

For example, TGF-β1 is released during inflammation, just as it is after injuries. That is why we see myofibroblasts in tissue during the first phases of wound healing that cause the so-called wound contraction (Gabbiani, 2004). The myofibroblasts that are produced in other inflammations, such as rheumatoid arthritis, also cause contraction of the tissue. However, in Dupuytren's contracture, there is usually no previous injury.

One explanation for the increased amount of TGF-β1 could be a local ischemia in combination with mechanical stress in the tissue (Wipff et al., 2007). Due to the ischemia and the subsequent contraction of tissue, the pressure on the vessels increases even more – leading to increased ischemia (Lee et al., 2010).

According to many authors, the most important factor in this process is the increased production of free radicals (Bayat et al., 2005; Murrell et al., 1987; Lee et al., 2010; Wipff et al., 2007; Perlemuter et al., 2005; Karabulut et al., 2002). Free radicals, or oxygen radicals (O_2^-), are produced in the mitochondria during energy-generating processes. Normally, these compounds are neutralized by antioxidants within the cells or within the interstitium. In the mitochondria, the enzymes Cu/Zn-SOD and Mn-SOD (SOD = superoxide dismutase) are responsible for this process. The following biochemical transformations take place in the mitochondria, in the cell outside of the mitochondria and outside of the cell (Karabulut et al., 2002):

$2 O_2^- + 2 H^+ \rightarrow H_2O_2 + O_2$ (under the influence of Cu/Zn-SOD or Mn-SOD).

Then, prompted by the enzyme catalase:

$2 H_2O_2 \rightarrow 2 H_2O + O_2$.

(Cu = cupper, Zn = zinc, Mn = manganese, H_2O_2 = hydrogen peroxide)

Through these reactions, the free radicals are neutralized. This is important because free radicals can attack and disturb the DNA of the mitochondria or the cell nucleus. If the DNA of the mitochondria is attacked, the mitochondria are destroyed. The more mitochondria that are destroyed, the less energy can be produced in the cell. This can lead to early cell death. That is why free radicals play such an important role in the aging process. If the DNA of the cell nucleus is attacked, tissue degeneracy, in the form of tumors, can develop.

Inagaki and coworkers (Inagaki et al., 1992) have demonstrated that in patients with Dupuytren's contracture or fibrosing diseases, the SOD concentration in the tissue is decreased, compared with that of healthy persons.

The next question that needs answering is: why is there an increase of free radicals? An explanation for this question could involve local ischemia, as well as other predisposing factors for Dupuytren's contracture, such as diabetes, smoking, alcohol abuse, barbiturate use, trauma, and possibly HIV infection (Lee et al., 2010; Burge et al., 1997). Interestingly, research suggests that alcohol abuse, in combination with heavy smoking, is the cause of many of the problems in Dupuytren's contracture (Lee et al., 2010; Burge et al., 1997).

Epidemiological factors reveal that the largest population group affected by Dupuytren's contracture consists of men older than 50 years. The ratio of males versus females with this condition is 7 to 15 versus 1. Furthermore, people from the northern part of Europe (e.g., Scandinavia, Scotland) are affected disproportionately highly, making up, for example, 40% of the elderly population with the condition (Kozma et al., 2007).

The disease typically begins in the fourth and fifth fingers with changes of the palmar fascia. As the disease progresses, changes of the skin can also take place (Wipff et al., 2007).

During the first stage of Dupuytren's contracture, the goal of therapy is to reduce the amount of free radicals by administering a high dosage of antioxidants (e.g., vitamins C and E, beta-carotene, selenium, zinc). Anti-inflammatory medications, such as corticosteroids, can also be helpful at this stage (Meek et al., 1999, 2002). Alternatively, one could try to decrease the inflammation with the supplementation of omega-3 fatty acids.

Mechanical stretching of the palmar fascia is counterproductive, though it is often recommended by medical doctors and performed by therapists. The reason that this intervention is counterproductive is that the stretching increases the mechanical stress on the tissue and on the cells, thereby worsening the ischemia. This probably leads, in turn, to an enhanced production of free radicals, making the problem increasingly severe.

Contracture phase

We will now examine the changes in the late phase of Dupuytren's contracture. Due to the contraction of the palmar fascia, there is the development of local thickening, in the form of nodules. The nodules are initially soft, but they gradually become firmer (Kozma et al., 2007).

Probably under the influence of free radicals, genetic changes take place within the fibroblasts and myofibroblasts. These changes finally cause morphologic and structural changes within the palmar fascia.

The following changes were found during the late phase of Dupuytren's contracture (Ulrich et al., 2009; Satish et al., 2008; Murrell et al., 1991; Lee et al., 2010; Meek et al., 1999; Kozma et al., 2007; Brickley-Parsons et al., 1981; Hinz et al., 2007; Wipff et al., 2007):

- increased liberation of TGF-β1 (transforming growth factor beta-1)

- increased liberation of BFGF (basic fibroblast growth factor)

- increased liberation of PDGF (platelet-derived growth factor)

- reduced MMP (matrix metalloproteinase) production

- increased TIMP (tissue inhibitor of matrix metalloproteinase) production

- increased fibroblast proliferation

- reduced liberation of collagen type I

- increased liberation of collagen type III

- increased amount of collagen types XIV and XV

- changes of dermatan sulfate

- increased amount of chondroitin sulfate

- changes of fibronectin

- increased amounts of fibronectin, tenascin, and laminin.

These changes suggest that the degradation of the matrix – in this case especially of collagen – is decreased by the reduced amount of MMP. The degradation of collagen is further decreased through inhibition by an increased amount of TIMP. By contrast, the production of collagen is increased. This all leads to a thickening of the palmar fascia. These changes take place under simultaneous contraction of the palmar fascia by myofibroblast activity.

The presence of collagen type XV in combination with the altered fibronectin and dermatan sulfate are apparently the prerequisite for this fibrosing process. These compounds allow for an increased adherence between the inflammatory cells (primarily lymphocytes and macrophages) and the endothelial walls of the vessels (Meek et al., 1999).

Due to the changes in dermatan sulfate, the fibrillogenesis becomes disturbed, and the cells bind less to the matrix and more to certain growth factors (Kozma et al., 2007).

In the nodules, there are numerous inflammatory cells but also much laminin and tenascin (Meek et al., 1999; Satish et al., 2008). The collagen shows a clear increase of soluble cross-links (Brickley-Parsons et al., 1981).

Laukkanen and colleagues report that higher amounts of paracetamol damage the liver, which is probably the result of increased production of free radicals in the liver (Laukkanen et al., 2001). The authors concluded that this was also the reason for the fibrosis of the liver (liver cirrhosis). Liver diseases are often associated with such factors as alcohol, smoking, oxidative stress, and lack of antioxidants.

Therapy in the late phase of Dupuytren's contracture is more challenging than in the early phase because of the many structural changes that have taken place. For this reason, stretching does not yield much of an effect. In this situation, the only effective treatment is probably surgery, though injections with collagenases in the palmar fascia may also be useful.

Besides treating the palmar fascia, it is also important to optimize the mobility of the finger joints (metacarpophalangeal, distal interphalangeal, and proximal interphalangeal). Large extension restrictions tend to arise in these joints. A major problem in patients with Dupuytren's contracture is that surgery is mostly performed at a very late stage. At that stage, the finger joints typically have large structural changes and thus mobilization of the joints does not produce any effect. This means that, even after surgery, the patient may still be unable to move the fingers or use the hand normally. Yet it is important that surgery is not performed too early, because the inflammation caused by the operation will stimulate the myofibroblasts even more.

Diseases such as Dupuytren's contracture are often associated with changes in the liver. It is important to understand the connections between changes in the liver and Dupuytren's contracture to determine the appropriate therapy.

Changes in the liver are often connected to alcohol abuse. It has been shown that alcohol abuse clearly leads to an increase of free radicals in the liver, as well as in the stomach, heart, nervous system, and very likely in the entire body (Manzo-Avalos & Saavedra-Molina, 2010). Alcohol abuse also causes reductions in the production of Cu/Zn-SOD and of mitochondrial Mn-SOD in the liver. This leads to damage to mitochondrial DNA and, eventually, to the destruction of the mitochondria. The end result is apoptosis of the liver cells and an alteration of the liver into nonfunctioning fatty tissue (Manzo-Avalos & Saavedra-Molina, 2010; Deshpande et al., 2013; Thome et al., 1997).

Due to these changes in the liver, there is also a reduced concentration of Cu/Zn-SOD in the erythrocytes and in the blood serum (Karabulut et al., 2002; Thome et al., 1997; Deshpande et al., 2013). The reduction of Cu/Zn-SOD in the circulating blood could be the most important connection between alcohol, liver disease, and Dupuytren's contracture. Shanmugan and colleagues (Shanmugam et al., 2011) have shown that the above-mentioned changes are far more severe in patients with diabetes.

References

Battié M. C., Videman T., Gill K. et al. Volvo Award in clinical sciences: smoking and lumbar intervertebral disc degeneration: an MRI study of identical twins. *Spine*. 1991;16:1015–1021.

Bayat A.,Walter J., Lambe H. et al. Identification of a novel mitochondrial mutation in Dupuytren's disease using multiplex DHPLC. *Plastic & Reconstructive Surgery*. 2005;115:134–141

Bergenstock M., Min W., Simon A. M., Sabatino C., O'Connor J. P. A comparison between the effects of acetaminophen and celecoxib on bone fracture in rats. *Journal of Orthopaedic Trauma*. 2005;Nov–Dec;19(19);717–723.

Bibby S. R., Jones D. A., Ripley R. M., Urban J. P. Metabolism of the intervertebral disc: effect of low levels of oxygen, glucose, and pH on rates of energy metabolism of bovine nucleus pulposus cells. *Spine*. 2005 Mar 1;30 (5):487–496.

Bibby S. R., Urban J. P. Effect of nutrient deprivation on the viability of intervertebral disc cells. *European Spine Journal*. 2004 Dec;13(8):695–701.

Birklein F., Weber M., Ernst M., Riedl B., Neundörfer B., Handwerker H. O. Experimental tissue acidosis leads to increased pain in complex regional pain syndrome (CRPS). *Pain*. 2000;87(2):227–234.

Bislo K., Tanelian D. L. Concentration-dependant effects of lidocaine on corneal epithelian wound healing. *Investigative Ophthalmology & Visual Science*. October 1992;33(11):3029–3033.

Black E., Vibe-Petersen J., Jörgensen L. N., Madsen S.M., Ägren M.S., Holstein P.E., Perrild H., Gottrup F. Decrease of collagen deposition in wound repair in type 1 diabetes independent of glycemic control. *Archives of Surgery*. 2003;138:34–40.

Brickley-Parsons D., Glimcher M. J., Smith R. J. et al. Biochemical changes in the collagen of the palmar fascia in patients with Dupuytren's disease. *Journal of Bone and Joint Surgery (Am)*. 1981;63:787–797.

Broadbent E., Petric K. J., Alley P. G., Booth R. Psychological stress impairs wound repair following surgery. *Psychosomatic Medicine*. 2003;65:865–869.

Brower M., Johnson M. Adverse effects of local anesthetic infiltration on wound healing. *Regional Anesthesia and Pain Medicine*. May/June 2003;28(3):233–240.

Burge P., Hoy G., Regan P. et al. Smoking, alcohol and the risk of Dupuytren's contracture. *Journal of Bone and Joint Surgery (Br)*. 1997;79–B:206–210.

Cole-King A., Harding K. G. Psychological factors and delayed healing in chronic wounds. *Psychosomatic Medicine*. 2001;63:216–220.

Currier D., Nelson R. *Dynamics of Human Biologic Tissues. 1st ed.* Philadelphia: F. A. Davis Company. 1992.

Darby I. A., Bisucci T., Hewitson T. D., MacLellan D. G. Apoptosis is increased in a model of diabetes-impaired wound healing in genetically diabetic mice. *International Journal of Biochemistry & Cell Biology*. 1997;29(1):191–200.

Deshpande N., Kandi S., Kumar P. V. B, Raman K. V, Muddeshwar M. Effect of alcohol consumption on oxidative stress markers and its role in the pathogenesis and progression of liver cirrhosis. *American Journal of Medical and Biological Research*. 2013;1(4):99–102.

Dormus M., Karaaslan E., Ozturk E., Gulec M., Iraz M., Edali N., Ozcan Ersoy M. The effects of single-dose dexamethasone on wound healing in rats. *Anesthesia & Analgesia*. 2003;97:1377–1380.

Dwivedi S., Kotwal P. P., Dwivedi G. Aortic atherosclerosis, hypertension, and spondylotic degenerative disease: a life-style phenomenon, coincidence, or continuum? *Journal, Indian Academy of Clinical Medicine*. 2003;4(2):134–138.

Ebrecht M., Hextall J., Kirtley L. G. et al. Perceived stress and cortisol levels predict speed of wound healing in healthy male adults. *Psychoneuroendocrinology*. 2004;29:798–809.

Ekmektzoglou K. A., Zografos G. C. A concomitant review of the effects of diabetes mellitus and hypothyroidism in wound healing. *World Journal of Gastroenterology*. 2006;12(17):2721–2729.

Finlayson G. R., Smith G. Jr., Moore M. J. Effects of chronic acidosis on connective tissue. *JAMA*. 1964;187:659–662.

Gabbiani G. The Evolution of the myofibroblast concept: a key cell for wound healing and fibrotic diseases. *Giornale di Gerontologia*. 2004;52:280–282.

Geiersperger K. Wundheilung und Ernährung. Master Thesis für der Universitätslehrgang für Sports

Physiotherapy. Paris Lodron Universität Salzburg – Abteilung Sportwissenschaften. 2009.

Gouin J. P., Kiecolt-Glaser J. K., Malarkey W. B., Glaser R. Influence of anger on wound healing. *Brain, Behavior & Immunity*. 2008;22(5):699–708.

Greenhalgh D. G., Sprugel K. H., Murray M. J., Ross R. PDGF and FGF stimulate wound healing in the genetically diabetic mouse. *American Journal of Pathology*. 1990;136(6):1235–1246.

Guimberteau J., Delage J., McGrouther D., Wong J. The microvascular system: how connective tissue sliding works. *Journal of Hand Surgery (Eur)*. 2010;35(8):614–622.

Guimberteau J., Sentucq-Rigall J., Panconi B. Introduction to the knowledge of subcutaneous sliding system in humans. *Annales de Chirurgie Plastique Esthétique*. 2005;50(1):19–34.

Hadley M. N., Reddy S. V. Smoking and the human vertebral column: a review of the impact of cigarette use on vertebral bone metabolism and spinal fusion. *Neurosurgery*. 1997;41(1):116–124.

Hinz B., Phan S. H., Thannickal V. J. et al. The myofibroblast: one function, multiple origins. *American Journal of Pathology*. 2007;170:1807–1816.

Hoff O. M., Midthjell K., Zwart J. A., Hagen K. The association between diabetes mellitus, glucose, and chronic musculoskeletal complaints. Results from the Nord-Trondelag Health Study. *Musculoskeletal Disorders*. 2008;2(9):160–167.

Holden-Lund C. Effects of relaxation with guided imagery on surgical stress and wound healing. *Researching in Nursing & Health*. 1988;11(4):235–244.

Holm S., Nachemson A. Nutrition of the intervertebral disc: acute effects of cigarette smoking. an experimental animal study. *Upsala Journal of Medical Science*. 1988;93(1):91–99.

Inagaki T., Katoh K., Takiya S. et al. Relationship between superoxide dismutase (SOD) and viral liver diseases. *Journal of Gastroenterology*. 1992;27:382–389.

Iwahashi M., Matsuzaki H., Tokuhashi Y., Wakabayashi K., Uematsu Y. Mechanism of intervertebral disc degeneration caused by nicotine in rabbits to explicate intervertebral disc disorders caused by smoking. *Spine*. 2002 Jul 1;27(13):1396–1401.

Kaftan H., Hosemann W. Systemic cortocoid application in combination with topical mitomycin or dexamenthasone. Inhibition of wound healing after tympanic membrane perforation. *HNO*. 2005;Sep;53(9);779–783.

Kauppila L. I. Atherosclerosis and disc degeneration/low-back pain – a systemic review. *European*

Journal of Vascular and Endovascular Surgery. 2009 June;37(6):661–670.

Karabulut A. B., Sömmez E., Bayindir Y. et al. A comparison of erythrocyte superoxide dismutase and catalase activity in patients with hepatitis C infection. *Turkish Journal of Medical Sciences*. 2002;32:313–316.

Kellum J. A., Song M., Li J. Science review: extracellular acidosis and the immune response: clinical and physiological implications. *Critical Care*. 2004;8:331–336.

Kiecolt-Glaser J. K., Marucha P. T., Malarkey W. B. et al. Slowing of wound healing by psychological stress. *The Lancet*. 1995;364:1194–1196.

Kozma E. M., Glowacki A., Olcyk K. et al. Dermatan sulfate remodeling associated with advanced Dupuytren's contracture. *Acta Biochemica Polonica*. 2007;54:821–830.

Kozma E. M., Glowacki A., Olcyk K., Glowacki A., Bobinski R. An accumulation of proteoglycans in scarred fascia. *Molecular and Cellular Biochemistry*. 2000;203:103–112.

Kumka M., Bonar J. Fascia: a morphological description and classification system based on a literature review. *Journal of the Canadian Chiropractic Association*. 2012;56(3):179–191.

Kurunlahti M., Tervonen Q., Vanharanta H., Ilkko E., Suramo I. Association of atherosclerosis with low back pain and the degree of disc degeneration. *Spine*. 1999 Oct;24 (20):2080–2084.

Ladhani S., Phillips S. D., Allgrove J. Low back pain at presentation in a newly diagnosed diabetic. *Archives of Disease in Childhood*. 2002;87:543–545.

Langevin H., Stevens-Tuttle D., Fox J. et al. Ultrasound evidence of altered lumbar connective tissue structure in human subjects with chronic low back pain. *BMC Musculoskeletal Disorders*. 2009;10(1):151–161.

Laukkanen M. O., Leppanen P., Turunen P. et al. EC-SOD gene therapy reduces paracetamol-induced liver damage in mice. *Journal of Gene Medicine*. 2001;3:321–325.

Lee S., Baytion M., Reinke D. L. et al. Surgery for Dupuytren contracture. 2015. http://emedicine.medscape.com/article/1238712-overview [accessed February 12, 2016].

Mäntyselkä P., Miettola J., Niskanen L., Kumpusalo E. Glucose regulation and chronic pain at multiple sites. *Rheumatology*. 2008a;47(8):1235–1238.

Mäntyselkä P., Miettola J., Niskanen L., Kumpusalo E. Chronic pain, impaired glucose tolerance and diabetes: a community-based study. *Pain*. 2008b;137(1):34–40.

Manzo-Avalos S., Saavedra-Molina A. Cellular and mitochondrial effects of alcohol consumption. *International Journal of Environmental Research and Public Health*. 2010;7:4281–4304.

Marsolais D., Cote C. H., Frenette J. Nonsteroidal anti-inflammatory drug reduces neutrophil and macrophage accumulation but does not improve tendon regeneration. *Laboratory Investigation*. 2003;83;991–999.

Marucha P. T., Kiecolt-Glaser J. K., Favagehi M. Mucosal wound healing is impaired by examination stress. *Psychosomatic Medicine*. 1998;60(3):362–365.

Meek R. M. D., McLellan S., Crossan J. F. Dupuytren's disease: a model for the mechanism of fibrosis and its modulation by steroids. *Journal of Bone and Joint Surgery (Br)*. 1999;81-B:732–738.

Meek R. M., McLellan S., Reilly J. et al. The effect of steroids on Dupuytren's disease: role of programmed cell death. *Journal of Bone and Joint Surgery (Br)*. 2002;27:270–273.

Murnaghan M., Li G., Marsh D. R. Nonsteroidal anti-inflammatory drug-induced fracture onunion: an inhibition of angiogenesis? *Journal of Bone and Joint Surgery (Am)*. 2006;88;140–147.

Murphy K. J., McPhee I., Tears of major tendons in chronic acidosis with elastosis. *Journal of Bone and Joint Surgery (Am)*. 1965;47-A(6):1253–1258.

Murrell G. A., Francis M. J., Bromley L. Free radicals and Dupuytren's contracture. *British Medical Journal (Clinical Research Ed.)*. 1987;295:1373–1375.

Murrell G. A., Francis M. J., Bromley L. The collagen changes of Dupuytren's contracture. *Journal of Hand Surgery (Br)*. 1991;16:263–266.

Muscará M. N., McKnight W, Asfaha S., Wallace J. L. Wound collagen deposition in rats: effect of an NO-NSAID and a selective COX-2 inhibitor. *British Journal of Pharmacology*. 2000;129;681–686.

Northcliffe S.-A., Buggy D. J. Implications of anesthesia for infection and wound healing. *International Anesthesiology Clinics*. Winter 2003;41(1):31–64.

Oda H., Matsuzaki H., Tokuhashi Y., Wakabayashi K., Uematsu Y., Iwahashi M. Degeneration of intervertebral discs due to smoking: experimental assessment in a rat-smoking model. *Journal of Orthopaedic Science*. 2004;9(2):135–141.

Perlemuter G., Davit-Spraul A., Cosson C. et al. Increase in liver antioxidantenzyme activity in non-alcoholic fatty liver disease. *Liver International*. 2005;25:946–953.

Peterson-Kim R., Edelman S. V., Kim D. D. Musculoskeletal complications of diabetes mellitus. *Clinical Diabetes*. 2001;19(3):132–135.

Pezeshki M. Z, Pezeshki S. Smoking and lumbar disc degeneration: a case-control study among Iranian men referring to lumbar MRI. *Research Journal of Biological Sciences*. 2007;2(7):787–789.

Ritzwoller D. P., Crounse L., Shetterly S., Rublee D. The association of comorbidities, utilization and costs for patients identified with low back pain. *Musculoskeletal Disorders*. 2006;7(72). http://bmcmusculoskeletdisord.biomedcentral.com/articles/10.1186/1471-2474-7-72 [accessed February 12, 2016].

Satish L., LaFramboise W. A., O'Gorman D. B. et al. Identification of differentially expressed genes in fibroblasts derived from patients with Dupuytren's contracture. *BMC Medical Genomics*. 2008;1(10). www.biomedcentral.com/1755-8794/1/10 [accessed February 12, 2016].

Scherb M. B., Courneya J.-P., Guyton G. P., Schon L. C. Effect of bupivacaine on cultured tenocytes. *Orthopedics*. 2009;32:26.

Seifter E., Rettura G., Padawer J., Stratford F., Kambosos D., Levenson S. M. Impaired wound healing in streptozotocin diabetes: prevention by supplemental vitamin A. *Annals of Surgery*. 1981;194(1):42–50.

Shanmugam K. R, Mallikarjuna K., Reddy K. S. Effect of alcohol on blood glucose and antioxidant enzymes in the liver and kidney of diabetic rats. *Indian Journal of Pharmacology*. 2011;43(3):330–335.

Sikiric P., Seiwerth S., Mise S., Staresinic M., Bedekovic V., Zarkovic N., Borovic S., Giurasin M., Boban-Blagiaic A., Batelia L., Rucman R., Anic T. Corticosteroid-impairment of healing and gastric pentadecapeptide BPC-157 creams in burned mice. *Burns*. 2003;Jun;29(4);323–334.

Silcox D. H., Daftari T., Boden S. D., Schimandle J. H., Hutton W. C., Whiteside T. E. The effect of nicotine on spinal fusion. *Spine*. 1995;20(14):1549–1553.

Singer I. I., Kawka D. W., Kazakis D. M. et al. In vivo co-distribution of fibronectin and actin fibers in granulation tissue: immunofluorescence and electron microscope study of the fibronexus at the myofibroblast surface. *Journal of Cell Biology*. 1984;98:2091–2106.

Solowiej K., Mason V., Upton D. Review of the relationship between psychological stress and wound healing, part 1. *Journal of Wound Care*. 2009;18(9):357–366.

Solowiej K., Mason V., Upton D. Psychological stress and pain in wound care, part 2: a review of pain and stress assessment tools. *Journal of Wound Care*. 2010a;19(3)110–5.

Solowiej K., Mason V., Upton D. Psychological stress and pain in wound care, part 3: management. *Journal of Wound Care*. 2010b;19(4) 153–155.

Soon K., Acton C. Pain-induced stress: a barrier to wound healing. *Wounds UK*. 2006;2(4):92–101.

Tabary J., Tabary C., Tadieu C. Physiological and structural changes in the cat's soleus muscle due to immobilization at different lengths by plaster casts. *Journal of Physiology*. 1972;149:231–244.

Thome J., Foley P., Gsell W., Davids E., Wodarz N., Wiesbeck G. A, Böning J., Riederer P. Increased concentration of manganese superoxide dismutase in serum of alcohol-dependent patients. *Alcohol & Alcoholism*. 1997;32(1):65–69.

Tokuda O., Okada M., Fujita T., Matsunaga N. Correlation between diffusion in lumbar intervertebral discs and lumbar artery status: evaluation with fresh blood imaging technique. *Journal of Magnetic Resonance Imaging*. 2006 Dec;25(1):185–191.

Tortland P. D. Sports injuries and nonsteroidal anti-inflammatory drug (NSAID) use. *Connecticut Sportsmed*. 2007;Winter;1–4

Turgut A., Sönmez I., Çakit B., Kosar P., Kosar U. Pineal gland calcification, lumbar intervertebral disc degeneration and abdominal aorta calcifying atherosclerosis correlate in low back pain subjects: a cross-sectional observational CT study. *Pathophysiology*. 2008 June;15(1):31–39.

Ulrich D., Ulrich F., Piatkowski A. et al. Expression of matrix metalloproteinases and their inhibitors in cords and nodules of patients with Dupuytren's disease. *Archives of Orthopaedic and Trauma Surgery*. 2009;129:1453–1459.

van den Berg F. *Angewandte Physiologie. Band 1: Das Bindegewebe des Bewegungsapparates verstehen und beeinflussen*. 3. Auflage. Stuttgart: Georg Thieme Verlag [*Applied Physiology Volume 1. 3rd edition. Stuttgart: Georg Thieme Publishers*]. 2011.

Vileikyte L. Stress and wound healing. *Clinics in Dermatology*. 2007;25(1):49–55.

Vormann J., Worlitschek M., Goedecke T., Silver B. Supplementation with alkaline minerals reduces symptoms in patients with chronic low back pain. *Journal of Trace Elements in Medicine and Biology*. 2001;15:179–183.

Weinman J., Ebrecht M., Scott S. et al. Enhanced wound healing after emotional disclosure intervention. *British Journal of Health Psychology*. 2008;13:95–102.

Wipff P. J., Rifkin D. B., Meister J. J. et al. Myofibroblast contraction activates latent TGF-beta1 from the extracellular matrix. *Journal of Cell Biology*. 2007;179:1311–1323.

Woo Y. C., Park S. S., Subieta A. R., Brennan T. J. Changes in tissue pH and temperature after incision indicate acidosis may contribute to postoperative pain. *Anesthesiology*. 2004;101:468–475.

Yugoshi L. I., Sala M. A., Brentegani L. G., Lamano Carvalho T. L. Histometric study of socket healing after tooth extraction in rats treated with diclofenac. *Brazilian Dental Journal*. 2002;13(21);92–96.

Zimmermann-Stenzel M., Mannuß J., Schneider S., Schiltenwolt M. Tabakkonsum und chronische Rückenschmerzen. *Deutsche Ärzteblatt*. 2008;105(24):441–448.

THE FASCIA AS THE ORGAN OF INNERNESS: A HOLISTIC APPROACH BASED UPON A PHENOMENOLOGICAL EMBRYOLOGY AND MORPHOLOGY*

Jaap C. van der Wal

Introduction: what about fascia?

In the article 'What is "fascia"? A review of different nomenclatures', Robert Schleip et al. make proposals to review the current terminology around fascia.[1] This issue also was a central item of the Second International Fascia Research Congress in 2009.[2,3] The necessity to review, for example, the nomenclature of fascial and connective tissue structures in the body, was argued based upon the widespread diversity and inconsistency of such terms and nomenclature. In fact, the anatomy of the human body is implicitly based upon the principle that names are given to discrete (meaning 'discernible' and 'dissectible') topographical structures and units in the body. Connective tissue structures, for example, are only recognized as anatomical structures if one is able to discriminate (again: dissect) them from other structures. It is for that reason that the British edition of *Gray's Anatomy* (this highly respected textbook of anatomy) defines fascia as 'masses of connective tissue large enough to be visible to the unaided eye'.[4] According to those authors, this apparently also indicates that no functional criterion is linked with the term 'fascia'. In principle, fascia was (is) considered to be a layer of connective tissue covering, enveloping, and separating discrete anatomical structures like muscles and bones. And that is how fascial layers are mostly still described today. If one, for example, describes and discriminates a fascia cruris, the definition is apparently topographical anatomical, saying this fascia is enveloping the (various anatomical elements of the) foreleg. The fascia colli (cervicalis media) is organized as a sheath around the so-called infrahyoid muscles. So in anatomical nomenclature names are given to fascial layers and structures based upon *where* they are situated and organized. The term or name does not say anything about *how* they are functionally and mechanically related to the underlying or neighboring tissue and structures.

If, however, one dissects the fascia cruris (or the analogous fascia antebrachii), one may observe and conclude that distally this fascia is loosely connected with (or should we say: 'dis-connectible' from) the underlying muscles. It therefore can be dissected easily as a separate layer or structure. In the proximal domain of the forelimbs, however, it is literally impossible to disconnect ('dis-sect') this fascia from underlying muscles. Here one has to separate with a sharp dissection procedure the underlying and inserting (!) muscle fibers from the fascia. Here it is apparent that the fascia is not a coverage layer but functions as a strong force transmission layer, like an aponeurosis. Aponeuroses, however, are well known and officially discernible anatomical structures, considered to be associated with given anatomical units like muscles, therefore recognized as auxiliary components of the related muscles. In *Gray's Anatomy* a kind of functional criterion is applied to discriminate between fascia and aponeuroses, in that 'in contrast to aponeuroses, fasciae are described as connective tissue structures with an "interwoven" arrangement of fibers'. One simple look at the architecture of the fibers of fascia

---

* 'It will emerge from this chapter that, in fact, 'organ of innerness' is a contradiction in terms. In this chapter it will be argued that our 'inner' or 'innerness' is actually *not* represented by or located 'in' a particular organ or region in the body, and definitely not in the brain, for example.

cruris, fascia lata, fascia antebrachii, and more makes it evident that for those parts of these fasciae that are organized within the context of force transmission, this criterion of fiber arrangement is not valid at all.[5]

It is apparent that this architecture should be considered as something other than anatomy and topography. In the context of the Second International Fascia Research Congress in 2009 the research community developed new criteria and formulated the definition of fascia as 'fibrous collagenous tissues which are part of a body wide tensional force transmission system'. This 'new' view on fascia is inspired by recent descriptions of the fascial net in terms of *tensegrity* structures.[6,7] Such a definition, however, tends to deviate in the opposite direction since it raises the question: how should we next consider and classify enveloping coverings like the cervical fascia? Or the visceral fasciae, as the mesothelial membranes covering viscera and inside body walls (like the peritoneum and pleura) are often called in the domain of osteopathy? Are those structures now no longer considered to be fascia or fasciae? Can we push such comments aside as being a purely semantic issue or are they related to a fundamental notion or even misunderstanding about the quality of the term 'fascia'? In particular, in the domain of osteopathy, the concept of fascia is on the one hand widespread and essential but on the other hand poorly defined, at least according to criteria of anatomy and topography ('where') as well as according to functional criteria ('how'). Moreover, in osteopathy the concept of fascia is more or less mystified, as in the often-cited quote of A. T. Still: 'The soul of man with all the streams of our living water, seems to dwell in the fascia of the body.'[8] What kind of organ is that which, on the one hand, is considered to be the bodily substrate of osteopathic treatment and manipulation, but, on the other hand, represents the functional substrate of a tensegrity system and – last but not least – is considered to be a kind of non- or trans-anatomical organ or system that is also considered to be a 'dwelling' for the soul? What kind of morphology and anatomy do we need to understand the functional architecture of such a multifunctional tissue or organ?

In this chapter the author will elaborate his strong conviction that only a phenomenological embryology and a holistic, morphological approach to the architecture of connective tissue will elucidate the aforementioned multifunctionality of the fascia. It may emerge that a thorough rephrasing of the substrate of fascia has to occur. First we will look at the functional embryology of connective tissue and fascia: where is the fascial tissue derived from, and in what terms and functional modalities should the morphology of it be understood? (See section A.) Then we will focus our attention on the inherent impossibility of describing the functional spatial relationship of fascia and its components in proper anatomical terminology. This chapter will present research that demonstrates that the proper way to describe the fascia is according to notions and terms of architecture and that this architecture is instrumental in the function of the fascia as organ of force transmission, movement, and sensing (section B). Next, again based upon a phenomenological embryological view, the model will be introduced that fascia as an organ may be best understood if the architecture of connective and muscular tissue is considered to be one integrated dimension of the human body in a broad sense (a so-called 'mesodermal' germ layer) and of the postural and locomotor[†] system in a narrow sense (tensegrity system) (section C). Last but not least, and interwoven into the considerations above, the phenomenological view will be presented that the meso(derm) represents the dimension of 'innerness' in the body, with the blood and the fascia as the main representatives of what could be considered as our 'innerness' or 'soul' (section D).

A. The embryonic origin and dynamic morphology of the fascia: a phenomenological approach

First we will examine the functional embryology of connective tissue and fascia: where is the fascial tissue derived from, and in what terms and functional modalities should its morphology be understood?

[†]Here the term 'postural and locomotor system' (apparatus) is preferred over 'locomotor system' because the activity of motion by means of our voluntary (skeletal) muscles is concerned with much more than locomotion. Indeed, a great deal of our so-called voluntary moving involves maintaining equilibrium and posture. The term 'system' is preferred over 'apparatus'. Whereas the term 'apparatus' represents the anatomical substrate of bones, joints, ligaments, and muscles, the term 'system' is applied to the functioning apparatus with elements of the (central) nervous system included.

To understand where fascia comes from, our attention should surely be addressed to the embryo. The first problem, however, is: how do we interpret the processes that lead to the formation of a body, an organism? In the view of the phenomenologist it is nonsense that we, as a whole, are built from or formed by elements and parts like cells and organs. From the first day of development we are an organism, a whole, and the parts, the tissues, and the organs result and originate from that whole (not the reverse). We originate from a germ, not from parts, elements, organs, or tissues.

So, differentiation is the leading principle of the developing embryo. Since genes are in this respect not active principles, the essential question about developing tissues and organs is: *where* do they come up? What are the metabolic and morphogenetic qualities of the domains and areas where cells, tissues, and organs are differentiated? The principle of the morphogenetic fields is developed from the domain of developmental biology. In this principle environmental conditions (metabolism, forces exerted on cells and tissues) are much more important for the process of differentiation then topographical or anatomical criteria.

The German embryologist Erich Blechschmidt (1914–1992) recognized this fully when he commented on the widely accepted notion that the primary differentiation of the human body is into two or three germ layers. He showed that differentiations are not only the result of a gene effect, but also are brought about through growth initiated by 'extragenetic' (occurring outside the gene) information. Without this 'extragenetic' (nowadays mostly called 'epigenetic') information, differentiation would not begin. First he recognized that the main criteria to define certain morphogenetic fields in the embryo were related to metabolic processes that, in their turn, are related to the forces that are exerted within or upon the cell populations and tissues. Many of the morphogenetic fields or units that he discriminated were based upon kinetic or biodynamic ('mechanical') principles like *densation*, *dilation*, and *retention*. Blechschmidt was also the first (and, as far as I know, the only) publishing embryologist who proposed to quit considering the three germ layers as three basically similar principles. Instead he discriminates between two *limiting tissues* on the one hand (ectoderm and endoderm) and *inner tissue* on the other hand, each having a different significance for growth and development.[9] So the three-layered germinal disc in the third week of human development is not actually three-layered but consists of a zone of inner tissue situated and functioning between two different layers of limiting tissue. The characteristic feature of inner tissue is that it is *in between* two limiting tissues. Inner tissue can therefore be identified as connective tissue and can best be described as undifferentiated connective tissue (mesenchyme). The formation of the mesoderm of the endocyst disc between the two gliding layers of ectoderm and endoderm is a repetition of an earlier event seen in the whole conceptus, where *mesoblast* was formed when *ectoblast* glided away from the more slowly growing endoblast.[7]

The essential difference between a limiting tissue and inner tissue is the existence of intercellular matrix and space. Limiting tissues, in principle, are epithelia. Between the adjacent and neighboring cells there exists no (or a virtual) intercellular space. Organs that are derived from such epithelial primordia therefore, in principle, do not have intercellular space between the constituting cells. The best example of this is the nervous tissue where the glia cells nowadays are considered to be a kind of cellular connective tissue with embedding quality for the actual nervous cells (glymphatic system).[10] The three (four) principal components of an inner tissue derivative, however, are cells (1); intercellular space filled with an intercellular substance like ground substance (2a, glycosaminoglycanes [GAGs] in proteoglycanes) and interstitial fluid (2b); and the fibers (3), consolidations of intercellular substances such as protocollagen. The cells of mesenchyme lack polarity (like epithelia) and can migrate easily in contrast to epithelial cells.

Phenomenologically therefore it is proposed here to cease using the term 'meso*derm*' and reserve the notion 'derm' for those tissues and organs that really have limiting quality and then to consider mesenchyme (mesoblast as well as 'mesoderm') as manifestations of the quality of '*meso*'. Incorporated with this notion are the characteristics of 'being in-between' and '(inter)mediation'. The latter quality may be mechanically and metabolically recognized in the quality of meso as the germ layer of 'shaping space as well as connecting'. Having said this, this may lead to a deeper understanding of the organization of our body. We are not constituted by and we are not the sum of parts and organs, and we are also not made up of the sum of three germ layers and their derivatives. Germ layers also represent functions – not only somatic functions but also, since our whole body is a psychosomatic substrate, psychological (or psychosomatic) dimensions.

What do such considerations mean for the functionality of the meso-domain? The three-layered germ disc in fact already represents the psychosomatic functional organization of our body, which is: two body walls, two limits and boundaries to the world, and our environment in between the meso-dimension as the dimension of 'interior' or 'innerness'. The notion 'inside' is deliberately avoided here because it is the endodermal (later visceral) dimension that is most often considered by anatomists to represent our 'inside dimension'. In the concept presented here, the anatomical 'inside' is not the same as 'innerness'. Most anatomists are convinced that the act of anatomical dissection essentially starts with the opening of the body and that by the dissection procedure the inside of the body is brought to light. Nowadays many surgical procedures are called and considered to be 'endoscopic' ('looking inside'), again suggesting that behind the outer body wall, mainly represented by the (ectodermal) skin, there is the 'innerness'. In the phenomenological concept of the body as presented here there are, however, two body walls, two 'outsides' with an 'in-between', so to speak. The first one (ectoderm) is dominated by the functional dimension of consciousness, perception, and communication with the environment and it acts as a border from or, on the psychosomatic level, separates us from that environment in terms of space and matter. The other one (endo-derm) is represented by the metabolic, interacting dimension of digesting, excretion, gas exchange and other substance exchange with the environment. The gesture here is 'bordering from' or, on the psychosomatic level, connecting us with that material environment. In this concept the dimension of meso, the in-between, is to be conceptualized as the 'real' innerness of our body. Anatomists go from outside (parietal body wall outside) to inside (visceral body wall inside) and pass, so to speak, the innerness. Our innerness, as we experience it, is not visible to anyone else; it is

an intimate experience that cannot by any means be made visible to or seen by an external observer. In our proprioceptive experience we perceive our body and its innerness as the 'obscure' and nonvisible 'inside'. It is always 'dangerous' and 'disturbing' when something of that inner comes to conscious perception by ourselves or an observer.

In such typical phenomenological considerations the meso is the best representative substrate of what we could describe as our proprioceptive innerness. In this context the notion that meso with its three constituents (cells, matrix, fibers) represents the in-between, easily comes together with the functional notion of meso as the dimension of three-dimensionality. While the two visceral and parietal body walls represent the two-dimensionality of the limiting tissue dimension, the three-dimensionality of 'meso' exhibits two functional characteristics: connecting and shaping space, centripetality and centrifugality respectively. These two characteristics are polarities and as polarities they are a unity,[11,12] a oneness, in the same way that inspiration and expiration, systole and diastole are one and always together. So meso has to be understood as the in-between, breathing in the two functional acts of separating and connecting.

This may throw new light on the notion 'connective tissue'. In psychology it is well-known that binding/attaching is one and is unthinkable without the dimension of detaching/releasing. In a similar way we have to realize that the primary function of mesenchyme and connective tissue is connecting *and* separating (not connection alone). In all mechanical notions related to meso(dermal) tissue one can perceive the same pattern. Likewise, therefore, muscles are not contractile organs letting skeletal elements, for example, approach each other; they must also be capable of relaxing and giving in and letting skeletal elements move away from each other. There exist two forces that play a role within the connective tissues and the skeletal system: traction and compression. Histologically, one can also discriminate in the meso the tendencies of compaction and loosening, resulting in massive organs and tissues on the one hand and body cavities, for example, on the other hand. This duality may be discriminated on all levels. Cartilage, for example, may connect by massification and compaction of the matrix (symphysis), but also it can actively create fissures as it does in articular joints. Also, the important body cavities, such as the peritoneal cavity, may be considered joint cavities where the meso actively creates gliding spaces for mobility. Connective tissue in the musculoskeletal system can connect two adjacent zones of muscular tissue, appearing as the functional dimension of intermuscular septa or aponeuroses meant to convey traction forces. However, loose areolar connective tissue layers may exist between two adjacent muscles, serving as gliding spaces like bursae or tendon sheaths in order to enable mobility.

To summarize, it may be noted that meso-tissue in the embryo always comes up in areas (fields) where a functional in-between-dimension is needed. In the third week of human development it is the *epiblast*-epithelium (in older embryology books called the ectoderm or ectoblast) that differentiates into meso as soon as it becomes interspersed between already present limiting tissue layers or becomes situated underneath a limiting layer. If, for example, neural crest cells (cells already differentiated towards neurogenic cells) reach the domain of the head, such cells will also ('have to') differentiate into a mesenchyme: the *head-mesenchyme*. Facial structures, skull elements, and other structures are derived from this as well as some types of glial cells. This derivative is often described as neuromesenchymal, which is nonsensical terminology in the context of the morphogenetic field concept.

B. Architecture of the fascia: not only 'where?' but also 'how?'

Next we will turn our attention to the inherent impossibility of describing the functional spatial relationship of fascia and its components in proper anatomical terminology. The following section presents research demonstrating that the proper way to describe the fascia is according to the notions and terms of the architecture, and that this architecture is instrumental in the function of the fascia as an organ of force transmission, movement, and sensing (proprioception).

Architecture instead of anatomy

In the traditional view of anatomy, muscles and ligaments are working *in parallel* (Fig. 10.1). In this model, ligaments are tough, passive, collagenous structures that run over a joint from one bone to the other. When the joint is bent toward the ligament, that ligament lies passively lax near the joint capsule. The muscles – farther out from the joint and dynamically controlled by the nervous system – stabilize the joint through its full range of motion. Only when the joint is at its full extent do the ligaments come into play, tightening suddenly to prevent further extension or damage at the end range of movement.

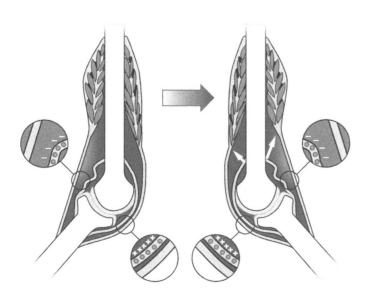

Figure 10.1
The traditional view of ligaments sees them arranged parallel to muscles, only coming into play when they are fully stretched at the end of the joint range

A simple example is the elbow: We expect the biceps and brachialis to control the stability of the joint through a preacher curl. Only when we let the weights back down to full extension would the ligaments be tightened to prevent further extension of the joint. As they tighten, the nerve endings in the ligaments communicate (sometimes quite loudly) to the spinal cord, which turns the muscles off or on to prevent damage to the joint.

In our attempt the make structural sense out of the mess that the human body presents to the dissector, we slipped our scalpel around the muscles, lifted them out and cleaned them off, and gave them names like biceps and brachialis. That pesky connective tissue binds everything together anyway; what we were looking for was a coherent picture of the organs within it – and the muscles numbered among those organs we separated out. In the example in Figure 10.1 (the supinator muscle in the elbow region) the supinator muscle is the force-conveying muscle and the annular and lateral collateral ligaments, for example, are the passive force-conveying ligamentous structures parallel to the muscles. So far, this is the traditional concept of maintaining joint stability.

If one, however, does not dissect structures (i.e. muscles and ligaments) but tries to dissect by means of a connective-tissue-sparing dissection[13,14] or (in the modern way) reconstruct the connective tissue apparatus in a joint region from a series of histological slices or MRI scans, another organization is revealed. One will be able to estimate the continuity of the connective tissue layers in such a region (1) and, moreover, unfold a more common organization of connective tissue layers and zones of muscular tissue *in series* (2). In the case of the current situation: there are *no* muscle fibers of the so-called dorsolateral extensor forearm muscles being inserted into the lateral epicondyle, as no supinator muscle fiber is doing so. Instead of that a connective tissue apparatus is revealed that conveys the muscle fibers (and therefore the tensile forces) to the lateral epicondyle. This apparatus appears to be the substrate of what in the usual 'correct' anatomical approach was considered to be intermuscular septa in the area plus fascia antebrachii, the lateral collateral ligament, and the annular

ligament. As for the example of the elbow, the situation appears to be like that presented in Figure 10.2.

This appears to be mechanically a much more 'logical' situation since now the periarticular connective tissue is organized *in series* with muscular tissue fibers and therefore may be capable of playing its mechanical role of conveying traction forces and its role as a substrate of mechanoreception (proprioception) in *all* positions of the joint! In other words, muscle contractions, which tense the muscle and its myofasciae (epimysium, perimysium, endomysium, and tendons but also its intermuscular septa and fascia antebrachii), also tense associated 'ligaments' because they are part of this same series of fascia in which the muscle was contracting.

This means that the ligaments, far from being active only at the moment of the greatest elbow extension in your preacher curl, are dynamically active in stabilizing the joint all through the movement, during both concentric and eccentric contraction. Such a 'muscle-ligament-combination' could be indicated as a 'dynament' (by a contraction of 'dynamic ligament'). It would be, however, another conceptual error to consider that the 'muscle man' of the anatomist now has to be replaced by a 'dynament-man'. There is nowadays much evidence that hardly at any functional level can the muscle be considered as a functional entity. Modern neuroscience, for example, has evaluated that 'the brain knows nothing about the muscles', indicating that our motion organization as regards task performance and also proprioception at the cortical cerebral level is not organized in anatomical units like muscles but in movements, patterns of movement, tasks, and actions. For example, expiration muscles do not only exist in the thoracic wall, all kinds of muscles (even the back muscles) can be mobilized in the process of expiration, depending on the body position and the force required to expire in a given situation. The ventral horn motor cells in the spinal cord actually represent the only and 'last' level where muscles are topographically represented in the central nervous system (CNS). Also, in a moving human being it is not true that the brain 'activates' or controls muscles, rather it indirectly controls motor units. The anatomy of motor units is a transmuscular

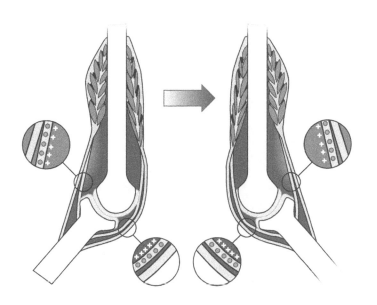

Figure 10.2
In this situation 'muscles' and 'ligaments,' as well as other periarticular connective tissue (fascial layers), are actually arranged in series and reinforce each other. This could be called a dynament arrangement

organization that is a functional hierarchy over the muscle units. In addition, it represents a functional suborganization of muscles. Actually, the motor units represent the physiological entity of muscle tissue.

So if we consider that one of the basic units of the postural and locomotor apparatus is, in principle, represented by the dynament, this entity is not to be considered as an anatomical but rather as an *architectural* unit. Architecture is the anatomical and functional principle of the fascia. In principle, the units via which traction forces can be conveyed over a joint are units of muscular tissue *in series* with two connective tissue layers connecting to the related skeletal elements. So we deal here not with an organization consisting of anatomical elements but rather with an *architectural* organization that is far more functional. Figure 10.3 indicates that with the conceptual model of a dynament, in principle, all the known 'anatomical' units of the postural and locomotor apparatus can be conceptualized, from 'typical' fleshy muscles to the ligament (as a 'dynament without muscular tissue'). The ligament is only there as a possible construction where the two opposite insertion points of the dense collagenous connective tissue structure in *all* positions of the related joint are at equal distance from each other. This makes the typical ligament rather an exception than a rule.

Considerations, such as those outlined opposite, redefine our whole concept of functional units within the postural and locomotor system (PLS). Take one area where this concept is already known to apply: the rotator cuff of the shoulder. The four muscles of the rotator cuff end distally in tendons blending with the ligamentous capsule around the shoulder. In dissection, it is quite hard to tell where the tissue stops being a tendon and starts being a ligamentous sleeve. If muscles are necessary to stabilize the loose, ligamentous capsule of the very mobile shoulder joint, extend that idea to the rest of the body. While there are ligaments that are not connected to the overlying muscles – the cruciate ligaments in the knee are a prime example of ligaments as we have always thought of them – most of our named ligaments are part of a continuous dynament construction.

Referring to what has been described here about the dual functionality of fascia (connectivity and continuity) one could state, for example, that in the forearm two functional architectural units may be discriminated. Distally there exist indeed parts of muscle tissue with a (central) tendon: here the fascia plays its disconnecting role in the form of gliding spaces and bursae with areolar connective tissue. The force-transmission connective tissue component of the fascia is represented here by a muscle unit with

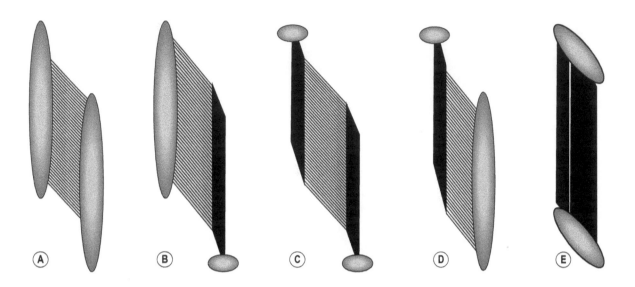

Figure 10.3
Dynament constructions. (A–D) Most 'ligaments' are in series in various configurations, i.e., bone–fascia–muscle–fascia–bone, as in hamstrings or rotator cuffs. (C) represents the most 'ideal' dynament situation: all types of muscle appearances can be conceptualized derived from that principle. (E) The pure (and rare) ligament, like the cruciate ligament, is represented on the right as bone–fascia–bone

a centrally organized tendon. This could be called a dynament arrangement with a centrally organised tendon. In the proximal forearm both the antebrachial flexor and extensor groups do not arise from the humeral epicondyle itself, but from 'layers' of fascia that arise from the condyle. These layers (intermuscular septa, muscle compartment walls, fascia antebrachii, and so on) form the origin of the muscular slips that passes down the arm toward the wrist, narrowing to individual tendons that are attached to more specific areas at the other end. Proximally, the fascia plays its connecting role and the units of force transmission are transmuscular units of muscle tissue architecturally connected with the fascia and intermuscular septa. The concept of the isolated 'muscle' makes more sense at the tendon end than it does back up at the meaty origin.

Take the erector spinae muscles, or the muscles of the lower arm and lower leg – all these complexes arise from complex layers (leaves) of heavy fascia (dense collagenous connective tissue) that join the muscles together with each other and with the ligaments beneath them.

The dynament is a much more functional way of thinking about how the body organizes movement. Even the hamstrings, those icons of singular muscles, are now understood to be both continuous with the sacrotuberous ligament, and to be complex dynaments with the string and membranes within them.

To cut a long story short: we simply cannot divorce the muscles and ligaments. They are linked in series and are part of *one* joint stabilizing and moving system. The relevant architecture of the fascia/muscle arrangement is the dynament, not the muscle.

The most important consequence of the methodological considerations above is that, in this respect again, a principle of twofoldness is to be associated with the fascia. The conclusion of the first part of this chapter (when considering the phenomenology of meso) was that mesenchyme and fascia reveal two principles: connecting and shaping space, continuity and connectivity. So it is with the fascia. There are *two* forces to be dealt with in posture and locomotion, i.e., traction and compression. In this way the triad of bones, joints (with capsules and ligaments), and muscles (or the triad of skeletal tissue, connective tissue, and muscular tissue) is 'reduced' to a far more logical and functional principle of duality or twofoldness. Dynaments as items of architecture instead of anatomy ('how' as well as 'where'), reconnect the classical anatomy again with the functionality of the fascia and meso. And notions like 'musculoskeletal system' in this context represent an odd and inadequate terminology.

Architecture is instrumental: fascia as the organizer of proprioception

Van der Wal[15] clearly demonstrated that it is not the anatomy of muscles versus ligaments and capsules that is instrumental in the organization of proprioception and that the organization of the substrate of proprioception can only be functionally understood in terms of architecture and force transmission.[16] Proprioception is a sense, not a sense organ. Proprioception sensu latu is the body sense as psychology deals with it: the perception and awareness of the body. Many various types of sense organs and receptors contribute to this sense, not only receptors in the fascia or in the elements and tissues of the postural and locomotor apparatus. Proprioception sensu strictu, however, is the awareness and perception of posture and motion, i.e the process of conscious and subconscious sensing of joint position or motion (statesthesia and kinesthesia). Encapsulated or unencapsulated mechanosensitive sensory nerve endings (so-called mechanoreceptors) together with the related afferent neurons provide the centripetal information needed for the maintenance of posture and for the control of locomotion. Considerations such as 'architecture versus anatomy (topography)' may mutatis mutandis also be applied to the spatial organization of those mechanoreceptors as the morphologic substrate for proprioception. To study the role and function of mechanoreceptors in the process of proprioception, it is important to know *where* they are located in such regions, but also *how* they are or are not connected with the related tissue elements. The actual spatial organization of such receptors can be better interpreted functionally when it is known how their topography is related to the architecture of the connective and muscular tissue, this means mutatis mutandis to the fascia.

The discrimination between so-called joint receptors and muscle receptors is an artificial distinction when function is considered. Mechanoreceptors, also the so-called muscle receptors (muscle and tendon spindles), are arranged in the context of force circumstances, that is, of the architecture of muscle and connective tissue rather than of the classical anatomic entities such as muscle, capsules, and ligaments. The receptors for proprioception appear to be concentrated in those areas where tensile stresses are conveyed over the related joint or where gliding and shearing forces exert compression or stretch on the mechanoreceptors. Those receptors should not and cannot be divided into either joint receptors or muscle receptors if muscular and collagenous connective tissue structures function *in series* to maintain joint integrity and stability. In vivo, those connective tissue structures are strained during movements of the skeletal parts, those movements in turn being induced and led by tension in muscular tissue. In principle, because of the architecture, receptors can also be stimulated by changes in muscle tension without skeletal movement, or by skeletal movement without change in muscle tension. A mutual relationship exists between structure (and function) of the mechanoreceptors and the architecture of the muscular and regular dense, connective tissue. Both are instrumental in the coding of proprioceptive information to the CNS. The conclusion of research like this may be that proprioception (sensu strictu) is also not a matter of anatomy but rather of architecture.

C. Meso, fascia, and tensegrity

Next, again based upon a phenomenological embryological view, the model will be introduced that fascia as an organ may be understood in the best way if the architecture of connective and muscular tissue is considered as one integrated dimension of the human body, in a broad sense (the so-called 'mesodermal' germ layer) as well as in the narrow sense of the postural and locomotor system (tensegrity system). To consider the dynament as the principal architectural unit of the postural and locomotor system is congruent with the modern concept of tensegrity (1) and it meets the observations on the development of that architecture in the human embryo (2).

'Tensegrity' (tensional integrity or floating compression) is a structural principle based on the use of isolated components in compression inside a net of continuous tension, in such a way that the compressed members (usually bars or struts) do not touch each other and the prestressed tensioned members (usually cables or tendons) delineate the system spatially. The term 'tensegrity' was coined by Buckminster Fuller in the 1960s as a portmanteau of 'tensional integrity'. Another term for tensegrity is *floating compression* or, as Tom Myers quoted at the International Congress on Osteopathy in Berlin 2014: 'The skeleton as islands of compression floated in a balanced sea of tension'.

Two elements are working in the tensegrity model. Earlier in this chapter, it was proposed that we replace the classical triad of bones, joints (with capsules and ligaments), and muscles with a functional twofoldness of skeletal elements (bones) versus dynaments. Now it becomes obvious that this fits much more closely with the concept of posture (and locomotion) in terms of a tensegrity system. Also, with robots at 'work' in our factories there are only two forces to control while moving and positioning the machine. These are tensile forces and compressive forces (and all variations of these, such as tangential or gliding forces). With the replacement of the muscle-man organization by the transanatomical-architectural organization of dynaments in relation to skeletal elements, harmony with the tensegrity model of posture and locomotion arises. To paraphrase, it could be stated that where the muscle man of the old anatomists was an obscure invention of a dissecting mind neglecting the architecture of fascia and connective tissue, it can now be stated that the postural and locomotor system as a tensegrity model can only be understood functionally if we consider the flexible architectural units of that system to be the dynaments that can adapt in any position of the stiff elements (the skeletal elements). Postural integration is the keyword for locomotion, no more or less than spatial and flexible adaptive architecture. Considering the postural and locomotor system as a tensegrity system values and is in harmony with the concept of the fascia as a bodywide, interconnected tensional network with continuity and connectivity.

In this context there exists amazing congruency with how the development of the limbs and other parts of the postural and locomotor apparatus takes place in the embryo according to the concepts of Blechschmidt. Again, in the spatial development of the postural and locomotor apparatus two principles are at work – this time the actions of concentration and dilatation, stretching and compression. Figure 10.4 shows the situation in a developing human foreleg in a fetus at five months old. On the one hand, there are relatively stiff elements, in this case cartilaginous skeletal elements, products of what Blechschmidt calls *densation* fields. They exhibit a piston-like effect in longitudinal direction on the surrounding mesenchyme. On the other hand, according to Blechschmidt, two types of fields may come up in such a stretched mesenchyme environment. And so here the qualities of muscle and (stress-conveying) connective tissue structures are developing.

According to Blechschmidt, the embryonic skeleton is formed by the loss of the intercellular liquid. Fluids diffuse, therefore the cell relations and connections are condensed. Such fields are *densation* fields. They most frequently lie deep within the inner tissue. Here the young cells are not stressed by pressure or tension in any preferred direction. They are therefore globular, forming primordial cartilage. The growing cartilage cells exhibit a so-called swelling growth. By its swelling growth each cartilage exerts a (piston-like) *distusion* function leading to stretching in the adjacent tissue. In such circumstances, *dilation* fields may come up. There cells are stressed by tension and dilated. These dilated cells develop into muscle cells. It is possible therefore to deduce schematically the position of muscles biodynamically from the distusion growth of the individual cartilaginous skeletal parts. This means that the development of muscles is always dynamically passive. The active partner in this process is the distusion growth of the swelling and elongating cartilaginous skeleton portions (or, for example, the expanding epithelial intestinal tube that acquires circumferential muscle fibers).

Studies on young embryos have revealed that the developing musculature functions not by active but by passive action. The fundamental movements of the developing musculature are not contractions but so-called growth dilations. It can be demonstrated in all early muscles that they are formed only where

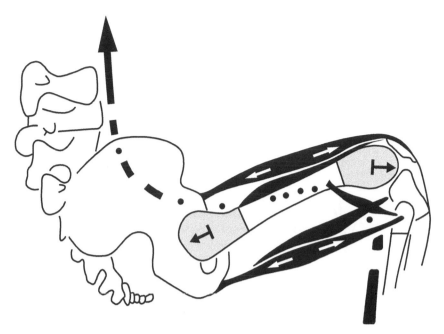

the spatial conditions exist for the preferred longitudinal growth in one chief direction, where there is room for lengthening, and where the necessary physical forces are right for the formation of muscle bulges and tendons. Muscles are not formed where we might perhaps use them later on for pragmatic reasons but in an early ordered basic structure, the *dilation* fields. The transition from dilatation to contraction is rhythmical. Shortly after the first dilatations, contractions start alternating with them as a living reaction to the initial dilation. Blechschmidt stated: 'if muscle was not stretched at first, it was not capable of shortening itself (contraction) in a later phase of the life cycle'. Inner tissue, constricted by cross-compression and stretched by tension perpendicularly to it, shows biodynamically similar signs. It exerts tensile resistance and thereby functions as a restraining structure. Metabolic fields where stretched tissue develops into a restraining apparatus represent *retension* fields. All tendons and ligaments in the human body, as well as the connective tissue-guiding structures of blood vessels, are such restraining structures.

Summarizing this indicates that again two principles are working in the mesenchyme environment. On the one hand concentration and centripetality (cartilage skeletal elements, *densation*), on the other hand stretching and centrifugality induced

by *distusion* of the same skeletal elements leading to muscles, tendons, and aponeuroses by means of the processes of *dilation* and *retension*. If one compares the architecture of a dilatation field of a muscle, according to Blechschmidt, including the related retension fields of the tendons, the analogy with the structure of a dynament is striking (see Figure 10.5). But also the congruency with the principle of tensegrity architecture of compressed members (usually bars or struts) not touching each other and prestressed tensioned members (usually cables or tendons) is evident. If our postural and locomotor system is organized as a tensegrity system then at least it concerns an apparatus in which the stiff components are connected with flexible connective elements (dynaments), so not by connective tissue alone. It also means that without muscle (and nerve) tissue, functional fascia is not conceivable!

D. The fascia as representative of the 'middle' and as the organ of innerness

Last but not least and interwoven into the considerations above, the phenomenological view will be presented that the meso(derm) represents the dimension of 'innerness' in the body, with the blood and the fascia as the main representatives of what could be considered as our 'innerness' or 'soul'.

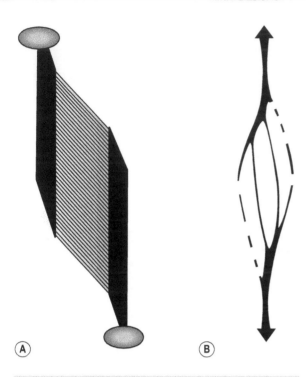

Figure 10.5

(A) Schematic representation of a dynament.
(B) Dilation field of a muscle in a longitudinal section according to Blechschmidt.[5] The diverging arrows indicate the main direction of the dilation stress

Fascia and the dimension of the 'middle'

In the second week of human prenatal development there is not a trace of meso or mesenchyme in the bilaminar disc in the center of the embryo, which is considered to be the substrate for the later actual body (or the 'proper' body). Of course there is mesenchyme active in the two-week-old human embryo, but it exists in between the *ectocyst* (the outer wall of the embryo derived from trophoblast) and the entity of the central bilaminar disc with yolk sac and amniotic sac (the so-called *endocyst*). As explained above, meso and mesenchyme may be considered as the functionality of mediation: connecting and shaping space. The two main derivatives of the meso (i.e., fascia and blood) exhibit this feature clearly in the way they are

organized. Fascial organization is typically matrix-like: fascia is in principle 'everywhere', be it connecting or disconnecting. It forms the matrix that embeds the organs as islands originating from ectodermal, endodermal, or ... mesodermal tissue. This concerns the fascia sensu strictu representing the connective tissue matrix of the body. As explained earlier in this chapter, the principle of fascia is architecture. This is also discernible in the dimension of the fascia as 'organizer', either in its often formative growth-resisting quality or as a pathway for the inductive organizing substances like signal proteins via the ground substance or interstitial fluid. There is evidence that in the process of differentiation and induction of tissues and organs the ground substance and interstitial fluid play an important role in the spatial creation of gradients and concentrations of inductive substances active in the process of organ differentiation. The inductive capacity of mesenchyme to induce the overlying and covering ectoderm and endoderm is well known.

The architecture also plays an instrumental role in force transmission as well as in the process of proprioception, as explained earlier. The twofoldness or duality of the fascia may also be recognized in the notion that the so-called postural and locomotor apparatus is composed of the two elements of a tensegrity system, i.e., stiff elements (here the cartilaginous or osseous skeletal elements) and the flexible adjustable elements (here the dynaments). One can consider the fascia sensu strictu, i.e., as the connective tissue matrix of the body, or sensu latu, i.e., as the whole constellation of skeletal and dynament elements, the postural and locomotor system or apparatus as a whole, and as a tensegrity system.

But if one extends the concept and configuration of mediation as a main function of meso and fascia, blood could also be considered as an exponent of meso (i.e., of fascia). In traditional histological categories blood was considered as a connective tissue derivative. At least the origin of blood is from the meso (derm) and the main morphological function of blood is connecting and shaping space. Blood is not a fluid; blood is an organ or a tissue that is capable of functioning as a fluid. Therefore the formation of the fluid cellular component of blood and the formation of vessels containing the 'fluid tissue' always go hand in hand. The matrix-aspect of the blood is discernible in the fact that the main and primary appearance of blood (i.e. the capillaries) does not have its own ('self-ish') anatomy but is an architectural principle: blood is everywhere and adapts its architecture to the structures and organs of the body. Unlike the fascia, which connects and shapes space between organs and body elements in a mechanical way, the blood does so in a dynamic and physiological way, which could lead to a typical phenomenological concept like: 'blood is everywhere and nowhere, always on the move'.

Also blood connects and shapes space: the appearance of blood in organisms makes it possible that distance between organs can be larger because the blood serves as the mediating organ or principle. The essential difference between plants and animals, for example, is the evident presence of 'something in there' that may react and from way back is recognized by us as 'soul' or 'innerness'. We have already seen that the dimension of innerness in the body is not synonymous with the inside (viscera, which, in principle, are body wall) but with the in-between. The animal is characterized by a psychological innerness, represented by a physiological innerness of organs and in the embryo characterized by the inner tissue, (i.e., the meso). It is not until the third week of development of the human embryo that one can discriminate a morphological representation of innerness by meso organized in between two limiting tissue or body walls. With the 'germ layer' of meso, innerness is going to be enabled.

Fascia as the organ of innerness?‡

In the work of A. T. Still a characteristic motto is that man is mind, matter, and motion: 'Osteopathy ... is the law of mind, matter, and motion'.[17] In his book *Interface*, R. Paul Lee argues that with this theme Still joins many other philosophers whose image of man is based upon a view of the human being known as 'triune' or 'threefold', like Swedenborg, Steiner, Sheldrake, and many others.[18] In such philosophies the human being is more than (only) a matter body – it also has a spiritual dimension ('mind') in the body trying to realize and manifest itself by means of that same body.

‡See footnote * on page 95.

Another characteristic feature is that for Still form (matter) and function (mind) are intertwined inseparably: 'I would say that the wisdom of God proved his highest point when it united soul and body, mind and matter, life and motion'.[19] So in this respect Still's view on the human organism could be interpreted as if we deal with a polarity ('mind' and 'matter') with a necessary interface domain in between ('motion'). In philosophies that practice similar threefold images of man (like anthroposophy) Mind (Spirit) and Matter are polarities and Soul represents the interface where the two are inseparably intertwined. The key word in the quoted motto of A. T. Still, however, is 'motion'. We learned here that indeed the central motif of meso is motion (intrinsic as well as extrinsic) and that the whole meso-dimension may be characterized as a dynamic in-between of breathing between the principles of connecting and disconnecting. Isn't this the theme of Life anyway? Life not as the duality (polarity) of Death but Life representing the breathing in-between between the two poles of Death that in the old Greek philosophy were characterized as Chaos and Cosmos and in the organism amongst others may be characterized as Form versus Process, Space versus Time? Respiration is inspiration as well as expiration, but, on the other hand, respiration as the middle of Life is neither inspiration nor expiration (which are the poles of Death).

The heart muscle and its function (which is *not* contraction alone!) make evident what is meant here: the extremes of systole (contraction) and diastole (relaxation) are the poles of Death in between which Life is manifest in the act of reversion and rhythm. Another triad comes into view in this way: between Mind and Matter the interface is Life itself, with Motion as functional manifestation, with the Middle as an organizational principle, and with Meso as the morphological representation of this quality! In the Middle, in the in-between, there the quality of Being, of Life is enabled! In such a context the aforementioned statement by A. T. Still ('The soul of man with all the streams of our living water, seems to dwell in the fascia of the body') becomes completely logical: there is no other place to be for the soul than the Middle and Meso! But for that it would be better to extend the concept of fascia as the system of connective tissue matrix to the fascia sensu latu, which then also includes the postural and locomotor system as well as blood, with, on every level, the theme of connecting and shaping space. In this case fascia becomes the 'organ' of meso, manifesting itself morphologically in the architecture of the connective tissues (including muscle, cartilage, and bone); physiologically in the principle of motion, in connecting and shaping space on all kinds of levels, in rhythm and breathing; and, last but not least, psychologically and mentally in the domain and function of 'soul'. Meso in general, fascia in particular enables innerness, the fascia therefore as the organ of innerness, being the domain that Still was referring to when he said 'The soul of man with all the streams of pure living water seems to dwell in the fascia of his body'.[20]

References

1. **Schleip R., Jäger H., Klingler W.. 2012.** What is 'fascia'? A review of different nomenclatures. *Journal of Bodywork and Movement Therapies.* 16(4):496–502. Available at: http://dx.doi.org/10.1016/j.jbmt.2012.08.001 [accessed February 15, 2016].

2. **Langevin H.M., Huijing P. A. 2009.** Communicating about fascia: history, pitfalls and recommendations. *International Journal of Therapeutic Massage and Bodywork.* 2(4):3–8.

3. **Findley T. W. 2009.** Fascia Research II: Second International Fascia Research Congress. *International Journal of Therapeutic Massage and Bodywork.* 2(3):4–9.

4. **Standring S. (ed.), 2008.** *Gray's Anatomy: The Anatomical Basis of Clinical Practice,* 40th ed., Elsevier, Edinburgh.

5. **van der Wal J. 2009.** The architecture of the connective tissue in the musculoskeletal system – an often overlooked functional parameter as to proprioception in the locomotor apparatus. *International Journal of Therapeutic Massage and Bodywork.* 2(4):9–23.

6. **Levin S. M., Martin D. C. 2012.** Biotensegrity: the mechanics of fascia. In: Schleip R., Chaitow L., Findley T. W., Huijing P. A. (eds) *Fascia – the Tensional Network of the Human Body. The Science and Clinical Applications in Manual and Movement Therapy.* Churchill Livingstone Elsevier, Edinburgh.

7. **van der Wal J. C. 2012.** Chapter 2.2 Proprioception. In: Schleip R., Chaitow L., Findley T. W., Huijing P. A. (eds), *Fascia – the Tensional Network of the Human Body. The Science and Clinical Applications in Manual and Movement Therapy.* Churchill Livingston Elsevier, Edinburgh, pp. 81–87.

8. **Lee R. P. 2005.** *Interface: Mechanisms of Spirit in Osteopathy,* Stillness Press, Portland, OR.

9. **Blechschmidt E., Freeman B. 2004.** *The Ontogenetic Basis of Human Anatomy: a Biodynamic Approach to Development from Conception to Birth.* North Atlantic Books, Berkeley, CA. pp. 62–63 & 85.

10. **Nedergaard M. 2013.** Sleep drives metabolite clearance from the adult brain. *Science.* 342 (6156): 373–377.

11. **van der Wal J. C. 2010.** Kontinuität und Konnektivität – die Architektur des Bindegewebes als Ergänzung der Anatomie der Faszien. In: Liem T., Dobler, T. K. (eds). *Leitfaden Osteopathie, Parietale Techniken,* 3. Auflage. Urban & Fischer. pp. 726–737.

12. **van der Wal J. 2003.** Dynamic morphology and embryology. In: Bie, G. van der, Machteld H. (eds). *Foundations of Anthroposophical Medicine.* Floris Books, Edinburgh. pp. 87–161.

13. **Mameren H. van, Drukker J. 1984.** A functional anatomical basis of injuries to the ligaments and other soft tissues around the elbow joint: transmission of tensile and compressive loads. *International Journal of Sports Medicine.* 5:88–92.

14. **van der Wal J. C. 1988.** The organization of the morphological substrate of proprioception in the elbow region of the rat. Thesis, University of Limburg, The Netherlands.

15. **van der Wal J. C. 2009.** The architecture of the connective tissue in the musculoskeletal system— an often overlooked functional parameter as to proprioception in the locomotor apparatus. *International Journal of Therapeutic Massage and Bodywork.* 2(4):9–23.

16. **van der Wal J. C. 2012.** Chapter 2.2 Proprioception. In: Schleip R., Chaitow L., Findley T. W., Huijing P. A. (eds), *Fascia – the Tensional Network of the Human Body. The Science and Clinical Applications in Manual and Movement Therapy.* Churchill Livingston Elsevier, Edinburgh, pp. 81–87.

17. **Still A. T. *Autobiography of Andrew T. Still.* Rev. ed.** Kirksville, MO: Published by the author; 1908. Distributed, Indianapolis: American Academy of Osteopathy, p. 229.

18. **Lee R. P. 2005.** *Interface: Mechanisms of Spirit in Osteopathy.* Stillness Press, pp. 97–98.

19. **Still A. T. [n. d.]** *Body and Soul of Man.* Personal collection of Elizabeth Laughlin, Kirksville, page 7.

20. **Still A. T. 1899.** *Philosophy of Osteopathy.* Kirksville, Missouri: A. T. Still, p. 165.

FASCIAL MECHANICS: THE PHYSICS OF ANATOMY AND FUNCTION

Serge Gracovetsky

Introduction

In the 1940s Bartelink was commissioned by the German Air Force to study the internal tissue forces that pilots ejecting from the new military jet airplanes were subjected to with sometimes very deadly consequences. During the course of his work, Bartelink suggested that the back muscles are the predominant structure that would control the trunk during simple tasks such as lifting weights. This idea was received with unabridged enthusiasm and, even to this day, many believe that this is the gospel of biomechanics. That this concept survived for so long against the contradictions it generated is a testimony to the unique ability of the art of medicine to keep an attractive idea alive in spite of a ruthless experimental annihilation.

In the 1860s, *Gray's Anatomy* described the presence of a very strong collagenous structure (the lumbodorsal fascia). For decades, no particular function was assigned to that important structure and its role was not understood until the 1970s when Harry Farfan was struck by the power difference between the hip extensors and the erector spinae.[1] In truth, Bartelink realized the discrepancy, and proposed that the internal abdominal pressure (IAP) would rise to push up the diaphragm during the lift.[2] Very few went on to calculate the level of IAP needed to lift 200 kg and even fewer were troubled by the fact that the calculated high pressure would result in having the hapless weightlifter explode during the exercise. Since people do not routinely explode while lifting heavy loads, I thought that a better explanation was needed.

Others noted that:

'comparative musculature anatomy between old world monkeys and modern humans suggests the presence of relatively smaller, and potentially weaker, lumbar extensor musculature in humans which may contribute to disuse atrophy of the lumbar extensors which, in turn, may explain the consistent association of their deconditioning in LBP [low back pain], and also predispose modern humans to the high prevalence of LBP.'

In other words, it was easier to dump the observed anatomical differences between species on a hypothetical pathological weakness of the human spine.

The power of the hip extensors cannot be transmitted to the upper extremities via the erector spinae because the erector spinae are not large enough to do the job. In addition, even if they were, their anatomical positioning would result in a compressive load that would crush the intervertebral joint. And instead of trying to explain this paradox, the expedient thinking of the time was to arbitrarily decide that our anatomy was deficient and responsible for the functional limitations leading to the dreaded LBP. Many went so far as to suggest that in a few million years our spine would evolve to eliminate the deficient lordosis and become straight: hence the label 'spinal column'. The minor difficulty with that popular argument is that monkeys already have a straight spine and, except for a few fortunate individuals especially in the field of politics, it was not obvious to me that we are evolving towards a monkey's stance. Again, a better explanation was needed.

Farfan thought that the attachment of the fascia to the tip of the spinous processes would permit the fascia to complement the erector spinae for an efficient transfer of loads, and speculated that the fascia would supply what he termed the 'missing moment', that is, the difference between what the hip extensors can provide and what the erector spinae can use.[3] That difference is not trivial as it can reach three to four times what the erector spinae can do.

In an elegant stroke, Farfan's simple idea gave justice to the optimality of human anatomy. Unfortunately, his suggestion was met with ferocious opposition, mainly from fossilized researchers that suddenly saw their pet theories being unceremoniously thrown out of the window. Farfan and I developed a model (based on the anatomical work of the Australian anatomist Nicolai Bogduk[4]) that conceptually and numerically explained what was observed.[5] The mathematical framework was the theory of optimum control that been recently been refined for the first flights to the Moon. The theory expressed that the force transfer throughout the spine will force a lordotic posture that will minimize and equalize the stress at all intervertebral joints,[6–9] but a direct measurement was needed to prove the validity of the approach. And so I decided in the 1980s to study the relationship between lordosis, the angle of trunk flexion, and the activity of the erector spinae. The protocol was as follows. A string of skin markers is placed over the spine of a volunteer together with a set of EMG surface electrodes at the L5 level. The volunteer's lordosis (or, equivalently, the curvature of a line drawn on the skin passing over the tips of the lumbar spinous processes) is measured simultaneously while the EMG activity of multifidus at L5, which is integrated (IEMG), is displayed (Fig. 11.1). The technology that assesses the

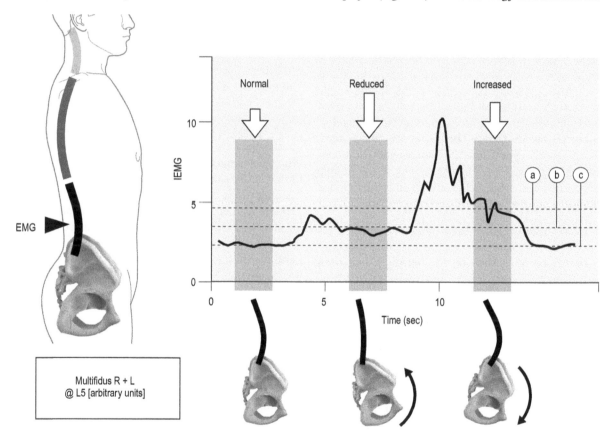

Figure 11.1

The integrated EMG activity is recorded bilaterally by superficial electrodes placed 2 cm to the right and left of the spinous process at L4. The raw EMG signal is band-filtered (5 Hz to 300 Hz), digitized at 1 kHz, rectified, averaged, and plotted. On this graph the signals from the right and left electrode on the multifidus have been added. The average levels corresponding to the most comfortable posture – normal (c), reduced (b) and increased (a) lordosis – are indicated by arrows

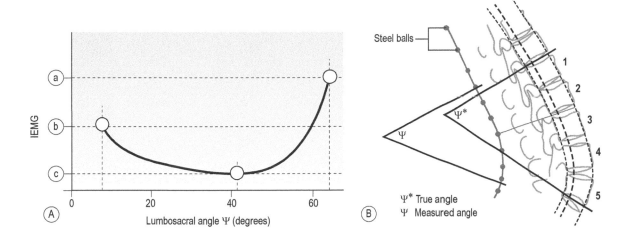

Figure 11.2
(A) Integrated EMG of the multifidus showing relative activity versus lumbosacral angle (lordosis).
(a) Corresponds to increased lordosis, (b) to decreased lordosis, and (c) to resting upright lordosis.
(B) Definition of the true lumbosacral angle Ψ* and its estimate Ψ

spine curvature using skin markers is described in *The Spinoscope User's Manual.*[8] From the tracking of the kinematics of the skin markers, an estimate of the lumbosacral angle Ψ is obtained which is linearly related to the true lordosis Ψ* (Fig. 11.2).

The volunteer is then asked to maintain the same posture (that is, the same general angle of forward flexion), but to first increase then decrease his lordosis by rotating his pelvis (nutation and counter nutation). The corresponding IEMG and lumbosacral angle Ψ are recorded as a function of lordosis (Figs 11.1, 11.2).

The average of the EMG signals corresponding to the three basic lordosis positions (normal, reduced and increased lordosis) are labeled (a), (b), and (c). This data will form the basis for the construction of the curve in Figure 11.2A and the surface shown in Figures 11.3 and 11.4.

This demonstrates that the most comfortable lordosis chosen by the subject corresponds to the minimum IEMG of multifidus at L5. This experiment can be repeated with the volunteer assuming a number of different angles of forward bending. For each angle of forward flexion, results obtained are similar to those shown in Fig. 11.2A. When all the IEMG versus lumbosacral angle Ψ curves are combined, the three-dimensional surface depicted in Fig. 11.3 is obtained.

Clearly, flexion-extension in the sagittal plane is not executed arbitrarily. The volunteer adjusts his lordosis according to the angle of forward flexion so that he remains at the bottom of the energy valley at all times, by minimizing the activity of his multifidus. In fact, the iliocostalis and longissimus lumborum exhibit exactly the same behavior. The subject prefers to do his movement by using the minimum amount of muscular energy or, in other words, the subject prefers to have the lumbodorsal fascia do the bulk of the force transfer from the hip extensors to the upper extremities.

It can be shown that when the muscular energy is minimized, the stress at the intervertebral joint is also minimized, thereby reducing the possibility of injury. This is what is meant by the optimization of spinal resources predicted by the mathematical model proposed in 1977. At that point it was reasonable to think that energy minimization was at least one desirable objective that the evolutionary process would follow

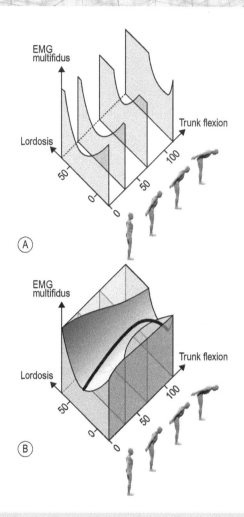

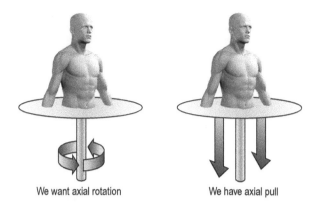

Figure 11.4
The fundamental issue in human locomotion is to convert the axial pull of the hip extensors into an axial torque driving the pelvis. There are no muscles capable of direct axial rotation of the pelvis. An indirect mechanism must be found. This is where the Earth's gravitational field, as a temporary storage element in the transfer of energy from the extensors to the pelvis, is so important for our species

Figure 11.3
(A) Assembly of the data collected in Figure 11.2(A) for four different angles of trunk flexion (in degrees). The axis labelled 'Lordosis' is the lumbosacral angle measured from the position of skin markers as shown in Figure 11.2 and is expressed in degrees. The IEMG is in arbitrary units. The meaning of this 3D image is apparent when the IEMG valley is highlighted as in Figure 11.3(B). (B) When all the individual curves are stacked together, a three-dimensional surface is obtained. Notice that the subject's preferred method of lordosis control for flexion–extension is in the bottom of the valley. This is an illustration of the principle of optimality in which the subject selects the strategy that minimizes his energy expenditure. Note the reduction in lordosis as the subject bends forward

in the design of the animal. But there was one more nagging, unresolved problem that was, again, first pointed out by Farfan in 1969.[10]

The human gait

After studying over 6,000 spine specimens, Farfan proposed that the existing pathological data was consistent with the existence of two families of degenerative patterns. Each family behaves with its own clinical manner and responds to its own different type of treatment. Specifically, the intervertebral joint was mainly injured from excessive compression (compression injury) and/or excessive axial rotation (torsional injury).[10]

This is not a semantic philosophical argument to get another paper published in a journal. A compression injury is a fracture of the cancellous bone of the vertebral endplates and as such heals relatively quickly.

A torsional injury implicates the integrity of the collagenous structure of the annulus fibrosus and is quite difficult to heal. Since both types of injury   AQ3 have a similar symptomatology, the clinician is confronted with some patients whose injuries are able to repair themselves quickly while other patients' symptoms become chronic. Hence the importance of recognizing the presence of torsional anomalies in an LBP subject early. This is the perfect illustration of when treating symptoms can lead to clinical mistakes.

That proposal was immediately subjected to heavy bombardment by those who at the time believed in good faith that a compression injury would damage the annulus fibrosus and start a cascade of events leading to LBP. The shells were essentially lobbed from Sweden where a brilliant man (Alf Nachemson) decided in the 1960s that excessive disk compression was the mother of all spinal diseases. Never mind that a few years earlier Virgin in 1951 demonstrated that an intervertebral joint in which he drilled a large hole was as good at supporting compression as an intact disk.[11] Farfan's data was guilty of confusing many with embarrassing facts and was therefore eagerly flushed out.

The resulting battle smoke could not hide a fundamental dilemma. On one hand, it was obvious to me that Farfan was right in exposing the predominance of torsional anomalies in subjects with chronic LBP. Had Nature given us a straight spine, that annoying torsional weakness would not be there and the theory of Nachemson would have prevailed. And so for many years, at every conference, Farfan and Nachemson slugged it out from their respective corners. But the success of the optimization procedure in explaining the lordosis variation during flexion and recovery from flexion convinced me that nature would not have permitted us to evolve with such a dangerous and potentially crippling design without a reason.

In other words, the risks represented by the possibility of torsional anomalies ought to be compensated for by a significant benefit for our species. Now the question was to find out what the significant evolutionary benefit could be that justified our species taking the risk of a torsional injury in a way that merged the significant work of Farfan and Nachemson, both rather strong-willed individuals, but delightful companions over a beer late at night in a Cambridge pub.

Human gait was the short answer. Note that there is a difference between bipedal locomotion (i.e., that of dinosaurs and the like) and human gait. Human gait requires the spine to support both compression and torsional forces. It is the need to exploit the Earth's gravitational forces, a constant resource all over the planet, which shaped the anatomy of our bipedal species and permitted Homo sapiens to colonize the entire planet from his humble African origins. Bipedalism is widely spread across species, but the unique feature and the extraordinary efficiency of our chosen locomotory mechanism dictated the need for axial rotation while the spine is subjected to large compressive pulses. And that in turn neatly explained the observed spinal pathology.

Simply put, human gait demands that the pelvis rotates in the horizontal plane. The problem is that there are no muscles in the horizontal plane that can do that (Fig. 11.4).

The only source of energy is produced by the powerful hip extensors, which are essentially perpendicular to the horizontal plane. A direct action would therefore be very inefficient. How can the axial pull of the hip extensors be converted efficiently into an axial torque driving the pelvis? This is what the theory of the spinal engine is all about (Fig. 11.5).[12] In short, there is a need to temporarily store the hip extensors' muscle energy in the gravitational field and recover that energy during heel strike.

The reader can convince himself of the role of gravity by trying to walk while his belly button is forced to remain in the horizontal plane. Surprise: it is not possible to walk and run that way since the interaction between the body and the gravitational field is prevented. This energy exchange is obvious in a runner that actually flies in the air at each step, forcing the center of gravity to move up and down, and in so doing betrays the exchanges between kinetic and potential energies. This is discussed at length by Gracovetsky.[9]

And so over the years a generalized concept of spinal function emerged based upon the laws of physics applicable to our home planet. It is hoped that formulating such an approach to normal function might encourage others to formulate a similar approach to the rehabilitation of a subject having abnormal function.

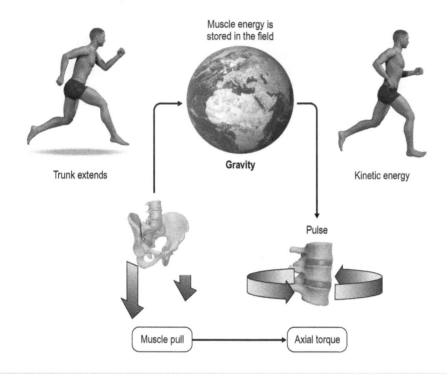

Figure 11.5

The spinal engine theory proposes that the hip extensors lift the body in the gravitational field, thereby converting the chemical energy liberated by the muscles in order for the energy to be recovered during heel strike. This is particularly obvious when both feet are off the ground, and it has long been noted that the center of gravity oscillates up and down during gait. During flight, the spine readjusts its geometry to prepare for landing. As the trunk descends, the potential energy is converted into kinetic energy. That kinetic energy is then recovered at heel strike in the form of a pulse that can be quite high (up to 19 times the body weight for runners in a 100m dash). The heel-strike pulse then travels up the leg, where it is mechanically filtered to compensate for the uneven ground surface. The resulting pulse emerging at the L5/S1 interface has the correct shape and timing that the spine can use to control the pelvis

In short, the ultimate purpose of this chapter is to encourage the structuring of manual medicine within a generalized and a unified perspective defendable from a basic science point of view. Indeed, it is becoming necessary to consider that the patient's pathology is independent of the clinician's training and hence the current plethora of treatments (chiropractic, osteopathic, physical therapy, yoga, etc.) must have some fundamental parts in common.

In particular, it can be expected that the various treatment philosophies are not independent and that some of the claimed differences might be simply a matter of semantics and communication. This could be resolved by developing a common language acceptable to everyone. If history is an guide, this step will probably be met with some resistance, since not everyone will be willing to renounce his/her beliefs, even if there is no scientific basis for continuing to adhere to them.

But the writing is on the wall. The funders of medical services, be they government agencies or private insurance companies, are asking for proof that what is being billed and paid for is actually working. And so there is a need to devise techniques to assess the efficacy of a rehabilitation procedure, in spite of the strenuous opposition of many providers who are not anxious to see an independent third party looking over their shoulder. In fact, many have argued that the relationship between patient and provider is so unique that no statistical blind study can ever be designed to assess the magic of the art. This is not a constructive position since it stifles innovation by preventing the research that is needed in order to move forward.

How to assess manual therapy

The purpose of medicine is to restore normal function in an impaired subject. But what is the normal spinal function that must be restored? For example, no cardiologist would attempt to interfere with the heart of his patient without first having done an electrocardiogram. Measuring the function of the organ is the first step in any intervention. Strangely enough, this strategy is rarely applied to the mechanical etiology of spinal disorders, and it is no wonder that the reha-

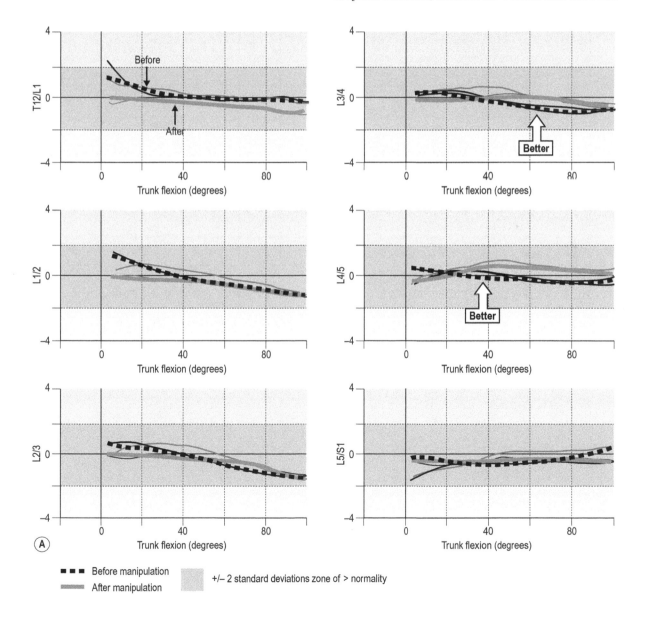

■ ■ ■ Before manipulation
▬▬▬ After manipulation

+/− 2 standard deviations zone of > normality

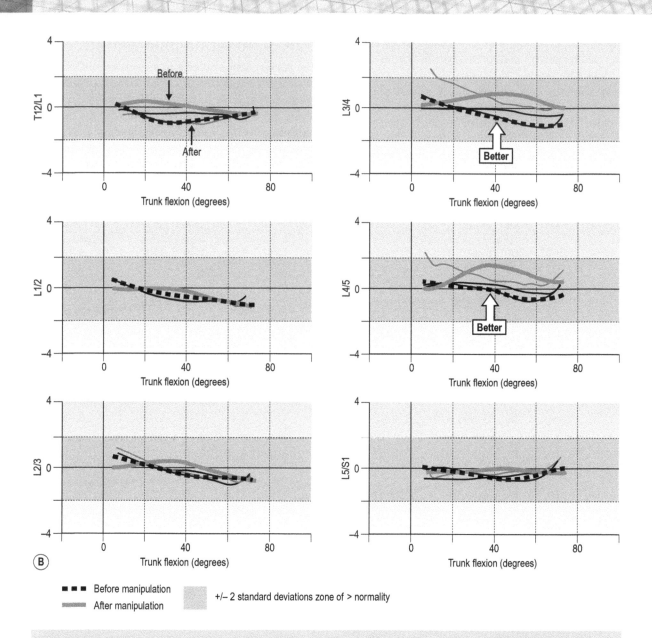

Before manipulation
After manipulation
+/− 2 standard deviations zone of > normality

Figure 11.6

The Z-score of the estimated motion of the intervertebral joints from T12/L1 to L5/S1 is plotted versus the angle of trunk flexion. The shaded zone is the (+/−2) standard deviation zone of normality. The subject has normal function in all joints before the manipulation in spite of complaints of pain. The dotted line is the premanipulation response for lifts of 0 lb and 9 lb. The subject was measured again just less than 20 minutes after a physical therapist had applied his manipulation (solid line) for both 0 lb and 9 lb lifts. The subject felt better and demonstrated a minor improvement at the L3/4 joint level. (A) Overlay of the data for the 0 lb lift before and after manipulation. (B) Overlay of the data for the 9 lb lift before and after manipulation

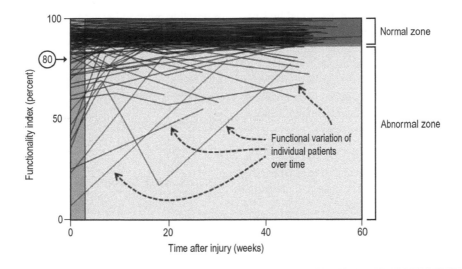

Figure 11.7
Variation in functionality for 100 subjects followed for over a year after their entry into a rehabilitation program for LBP. Note that about 80% of the subjects are functionally normal to begin with and remain essentially normal (unchanged) during the treatment. The remaining 20% of the subjects enter the program as functionally abnormal and experience various degrees of improvement over time

bilitation of subjects with LBP is mainly a matter of trial and error.

In truth, it is very difficult to assess a subject with LBP. A landmark study conducted in 1992 by the Quebec Workers' Compensation Board with the guidance of McGill University and the University of Montreal demonstrated that for benign LBP, the clinician does not have the ability to see beyond what the patient is willing to tell him. In other words, the physical examination is ineffective. The sobering results can be found in *Non-Invasive Assessment of Spinal Function* by Gracovetsky.[9] As expected, a considerable amount of ferocious and unsolicited criticism greeted the news.

But if the sensory equipment of the clinician does not permit an assessment, then to what extent can technology assist the clinician in compensating for his natural limitations?

There is no magic bullet here. The days when all data (radiological, pain, clinical examination, etc.) is integrated by a machine are still a long way off, but partial data can be generated that can be of assistance in specific cases.

Before going into how it can be done, let us revisit the concept of normality as it applies to spinal function. It is proposed that normality be defined by the ability of the musculoskeletal system to function at minimum energy expenditure in such a way that the stress on all structures is as low as possible. That is another way to express the fundamental idea of survival of the species brilliantly exposed by Darwin over a century ago. This is also a very general concept applicable to many other biological systems. In short, a person is said to be normal if he/she is able to use his/her resources optimally.

Mathematics allows us to go one step further. To function at minimum energy expenditure demands a very specific coordination between pelvis and spine so that muscles and fascia are able to complement each other for the benefit of the whole musculoskeletal system. A suitable motion analysis system will be able to pick up that coordination, and a proper expert system will then interpret the objective kinematic data into pathological findings digestible by the clinician in charge of rehabilitating the patient.

That is what has been done and described by Gracovetsky.[8,9] To illustrate the application of the technology, consider the changes in the spine function of a subject that has been manipulated by a physical therapist. This experiment consisted of measuring the estimated motion of the lumbar intervertebral joints before and 20 minutes after a single manipulation. The results are given in Figure 11.6.

Since the system can detect changes after one manipulation, it should be possible to measure the changes after a longer period of repeated manipulation. This experiment was done by tracking the functional changes of 100 consecutive patients over a 60-week period while they were enrolled in a rehabilitation program following complaints of LBP. The results are in Figure 11.7.

This limited experiment shows that the measure for the success of a rehabilitation program is not a simple matter of physical performance. It also raises the issue of determining what the ingredients are that benefit the patients, including the impact of the so-called placebo effect.

Conclusion

This short chapter is an attempt to explain the thought processes that guided this author in the study of the function of the human spine. I have proposed a unified theory that could be generalized to apply to the entire musculoskeletal system. In so doing I have developed some equipment that has led to a technique to assess that function and hence to a possible method for assessing the benefits of rehabilitation.

References

1. **Farfan H. F (1975)** Muscular mechanism of the lumbar spine and the position of power and efficiency. *Orthop Clin North Am*. 6:135–144.

2. **Bartelink D. L. (1957)** The role of abdominal pressure in relieving the pressure on the lumbar intervertebral discs. *J Bone Joint Surg*. 39-B(4): 718–725.

3. **Farfan H. F. (1978)** The biomechanical advantage of lordosis and hip extension for upright activity: man as compared with other anthropoids. *Spine*. 3:336–342.

4. **Bogduk N., Twomey L. (1987)** *Clinical Anatomy of the Lumbar Spine*. Churchill Livingstone.

5. **Gracovetsky S., Farfan H. F. (1986)** The optimum spine. *Spine*. 11:543–573.

6. **Gracovetsky S., Farfan H. F., Lamy C. (1977)** A mathematical model of the lumbar spine using an optimization system to control muscles and ligaments. *Orthop Clin North Am*. 8(1):135–154.

7. **Gracovetsky S., Farfan H. F., Lamy C. (1981)** The mechanism of the lumbar spine. *Spine*. 6:249–262.

8. **Gracovetsky S. (2010a)** *The Spinoscope User's Manual*, Lulu Press.

9. **Gracovetsky S. (2010b)** *Non-Invasive Assessment of Spinal Function*. Lulu Press.

10. **Farfan H. F. (1969)** Effects of torsion on the intervertebral joints. *Can J Surg*. 12:336–341.

11. **Virgin W. (1951)** Experimental investigations into the physical properties of the intervertebral disc. *J Bone Joint Surg*. 33B(4):607–611.

12. **Gracovetsky S. (2008)** *The Spinal Engine*, Lulu Press. pp.103–239.

TENSEGRITY IN THE CONTEXT OF THE MYOFASCIAL NETWORK: ITS RELEVANCE TO OSTEOPATHIC PRACTICE

David J. Hohenschurz-Schmidt

Introduction: biotensegrity principles

Tensegrity structures constitute a fascinating way of integrating the demands of stability and mobility, while remaining energy-efficient and light. Compressive elements such as rods or bones are balanced in a continuity of tensile structures, so that the overall configuration integrates all parts into a unified whole – very much like the body, where the connective element is almost synonymous with fascia. For clinicians, tensegrity offers an inclusive biomechanical theory along with a model that can be touched and felt (Fig. 12.1).

The development of the biotensegrity concept by S. Levin has marked the application of tensegrity principles to the human form. Biotensegrity is often contrasted with 'traditional lever-based mechanics'. The argument in favour of tensegrity is twofold. Firstly, geometrical considerations require triangulated structures if the overall structure is to have mobile joints and be simultaneously stable. The angles of triangles can shift without a compromise in the stability of the overall structure. Triangles are the only geometrical structures where this holds true – cubes, for example, lose stability if their centre of gravity is shifted away from the center.

Secondly, mathematical calculations and experimental evidence show that indeed skeletal components could not withstand the forces calculated with compressive lever-based mechanics alone. A lumbar vertebra, for example, would crush even under a light weight without the force being dissipated laterally (Gracovetsky, 1988; Levin, 2002). Thus, a new way of modeling biomechanical reality was needed and tensegrity provides both lateral force distribution and triangulation. Recent research supports the notion

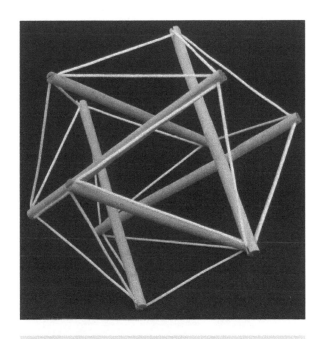

Figure 12.1

In a tensegrity structure, a configuration of distinct ('hard') structures is connected by any given arrangement of tensioned strings or membranes (Skelton & de Oliveira, 2009). This model is made up of six compressive rods and 30 tensile strings, constituting an icosahedron: a platonic solid with 20 equilateral triangular surfaces and 16 vertices. Tensegrity icosahedron reproduced with permission from Mr Graham Scarr

that the myofascial network plays a crucial role in this dissipation of force (Han et al., 2012; Rohlmann et al., 2009). Basic computational models using tensegrity frameworks produce values of the same magnitude as measured in vivo (Siemsen & Dittrich, 2009).

Tensegrity structures are advantageous for biomechanical modeling. Biological structures have evolved to surprising degrees of energy efficiency and resiliency, and tensegrity can account for most of such properties. Being essentially triangulated, tensegrity structures allow for movement at the joints while remaining stable and light overall. The tetrahedron, octahedron, and icosahedron are fully triangulated, three-dimensional structures that can be built from tension and compression elements. With its 20 triangular surfaces, the icosahedron is the most suitable for biological modeling, being omnidirectional, stable and having the largest volume–surface ratio and the closest packing properties (Levin & Martin, 2012). Additionally, icosahedrons can also be arranged in a hierarchical manner, with similar forms repeating themselves at different levels of scale. This feature of self-similar hierarchy is essential for many biological structures (Ingber, 2003; Weibel, 2009) (Fig. 12.2).

How do these geometrical considerations connect the tensegrity model to the human body? According to Turvey & Fonseca (2014), the human body and the

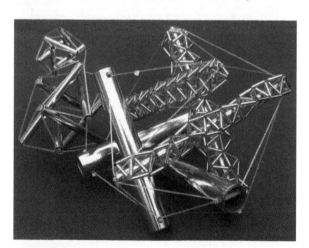

Figure 12.2

Within the internal skeleton of this large tensegrity structure, the compressive rods are themselves made up from smaller tensegrity structures: a hierarchical arrangement. Brass tensegrity model reproduced with permission from Mr Graham Scarr

tensegrity model share both morphological (what they look like) and physiological (how they work) features (Turvey & Fonseca, 2014). Donald Ingber demonstrated this on a microscopic level. The cytoskeleton consists of individual compressive elements, which are connected by a tensile network of microfilaments. These microfilaments in turn connect several cells to each other via membrane proteins and, at the same time, transmit mechanical forces (or 'information') right down to the level of the nucleus – making the cell more like an icosahedron with an internal tensegrity system than a fluid-filled balloon. By this mechanism, termed mechanotransduction, cell physiology can respond to mechanical stresses (Ingber, 2008; Stamenovi & Ingber, 2009). The principles of force transmission that could thus be demonstrated at cellular level are likely to hold true on a larger scale as well, even though they become much more complex and less easy to observe.

For osteopaths, the question with regard to tensegrity is really: how can it inform my practice? Given the fundamental nature of the aforementioned considerations, tensegrity can certainly be seen to constitute part of the scientific underpinning of manual therapies. It describes how forces are distributed throughout the body, thereby taking into account the global fascial network. On a cellular level, it accounts for modifications in cell physiology and gene expression in response to mechanical forces. The validity of tensegrity on all such levels of scale may be part of the explanation of how osteopaths may be able to influence physiological processes by the superficial application of force (Hohenschurz-Schmidt et al., 2016). So, yes, there is a relevance at a theoretical level. But in practice? Hands-on?

Tensegrity and fascia

Fascia is everywhere. If the body is indeed a tensegrity-like structure, what is the role of fascia?

The myofascia constitutes the tensile network of the body. Tension produced by muscle is not just transmitted linearly to its tendon, but also laterally through the connective tissue matrix (Huijing et al., 2011). With its structural and mechanical continuity, the myofascial net has been compared to the tensile component of a tensegrity structure (Hohenschurz-Schmidt, 2014). Fascia invests every structure of the body on all levels of scale and is therefore comparable to the strings in a tensegrity toy model. Of course, the human body is infinitely more complex and comparison with a tensegrity model can only be a simplification. Models are never more than an approximation of reality, but using them in this way can be useful to clinical practice. The notion that bones provide the compressive elements while the connective tissues are the 'continuous tension network' of a whole-body tensegrity structure is one such a simplification that may be useful in clinical practice. This idea is complemented by the fact that the body is built in a fractal-like manner, with similar shapes repeating themselves on different levels of scale. This idea conforms with essential tensegrity ideas, where individual parts of the structure can themselves have an internal tensegrity arrangement (Scarr, 2014; Scarr 2015). The implication is, for example, that bones, even though functioning largely as compressive elements on the macro level, can be looked at as internally balancing tension and compression and as tensegrity structures in their own right (Huang & Ogawa, 2010; Kardas et al., 2013).

Another key feature of tensegrity structures is their 'shape-memory'. Within limits, energy stored in the pre-tensed network of strings will return the structure to its original shape after being deformed (Ingber, 1998). Fascia has similar elastic properties and can thus support smooth movement in an energy-efficient manner (Schleip & Müller, 2013).

Whether the whole body is a tensegrity structure in a literal sense is open to debate, but the fact that human biomechanics are to a greater part tension-dependent is not. Perceiving the body as a tensegrity structure has certain clinical benefits. Considering the myofascia to be the tensile component of a whole-body tensegrity appears especially sensible due to its analogous features of network-like tension and its unifying and integrating role in the body. Similar to tensegrity toy models, where a focal concentration of tension alters the overall shape and restrains mobility, focal adhesions in the myofascial web may influence the healthy function of distant parts.

Myers' concept of myofascial meridians is also useful in this context, as it provides the practitioner with a broad map of typical lines of force transmission,

which can be linked to the tensile cables of a tensegrity (Myers, 2012). In a functional context, these meridians have to be understood *in motion* as pre-tensing structures for efficient movement. The tensile lines of a body tensegrity are thus also spring-like 'storers' of mechanical energy, due to the viscoelastic properties of the myofascial system (Stecco et al., 2014). An excessive storage or a failure to release the accumulated energy could then lead to dysfunction either locally or elsewhere in the tensegrity through a shift in the overall pattern (Willard et al., 2012; Klingler et al., 2014). Such dysfunction can manifest either as straightforward tissue damage and pain, or it may be of a functional nature, preventing the individual from fulfilling their needs or expectations.

When we consider the analogy between tensegrity models and the human body, the implications for manual therapy practice start to become apparent

Tensegrity in a manual therapy context: osteopathic relevance

Tensegrity appears to naturally appeal to osteopaths – somehow it just *feels* right. There is an abundance of literature in the fields of osteopathy and manual therapy published in the last few years, which give significant attention to tensegrity (e.g., Stone, 1999; Parsons & Marcer, 2006; Swanson, 2013). The model is often mentioned in lectures and courses on, for example, myofascial and even cranial techniques.

A recent qualitative study conducted with manual therapists attempted to explore the affection in which practitioners hold this model. It appears that it may be grounded in several reasons. Tensegrity appears to match the way in which some practitioners have perceived the body, even before learning about tensegrity. Now, they feel their perception is supported by a scientifically sound model. Moreover, it provides osteopaths with a visible and intelligible model for their palpation, even distant palpation. Others found that tensegrity resonates with osteopathic principles such as holism and the interrelatedness of parts. On a biomechanical level, a tensegrity can be balanced. For some osteopaths, a balanced human tensegrity allows for bodily self-reorganization, and is thus in accord with the osteopathic tenet of the innate self-healing capacity of the body (Hohenschurz-Schmidt, 2014; Hohenschurz-Schmidt, 2016).

Conceptual role: a different way of looking at the body

Nowadays, scientists studying biomechanics no longer think that the spine, for example, is a compressive pillar of blocks. Tensile forces are integrated into every modern biomechanical analysis. In this context, the benefit of tensegrity is that it connects this concept of tension and compression to a scientifically sound model and, at the same time, provides us with a picture: rods or blocks balanced by tension cables, or even sheaths of tense material. Tensegrity therefore provides the manual therapist with knowledge about the way biomechanics work, and with an experience of how it may feel. For this purpose, tensegrity toy models are useful. The tensegrity model is a rather inclusive way of looking at the body, attempting to simultaneously appreciate compressive and tensile structures and on different levels of scale. As such, tensegrity can be called a holistic biomechanical model, an explanation that ties in well with traditional osteopathic principles. Research by Ingber, who demonstrated the effects of mechanical tissue properties on cellular physiology, showed that tensegrity can seemingly also account partially for the osteopathic link between structure and function: anatomy or biomechanics and physiology.

A dysfunctional tensegrity

Tensegrity models will always balance themselves in a state of optimal tension distribution. This becomes clear when handling a tensegrity model. If left alone, every string is under the same amount of tension. If any part is compressed or stretched by external application of force, all other parts will have to adapt. Homeostasis means that the human body has a similar tendency to equilibrate, be it on biomechanical, biochemical, or even spiritual levels. An excessive or prolonged departure from such a state of dynamic equilibrium can be seen as the origin of dysfunction and ill health. In the model, it is a question of whether the material can cope with the amount or duration of excessive stress. The situation in the body is comparable: how much strain can the system cope with, and does the necessary adaptation compromise overall

function? Osteopathic physicians thus search for areas of such restriction in the sense of a dysfunction that prevents the return to a balanced state of tension and compression.

This is often more complex when systemic states are thought to be affected. More heed needs to be paid to psychological, neurological, and biochemical considerations. On a practical level, however, it is often a mechanical pattern that the physician tries to balance – similar to that of a tensegrity toy model.

Application to practice

Arguably, for the tensegrity model to be applicable in (osteopathic) practice, a number of prerequisites are necessary. Firstly, the practitioner requires detailed knowledge of the human form and its function. Similarly, the theoretical basis of tensegrity and its biological context need to be understood in quite some detail (see Scarr, for example, Scarr, 2014; Scarr 2015). Just as biomechanical principles need to be acquired through dedicated study, the informed palpation of normal and abnormal variants of the human body and its tissues requires practice.

The qualitative study mentioned earlier in this chapter showed that some manual therapy practitioners already use the tensegrity model during treatment to visualize tensional patterns under their hands. Doing so seems to assist cognitive processing of palpatory experiences. Palpated tension patterns evoke mental images, which can be linked to the knowledge of tensegrity (Hohenschurz-Schmidt, 2014; Hohenschurz-Schmidt, 2016).

The individual practitioner will integrate this theoretical knowledge of the model and the palpated information with their personal experience and beliefs as an osteopath. The tensegrity model is, as many concepts in osteopathy are, as dependent on its theory as on the practitioner who applies it. It can provide the interested practitioner with an individualized tool for observing and understanding the body (Fig. 12.3).

In practice, the practitioner who is knowledgeable about the tensegrity model can perceive the human body in a different way. A patient's hip problem, for example, can be understood in the context of tensile and compressive structures constituting and related to the

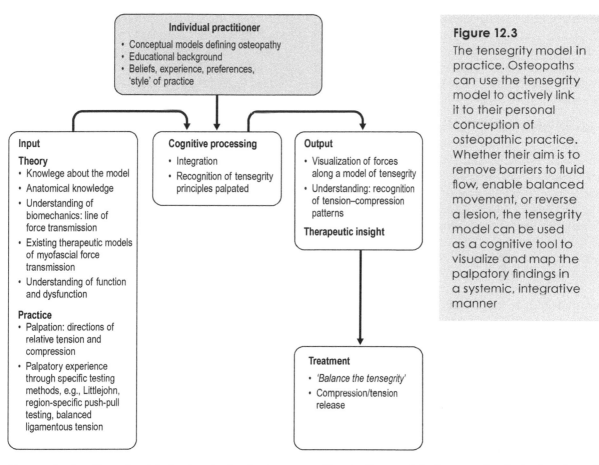

Individual practitioner
- Conceptual models defining osteopathy
- Educational background
- Beliefs, experience, preferences, 'style' of practice

Input

Theory
- Knowlege about the model
- Anatomical knowledge
- Understanding of biomechanics: line of force transmission
- Existing therapeutic models of myofascial force transmission
- Understanding of function and dysfunction

Practice
- Palpation: directions of relative tension and compression
- Palpatory experience through specific testing methods, e.g., Littlejohn, region-specific push-pull testing, balanced ligamentous tension

Cognitive processing
- Integration
- Recognition of tensegrity principles palpated

Output
- Visualization of forces along a model of tensegrity
- Understanding: recognition of tension–compression patterns

Therapeutic insight

Treatment
- *'Balance the tensegrity'*
- Compression/tension release

Figure 12.3
The tensegrity model in practice. Osteopaths can use the tensegrity model to actively link it to their personal conception of osteopathic practice. Whether their aim is to remove barriers to fluid flow, enable balanced movement, or reverse a lesion, the tensegrity model can be used as a cognitive tool to visualize and map the palpatory findings in a systemic, integrative manner

hip complex locally, and a global network of such structures integrating the joint into the whole organism. For practical purposes, body structures are regarded as either tensile or compressive in nature. Nonetheless, the hierarchical features and issues of complexity, as already discussed, are acknowledged. This structural and functional perception of anatomy will add to the practitioner's palpatory experience and potentially provide a framework for diagnosis and treatment. If, for example, a barrier in the transmission of tensile forces is detected in an area where such transmission should normally be possible due to the 'normal' anatomical arrangement, this could indicate a dysfunctional element in the global tensegrity system. Similarly, an excessive accumulation of compression – be it intraosseous or in a number of spinal segments – may compromise the energy-efficient force transfer the body tensegrity was designed to provide. In this way, a seemingly abstract biomechanical model becomes relevant in the practical context of manual diagnosis and treatment.

Eventually, models have only limited value if they cannot influence practice. By influencing our thoughts, the tensegrity model can eventually affect what our hands do. By understanding how a tensegrity toy model will behave in our hands, the palpatory subtleties of manual therapy gain new meaning. If, for example, a tensegrity icosahedron (see Figure 12.1) is compressed at two opposing ends, the part in between will become more 'loose'. Similarly, the thoracic diaphragm has more 'space' if the manual therapist laterally compresses the thoracic cage near its attachments. The ribs and the central tendon of the diaphragm could, for this practical purpose, be considered as compressive elements floating in a tensile myofascial web, including the diaphragm itself. Using constant palpatory feedback, the structures can be moved in a way that provides an optimal balance between global forces of tension and compression, so that, eventually, the thoracic diaphragm may relax. This example may help with the conceptualization of so-called 'balanced ligamentous tension techniques': On a therapeutic level, a careful application of force or following into the direction of least resistance aims to rebalance what is perceived as tensegrity structure – a balance is reached at the point when *the body can do the rest*.

The therapeutic effect is arguably more potent the less abstract the application of the tensegrity model to the human form, meaning that biomechanical analysis is necessary for insight into the compressive or tensile nature of anatomical structures (science). Also, the deeper our understanding of model and reality (knowledge) and the more precise our palpation (practice), the more applicable the tensegrity idea becomes. Ultimately, appreciation of tensegrity ideas should facilitate conceptualization of function and dysfunction, enable the practitioner in his/her physical assessment to link palpatory experience to a scientific model and osteopathic concepts, and, eventually, prompt the choice of techniques for more effective treatment.

Existing theories

The tensegrity model could arguably be integrated with several existing theories from osteopathy and other manual medicine modalities.

On examination, traditional osteopathic concepts, such as Sutherland's tension-dependent reciprocal tension membrane and even Littlejohn's spinal triangles, contain aspects that can be linked to tensegrity. They are descriptions of a compression–tension system, characterized by a unified mechanical response to external or internal perturbations of force. A detailed analysis of this is beyond the scope of this chapter.

The only certain prediction the tensegrity model can offer is that the *whole* will adapt to dysfunction, not just parts. By understanding existing therapeutic theories in the light of tensegrity, they gain in scientific credibility. Conversely, the tensegrity idea becomes more meaningful in a clinical context as these holistic approaches provide an anatomical context for the body tensegrity.

The recent surge of fascia research adds therapeutic models (e.g., Myers' myofascial trains) and treatment approaches (e.g., Schleip's myofascial training) to the discussion. A consideration of 'dynamic tensegrity', *tensegrity in motion*, is implicit. A consideration of the myofascia as the tensile component of a whole-body tensegrity appears to be especially sensible due to its analogous features of networklike tension and its unifying and integrating role in the body. Moving the body tensegrity requires muscles and fascial energy storage, so a detailed study of the myofascial system is crucial to understanding how tensegrity applies to everyday or high-performance biomechanics.

Altogether, the idea of tensegrity is in itself a useful concept of the body. It adds substance to existing clinical models, and it also needs to be used with existing models to acquire a certain clinical predictability.

Conclusion

Initially, tensegrity may seem to be simply an interesting idea. On closer examination, however, we have seen that tensegrity is more than a curious side note worth a few slides in a lecture on cranial or myofascial techniques. It is part of the scientific foundations on which the osteopathic house is built. It can provide practitioners with a conceptual basis for their palpation and could probably play a role in the teaching of palpation. Moreover, its practical and clinical application is open to individual experiment. The body tensegrity can mean something different to each and every osteopath. It will feel different and it can be worked with in many ways, but for the tensegrity model to develop in a therapeutic context, practitioners will need both knowledge of the model and the disposition to let it influence their thoughts.

References

Gracovetsky, S., 1988. *The Spinal Engine.* Springer-Verlag, New York.

Han, K.-S., Zander, T., Taylor, W. R., Rohlmann, A., 2012. An enhanced and validated generic thoracolumbar spine model for prediction of muscle forces. *Med Eng Phys.* 34, 709–716.

Hohenschurz-Schmidt, D., 2014. Tensegrity and manual therapy practice: a qualitative study. [Unpublished Master in Osteopathy]. British School of Osteopathy, London, UK.

Hohenschurz-Schmidt, D. J., Esteves, J. E., Thomson, O. P., 2016. Tensegrity and manual therapy practice: a qualitative study. Int *J Osteopath Med.* 21, 5–18.

Huang, C., Ogawa, R., 2010. Mechanotransduction in bone repair and regeneration. *FASEB J.* 24, 3625–3632.

Huijing, P. A., Yaman, A., Ozturk, C., Yucesoy, C. A., 2011. Effects of knee joint angle on global and local strains within human triceps surae muscle: MRI analysis indicating in vivo myofascial force transmission between synergistic muscles. *Surg Radiol Anat.* 33, 869–879.

Ingber, D. E., 1998. The architecture of life. *Sci Am.* 278, 48–57.

Ingber, D. E., 2003. Tensegrity I. Cell structure and hierarchical systems biology. *J Cell Sci.* 116, 1157–1173.

Ingber, D. E., 2008. Tensegrity and mechanotransduction. *J Bodyw Mov Ther.* 12, 198–200.

Kardas, D., Nackenhorst, U., Balzani, D., 2013. Computational model for the cell-mechanical response of the osteocyte cytoskeleton based on self-stabilizing tensegrity structures. *Biomech Model Mechanobiol.* 12, 167–183.

Klingler, W., Velders, M., Hoppe, K., Pedro, M., Schleip, R., 2014. Clinical relevance of fascial tissue and dysfunctions. *Curr Pain Headache Rep.* 18, 1–7.

Levin, S. M., 2002. The tensegrity-truss as a model for spine mechanics: biotensegrity. *J Mech Med Biol.* 02, 375–388.

Levin, S., Martin, D. C., 2012. Biotensegrity: the mechanics of fascia. In: Schleip, R., Findley, T. W., Chaitow, L., Huijing, P. A. (Eds), *Fascia: The Tensional Network of the Human Body*. Churchill Livingstone Elsevier, London, pp. 137–142.

Myers, T., 2012. Anatomy trains and force transmission. In: Schleip, R., Findley, T. W., Chaitow, L., Huijing, P. A. (Eds), *Fascia: The Tensional Network of the Human Body*. Churchill Livingstone Elsevier, London, pp. 131–136.

Parsons, J., Marcer, N., 2006. *Osteopathy: Models for Diagnosis, Treatment and Practice*. Churchill Livingstone, Edinburgh; New York.

Rohlmann, A., Zander, T., Rao, M., Bergmann, G., 2009. Applying a follower load delivers realistic results for simulating standing. *J Biomech.* 42, 1520–1526.

Scarr, G. M., 2014. *Biotensegrity: The Structural Basis of Life*. Handspring Publishing.

Scarr, G., 2015. *Biotensegrity: the Architecture of Life*. Handspring Publishing.

Schleip, R., Müller, D. G., 2013. Training principles for fascial connective tissues: scientific foundation and suggested practical applications. *J Bodyw Mov Ther.* 17, 103–115.

Siemsen, C.-H., Dittrich, H., 2009. Kräfteverteilungen im Körper des Menschen am Beispiel von Gewichthebern – Tensegrity als Erklärungsmodell. *Osteopat Med Z Für Ganzheitliche Heilverfahr.* 10, 14–18.

Skelton, R. E., de Oliveira, M., 2009. *Tensegrity Systems*. Springer, London.

Stamenović, D., Ingber, D. E., 2009. Tensegrity-guided self assembly: from molecules to living cells. *Soft Matter.* 5, 1137–1145.

Stecco, C., Pavan, P., Pachera, P., De Caro, R., Natali, A., 2014. Investigation of the mechanical properties of the human crural fascia and their possible clinical implications. *Surg Radiol Anat.* 36, 25–32.

Stone, C., 1999. *Science in the Art of Osteopathy: Osteopathic Principles and Practice*. Stanley Thornes, Cheltenham.

Swanson, R. L., 2013. Biotensegrity: a unifying theory of biological architecture with applications to osteopathic practice, education, and research—a review and analysis. *JAOA J Am.* 113, 34–52.

Turvey, M. T., Fonseca, S. T., 2014. The medium of haptic perception: a tensegrity hypothesis. *J Mot Behav.* 46, 143–187.

Weibel, E. R., 2009. What makes a good lung? *Swiss Med Wkly.* 139, 375–386.

Willard, F. H., Vleeming, A., Schuenke, M. D., Danneels, L., Schleip, R., 2012. The thoracolumbar fascia: anatomy, function and clinical considerations. *J Anat* 221, 507–536.

THE MYOFASCIAL SYSTEM AND FORCE TRANSMISSION IN THE FASCIA

Peter A. Huijing

Introduction

In seventeenth-century London, surgeon William Molins published a book on anatomical dissection of muscles for his fellow surgeons and their students. The title page is reproduced in Figure 13.1. Note particularly the subtitle: 'Muscles ... as they arise in Dissection ....' If one takes this text literally, it indicates that muscles are not only distinguished, but also 'constructed' by dissectors in the process of dissection.

Many modern anatomists and, to an even greater extent, modern scientific and clinical users of anatomical information, have lost such a lucid view of anatomical information. The situation is actually worse: many inferences regarding muscle function in health and disease are still based on a concept that muscles operate as if they were fully dissected, that is, fully independent of each other and of surrounding tissues.

The aim of this chapter is to show that there is growing experimental evidence indicating that, when considering the human form, movement and muscular function, one has to take into account the natural connections that exist between muscle and its surrounding tissue (for readers having command of German, a presentation some of the ideas of this chapter are also available in that language).[1]

Intramuscular myofascial force transmission: two parallel paths

Muscular force is generated intracellularly within each muscle cell (myofiber). In the classical view, such force is exerted at the myotendinous junction located at each end of myofibers and is exerted on an aponeurosis or tendon. In such a view, movement is caused in

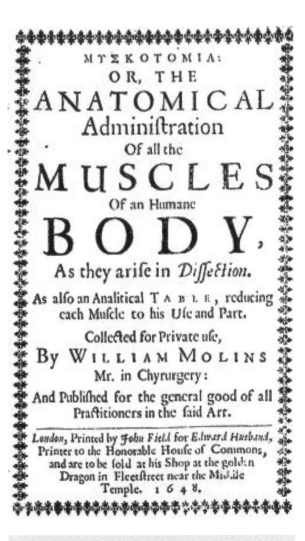

Figure 13.1

Title page of *The Anatomical Administration of all the Muscles* by William Molins a fairly simple way, because the tendon is connected to bone and, if unopposed, the force exerted will move the bone, and bodily movement will ensue.

However, each myofiber is active within a connective tissue tube, made up of its endomysium, and is actually linked elastically to the wall of that tube. A set of such tubes makes up a fascicle, which itself is enveloped by a larger tube (perimysium). In turn, the set of interconnected perimysial tubes is enveloped by the muscular fascia (epimysium). All these intramuscular, interconnected tubes together are called the muscular stroma. This stroma itself is also connected to tendons or aponeuroses, or for muscles that have a bony origin or insertion, via the periosteum directly to bone. This means that within each muscle there are two parallel paths connecting sarcomeres to bone:

1. From sarcomere to in-series sarcomere to the myotendinous junction and via the tendon to bone.

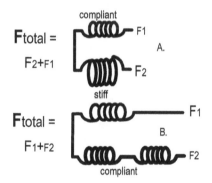

2. From sarcomere to parallel sarcomere to the muscular stroma. Thus the muscular stroma may act as an integrator (place for addition) of muscular and other forces exerted on the stroma.

In the case of a parallel path for force transmission, physics teaches us that force is divided over such available paths on the basis of their stiffness: The stiffest path will transmit most force. This is a crucial rule, but for most people not intuitive. Checking this principle can be done quite simply by connecting two elastic bands, one stiff (e.g., thick or short) and one compliant (e.g., thin or long), in parallel. With the use of a few extra hands, the validity of this rule is easily established (Fig. 13.2). By sensing forces exerted after stretch it will be quite clear that the stiffest part transmits most of the force.

It is a major advantage to have such parallel paths, because if there were only one path and if that path were damaged, force transmission would cease.

Discovering important principles in animal experiments

As a single (i.e., fully isolated) myofiber working within its endomysium can still exert substantial force at its myotendinous ends, even when all parallel sarcomeres are broken at some locations between the two endpoints,[2] it is obvious that such force has to be transmitted via its endomysial tube.

Results yielding similar conclusions for isolated fascicles are available as well.[3] With an experiment on maximally dissected rat extensor digitorum muscle (Fig. 13.3), we showed that with cut myotendinous connections to bone (by tenotomy), for 45% of its myofibers, the muscle is still able to exert approximately 85% of its maximal force.[4]

In experiments such as those described above, force transmission was necessarily limited (by different degrees of dissection) to the morphological unit selected and created for the experiment. Nevertheless, comparison of the three types of results yields the conclusion that if one places a selected unit at a higher level of organization (e.g., a fascicle within a muscle), one has to deal with the mechanical interaction between the unit under study and its connective

Figure 13.2
Illustration of a major principle of force transmission via two parallel paths having different stiffness properties. The highest force is transmitted via the stiffest path. The size of the springs indicates higher or lower stiffness. Similarly, the fraction of the force transmitted via each of the parallel paths is indicated by the size of 'F1' and 'F2.' Since there are only two parallel paths, the total force is always equal to F1+F2. (A) In this case a relatively stiffer path is created by a spring of equal length, but made of stiffer materials. (B) All springs are made of the same materials, but a more compliant path (i.e., less stiff) is created

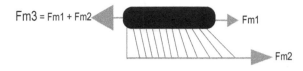

$$Fm3 = Fm1 + Fm2 \qquad Fm1$$
$$Fm2$$

Figure 13.3

A schematic of myofascial force transmission between a muscle and fascial structures. The muscle is indicated by the solid shading. In this example the myofascial connections are directed to the right and transmit force in that direction. As a consequence, that force is not exerted at the muscle's tendon on the right. Within the muscle, force Fm1 and Fm2 to be exerted together at the tendon on the left. Note that, if the myofascial connections were oppositely directed, which could be obtained by moving exclusively the muscle to the right (not drawn), the effects would be opposite and the sign of the difference in forces exerted at the tendon would be opposite as well

tissue surroundings. Such interaction may cause important changes of functional properties.

The question arises: will a muscle that is passive or active within its physiological connective tissue or fascial context be similarly affected?

Inter- and extramuscular myofascial force transmission

Muscular stromata of neighboring muscles are connected directly, and this connection connection also exists between a muscle and nonmuscular structures within a limb. If force is transmitted over any such paths we call it epimuscular myofascial force transmission (because force has to pass via the epimysium). The fact that there are inter- and extramuscular connections (from muscle to nonmuscular tissues) is less important than how stiff these connections actually are. Intuitively, one might think that the strength of the connections (i.e. at what level of force do they break?) is important, and it is true that if the linkages were not strong they would soon lose their functionality. But again it is the stiffness of a particular connection that determines

its functionality. This sounds simple, but the stiffness of any connection is not a given value, but determined by the actual conditions under which it is working, with major functional implications (see below).

First, however, let us consider what happens in a muscle that has links to other structures. As part of the force generated within the muscle is transmitted sideways out of the muscle, the muscle force will not be exerted fully at one of the tendons, and as a consequence a proximo-distal force difference will be present. The occurrence of such differences constitutes absolute proof of epimuscular myofascial force transmission taking place.

The classical view is that one function of connective tissues is to allow sliding of different tissue layers over each other. For example, if one muscle shortens and a neighboring muscle does not, or not to the same degree, the muscles need to slide with respect to each other. If myofibers of two muscles were directly and tightly connected, movement would not be possible. However, it is often overlooked that as muscles show relative movement, the connections will be stretched and increase in stiffness, and become increasingly important as force-transmitting paths. Therefore, as muscles slide with respect to each other, or with respect to nonmuscular tissues, the paths of force transmission will also change in stiffness relative to each other, so that some paths become more important and others less important. Several experiments aimed at moving a muscle through its intact natural context of connective tissues without changing its length have been recorded.[5-7] This was done for the extensor digitorum longus (EDL) muscle of the rat, which is a biarticular muscle in that species, for example, by stretching it at its proximal end and shortening it an equal distance at its distal end so the muscle–tendon complex is kept at a constant length. Figure 13.4 illustrates an example of the results of such experiments for maximally active muscle. Note that if no myofascial force transmission is present, the force exerted at both tendons should be equal and constant, regardless of relative position. However, forces exerted at proximal and distal tendons vary continuously as a function

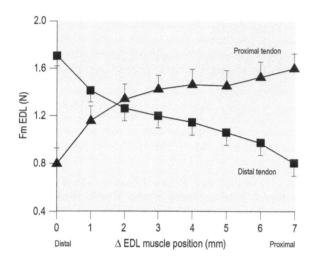

Figure 13.4

Superimposed plots of proximal and distal isometric forces exerted by maximally active rat extensor digitorum longus (EDL) muscle kept at constant length, but moved through different positions relative to its connective tissue context (actual experimental results). As the length is kept constant, all changes in force must be ascribed to the altered relative positions of the FDL muscle with respect to its surroundings

of position. Note also that the direction of force transmission is changed: at distal positions distal force is higher, whereas at more proximal positions proximal force dominates. It should be noted that the conditions created here are aimed at showing the phenomenon in its clearest form. Such conditions are not very likely to occur often in vivo. It is important to realize that in real-life conditions, effects of length and position will be present simultaneously, however, the principle of relative position may be quite important for manual therapies, and also osteopathic manipulation. This is because by handling the tissues, relative positions of muscle (parts) are altered, affecting the paths of force transmission acutely. Which tissues are manipulated depends on the stiffness of the connections and, as the tissues are dependent on the condition of several joints and muscles (see below), they are potentially highly variable.

Force transmission between antagonistic muscles

Up to this point we have focused on force transmission to relatively nearby structures (e.g., synergistic muscles within one compartment), however, a whole set of experiments proves that similar principles also apply for structures that are located further away.[8,9] This means that even antagonistic muscles cannot be considered as being mechanically independent of each other, because they will show very significant interaction if their connections are stiff enough. Note also that for in vivo movement the changes in relative position of antagonistic muscles are huge, since if a flexor muscle (group) is stretched, simultaneously the extensor is shortening.

An important consequence of such interaction is that force generated within the myofibers of a muscle may, depending on conditions of relative muscular position and the properties of the connective tissues linking them, be exerted at one of the tendons of its antagonistic muscle. This means also that some of the sarcomeres in the first muscle are arranged in series with some of the sarcomeres in the second muscle. Note that this a conclusion that challenges the very concept of antagonistic muscles. It also has widespread consequences for manual therapies. The effects locally will be determined also by the conditions of muscles at a distance.

It is clear that we will have to change our concept of a limb and see it not as separate muscle and connective tissue, but more as a whole and a continuum.

Confirmation of principles in experiments on humans

As control over experimental conditions in most experiments involving humans is much more difficult than for experiments involving animals, it is difficult to discover and prove the principles described in the previous paragraphs. However, once one understands the principles of myofascial force transmission, experiments can be performed on human subjects and patients with the aim of recognizing the effects described.

Invasive conditions

In exceptional cases, the principle of myofascial force transmission can be demonstrated invasively during surgery, for example, in patients with a spastic movement disorder on whom tendon transfers are performed in an effort to alleviate nonfunctional positions of the hand.[10–13] In patients undergoing this type of surgery for transfer of the flexor carpi ulnaris (FCU) muscle to an extensor site, we found phenomena that cannot be explained without involving the aforementioned principles of epimuscular myofascial force transmission. After a tenotomy of the FCU the muscle–tendon complex retracted in a proximal direction, indicating that prestretch of the myofascial system may be a normal condition. A simple example of the special effects that occur is if the surgeon moves the hand of the deeply anesthetized patient (with no acute effects of spasticity) repeatedly between palmar and dorsal flexion, the FCU is repeatedly lengthened and shortened, even though, due to the tenotomy, that muscle no longer crosses the wrist. In fact, such length changes constitute 89% of those occurring before tenotomy with an identical wrist movement. Full dissection of the FCU in a proximal direction for 33–50% of its length, necessary to allow later smooth transfer of the FCU to a new extensor insertion on the hand, removed most but not all of this effect, with 7.2% of the length changes remaining.[14] The explanation for this phenomenon is that muscular and nonmuscular structures still crossing the wrist are stretched on dorsal flexion and, because of epimuscular myofascial force transmission, the FCU is pulled along. With the opposite movement of the hand, elastic recoil, possibly in combination with force-transmission effects, allows the FCU to shorten again to its post-tenotomy initial position.

Noninvasive: in vivo conditions

A second experiment was noninvasive in character and performed on healthy volunteers. The subjects were placed within the bore of a magnetic resonance imaging (MRI) machine, with an orthosis keeping the ankle at a fixed position (foot at 90° to the tibia), and images of a segment of the lower leg were recorded. Subsequently, a box was placed under the subject's chest, affecting hip and knee joint angles but not the ankle (knee angle changed from mean

$173° \pm 3°$ to $150° \pm 6°$), and a new set of images was recorded.

In these conditions, one expects the length of the gastrocnemius muscle to change because of the changes in knee angle imposed. On the basis of experimental work on human cadavers it was judged that the gastrocnemius muscle tendon length would change by approximately 1.5% (expressed as fraction of individual tibia length).

In contrast, advanced image analysis, performed by my engineering colleagues, allowed calculation of very local length changes within this muscle tissue (Fig. 13.5). On average such length changes were approximately 10% (expressed as fraction of the initial length of the structure involved). This makes it clear that local normalized length changes to the muscle can be much higher than globally imposed ones. This is important if one thinks about the effects on the stiffness of linking structures. Note, however, that not only were length changes seen with the same characteristics (stretching or shortening) as the globally imposed ones, but also with opposite characteristics (+10% lengthening combined with shortening of -10% at nearby locations). In addition, note that in Figure 13.5 the monoarticular soleus muscle did not change its muscle–tendon complex length between conditions. Lengthening and shortening of similar magnitudes were encountered, indicating mechanical interaction between synergistic healthy human muscles. It has also been shown that that similar changes also occur further away[15] within muscles antagonistic to the gastrocnemius muscle (within the deep flexor, peroneus, and anterior crural muscle groups, i.e., within all other muscle groups of the lower leg) and that local lengthening and shortening encountered there are only somewhat smaller (absolute values ranging ≈ ± 7–9%) than those within the gastrocnemius.

Some further consideration of particular joint positions in spastic paresis

Personally, I have asked many people why, for example the hands and feet of patients with spasticity are in such characteristic positions, but I have never received answers that I found convincing and satisfying.

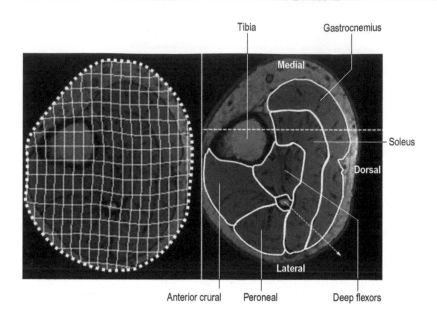

Figure 13.5
Examples of magnetic resonance images made and deformation of lower leg tissues calculated (left panel). A sketch of the outlines of the soleus and gastrocnemius muscles, as well as all other muscle groups, is superimposed on the right panel. Originally the grid imposed was made up of squares, so that the deviation from that form (left panel) indicates the calculated deformation ascribable to altered hip and knee joint angles. Note that deformations are to be seen throughout the cross-section. For details on methods and results, see Yaman et al.[15]

The spastic contraction itself is a muscle-spindle-mediated reflex in reaction to rapid stretching of the spastic muscle. So why are patients not able to change the hand position slowly? Length–force characteristics of the spastic FCU measured after partial dissection show nothing that could explain the peculiar joint position of the wrist.[12] In ongoing work on mechanical, histological, and histochemical analysis of small samples of spastic and control human FCU, we can find no general changes (such as changes in fiber dimensions or an increase in intramuscular connective tissues, etc.). These findings, taken together, suggest that the particular wrist position is somehow related to interaction of the FCU with its connective tissue surroundings.

Even if a spastic muscle was somewhat overactive, it would be active at low lengths and exert low forces because of length effects, while antagonistic muscles are active at more favorable lengths for force exertion. Why is it not possible to excite antagonistic muscles

a bit more to change the position of the hand or foot? Practically, we know it is not possible, but we do not understand why.

The nomenclature used to describe such effects often suggests that we understand the mechanisms, but in fact it means nothing more than that the patient finds it very difficult to move his hand away from the flexed and adducted position or the feet from a plantar flexed position. However, it seems likely that some form of intermuscular myofascial force transmission is involved.

Myofascial force transmission as potential mechanism yielding explanation: antagonistic muscles interacting

The principles of force transmission described earlier suggest a surprising new idea.[16] Before presenting such an idea it needs to be pointed out that it is only a hypothesis (i.e., it needs to be tested experimentally). It is clear that the relative positions of muscles in a person suffering from spastic paresis deviate from the physiological positions of healthy people. One factor contributing to this is deformations of the joints involved (e.g., flat feet, subluxation, etc.). We have shown recently[17] that the angle of the sole proved to be an invalid estimator of talocrural joint angle. In children with cerebral paresis of calf muscles, as the ankle is dorsiflexed at relatively low moments, up to half of the movement of the foot sole may originate from deformation within the foot, rather than from movement at the ankle joint (affecting calf muscles). Note that this finding has severe consequences for clinicians who use the angle of the sole in diagnoses, as well as for scientists who try to describe movement at the ankle and its consequences. Similar effects, albeit at higher moments, have been described by Iwanuma et al. for healthy subjects.[18]

Therefore, it is likely that muscular positions are altered in such a way that forces maintaining the characteristic joint position, such as equinus at the ankle in club foot, may not originate exclusively from the triceps surae muscle, but could at least in part originate from antagonistic muscles. This would mean that, as a patient tries to exert force with nonspastic antagonistic muscles to bring the foot more towards dorsal flexion, (part of) such force is transmitted to the triceps surae and contributes to the plantar flexion moment exerted at the ankle. It could mean that the harder the patients tries to attain dorsal flexion, the higher the plantar flexion moment would be. Alternatively, it could be that connections between bone and muscle lead to high local sarcomere lengths and enhanced muscular stiffness.

Conclusion

In this chapter only the most simple examples have been selected to introduce and clarify the major principles involved. In actual fact, conditions of epimuscular myofascial force transmission are much more complex, for example, multiple myofascial loads on each muscle, having either similar or different directions. In such cases, the simple examples in this chapter provide only indications of the net results of such multiple processes of force transmission.

Having an integral fascial network fit for transmission of forces within the human body creates a huge potential for mechanical clinical interventions as used in osteopathy, for example. One should realize, however, that such a system requires a much more detailed description of actual conditions involving several joints and muscles (agonistic, synergistic, and antagonistic) to adequately diagnose and treat local tissues.

References.

1. Huijing, P. A., Prinzipien der myofaszialen Kraftübertragung bei spastischer Parese in der Physiotherapie sowie in manuellen Therapien. Physiotherapia Paediatrica, Bulletin, 2013. [s.v.](Nr. 30 (juni)):18–24.

2. Street, S. F. and R. W. Ramsey, Sarcolemma transmitter of active tension in frog skeletal muscle. Science, 1965. 149:1379–1380.

3. Street, S. F., Lateral transmission of tension in frog myofibres: a myofibrillar network and transverse cytoskeletal connections are possible transmitters. Journal of Cellular Physiology, 1983. 114:346–364.

4. Huijing, P. A., G. C. Baan, and G. Rebel, Non myo-tendinous force transmission in rat extensor digitorum longus muscle. Journal of Experimental Biology, 1998. 201:682–691.

5. Huijing, P. A. and G. C. Baan, Myofascial force transmission: muscle relative position and length determine agonist and synergist muscle force. Journal of Applied Physiology, 2003. 94:1092–1107.

6. Maas, H., G. C. Baan, and P. A. Huijing, Muscle force is determined also by muscle relative position: isolated effects. Journal of Biomechanics, 2004. 37(1):99–110.

7. Maas, H., G. C. Baan, P. A. Huijing,et al., The relative position of EDL muscle affects the length of sarcomeres within muscle fibers: experimental results and finite-element modeling. Journal of Biomechanical Engineering, 2003. 125(5):745–753.

8. Huijing, P. A., ISB Muybridge Award lecture 2007: Epimuscular myofascial force transmission, its ubiquitous presence across species and some of its history, effects and functional consequences. Journal of Biomechanics, 2007. 40(supplement 2):S22–S22.

9. Huijing, P. A., ed. Special Section: Myofascial force transmission and spastic paresis. Journal of Electromyography and Kinesiology, 2007. 17(6) (December):643–724.

10. Kreulen, M., M. J. Smeulders, J. J. Hage, and P. A. Huijing, Biomechanical aspects of surgical

muscle dissection in a tendon transfer procedure. Journal of Hand Surgery, 2002. 27B-Suppl.1:55.

11. Smeulders, M. J., M. Kreulen, J. J. Hage, et al., Progressive surgical dissection for tendon transposition affects length-force characteristics of rat flexor carpi ulnaris muscle. Journal of Orthopedic Research, 2002. 20(4):863–868.

12. Smeulders, M. J., M. Kreulen, J. J. Hage, et al., Overstretching of sarcomeres may not cause cerebral palsy muscle contracture. Journal of Orthopaedic Research, 2004. 22(6):1331–1335.

13. Smeulders, M.J., M. Kreulen, J. J. Hage, et al., Intraoperative measurement of force-length relationship of human forearm muscle. Clinical Orthopaedics and Related Research, 2004(418):237–241.

14. Kreulen, M., M. J. C. Smeulders, J. J. Hage, and P. A. Huijing, Biomechanical effects of dissecting flexor carpi ulnaris. Journal of Bone and Joint Surgery Br., 2003. 85(6):856–859.

15. Yaman, A., C. Ozturk, P. A. Huijing, and C. A. Yucesoy, Magnetic resonance imaging assessment of mechanical interactions between human lower leg muscles in vivo. Journal of Biomechanical Engineering, 2013. 135(9).

16. Huijing, P.A., Epimuscular myofascial force transmission between antagonistic and synergistic muscles can explain movement limitation in spastic paresis. Journal of Electromyography and Kinesiology, 2007. 17(6 December):708–724.

17. Huijing, P. A., M. R Bénard, J. Harlaar, et al., Movement within foot and ankle joint in children with spastic cerebral palsy: a 3-dimensional ultrasound analysis of medial gastrocnemius length with correction for effects of foot deformation. BMC Musculoskeletal Disorders, 2013. 14:365.

18. Iwanuma, S., R. Akagi, S. Hashizume, et al., Triceps surae muscle–tendon unit length changes as a function of ankle joint angles and contraction levels: the effect of foot arch deformation. Journal of Biomechanics, 2011. 44:2579–2583.

THE LIGAMENTOUS–MYOFASCIAL SYSTEM

Michael J. Decker, Bradley S. Davidson

Introduction

A considerable amount of load transfer between the upper and lower body occurs through the sacroiliac (SI) joint. The nearly vertical orientation of the flat SI joint surfaces makes it vulnerable to shear forces during mechanical load transfer. These large shear

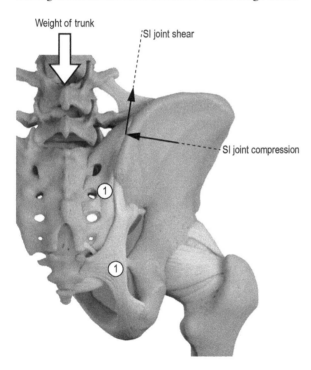

Weight of trunk

SI joint shear

SI joint compression

forces tend to produce positional and movement abnormalities of the SI joint, leading to painful stimuli from the articular surface and adjacent soft tissues (Rupert et al., 2009). The concerted tensing actions of the ligaments, thoracolumbar fascia (TLF), and muscles provide a compression force on the SI joint (force closure) to counteract the influence of the shear force and promote stability for proper load transfer through the lumbopelvic region (Fig. 14.1).

Muscles provide the greatest contribution to force closure of the SI joint (Wingerden et al., 2004). Patients with SI joint pain demonstrate alterations in muscle activation characteristics yet limited information is available describing which structures provide the greatest contributions of proprioceptive feedback for the control of force closure. With regard to the SI joint, proprioceptive feedback from sensory receptors in the muscles, ligaments, and fascia provides the central nervous system (CNS) with information about the joint's mechanical state, and this information is used to shape muscle activation patterns. Given that motor control impairments often describe patients with SI joint pain, we suggest that an important motor control strategy is to finely tune the control of SI joint stability for effective load transfer between the lower extremities and spine during weight-bearing activities.

SI joint ligaments

A system of strong ligaments spanning the dorsal and ventral sides of the SI joint serves an important role in SI joint stability by limiting the forward (nutation) and backward (counternutation) sagittal plane rotations and translations of the sacrum relative to the ilium. The long dorsal sacroiliac, sacrotuberous, and iliolumbar ligaments are reported to be the most commonly injured ligaments that cause SI joint pain (Sims et al., 1996; Vleeming et al., 1996). Counternutation

Figure 14.1
Posterior view of the pelvis and a simplified model of the directions of force exerted by the right ilium through the SI joint as a reaction to weight of the trunk. The sacroiliac (1) and sacrotuberus (2) ligaments span the SI joint and assist force closure and joint stability

creates tension in the long dorsal sacroiliac ligament, whereas nutation causes tension in the sacrotuberous ligament (Vleeming et al., 1996). Counternutation with lumbar flexion (i.e., slouching posture) causes tension in the iliolumbar ligament (Pool-Goudzwaard et al., 2004). These joint motions lengthen the ligaments that span the SI joint, resulting in the delivery of tension that contributes to SI joint, compression. This compression combats the destabilizing effect of SI joint shear forces, thus facilitating effective load transfer between the trunk, pelvis, and legs (Snijders et al., 1993; Vleeming et al., 2012).

Ligamentous–fascial system

The TLF consists of three dense connective tissue layers and is an integral component of the load transfer system of the lumbopelvic region. Each layer has different directions of pull, and loss of independent gliding of adjacent connective tissue layers has been implicated in low back pain (LBP) (Langevin et al., 2011). The TLF attaches to both the sacrum and iliac bones and is anatomically continuous with the long dorsal sacroiliac, sacrotuberus, and iliolumbar ligaments, hence tension produced in the TLF is transmitted to these ligaments (Vleeming et al., 1995; Vleeming et al., 1996; Benjamin, 2009). Although the TLF and SI joint ligaments contribute compression force to the SI joint, it is unlikely to adequately enlarge the compression force to stabilize the SI joint where the transfer of large loads is expected. Because these structures contain an ample amount of mechanoreceptors, they are well suited to monitor SI joint motion and provide afferent information to the CNS for the development of a muscular response pattern (Panjabi, 2006; Schleip et al., 2006; Willard et al., 2012).

The anatomical continuity of the ligamentous–fascial system in the lumbopelvic region offers a source of redundant sensory information for the CNS to finely tune SI joint stability. Deformation, mechanical stress, adhesions, or injury to the ligamentous–fascial system and the embedded mechanoreceptors may modify or interfere with sensory and motor responses of particular muscles (Solomonow, 1998). Patients with SI joint pain demonstrate delayed onset timing of the primary muscles that provide SI joint stability, including the multifidus, gluteus maximus, erector spinae, and biceps femoris muscles (Hungerford et al., 2003; Shadmehr et al., 2012). These muscles interact with the ligamentous–fascial system due to their influence on SI joint motion from their bony muscular attachment sites on the sacrum and ilium and anatomical continuities with the TLF and the sacrotuberus or long dorsal sacroiliac ligaments.

Thus, it is plausible that sensory projections exist between the ligamentous–fascial system and the lumbopelvic muscles. Damage to any component of the ligamentous–fascial system will predictably influence muscle activation characteristic of the lumbopelvic region and impair the fine tuning of SI joint stability.

Ligamentous–myofascial system

A key feature of the proprioceptive function in the musculoskeletal system is the combined architecture that the ligamentous–fascial system creates with the muscles. van der Wal (2009), introduced a paradigm-shifting model that places the muscle in series with the ligaments instead of the traditionally parallel arrangement taught in virtually all anatomy texts. Two key observations based on the presence and continuous nature of fascia support an in-series arrangement: 1) ligaments are not simply a passive force-guiding structure that acts alongside a force-producing structure, and 2) anatomically, structures cannot be divided into joint receptors and muscle receptors. As a result the fascia, ligament, and muscles can be considered as a single system: the ligamentous–myofascial system.

Sensorimotor control of SI joint stability

The framework of sensorimotor control provides a well-defined template with which we can interpret the importance of the interactions of the ligamentous–myofascial architecture to achieve SI force closure. Regardless of the location in the body, sensorimotor control is the integration of afferent sensory information from multiple sources within the central nervous system and generation of efferent motor commands to achieve the desired anatomic movement (Fig. 14.2). A well-studied example is the

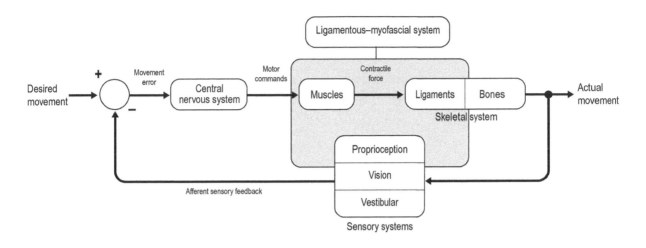

Figure 14.2
Schematic of sensorimotor, closed-loop control where the CNS regulates movements by issuing motor commands based on feedback from multiple sensory systems. The ligamentous–fascial system (gray-shaded area) spans across pathways due to its architecture and plays a large role in the sensorimotor control system. In SI joint function, it composes the entirety of afferent sensory feedback in the form of proprioception

fusion of sensory feedback from the visual, vestibular, and somatosensory structures to achieve standing balance (Horak, 2006). Somatosensory feedback includes both proprioceptive and haptic cues (Berryman et al., 2006). Afferent signals for SI force closure, however, are primarily proprioceptive given the lack of haptic interaction with the external environment and the long distance to the eyes (visual) and inner ear (vestibular).

The structure of the ligamentous–myofascial system across the SI joints allows proprioceptive information for afferent feedback in sensorimotor control of SI joint force closure and stability. Because the in-series arrangement of the ligamentous–myofascial system remains intact posterior and anterior to the SI joint, the proprioceptive afferents that arise from mechanoreceptors in active and passive tissue provide rich information about SI joint position, motion, and loading. The approximate superior to inferior arrangement of the posterior ligamentous–myofascial system across the SI joint is: multifidus, deep layers of the thoracolumbar fascia, posterior ligaments (interosseous sacral, posterior sacroiliac, sacrotuberous), gluteus maximus, and biceps femoris long head. The

approximate superior to inferior arrangement of the anterior ligamentous–myofascial system across the SI joint is: the iliolumbar ligament, transversalis fascia, lumbosacral ligament, anterior sacroiliac ligament, iliac fascia, piriformis plus piriformis fascia, sacrospinous ligament, and the obturator internus plus obturator internus fascia. The proprioceptive influence of in-series anatomical elements distal to the SI joint (i.e., latissimus dorsi, serratus anterior) is currently unclear but is contained within the framework of sensorimotor control.

Within this framework of sensorimotor control, proper force closure is highly dependent on the integrity of the ligamentous–myofascial system because it completely contains both the afferent and efferent structures in the system. This observation calls into question the application of the three-subsystem model of independent passive, active, and CNS control (Panjabi, 2006) as applied to the SI joint. The theory of ligament subfailure assumes a parallel configuration of the passive and active subsystems, which does not correspond to the serial arrangement of the ligamentous–myofascial system. Therefore, SI joint dysfunction, whether laxity or immobilization, may be linked directly to proprioceptive deficiencies that occur somewhere in the ligamentous–myofascial system.

The role of the ligamentous–myofascial system supports a treatment model of regional interdependence. The current model of treatment is the 'biomedical model', which requires initial identification of the underlying mechanism of dysfunction and prescribes the corresponding treatment. In contrast, regional interdependence provides a foundation on which a patient's primary complaint is related to an impairment elsewhere in the body (Wainner et al., 2007; Wainner et al., 2001). The rich interaction of so-called passive and active tissues within the ligamentous–myofascial system almost completely eliminates the ability to identify the underlying mechanism of dysfunction. As a result, the 'proper' treatment for SI joint dysfunction and LBP is often determined by trial and error. In addition, the ligamentous–myofascial system provides the missing link that connects these seemingly disparate anatomic regions through a continuum of fascia, ligaments, and muscle.

A sensorimotor framework that includes the ligamentous–myofascial system can assist our limited understanding of the underlying mechanisms of regional interdependence. Several clinical trials have demonstrated support for regional interdependence of the hip, pelvis, and low back (Childs et al., 2004; Whitman et al., 2006). In addition, clinical tests have emerged that support regional interdependence such as the active straight leg raise test for pelvic pain and altered regional muscle recruitment (Hungerford et al., 2003) and the active side-lying hip abduction test for prediction of LBP (Nelson-Wong & Callaghan, 2010; Nelson-Wong et al., 2009). Analyzing these clinical outcomes and tests within the paradigm of the ligamentous–myofascial system (in a series that spans multiple joints) may provide additional insight into connections between tests, treatments, and mechanism.

Experimental and computational biomechanics research of spine stability will also be greatly affected by the ligamentous–myofascial system paradigm and regional interdependence. The overwhelming majority of biomechanical testing aimed at LBP focus testing and interpretation on the lumbar spine in isolation (Moorhouse & Granata, 2007; van Dieën et al., 2003). Although these provide a window into lumbar spine integrity, without considering pelvic interaction, a complete picture of core proprioception is unavailable.

The unstable sitting test (Fig. 14.3) provides an opportunity to investigate mechanisms of core stability while considering regional interdependence

Figure 14.3
Participant performing an unstable sitting task (A), which is composed of a chair resting on a hemisphere (B) while an adjustable 12kg counterweight is attached to the foot plate of the chair (C) to offset the mass of the feet and legs

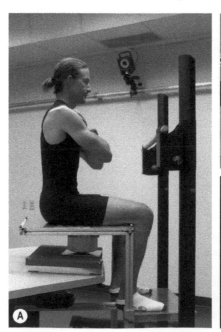
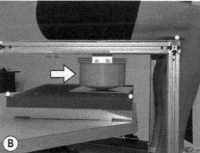
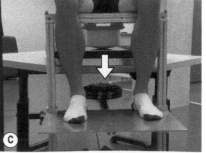

and the ligamentous–myofascial system. Since its introduction by Cholewicki et al. (2000), sway during unstable sitting has been used primarily as a performance variable to discriminate patient groups with LBP (Radebold et al. 2001; van Dieën, 2010) and the influence of visual input (Silfies et al. 2003). Recently, investigators have characterized movement adaptations in patients with LBP using the unstable sitting test (Freddolini et al., 2014). However, interpretation has focused only on the lumbar spine, and the underlying causes of differences measured have not been established.

We recently used the unstable sitting test for initial hypotheses testing of regional interdependence of the hip and lumbar spine. The results demonstrated an association of hip abductor strength asymmetries with unstable sitting (Myers et al., 2013) and an effect of external hip abductor support on unstable sitting (Myers et al., [in review]). In addition, adopting the paradigm of the series arrangement of the ligamentous–myofascial system provides an interpretive lens through which to examine changes in unstable sitting with LBP. Given the important role played by the ligamentous–myofascial system across the pelvis and lumbar spine in providing proprioceptive feedback for a task that is based on sensorimotor control, these measurements may be directly linked to quality of proprioceptive feedback in the pelvis. Although ligament injury and subfailure is still the most commonly cited reason for LBP and pelvic dysfunction, the ligamentous–myofascial system paradigm calls this standard interpretation into question because forces are transmitted through each element within the ligamentous–myofascial system. An investigation on trunk muscle recruitment concluded with similar questions about the origin of LBP always being connected to ligament subfailure (Silfies et al., 2005). Future research based on the ligamentous–myofascial system will provide more details of how this system as a whole and the individual elements contribute to stabilization based on sensorimotor control.

Conclusion

In summary, the continuous nature of the ligamentous–fascial system gives it a critical role in SI joint stability. The high concentration of mechanoreceptors in series within the ligamentous–myofascial system creates an environment of rich proprioceptive signaling for effective sensorimotor control for SI force closure. The series architecture of the ligamentous–myofascial system provides a framework by which regional interdependence of the hip, pelvis, and spine can be examined. These principles form the basis for clinical and basic science investigations that will ultimately lead to more effective treatment of LBP.

References

Benjamin, M., 2009. The fascia of the limbs and back: a review. *J Anat.* 214, 1–18.

Berryman, L. J., Yau, J. M., Hsiao, S. S., 2006. Representation of object size in the somatosensory system. *J Neurophysiol.* 96, 27–39.

Childs, J. D., Fritz, J. M., Flynn, T. W., Irrgang, J. J., Johnson, K. K., Majkowski, G. R., Delitto, A., Childs, M. J. D., Johnson, M. K. K., 2004. A clinical prediction rule to identify patients with low back pain most likely to benefit from spinal manipulation: a validation study. *Ann Intern Med.* 141, 920–8.

Cholewicki, J., Polzhofer, G., Radebold, A., 2000. Postural control of trunk during unstable sitting. *J Biomech.* 33, 1733–1737.

Freddolini, M., Strike, S., Lee, R., 2014. Dynamic stability of the trunk during unstable sitting in people with low back pain. *Spine.* 39, 785–90.

Horak, F. B., 2006. Postural orientation and equilibrium: what do we need to know about neural control of balance to prevent falls? *Age Ageing.* 35, Suppl 2, ii7–ii11.

Hungerford, B., Gilleard, W., Hodges, P., 2003. Evidence of altered lumbopelvic muscle recruitment in the presence of sacroiliac joint pain. *Spine.* 28, 1593–1600.

Langevin, H. M., Fox, J. R., Kopituch, C., Badger, G. J., Greenan-Naumann, A. C., Bouffard, N. A., Konofagou, E. E., Wie-Ning, L., Triano, J. J., Henry, S. M., 2011. Reduced thoracolumbar fascia shear strain in human chronic low back pain. *BMC Musculo Dis.* 12, 203. http://www.biomedcentral.com/1471-2474/12/203 [accessed February 21, 2016].

Moorhouse, K. M., Granata, K. P., 2007. Role of reflex dynamics in spinal stability: intrinsic muscle stiffness alone is insufficient for stability. *J Biomech.* 40, 1058–65.

Myers, C. A., Decker, M. L., Shelburne, K. B., Davidson, B. S, 2013. The relationship between hip function and core proprioception. American College of Sports Medicine Annual Meeting, Indianapolis, IN, May 28–June 1, 2013.

Myers, C. A., Decker, M. J., Shelburne, K. B., Davidson, B. S., [in review] Effects of external core support on proprioception and dynamic stability *J Sports Sci.*

Nelson-Wong, E., Callaghan, J. P., 2010. Is muscle co-activation a predisposing factor for low back pain development during standing? A multifactorial approach for early identification of at-risk individuals. *J Electromyogr Kinesiol* 20, 256–63.

Nelson-Wong, E., Flynn, T., Callaghan, J., 2009. Development of active hip abduction as a screening test for identifying occupational low back pain. *J Orthop Sports Phys Ther.* 9, 649–657.

Panjabi, M. M., 2006. A hypothesis of chronic back pain: Ligament subfailure injuries lead to muscle control dysfunction. *Eur Spine J.* 15, 668–76.

Pool-Goudzwaard, A., Kleinrensink, G. J., Snijders, C. J, Entius, C., Stoeckart, R., 2001. The sacroiliac part of the iliolumbar ligament. *J Anat.* 199, 457–463.

Radebold, A., Cholewicki, J., Polzhofer, G., Greene, H., 2001. Impaired postural control of the lumbar spine is associated with delayed muscle response times in patients with chronic idiopathic low back pain. *Spine.* 26, 724–730.

Rupert, M., Lee, M., Manchikantio, L., Datta, S., Cohen, S., 2009. Evaluation of sacroiliac joint interventions: a systematic appraisal of the literature. *Pain Physician.* 12, 399–418.

Schleip, R., Klingler, W., Lehmann-Horn, F., 2006. Fascia is able to contract in a smooth muscle-like manner and thereby influence musculo-skeletal mechanics. In: Liepsch, D. Proceedings of the 5th World Congress of Biomechanics, Munich. pp. 51–54.

Shadmehr, A., Jafarian, Z., Talebian, S., 2012. Changes in recruitment of pelvic stabilizer muscles in people with and without sacroiliac joint pain during the active straight-leg-raise test. *J Back Musculoskelet Rehabil.* 25, 27–32.

Silfies, S.P., Cholewicki, J., Radebold, A., 2003. The effects of visual input on postural control of the lumbar spine in unstable sitting. *Hum Mov Sci.* 22, 237–252.

Silfies, S. P., Squillante, D., Maurer, P., Westcott, S., Karduna, A. R., 2005. Trunk muscle recruitment patterns in specific chronic low back pain populations. *Clin Biomech* 20, 465–473.

Snijders, C., Vleeming, A., Stoeckart, R., 1993. Transfer of lumbosacral load to iliac bones and legs. Part 1 : Biomechanics of self-bracing of the sacroiliac joints and its significance for treatment and exercise. *Clin Biomech.* 8, 285–294.

Sims J. A., Moorman S. J. 1996. The role of the iliolumbar ligament in low back pain. *Med Hypotheses.* 46(6):511–515.

Solomonow, M., Zhou, B. H., Harris, M., Lu, Y., Baratta, R. V., 1998. The ligamento-muscular stabilizing system of the spine. *Spine.* 23, 2552–2562.

van der Wal, J., 2009. The architecture of the connective tissue in the musculoskeletal system: an often overlooked functional parameter as to proprioception in the locomotor apparatus. *Int J Ther Massage Bodywork.* 2, 9–23.

van Dieën, J. H., Cholewicki, J., Radebold, A., 2003. Trunk muscle recruitment patterns in patients with low back pain enhance the stability of the lumbar spine. *Spine.* 28, 834–841.

van Dieën, J. H., Koppes, L., Twisk, J., 2010. Low back pain history and postural sway in unstable sitting. *Spine.* 35, 812–817.

Vleeming, A., Pool-Goudzwaard, A. L., Hammudoghlu, D., Stoeckart, R., Snijders, C. J., Mens, J. M., 1996. The function of the long dorsal sacroiliac ligament: its implication for understanding low back pain. *Spine.* 21, 556–562.

Vleeming, A., Pool-Goudzwaard, A. L., Stoeckart, R., van Wingerden, J.P., Snijders, C.J., 1995. The posterior layer of the thoracolumbar fascia. Its function in load transfer from spine to legs. *Spine.* 20, 753–758.

Vleeming, A., Schuenke, M. D., Masi, A. T., Carreiro, J. E., Danneels, L., Willard, F. H., 2012. The sacroiliac joint: An overview of its anatomy, function and potential clinical implications. *J Anat.* 221, 537–567.

Wainner, R., Flynn, T., Whitman, J., 2001. *Spinal and Extremity Manipulation: The Basic Skill Set for Physical Therapists.* Manipulations, Inc., San Antonio, TX.

Wainner, R. S., Whitman, J. M., Cleland, J. A., Flynn, T. W., 2007. Regional Interdependence: a musculoskeletal examination model whose time has come. *J Orthop Sports Phys Ther.* 37, 658–660.

Whitman, J. M., Flynn, T. W., Childs, J. D., Wainner, R. S., Gill, H. E., Ryder, M. G., Garber, M. B., Bennett, A. C., Fritz, J. M., 2006. A comparison between two physical therapy treatment programs for patients with lumbar spinal stenosis: a randomized clinical trial. *Spine.* 31, 2541–2549.

Willard, F. H., Vleeming, A., Schuenke, M. D., Danneels, L., Schleip, R., 2012. The thoracolumbar fascia: anatomy, function and clinical considerations. *J Anat.* 221, 507–536.

Wingerden, J. P., Vleeming, A., Buyruk, H. M., Raissadat, K., 2004. Stabilization of the sacroiliac joint in vivo: verification of muscular contribution to force closure of the pelvis. *Eur Spine J.* 13, 199–205.

Anatomy and structure of fascia | 3

3

INTRODUCTION

Paolo Tozzi

This section offers an extensive overview of fascial anatomy and organization throughout the different body layers from superficial to deep. A foundation for informed awareness of fascial structures in various body regions is provided in detail with an emphasis on fascial anatomical continuity and its ubiquitous distribution. The reader should note that there is not a current international agreement about what the word 'fascia' should or should not include, since different definitions of it have been proposed throughout the years, with corresponding different structures under each definition. However, the editors have chosen to include in the so-called 'fascial system' the superficial subcutaneous fascia, the meningi, the perineurial and perivisceral connective tissue, and the diaphragmatic elements, since they all represent distinct fascial differentiation of a body-wide structural 'net', extending from the macroscopic to the cellular depth and sharing a common embryological origin. Therefore, despite local differences in structure and form, including fiber arrangement, direction and density, the fascia shows a hierarchical continuity at different levels of complexity that truly makes it a system between and within the body systems.

GENERAL ANATOMY OF FASCIA

Jean-Claude Guimberteau

Observations made of living matter with an intratissular endoscope allow us to understand the world under the skin with stunning, realistic perspective, suggesting new explanations for the tissue characteristics of flexibility and elasticity, poorly explained until now.

Science's biomechanical explanations have been limited: vague with regard to notions of elasticity, and lacking evidence with regard to loose connective tissue as stratified, hierarchical layering planes with a more or less a virtual space. Yet these concepts of the last century have never been debated and are viewed as accepted fact. The classic doctrine is: connective tissue is connective and is the link between the vital organs. As this tissue seems to be mobile, it is self-evident that it ensures mobility and thereby elasticity.

Perhaps the problem is that, for over 50 years, scientific research has been focused on the microscopic level while putting to one side general anatomy at the mesoscopic level. Furthermore, connective tissue has been considered unimportant, neglected by surgeons and anatomists due to its fragility in dissection and its appearance of consisting of nothing but insignificant fibrous structures.

Surgical dissection used in these areas, such as separation or undermining, are easiest. During an operation the surgeon will often demolish the fibrous webbing to gain access to bony or organ structures beneath. Consequently, what we call surgical planes are only created by excavation with the surgeon's scissors. Physically these planes do not exist, as observation at the mesoscopic level in living tissue proves. In fact, careful mesoscopic observation reveals total tissue continuity (Fig. 15.1). It is this notion of tissular intracorporeal continuity, as

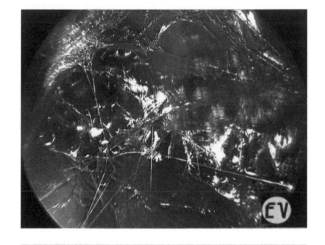

Figure 15.1
Careful observation reveals that connections are a real connective tissue histological continuity without any clear separation. Tissue continuity is total

opposed to spare parts attached to each other, that constitutes the keystone for an understanding of fascial anatomy.

I studied connective tissue organization for 15 years in search of a deeper understanding founded on reproducible science. During countless hours of surgical observations using contact endoscopy, taking video sequences at high resolution of the connective tissue and sliding systems, I came to realize that this too-neglected connective tissue is essential as well as structural. It is not, as traditionally thought, just a secondary tissue – a filling between organs without essential function, or just a simplistic packaging tissue as implied when it is described as an 'envelope' (Fig. 15.2).

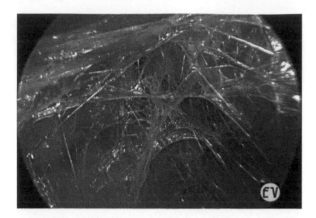

Figure 15.2
The connective tissue is not just a secondary tissue. It is not a filling between organs without essential function, or just a simple packaging tissue as traditionally thought

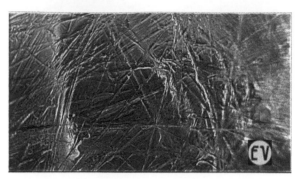

Figure 15.3
The interior architecture does not exhibit the kind of regular order that we might expect to find. It is made up of myriads of collagen fibrils framed in an irregular and fractal manner, interwoven in three dimensions

Instead, I found a world of fibers and fibrils of different diameters and forms, appearing as ropes, veils, cables, and sails. I called this fibrillar scaffold the multimicrovacuolar collagenic absorption system (MVCAS), because it permits sliding while diffusing applied forces, and does so without breaking.

Through intratissular endoscopic technology, it can be seen that this MVCAS system operates far from traditional mechanical analysis. The world under the skin does not exhibit the kind of regular order that we might expect to find (Fig. 15.3). Instead, our interior architecture is composed of myriads of collagen fibrils woven into three-dimensional microspaces that are more or less cellularized and functionalized: the pivotal 'microvacuole', whose shape is polyhedral, irregular, and fractal and that provides an explanation for the movement of water and other biological fluids found within (Fig. 15.4).

From a biomechanical point of view, this network has interconnections whose behavior is nonlinear and that allow optimum adaptation to mechanical stress. The distribution seems chaotic, but is not arranged by chance, for this architecture allows for the optimal occupation of space. This notion of a microvacuole is fascinating because it helps to explain the ability to

fill the intracorporeal space. Indeed, the organization of the fibrillar scaffold is irregular and fractal, with an unpredictable mobility, but in a dynamic sense that is not meaningless. The introduction of the irregularity, chaos, and unpredictability, is almost a form of intellectual violence when we know that it affects the living. We have to reconcile chaos and efficiency.

The microvacuoles, filled with glycosaminoglycans, with varying pressure but stable volume, and found throughout the human body, serve as a stress-absorbing

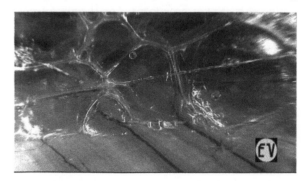

Figure 15.4
Between each intertwining of this system arises a small volume – the functional unit – the microvacuole whose shape is fractal, irregular, and polyhedral

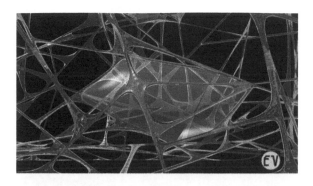

Figure 15.5
The microvacuoles are filled with glycosaminoglycans, serving more as an absorbing system with varying pressure, but with stable volume, and found throughout the human body

system (Fig. 15.5). This system has its own dynamic behavior. It uses very specific movements between fibrils: stretching, dividing, and sliding to create and sustain an extendable and mobile interior architecture (Fig. 15.6).

How do we make sense of this irregular architecture that exists throughout the body at all levels?

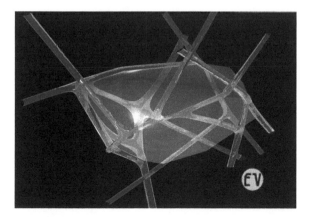

Figure 15.6
The microvacuoles are the result of the intertwining of the fibers into three-dimensional microspaces

The dynamic behavior of this multimicrovacuolar structure, through different degrees of preconstraint and fusion–fission–division of the molecular system, allows all the possibilities of movement within the body, combining mobility, speed, interdependence, and adaptability.

Our body is like a perfect interlocked pattern made up of fibers, fibrils, microfibrils, and microvacuolar spaces, fractal, and more or less cellularized, all of which provide a structural coherence (Fig. 15.7). Sliding tissue, connective tissue, seems to be the structuring and global framework; it is not only connective, it also appears to be the *constitutive* tissue. This thinking gives rise to a new structural ontology based on the functional unit that is the microvacuole – an

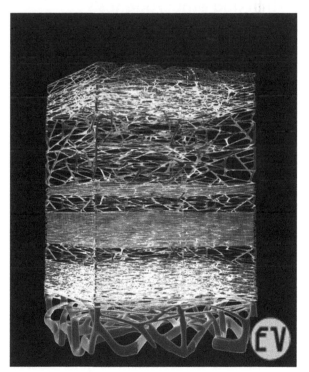

Figure 15.7
The fibrillar continuum from the surface of the skin to the cell – depending on functional adapted densifications – can be defined as the global fascial network of the body, – linking from the top of the head to the toes, from the surface to the deepest areas

intrafibrillar microvolume responsible for shape and dynamic behavior. This basic unit of volume, the microvacuole, is not a fixed entity, nor is it strictly defined; it is transitional and may change, disappear, or recover based on fibrillar games and in a whole, nonlinear but coherent ballet, and needs to be viewed holistically in order to be fully understood.

Acceptance of the microvacuolar concept helps to define the states of matter in pathological circumstances, such as in edema, inflammation, obesity, growth, and aging. It also helps us to understand the healing response and opens new avenues for improving our techniques for optimizing tissue flexibility while limiting adhesions and scars.

Rethinking embryogenesis

Let us now consider new ideas and areas for further research in the light of our observations, which demonstrate the importance of the role of the extracellular matrix through its architectural organization, its physicochemical influence and, in particular, in embryogenesis.

Traditionally, we are taught that the two components of the skin are formed from two different embryonic layers. Their development is considered distinct in both time and space. This concept is based on the supposition that the dermis and epidermis are separate. However, a detailed study of the global dynamics of the skin demonstrates a very close relationship between the dermis and the epidermis, which completely contradicts the concept of two separate and distinct layers. Is the hypothesis of the three distinct embryonic layers – ectoderm, endoderm, and mesoderm – still valid in the light of these new observations? Do these layers really exist? Does this tissue hierarchy, if it exists, continue during the growth and development of the form? Must we always separate the body into layers, lamellae, sheaths, and folds?

This no-separation idea evolved gradually, but was reinforced by in vivo observations of the mobility of the adipocytes inside a fatty lobule when subjected to light pressure (Fig. 15.8). I immediately thought of the coordinated, choreographic, seamless movement of a shoal of fish, and of the shared spontaneity of the whole shoal moving as one. This synchronized

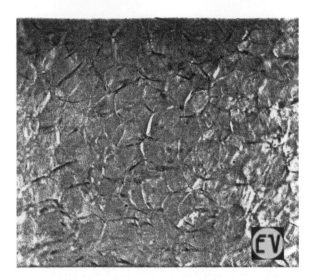

Figure 15.8

The mobility of the adipocytes inside a fatty lobule when subjected to light pressure looks like a coordinated, choreographic, seamless movement of a shoal of fish, with the shared spontaneity of the whole shoal moving as one

movement within the global movement is associated with the unique movement of each adipocyte. The adipocytes are stretched and compressed. They twist, rotate, flatten, or round out, etc.

The links between the cells and the extracellular system are well documented. They are composite structures that consist of molecules entangled by their physicochemical affinities and that react to basic physical forces.

In my opinion, the three embryonic layers cannot exist without close links between them. Before differentiation occurs, the layers are present and are closely connected. Eric Blechschmidt, a German gynecologist, was a leading authority in the field of human embryo research. He studied each stage of the development of the human embryo and his research was carried out under exceptional conditions with very well-preserved tissue samples of excellent quality. He observed that the differentiation between the three supposed embryonic layers begins with characteristic cellular deformation involving biodynamic relationships. These are *forces*, not biochemical substances.

He stressed that blastocysts are linked kinetically by an intercellular substance that forms links that can be localized and in which metabolic movements take place. These links are not simple partitions that separate individual blastocysts. The structure of the nuclei remains unchanged during the process of ontogenic evolution, but cell membranes and the cytoplasm are significantly modified. It seems that physical stimuli play a decisive role in the differentiation of the organism, perhaps as a result of physicochemical disturbances of the metabolism. Genes seem to play a role in the formation of various proteins, but do not appear to be involved in the process of differentiation. From the outset, the stimuli are mainly external. They come from outside the cell, not the nucleus. The cell membranes undergo constant destruction and reconstruction with involvement of the cytoplasm. The biokinetic information transmitted by the cell membranes seems to be a conditioning factor in the process of differentiation, and it is the difference between the internal and external influences that creates a reaction in the metabolic field of the cytoplasm.

Many doctors and scientists, having carried out serious research, speak of the concepts of metabolic fields, morphomagnetic fields, and the theory of hydrodynamics. These ideas have arisen from the observation of cells moving together at the same time toward a common destination (Fig. 15.9). The term 'sphere of influence' is poorly understood and its interpretation can be misleading, but cell polarity exists and ionic attraction or repulsion is an indisputable fact. These polarities can also exist in the extracellular environment, and they may generate forces.

Meiosis, with bipartition of complementary polarities, evolves towards successive mitotic division. Each chromosome in the nucleus splits into two daughter chromosomes. Irregularity is already present at the blastula stage of embryonic development. The germ cells are different. This observation alone requires us to address the issue from a different perspective than that of the traditional view in which development takes place in different 'workshops', each producing separate body parts.

On day three a vesicle appears. Cells produced by cleavage are called blastomeres (blastocytes). The daughter cells are smaller than those produced by the

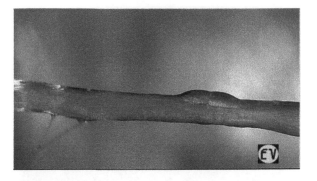

Figure 15.9
The concepts of metabolic fields, morphomagnetic fields, and the theory of hydrodynamics have arisen from the observation of cells moving together at the same time towards a common destination

initial divisions. The intercellular substance occupies more space than it did at the beginning of the process. Furthermore, study of the blastomeres reveals that they do not stain in the same way, which is proof of different metabolic activities. The blastomeres arrange themselves at the periphery and do not have the same relationship with the walls of the blastocyst, which will thicken differently and irregularly.

The ovum attaches to the mucous membrane of the uterus at the place where its lining is the thickest. The two metabolic fields come into contact. This has a polarizing effect on the whole of the ovum. Again, we see an association between the link; movement; and the separate, well-differentiated and delineated structures. The link is there from the beginning and remains during the process of development.

At the stage of the gastrula, why should we not assume strong links between the different germ cells?

Thereafter, growth requires cell multiplication and the expansion of the extracellular network. Existing polarization will get underway, but the link will remain. It is therefore possible, in the light of what we have observed, to suggest that these polarized embryonic cells, of which there are so few at the beginning, gradually find their place in the gastrula while maintaining their links with neighboring cells. The identification of the epidermis and the dermis, the ectoderm

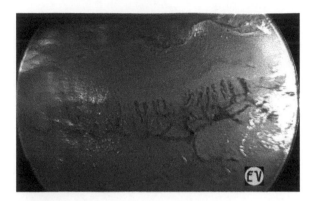

Figure 15.10
The links that we observe between the dermis and the epidermis are too dense, and their relationship too intimate, for their origins to be different, unconnected, and geographically distant

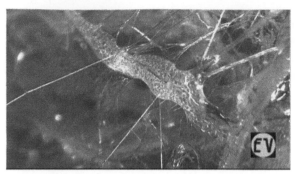

Figure 15.11
The extracellular matrix transmits mechanical stimuli, directing cellular responses both in space and time and in accordance with the physical demands of the princeps architecture

and the mesoderm, cannot break this permanence of diverse links, including vascular and nerve connections. The links that we observe between the dermis and the epidermis are too dense and their relationship too intimate for their origins to be different, unconnected, and geographically distant (Fig. 15.10).

During the process of cell migration into the folds and invagination of the embryo, some cell groups must grow faster than other groups that are less mobile and remain attached to each other.

This tissue mobility is surprising, but anatomical specification cannot break the individual links and the overall cohesion. However, we must also accept the facts. We cannot simply ignore all the work that has been carried out during the past century. The three germ layers may exist, but they must be interrelated, and their development cannot take place independently.

The role of the extracellular matrix

What role does the extracellular matrix play in the process of cell migration? Does the extracellular matrix contain the blueprint?

Endoscopic exploration has revealed that cells are not present everywhere. They tend to group together to form structures and clusters. They are rarely scattered. They are surrounded by the fibrils and microfibrils of the extracellular matrix. There are large areas between tendons, nerves, arteries, and muscles that are practically devoid of cells, but are occupied by the sliding system previously known as connective tissue. Furthermore, there are areas in which it is difficult to ascertain what type of cell performs the function. A good example is the area of attachment of a tendon to the periosteum.

The cytoskeleton with its framework of microfibrils transports procollagen for the fabrication of microfibrils and fibrils. These organize themselves to form tendons, fascia, and aponeuroses. These fibrils do not all orient themselves in the same direction as they leave the cell membrane. They migrate in different directions. Are the extracellular spaces responsible for the orientation and assembly of these fibrils, as well for as their migration? The extracellular matrix transmits mechanical stimuli and directs cellular responses both in space and time and in accordance with the physical demands of the princeps architecture (Fig. 15.11).

Conclusion

Finally, I would simply like to reiterate the fact that the completion of 'the form' cannot take place without the extracellular matrix that accompanies the cells during their migration. The plasticity of the extracellular matrix allows for permanent intercellular proximity and cell differentiation as well as for the efficient use of space during growth. We must keep in mind the fact that the final form must conform to the blueprint and comply with the basic principles of living organisms: movement, adaptability, supply, and morphological stability. The exploration of living tissue is at its beginning; endoscopic technological improvements will bring new discoveries and will challenge old dogmas. However, we must first accept that the Cartesian order, rationalism, and positivism are not the only effective views.

THE SUPERFICIAL FASCIA

Antonio Stecco, Carla Stecco, Luigi Stecco

Introduction

The superficial fascia is still the subject of debate. While some authors admit the existence of a membranous layer separating the subcutaneous tissue into two sublayers, some do not acknowledge it, and others describe multiple layers (Wendell-Smith, 1997).

The ancient anatomists (Fabrici, Casseri, Spiegel, Bartholin, Vesling), following the teachings of Vesalius (1543), described the subcutis as having an adipose and a carnosus layer. They knew that cutaneous musculature was present throughout the body in animals, but in humans it was limited to the neck, forehead, occiput, and a few other regions. Under these layers they recognized the 'membrana musculorum communis', independent of muscles. The term 'superficial fascia' appeared only at the end of the nineteenth century, when Camper (1801), Colles (1811), and Scarpa (1809; 1819), studying the formation of inguinal hernias, described a fibrous layer inside the hypodermis of the abdominal and pelvic regions. This layer was designated the superficial fascia, to distinguish it from the term 'deep fascia'. In 1825 Velpau affirmed that 'the superficial fascia is a fibrous layer present throughout the body, not just in the abdomen and pelvis'. Unfortunately, no other research was conducted, thus the confusion about the terminology and organization of the subcutis remained. According to the French school guided by Testut (1899), the subcutis consists of two fibrous sublayers. The first is just under the dermis and the second is near the deep fascia. Both are separated by a thin layer of loose connective tissue. But according to the Italian and German schools, the superficial fascia is a fibrous layer that divides the subcutis into a superficial and deep adipose layer that is loosely organized. Velpau agreed with the latter description of the subcutis and described a superficial layer (the *couche areolaire*), and a deep layer (the *couche lamellare*), but his description was abandoned in favour of Testut's interpretation (Testut, 1899).

It is interesting to note that the meaning of the terms panniculus adiposus and superficial fascia differs in English-, French- and German-speaking countries. For example, the fibrous lamina dividing the subcutis is called 'textus connectivus compactus' by the Federative Committee on Anatomical Terminology (FCAT), 'fascia superficialis' by Italian and French anatomists, 'membranous layer' by English anatomists, '*straffen Bindegewebe*' by German authors, and 'subcutaneous fascia' or 'tela subcutanea' by Wendell-Smith (1997). We suggest that the adipose tissue be clearly differentiated from the connective tissue for anatomical and clinical reasons. Nowadays many authors suggest simply using the term 'hypodermis' or 'subcutis' without further elaboration, and even the *Nomina Anatomica* of 1998 uses the general term 'hypodermis' instead of superficial fascia, but this nomenclature can cause confusion when a radiologist is describing the obvious intense line present inside the subcutaneous fat, or a clinician wants to affect the elasticity of the subcutaneous connective tissue.

Overview

Over the last 15 years our group has performed dissections of the entire human body in order to schematize and summarize the macroscopic and microscopic morphology, taking into account the possible local differences. The dissections, performed layer by layer on fresh cadavers, revealed that the subcutis is divided by fibrous lamina in two sublayers, each with distinct features (Fig. 16.1). In light of the results of

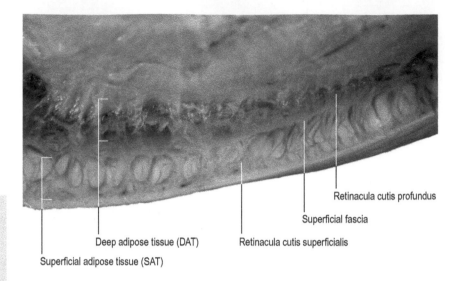

Retinacula cutis profundus

Superficial fascia

Deep adipose tissue (DAT)

Retinacula cutis superficialis

Superficial adipose tissue (SAT)

Figure 16.1

Anatomical dissection of the lateral side of the abdominal wall in an embalmed body

our research we have decided to call the superficial sublayer 'superficial adipose tissue' (SAT) and the deep layer 'deep adipose tissue' (DAT). These two layers are separated by a fibrous lamina in the middle – the 'superficial fascia'. We employ the term superficial fascia, after the description by Professor Sterzi (1910). The *Terminologia Anatomica* defines fascia as a sheath, a sheet, or any number of other dissectible aggregations of connective tissue. The superficial fascia is connected to the skin (retinaculum cutis superficialis) and to the deep fascia (retinaculum cutis profundus) by fibrous septa, which impart specific mechanical properties to the subcutis (Nash et al., 2004). The analysis of a small portion of the subcutis can reveals what appear to be multiple fibrous laminae because some septa are very oblique. But if we dissect larger areas, we find that these laminae finally merge in the same structures: superficial fascia in one direction and deep fascia or skin in the other. These conclusions were confirmed by imaging (CT scan, ultrasonography) and histological examination. It is evident that the subcutis is uniformly structured, with specific features that differ by region of the body. In some areas of the body the fibrous component is prevalent, in other areas the adipose component is prevalent. This defines the mechanical and biological features of the subcutis and explains some possible clinical implications such as localization of edema as well as identifying the most effective body areas for application of manual treatment.

The features of the subcutaneous tissue vary throughout the body. In particular the SAT and DAT differ in thickness, form, and disposition of the adipose lobes and fibrous septa. The retinacula cutis superficialis (known as skin ligaments in English textbooks) are usually almost perpendicular (Fig. 16.2). The retinacula cutis profundus are usually more oblique, thinner, and more elastic than the superficial septa. They create a clear separation of the superficial fascia from the deep fascia. For instance, during the typical 'pinch-and-roll' test the retinacula cutis profundus is more elastic than the superficial fascia. Where the superficial and deep retinacula cutis insert into the superficial fascia, they typically show a large area of attachment, similar to a fan or a cone. In these areas the superficial fascia appears thicker. It is probable that the arrangement of these septa have contributed to the great variability in the fascial thickness values reported in the literature.

The superficial fascia and the retinacula cutis form a three-dimensional network between the fat lobules of the hypodermis, like a beehive. This arrangement permits a flexible and yet resistant mechanism of transmission of mechanical loads from multidirectional forces. According to Li & Ahn (2011) the superficial and deep retinacula cutis and superficial fascia (which they call altogether subcutaneous fascial bands') could be considered as structural bridges that mechanically link the skin, the subcutaneous

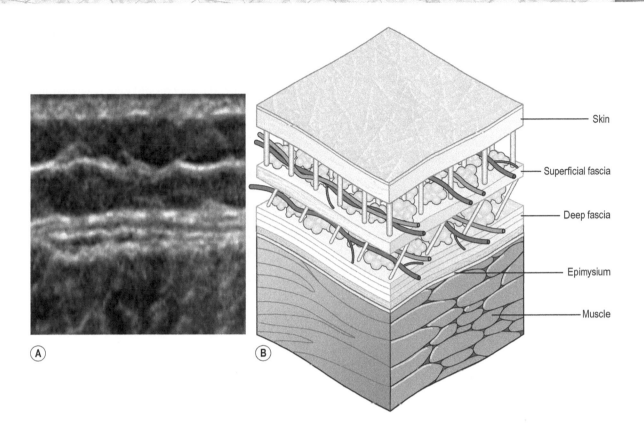

Figure 16.2
(A) Ultrasonography imaging. (B) The subcutis area

layer, and deeper muscle layers. Their quantity and morphological characteristics vary according to the region of the body. For example, in the thigh and calf the area occupied by the retinacula cutis with respect to the subcutaneous tissue is thicker than in the arm. The thigh has the highest average number of retinacula cutis while the greatest average retinacula cutis thickness is seen in the calf. Regional variations determine the differences in mobility of the skin with respect to underlying tissues and may reflect the composite mechanical forces experienced by the body part. For example, in the eyelids, the penis, and the scrotum the adipose tissue and the retinacula cutis are absent, and so the skin shows an increased mobility with respect to the underlying planes. Other examples are the palm of the hand and the plantar surface of the foot, where DAT is absent. In these areas the superficial fascia adheres to the deep fascia,

and in SAT the skin ligaments are very thick and densely packed, strongly connecting the skin with the underlying planes. On bony prominences and at some ligamentous folds the superficial fascia adheres to the deep fascia.

The superficial fascia (fascia superficialis)

The superficial fascia is a fibrous layer of connective tissue formed by loosely packed, interwoven collagen fibers mixed with abundant elastic fibers. It is the equivalent of the cutaneous muscle layer (panniculus carnosus) found in other mammals. This muscular layer is rare in humans. It is well developed in many lower mammals where muscular fibers remain in a thin sheet of striated muscle lying within or just beneath the superficial fascia, serving to produce local movement of the skin. This is rare in humans and, when found, assumes a precise muscular structural arrangement primarily in the neck (platysma muscle), in the face (the superficial muscular aponeurotic system or SMAS), in the anal region (external anal sphincter), and in the scrotum (the dartos). While muscle fibers can be found in all superficial fascia, all that remains that corresponds to mammalian panniculus carnosus in most parts of the human body is a fibrous layer in the middle of the hypodermis.

The superficial fascia is present throughout the body and, according to Abu-Hijleh et al. (2006), its arrangement and thickness vary according to body region, body surface, and gender. It is thicker in the lower than in the upper extremities, on the posterior rather than the anterior aspect of the body, and in females more than in males. Sterzi (1910) describes the superficial fascia as thicker and more resistant in sturdy individuals with well-developed muscles. In humans the superficial fascia becomes very thin at the distal ends of the limbs, and it is impossible to separate it out as a distinct fibrous layer. It is, however, always possible to distinguish the SAT and DAT. In mammals like the rabbit, for instance, the panniculus carnosus (cutaneous muscle layer) is absent in the distal portion of the limbs, and only a thin fibrous layer continues up to the carpus and tarsus. This explains why it is so easy to skin these animals, except in the paws, tail, ears, and around the muzzle.

In the abdomen the superficial fascia has a mean thickness of $847.4 \pm 295\,\mu m$, increasing in a proximocaudal direction with a mean value of $551\,\mu m$ in the epigastrium and $1045\,\mu m$ in the hypogastrium. The thickness of the superficial fascia varies significantly among different subjects and in various regions of the body. Abu-Hijleh et al (2006) found that the mean thickness of the superficial fascia on the dorsal aspects of the foot, thigh, and back is significantly higher in females than in males. The mean thickness of this layer on the dorsal aspect of the hand and arm is significantly higher in males than in females. On the other hand, the mean thickness of the superficial fascia on the anterior aspect of the thigh and periphery of the breast is significantly higher in females than in males. On the anterior aspect of the leg the mean thickness of the layer is higher in males than in females. In the obese the superficial fascia is usually stuffed with fat cells and shows a thickness increase of 50%.

Histologically, the superficial fascia is formed by a net of collagen and elastic fibers arranged irregularly. Macroscopically, the superficial fascia appears and can be isolated as a well-defined membrane, but microscopically its structure is better described as multilamellar, or like a tightly packed honeycomb. The various sublayers have a mean thickness of $66.6 \pm 18.6\,\mu m$. Many points of interconnection between the sublayers can be distinguished. Irregular islands of fat cells (mean thickness $83.87 \pm 72.3\,\mu m$) may be deposited between sublayers of collagen fibers.

Inside the superficial fascia there are many nerve fibers. In some regions the superficial fascia splits, forming special compartments. This occurs particularly around major subcutaneous veins (Caggiati, 1999) and lymphatic vessels with fibrous septa that extend out to attach to vessel walls.

Functionally, the superficial fascia plays a role in the integrity of the skin and supports subcutaneous structures, particularly the veins, ensuring their patency. The superficial fascia together with the retinacula cutis support and help organize the position of fat tissue. Finally, the superficial fascia separates the skin from the musculoskeletal system, allowing normal sliding of the muscles and skin upon each other.

The normal anatomical features of the retinacula cutis allow the autonomy of skin with respect to deep fascia. This is important for the protection of nerves and vessels that cross the deep fascia. Notably, they ensure that the receptors inside the deep fascia will not activate during normal stretching of the skin.

Mechanical behavior

The superficial fascia is a fibroelastic layer that may easily be stretched in various directions and then return to its initial state due to its rich concentration of elastic fibers.

The mechanical behavior of the superficial fascia cannot be understood without considering the superficial and deep retinacula cutis, because they are strongly connected with the superficial fascia and form with it a three-dimensional network. This structure of the subcutis supports the fatty tissue and anchors the skin to the deep anatomical planes. At the same time, it permits some independent movement of the skin and muscles. During skin movement the subcutaneous tissue also moves, but SAT glides more than DAT. Retinacula that are short, strong, and vertical strongly connect the skin with the underlying planes, allowing stress to the skin to be more directly transmitted to deeper planes. However, they have a great capacity for muting mechanical stresses applied to the deep fascia by way of the skin. The deep fascia is also involved in the displacement of the skin to a minor extent because of the adaptation of the retinacula cutis and superficial fascia. Both the retinacula cutis and superficial fascia are elastic and they progressively mitigate the shifting.

In addition to muting skin stresses to subcutaneous tissues, the superficial fascia and retinacula also help prevent the harmful effects of muscular contraction on the skin. Normally, when muscles contract they slide easily under the subcutaneous tissue and the skin is not involved. This occurs because, while muscle movement always stretches specific portions of the deep fascia, their action into the skin is mitigated by the retinacula cutis and by the mutual movement of the superficial fascia with respect to the deep fascia. According to Nakajima et al. (2004), the two adipose layers of the subcutis differ in mechanical and functional aspects. The SAT forms a solid structure and is understood to protect against external forces. The DAT forms a mobile layer and is understood to lubricate musculoskeletal movement.

Scar tissue analysis reveals that scars have lost the ability to mute stress since the entire subcutis is transformed into fibrous tissue that creates a rigid connection between skin and deep fascia. Every time mechanical stress is applied to scar tissue the deep fascia is also stressed, causing activation of its receptors. Whenever a muscle is activated the deep fascia receptors in this area will be activated, along with the receptors within the locally stretched skin. This may explain why stressing scars can result in confusion of

afferentation and probable overstimulation of certain receptors resulting in oversensitive and painful scar tissue areas.

The mechanical behavior of the retinacula cutis and superficial fascia supports the skin and subcutaneous fat. Tsukahara et al. (2012) show a relationship between the depth of facial wrinkles and the density of the retinacula cutis in the subcutaneous tissue of the skin. In particular, these authors demonstrate that facial wrinkles seem to develop above the sites of reduced retinacula cutis density. As wrinkles increase, the density of the retinacula cutis decreases even more.

In the young, the superficial fascia is very elastic, permitting the subcutis to adapt to stress in all directions and then spring back to its original state. With age, the superficial fascia and retinacula cutis lose their elasticity. This could explain the eventual ptosis of the skin, formation of wrinkles, and the general hypotonicity of the subcutis.

Using ultrasound imaging Ahn & Kaptchuk (2011) demonstrated the spatial anisotropy of subcutaneous tissues. In particular, the calf was significantly associated with greater anisotropy compared with the thigh and arm. Anisotropy was significantly increased with longitudinally oriented probe images compared with transversely orientated images. Maximum peaks in spatial anisotropy were frequently observed when the longitudinally oriented ultrasound probe was swept across the extremity, suggesting that longitudinal channels with greater tension exist in the subcutaneous layer. These results suggest that subcutaneous biomechanical tension is mediated by collagenous/echogenic bands, greater in the calf than in the thigh and arm. The tension is increased in thinner individuals and is maximal along longitudinal trajectories parallel to the underlying muscle. Spatial anisotropy analysis of ultrasound images has yielded meaningful patterns and may be an effective means of understanding the biomechanical strain patterns within the subcutaneous tissue of the extremities. Isolated superficial fascia shows strong anisotropy and great variation of its mechanical properties depending on the different regions analyzed. It is possible that spatial anisotropy can be used as an effective surrogate for the summative tensile forces experienced by subcutaneous tissues.

Conclusion

The anatomical variations of the superficial fascia should be take into consideration every time a patient is assessed. The knowledge of the localization of the areas with less gliding will permit the physician to better understand the clinical situation of the patient.

The structural organization of the subcutis and the mechanical behavior of the superficial fascia and retinacula cutis in the different regions of the body may also influence the modality of manual treatment of the superficial and deep fascia. It is evident that in areas with loose and thin retinacula cutis, superficial massage to the skin will be unlikely to affect the deep fascia (except for possible indirect effects). To mechanically affect the deep fascia the subcutaneous fatty tissue must be displaced, so it is necessary to use a small-surface localized contact and to point directly into the deeper planes.

References

Abu-Hijleh M. F., Roshier A. L., Al-Shboul Q., Dharap A. S. Harris P. F. (2006) The membranous layer of superficial fascia: evidence for its widespread distribution in the body. *Surg Radiol Anat.* 6:606–619.

Ahn A. C., Kaptchuk T. J. (2011) Spatial anisotropy analyses of subcutaneous tissue layer: potential insights into its biomechanical characteristics. *J Anat.* 219:515–24.

Caggiati A. (1999) The saphenous venous compartments. *Surg Radiol Anat.* 21:29–34.

Camper P. (1801) *Iconesherniarumeditae a S. T. Soemmering.* VarrentrappetWenner, Frankfurt am Main.

Colles A. (1811) *A Treatise on Surgical Anatomy.* Gilbert & Hodges, Dublin.

Federative Committee on Anatomical Terminology (FCAT) (1998) *Terminologia Anatomica: International Anatomical Terminology.* Thieme, Stuttgart.

Li W., Ahn A. C. (2011) Subcutaneous fascial bands—a qualitative and morphometric analysis. *PLoS One.* 6:e23987.

Nakajima H., Imanishi N., Minabe T., Kishi K., Aiso S. (2004) Anatomical study of subcutaneous adipofascial tissue: a concept of the protective adipofascial system (PAFS) and lubricant adipofascial system (LAFS). *Scand J PlastReconstr Surg Hand Surg.* 5:261–266.

Nash L. G., Phillips M. N., Nicholson H., Barnett R., Zhang M. (2004) Skin ligaments: regional distribution and variation in morphology. *Clin Anat.* 4:287–293.

Scarpa A. (1809) *Sull'erniememorieanatomo-chirurgiche (1st ed.).* RealeStamperia, Milano.

Scarpa A. (1819) *Sull'erniememorieanatomo-chirurgiche (2nd ed.).* StamperiaFusi e Compagno, Pavia.

Sterzi G. (1910) *Iltessutosottocutaneo (telasubcutanea).* Luigi Niccolai, Firenze. Caggiati, 2000.

Testut L. (1899) *Traité d'anatomie humaine.* Gaston Doln and Cie, Paris.

Tsukahara K., Tamatsu Y., Sugawara Y., Shimada K. (2012) Relationship between the depth of facial wrinkles and the density of the retinacula cutis. *Arch Dermatol.* 148:39–46.

Vesalius A. (1543) *De humani corporis fabrica (On the Structure of the Human Body).* Ex officina Joannis Oporini.

Wendell-Smith C. P. (1997) Fascia: an illustrative problem in international terminology. *Surg Radiol Anat.* 5:273–277.

FASCIAL ANATOMY OF THE TRUNK

Peter J. Brechtenbreiter

The deep fascia of the trunk is made up of dense, braid-twist scaffold conjunctive tissue. It originates from the embryonic mesenchyme and runs from the head to the pelvis. The deep fascia of the trunk is located directly beneath the superficial fascia and both are frequently coalesced. The deep fascia expands deep into the body and encloses the front and the back muscles of the vertebral column. It is frequently double layered, to invest muscles that evolve from the deep fascia of the trunk, such as the latissimus dorsi, major pectoralis, and gluteus maximus muscles. It is not only skeletal muscles that originate from its substance but also tendons, ligaments, aponeuroses, and joints. Hence the deep fascia of the trunk is hard to distinguish from the corresponding epimysium of a specific muscle (Skandalis et al., 2006).

The deep fascia of the trunk can be separated into three layers: the superficial or investing layer, the middle or intermediate layer, and the deep layer. Each layer is split bilaminally to enclose the corresponding muscles.

The three layers of the deep trunk fascia

The superficial or investing layer

The superficial layer separates at the neck to cover the sternocleidomastoid and trapezius muscles. Caudally it extends via the pectoral fascia, the latissimus dorsi fascia, and the gluteus maximus fascia.

The middle or intermediate layer

In the area of the neck the middle layer surrounds the infrahyoidal muscles and elongates caudally in the clavipectoral fascia, the serratus anterior fascia, and the oblique abdominal muscles.

The deep layer

The prevertebral and paravertebral muscles are enclosed by the deep layer, which caudally surrounds the erector spinae and also the iliopsoas muscles.

Deep cervical fascia (DCF)

At the neck the deep fascia is subdivided in several laminae known as superficial or investing lamina (in the superficial layer), pretracheal lamina (in the middle layer), and prevertebral lamina (in the deep layer).

Superficial or investing lamina of the DCF

The superficial lamina covers the neck completely apart from the platysma muscle, which lies on top of it. It is split up to enclose the sternocleidomastoid and the upper trapezius muscles.

The epimysium of these muscles is completely fused with the superficial lamina of the neck fascia. The cranial attachment sites of the superficial lamina are the superior nuchal line and the external occipital protuberance; the two mastoid processes; and the angles and the horizontal portion of the mandible. Caudally the superficial lamina is attached to the manubrium, the clavicles, the acromions, and the spine of the scapula. Inferiorly it extends ventral to the superficial lamina of the pectoralis major muscles, posterior to the lower trapezius muscles, and lateral to the deltoid muscle fascia.

Anteriorly, where it is covered with the platysma muscle, the superficial lamina is thin and is further attached to the hyoid bone. Under the hyoid bone it adheres to the manubrium and to the middle layer, (i.e., the pretracheal lamina). Laterally and posteriorly the superficial lamina is denser than anteriorly.

Posteriorly, after enveloping the trapezius muscles, it unites again and inserts at the posterior tubercle of the atlas and the spinous processes of the cervical vertebrae.

Middle or pretracheal lamina of the DCF

The pretracheal lamina is located in the anterior part of the neck. Triangle-shaped, it runs from the hyoid bone caudally to the upper and the back margins of the manubrium, over two-thirds of the clavicle, following the inferior belly of the omohyoid muscle, which, together with the superior belly of the omohyoid muscle, forms the lateral borders of the pretracheal lamina. Here it coalesces laterally with the superficial lamina. The pretracheal lamina envelops the infrahyoidal muscles (sternohyoid, sternothyroid, thyrohyoid, and omohyoid muscles) and abuts them on each side. Ventrally it is also fused with the superficial lamina. Caudally the pretracheal lamina continues into the subclavia and the endothoracic fascia.

Deep or prevertebral lamina of the DCF

The prevertebral lamina sheathes cylindrically the prevertebral and paravertebral muscles. It inserts at both sides of the nuchal ligament and encloses the deep erector spinae muscles, all the scalenus muscles, as well as the prevertebral muscles (longus capitis, longus colli, rectus capitis lateralis, and anterior). There the prevertebral lamina attaches anteriorly to the ventral surfaces of the transverse processes and the vertebral bodies from C1 to C7. Cranially it is circularlly attached to the cranial base, from the basilar part of the occipital bone over the mastoid processes to the superior nuchal line with the external occipital protuberance. Ventral between both transversal processes and the prevertebral muscles the prevertebral lamina separates, up to its insertion at the first thoracic vertebrae into a superficial and deep lamina, filled with loose connective tissue. The superficial lamina is also termed alar fascia. Beginning at the first thoracic vertebral body the prevertebral fascia descends and blends into the endothoracic fascia. At the caudal cervical region the prevertebral lamina forms a sheath for the brachial plexus and the subclavian artery and vein, where it fuses with the axillary fascia. Laterally to the prevertebral lamina the carotid sheath is located, formed by all laminae of the deep neck fascia. Within the carotid sheath runs the common carotid artery, the internal jugular vein, the vagus nerve, and the deep cervical lymph nodes (Fig. 17.1).

Beginning at the sternum, the clavicles, and the scapular spines, the deep cervical layers continue into the thoracic extension of the trunk fascia, as well as in the fascia of the upper extremity. The trunk fascia descends internally and externally. Internally it is called endothoracic fascia and in its elongation it is called transversalis fascia, iliac fascia, and the psoas major muscle fascia. Externally it encloses the pectoral, trapezius, latissimus dorsi, and lumbosacral muscles, as well as muscle fascia of deeper-located muscles, such as the external intercostal, serratus anterior, quadratus lumborum, and the autochthonous back muscles.

Figure 17.1
Prevertebral lamina

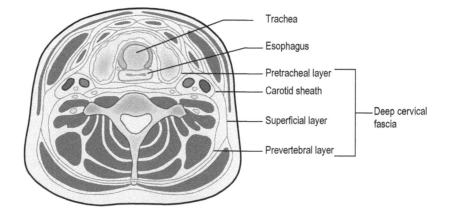

- Trachea
- Esophagus
- Pretracheal layer
- Carotid sheath
- Superficial layer — Deep cervical fascia
- Prevertebral layer

Endothoracic fascia (ETF)

As pointed out earlier, the pretracheal lamina continues anteriorly and the prevertebral lamina posteriorly into the ETF. The ETF lines the rib cage and the internal intercostal muscles, the latter merged with their fiber structures. It not only lines the inner chest wall but also covers the pleural domes, where it is termed suprapleural membrane or Sibson's fascia, and also the diaphragm, where it is termed phrenicopleural fascia. The ETF consists of loose, subserous connective tissue, sporadically it is just one-layered and forms the border with the underlying parietal pleura. Posteriorly it is more of dense and ligamentous structure and adheres with the thoracic ribs. In the region of the first rib, the ETF is attached to the anterior vascular sheath of the subclavian artery and here the cervicothoracic diaphragm is located – a fibrous septum that is also termed fascia or Bourgery's diaphragm. Here is the location of the Cooper's ligaments or suspensory ligaments (costopleural, transversopleural, and vertebropleural ligaments), which are connective tissues that help to maintain the structural integrity of the ETF and the pleura. Anteriorly and posteriorly the ETF is attached to the mediastinal connective tissue. It descends and continues in the transversalis fascia, which will be discussed later in this chapter.

Pectoral fascia (PF)

The major pectoralis muscle is enclosed by a superficial and a deep lamina. The superficial lamina is the elongation of the deep neck fascia. The deep lamina is firmly attached to the periosteum of the clavicle bone and medially to the periosteum of the sternum. The superficial stratum crosses the sternum to fuse with the PF from the other side. The PF is made up of curly collagen fibers that increase in number from cranial to caudal, having an average diameter of 151 μm. The PF runs more or less at a right angle to the muscle bellies. In the mamma area the collagen fiber diameter rises up to 578 μm on average. Intramuscular septa, rising interiorly from the fascia, separates the muscle into fascicles, thus strengthening the fascia. Distally the PF is strengthened with the fibrous offshoots of the rectus sheath and the fascia of the contralateral external oblique muscle. Due to this reinforcement the fibers in the xyphoid process emerge in a specific,

woven pattern. Laterally the PF continues along with the sublayered clavipectoral fascia (CPF) as the axillar fascia.

Clavipectoral fascia (CPF)

The CPF is a strong fibrous sheet, originating from the clavicle bone and enclosing the subclavius and minor pectoral muscles. Cranially the subclavius muscle sheath is reinforced with the coracoclavicular ligament. Ventral of the CPF to the major pectoral muscle arises a thick gap filled with loose connective tissue, enabling locomotion between the pectoral muscle and the CPF. Laterally the CPF fuses with the pectoral muscle and the axillar fascia. Via its attachment with the minor pectoral muscle to the coracoid process the CPF continues in the coracobrachial fascia. From the coracoid process to the first rib, the lateral sheath of the minor pectoral muscle is reinforced with the costocoracoid ligament, thus shaping the border of the ventral thoracic wall to the axilla.

The deep fascia of the abdominal wall

The thoracic fascia descends ventrally and laterally from the abdomen to the transverse processes of vertebral bodies via the oblique and transverse abdominal muscles and the sheath of the rectus abdominis muscle. The PF continues into the fascia of the external oblique abdominal muscle, which (as the most superficial of the three oblique abdominal muscles) lies beneath the superficial abdominal wall fascia, Scarpa's fascia. Its muscle fibers run downward, in a cranial-lateral to caudal-medial direction. Muscle fascia separates the external and internal oblique abdominal muscles, as well as the transversus abdominis and the rectus abdominis muscles, from each other. These fascia are very thin, except the transversalis fascia, which encloses the transverse abdominal muscle. Ventrally the muscles continue to flat, broad tendons, also called aponeuroses, which cross the body midline and fuse with the aponeuroses from the other side, intertwining with each other. In this way the linea alba is built, which runs from the xiphoid process to the symphysis pubis. Around the umbilicus the crossing collagen fibers are circularly arranged and circularly reinforced. The external oblique muscle builds the inguinal ligament between its attachments to the anterior superior iliac spine and to the pubic tubercle.

Laterally from the linea alba the aponeuroses of the three abdominal muscles make up the rectus sheath of the rectus abdominis muscle. The external oblique muscle aponeurosis and the ventral lamina of the internal oblique muscle aponeurosis comprise the front side of the rectus sheath. In the lower quarter of the rectus sheath, at the arcuate line, the transverse abdominal muscle aponeurosis comes to the front, which means that thereafter all three aponeuroses are at the front. Thus, just the transversalis fascia (TF) makes up the dorsal border of the rectus sheath. Above the arcuate line the dorsal lamina of the rectus sheath is composed of the dorsal lamina of the internal oblique muscle aponeurosis, the transversus muscle aponeurosis, and the TF.

Lateral to the abdominal wall, ascending from the iliac crest along the lateral border of the erector spinae muscle, spans a dense raphe, the lateral raphe (Bogduk & Mackintosh, 1984). It is the origin of the internal oblique and the transversus abdominis muscles and in this way it is indirectly coalesced with the thoracolumbar fascia (TLF), which will be described later on.

Transversalis fascia (TF)

The TF is intimately merged with the transversus abdominis muscle and thus indistinguishable from its epimysium. Inferior to the arcuate line the TF separates from the transversus abdominis muscle to shape the dorsal wall of the rectus sheath. The TF internally coats completely the abdominal wall and the transversus abdominis muscle. At the top it covers the diaphragm caudally forming the diaphragm fascia. Posteriorly, where the transversus abdominis and the internal oblique muscle originate from the TLF via the lateral raphe, the TF covers the quadratus lumborum and the psoas muscles. Laterally from the iliac crest the TF merges into the iliac fascia (IF).

Iliac fascia (IF)

The IF sheathes the iliac muscle, the whole internal iliac fossa, and envelops the psoas muscle from its origin downward to its insertion at the minor tro-

chanter. The IF also coats the lumbar plexus. Medially it attaches at the vertebral bodies of the lumbar spine and the basis of the sacrum, caudally to the internal labium of the iliac crest and the inguinal ligament. From the inguinal ligament fibers, the IF continues dorsomedially orientated to the iliopubic eminence and forms the iliopectineal arch, subdividing the area inferior to the inguinal ligament into a medial vascular lacuna and a lateral muscular lacuna. At the top the IF is thin and in the course of descending it increases in strength.

Thoracolumbar fascia (TLF)

The TLF is a construction containing aponeurotic and fascial parts, which are united in order to enclose the paraspinal muscles and stabilize the lumbosacral spine. The transmission of the load of the trunk to the legs is aided by the robust structure of the TLF.

The TLF covers the back muscles of the trunk, starting at the sacrum and extending along the thorax up to the nuchal fascia, acting as origin and insertion locations for muscles.

The posterior layer consists of copious layers of aponeuroses and fascia, originating from numerous muscles. In this way the TLF acts as a retinaculum surrounding the paraspinal muscles of the lumbar and sacral region and extends within the thorax and the neck as the paraspinal fascia, where several trunk and extremity muscles insert. In this way a myofascial belt is created, which is substantially a sophisticated entity of multilayered fascial layers and aponeuroses that embraces the trunk and affects posture, force transmission, and also the external respiration process.

At the lower trunk these aponeurotic tissue layers are shaped in a firm brace, which spreads between the posterior superior iliac spine and extends down to the ischial tuberosities. Several models of the TLF are mentioned and a variety of nomenclatures emerge. Bogduk & Macintosh (1984), Vleeming et al. (1995) and Barker et al. (2007) postulate the TLF as a three-layered model in contrast to other authors in earlier years, such as Gray & Spalteholz in 1923 and Clemente in 1985, who suggest a two-layered model (Willard et al., 2012).

Three-layered model	Two-layered model
Posterior layer	Posterior layer
Medial layer	Anterior layer
Anterior layer	Transversalis fascia

Table 17.1
Models of the thoracolumbar fascia

In both models the posterior layer is identical. The medial layer of the three-layered model corresponds with the anterior layer of the two-layered model. The anterior layer of the three-layered model is the TF of the two-layered model (Table 17.1).

The employment of these two different models often causes confusion, so in this chapter we will refer to the three-layered model as it is the most commonly applied model in research.

The posterior layer consists of two laminae, the superficial and the deep. The superficial lamina is made up of the latissimus dorsi muscle aponeurosis. The deep lamina covers the paraspinal muscles from behind. At the level of L4 the serratus posterior inferior muscle aponeurosis lies in between these two laminae and blends into the superficial lamina.

The medial layer separates the paraspinal and quadratus lumborum muscles.

The anterior layer separates the quadratus lumborum and the psoas muscles and is also considered to be an elongation of the TF. But the anterior layer is much more than just the thin TF; otherwise it would be incapable of withstanding the tension transmission from the abdominal muscles to the TLF.

In this way the paraspinal muscles run through an osteofibrous compartment formed by the vertebral lamina and the deep lamina of the posterior layer of the TLF, which itself is attached to the middle of the spinous processes and is anterior lateral to the transverse processes.

Superficial lamina of the posterior layer

The superficial lamina has a thickness of 0.68 mm and is made up of three collagenous fiber-bundled sublayers: the thin epimysium of the latissimus dorsi muscle, its aponeurosis; and the aponeurosis of the serratus posterior inferior muscle (Willard et al., 2012). Along the thoracic region it declines substantially in thickness. The superficial lamina ascends underneath the trapezius and the rhomboid muscles (being attached to them) and continues cranially in the nuchal fascia. In descending it is attached to the posterior superior iliac spine and merges with the serratus posterior inferior muscle aponeurosis together with the origin of the gluteus maximus muscle. The lateral border of the superficial lamina is built by the continuation of the latissimus dorsi muscle. Its fibers spread into the gluteus maximus and latissimus dorsi muscles, with small parts spreading into the aponeuroses of the oblique external and trapezius muscles. These fibers, for the most part, come from the aponeurosis of the latissimus dorsi muscle, run more horizontally in the superior area, and become more diagonal up to nearly 20–40° from cranial-lateral to caudal-medial direction to its medial attachments at the supraspinal ligament and the spinous processes down to L4.

Under L4/L5 the superficial lamina is loosely attached to the supraspinal ligament, the spinous processes, and the medial sacral crest. Here the fibers cross over the midline of the sacrum and are attached at the sacral bone, the posterior inferior iliac spine, and the iliac crest of the contralateral side. At the sacral area the superficial fascia of the posterior layer continues in the fascia of the gluteus maximus muscle, with the fibers in a crosswise direction, orientated cranial–medial to caudal–lateral, and ends at the medial sacral crest. However, under L4/L5 some fibers cross over the midline and are attached to the posterior superior iliac spine and the iliac crest of the contralateral side. In the area of the iliac crest some fibers are firmly blended into the lateral raphe. Particularly at the level of L4/L5 and sometimes further down, the fibers of the superficial lamina and the gluteus maximus muscle fascia display in a crosswise direction (Fig. 17.2).

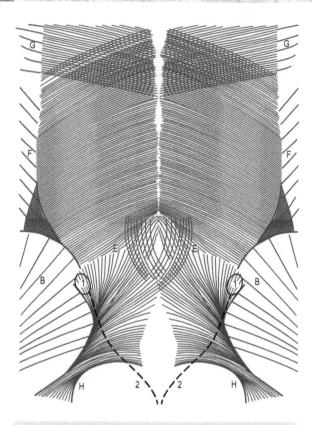

Figure 17.2
The deep layer of the TLF and its attachments. The deep layer of the TLF is a good example of tensional continuity of the myofascial system. This fascia attaches to: **B** gluteus medius; **E** attachments between the deep layer and the erector spinae muscle; **F** the internal oblique; **G** serratus posterior inferior; **H** the sacrotuberous ligament; **1** PSIS; **2** sacrum. Reproduced from Chaitow L., 2014, *Fascial Dysfunction: Manual Therapy Approaches*, by kind permission of Handspring Publishing

Deep lamina of the posterior layer

The deep lamina is attached to the spinous processes of the lumbar vertebrae, the sacrum, and the supraspinal ligament, extending laterally it coats the paraspinal muscles to form a paraspinal retinaculum sleeve (Schuenke et al., 2012). The deep lamina envelops anteriorly up to the lateral edge to join the middle layer, which separates the paraspinal muscle from the quadratus lumborum muscle. Other attachments of the deep lamina are the posterior superior iliac spine, the iliac crest, and the posterior sacroiliac ligament. Laterally the deep lamina fuses over the iliac crest with the gluteus medius muscle aponeurosis. It is located just below the superficial lamina and medial to the posterior superior iliac spine. Both fuse together forming an intermuscular septum to which the gluteus maximus muscle is attached in a bilaterally pennated way, with some fibers crossing over the midline at the level of L5/S1 and continuing in the sacrotuberous ligament (Vleeming et al., 1995). At the sacral area the fibers increase in thickness. Cranially the deep lamina thins out, merging with the posterior inferior serratus muscle aponeurosis at the lower thoracic levels. Overall the deep lamina fibers are orientated from cranial–medial to caudal–lateral with 20–30° relative to horizontal.

The middle layer of the TLF

The middle layer is situated between the quadratus lumborum and the paraspinal muscles. It is a thick, strong aponeurotic tissue originating medially from the tips of the transverse processes, more precisely from their lateral rims. Near the transverse processes the middle layer is approximately 0.63 mm thick, and in other locations it ranges from 0.11 to 1.34 mm (on average 0.56 mm). Cranially the middle layer is attached to the 12th rib. Between the 12th vertebral body and the transverse processes of L1 and L2 it is reinforced by the lumbocostal ligament. Caudally the middle layer is attached to the iliolumbar ligament and the iliac crest. Ascending laterally from the iliac crest up to the 12th rib it merges with the transverse abdominal muscle aponeurosis, where it is joined caudally by the internal oblique muscle. Most of the collagen fibers of the middle layer run in a caudal–lateral direction at 20–30° relative to the horizontal (Barker et al., 2007). Between the transverse processes the collagenous bundles consist of a fiber-free zone, through which the posterior rami of the spinal nerves penetrate.

The anterior layer of the TLF

The anterior layer runs from the lateral raphe to the medial, covering the quadratus lumborum muscle at the front, and proceeding to the distal ends of the transverse processes of the lumbar vertebral bodies and further down between the sides of the psoas and quadratus lumborum muscles. The anterior layer consists of a thin, almost membranous structure, with an average thickness of 0.10 mm (Barker & Briggs, 1999; Barker et al., 2007). Caudally it is attached to the iliac crest. At the cranial end the anterior layer forms the arcuate lateral ligament, to which the diaphragm is attached.

Conclusion of the TLF

The TLF forms the keystone of the lumbar region and the sacroiliac joints for load transmission between the spine and the legs. Through the attachments of latissimus dorsi and gluteus maximus muscles at the posterior layer of the TLF, forces can be transferred to the opposite side.

The middle layer has an important force-transmission function due to the attachment of the transverse abdominal muscle as well as the internal oblique muscle. Through the interaction of the aforementioned muscles, together with others, the TLF features prominently in mastering the force transmission in cranial, caudal, transversal, and diagonal directions.

References and further reading

Anderhuber, F., Fanghänel, J., Nitsch, R., Pera, F., Waldeyer, A. (2012) *Waldeyer – Anatomie des Menschen. 19., Aufl.* Berlin: de Gruyter (de Gruyter: Studium).

Barker, P. J., Hapuarachchi, K. S., Ross, J. A., Sambaiew, E., Ranger, T. A., Briggs, C. A. (2014): Anatomy and biomechanics of gluteus maximus and the thoracolumbar fascia at the sacroiliac joint. *Clinical anatomy.* 27(2):234–240.

Barker, P. J., Briggs, C. A. (1999) Attachments of the posterior layer of the lumbar fascia. *Spine.* 24(17):1757–1764.

Barker, P. J., Urquhart, D. M., Story, I. H., Fahrer, M., Briggs, C. A. (2007): The middle layer of lumbar fascia and attachments to lumbar transverse processes: implications for segmental control and fracture. *Eur Spine J.* 16(12):2232–2237.

Bogduk, N., Macintosh, J. E. (1984): The applied anatomy of the thoracolumbar fascia. In: *Spine.* 9(2):164–170.

Kumka, M., Bonar, J. (2012) Fascia: a morphological description and classification system based on a literature review. *J Can Chiropr Assoc.* 56(3): 179–191.

Leuffen, Sascha (2014) *Intrathorakale faszien und das sympathische nervensystem.* [S.l.]: Av Akademikerverlag.

Schleip, R., Findley, T. W., Chaitow, L., Huijing P. A. (2012) Fascia: The Tensional Network of the Human Body: The Science and Clinical Applications in Manual and Movement Therapy, Churchill Livingstone.

Schuenke, M. D., Vleeming, A., Van Hoof, T., Willard, F. H. (2012) A description of the lumbar interfascial triangle and its relation with the lateral raphe: anatomical constituents of load transfer through the lateral margin of the thoracolumbar fascia. *Journal of Anatomy.* 221(6):568–576.

Skandalakis, P. N., Zoras, O., Skandalakis J. E., Mirilas, P. (2006) Transversalis, endoabdominal, endothoracic fascia: who's who? *Am Surg.* 72(1):16–18.

Stecco, L., Stecco, C., Day, J. A., Schleip, R. (2009) *Fascial Manipulation. Practical Part.* Padova: Piccin.

Vleeming A. et al. 1995. The posterior layer of the thoracolumbar fascia: its function in load transfer from spine to legs. *Spine.* 20:753–758.

Willard, F. H., Vleeming, A., Schuenke, M. D., Danneels, L., Schleip, R. (2012) The thoracolumbar fascia: anatomy, function and clinical considerations. *Journal of Anatomy.* 221(6):507–536.

FASCIAL ANATOMY OF THE LIMBS

Andrzej Pilat

Introduction

In classical anatomy textbooks the topographic description of the fascia prevails and fascia is named specifically in relation to the other structures (mainly muscles, e.g., latissimus dorsi fascia, deltoid fascia, bicipital fascia) with which it is associated topographically. Although this analysis is topographically accurate, at the same time it is abstract, isolated, and has a limited functional correlation between anatomical elements. Anatomical studies on embalmed cadavers do not allow us to fully understand the conditions, connections, and continuity of the fascia and its biomechanical interrelationships. This chapter focuses on the continuity of the fascial system in the extremities and discusses the most relevant anatomical aspects. For a complete topographical analysis it is advisable to consult the classic anatomy texts. All the photographs of anatomical samples presented in this chapter were taken in the course of dissections carried out on cadavers that had not been embalmed.

Fascia taxonomy

From a clinical approach, it is suggested that fascia be described as a system of anatomical and functional continuity, interconnection, and integration. Thus, fascia can be related to movements within and between muscles, including the vascular and neural structures with which the fascial system acts as an uninterrupted communicational network. Considering the basic functional analysis, we recognize the existence of the superficial and deep fascia. The deep fascia can be subdivided into myofascia, viscerofascia, and meninges. The anatomical descriptions in this chapter focus on the functional aspects of the myofascia.

Superficial fascia: construction and mechanics

The superficial fascia is known by different names: subcutaneous fascia (Rouviere & Delmas, 2005), cellular cutaneous tissue (Testut & Latarjet, 2007), or subcutaneous adipofascial tissue (Avelar, 1989). Its characteristics are analyzed mainly in connection with plastic surgery and the skin-healing process (Congdon et al., 1946; Markmann et al., 1987; Avelar, 1989). The superficial fascia is the major anatomical structure, though the lack of an exhaustive anatomical and biomechanical analysis makes it difficult to clarify its precise role in body movements. Superficial fascia has the following key features:

- firm attachment to the skin
- forms a functional whole of protection, lubrication, and motion control
- traps and controls superficial fat
- acts as a store of nutrient reserves in the fat nodules
- fills irregularities at subcutaneous level (wrinkles, cellulitis) (Kapandji, 2012)
- has anatomy that differs depending on gender, amount of fat, and body region
- represents a continuous network extending from subdermal level to the deep (muscles) fascia
- construction consists of two continuous layers – superficial and deep (Fig. 18.1) (Fernández-de-las-Peñas & Pilat, 2012; Nakajima et al., 2004).

Deep fascia: construction and mechanics

Deep fascia has the following key features:

- contains collagen fibers organized in the form of undulating bundles

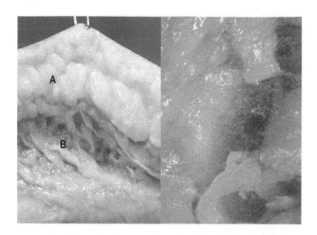

Figure 18.1
A close-up image of superficial fascia in the anterior aspect of the thigh in an unembalmed cadaver dissection of a person with a high percentage of body fat. Left: **A** superficial layer of superficial fascia (honeycomb fascia) with a large amount of fatty nodes; **B** deep layer of superficial fascia with flat fatty nodes. Right: close-up of fascial connections inside the deep layer. Note the continuity of the fine network of fascial tissue that includes the fat nodes

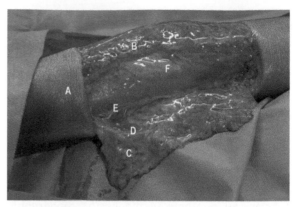

Figure 18.2
Cubital fossa region. **A** skin; **B** superficial fascia with fat nodes; **C** superficial fascia with fat nodes (inner view). Note the fascia connection between fat nodes; **D** cutaneous vein; **E** cutaneous nerve; **F** deep fascia. Note the morphological differences between the superficial and deep fascia

Anatomical considerations relating to the continuity of the fascial system of the upper extremity

Introduction

The anatomical continuity of the fascial system of the upper limb, initiating at the cervical area, can be observed at the superficial and deep layers.

Superficial fascia

The superficial layer is located just below the skin (Fig. 18.3). At the anterior aspect it involves the neck and continues up to the hand without any interruption. Along the shoulder and arm region its fat level is high, particularly in women. In the forearm, the fat level varies depending on the build of the individual, and it gradually reduces along its span. In the hand's dorsal region the fascia is loose and thin, which enables considerable mobility for flexing the fingers in their manipulative functions. The fascia of the palmar region adheres firmly to the skin, though as it runs through the thenar and hypothenar eminences, the superficial fascia is looser and thinner. That distribution facilitates the manipulative and gripping action

- also contains elastic fibers
- consists of several layers
- density and direction of fiber varies between layers and also between different parts of the same layer
- layers are separated by loose connective tissue that contains thin fat nodes – this structure allows all layers to slide.

Morphological and biomechanical characteristics

Figure 18.2 shows morphological differences between the superficial and deep fascia on the upper extremity. The superficial fascia is characterized as a highly hydrated structure with large amounts of fat nodes. In the deep fascia the fibrous structure stands out. The relationship between fascia, blood vessels, and nerves can also be observed.

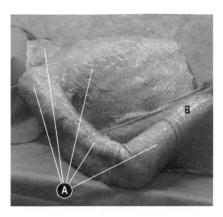

Figure 18.3
Superficial fascia continuity over the cervical, pectoral, deltoid, brachial, and antebrachial area. **A** superficial fascia with fat nodes; **B** the skin (inner view)

of both eminences. There is no movement between the skin and the superficial layer (Pilat, 2015).

Deep fascia

The main dynamic fascial link, between the cervical region and the upper limb, is created through the deep cervical fascia that, in its lower span, extends the length of the upper limb (Fig. 18.4) (Pilat, 2015).

Shoulder girdle fascial system

Anatomical attachments

Anteriorly from the cervical area, the deep fascia is continuous across the clavicle, then becomes thinner toward the pectoralis major area and surrounds the pectoralis major muscle. In its medium span it is firmly inserted into the sternum and continues, covering the front of the pectoralis major muscle, enfolding the lower edge, and supporting the inner face (see Fig. 18.4). Caudally, the pectoralis major fascia is continuous with the fascia of the anterior abdominal wall and toward the axilla it merges with the fascia of the latissimus dorsi muscle. In the intermediate plane, below the clavicle, fascia enfolds the subclavius muscle, continuing as clavipectoral fascia (Fig. 18.5), which is suspended on the front edge of the clavicle, the coracoid process, and the coracoclavicular ligament. It continues over the front part of the sternum and joins the deltoid fascia laterally. Caudally, it expands from its lower edge to enfold the pectoralis minor muscle, and in its deep span it is firmly integrated into the intercostal muscles and the ribs (see Fig. 18.5). Its lower end continues to the axillary fossa where it joins the deep sheet of the pectoralis fascia. Below the lower edge of pectoralis major, fascia becomes the serratus anterior fascia, which manifests as a very thin structure, evenly covering the entire muscle surface (see Fig. 18.5). Laterally, it is continuous with the axillary fascia, which in turn becomes the fascia of the latissimus dorsi muscle.

Morphological and biomechanical characteristics

The pectoralis fascia forms a thin sheet, which is firmly attached to muscle belly and deployed over the front of the thorax. From the front sheet intermuscular septa emerge and penetrate the muscle belly, creating spaces for muscle fascicles. The clavipectoral fascia is perforated

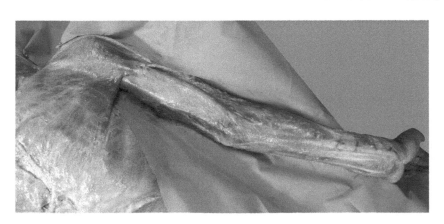

Figure 18.4
Deep fascia continuity over the cervical, pectoral, deltoid, brachial, and antebrachial area in an unembalmed cadaver dissection

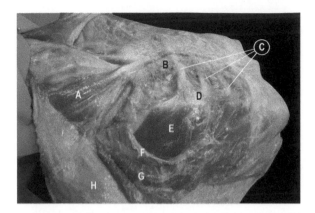

Figure 18.5
Deep fascia continuity over the cervical and pectoral areas. **A** cervical fascia; **B** sternum; **C** ribs; **D** intercostal space; **E** pectoralis minor; **F** clavipectoral fascia; **G** pectoralis major (inner view); **H** superficial fascia (inner view)

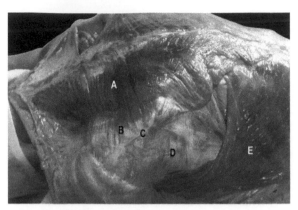

Figure 18.6
Deep fascia at the dorsal aspect of the shoulder girdle. **A** trapezius; **B** supraspinatus fascia; **C** spine of the scapula; **D** infraspinatus fascia; **E** latissimus dorsi

by a lower pectoral nerve, cephalic vein, and thoracoacromial artery (branch of axillary artery).

Axillary fascia

Anatomical attachments

Axillary fascia forms the axillar base. Throughout its surface it spans the lower border of the pectoralis fascia toward the lower end of the teres major and latissimus dorsi muscles. Its forms a sort of square, suspended from the lower border of the pectoralis minor, running through the axillary edge of the scapula, entering the insertions of the subscapularis, teres major, and teres minor and finally approaching the glenoid cavity. In its medial span, it approaches the serratus anterior (Testut & Latarjet, 2007; Bochenek & Reicher, 1997; Rouviere & Delmas, 2005).

Axillary fascia compartments

At the posterior aspect, the superficial fascia surrounds the shoulder girdle area and continues over the trunk. At the deep layer the cervical fascia continues toward the spine of the scapula, the acromion process, then links toward the deltoid, the trapezius, the infraspinatus, the teres minor, the teres major, and the latissimus dorsi muscles (Fig. 18.6). Over the trapezius muscle, fascia is continuous with the superficial sheet of the deep cervical fasciae in its posterior length. From the spine of the scapula, it becomes the trapezius fascia and covers middle and lower fibers. The deepest layer involves the supraspinatus, levator scapulae, rhomboid, and subscapularis. The supraspinatus fascia enfolds the supraspinatus muscle, enclosing it together with the osseous channel of the supraspinatus fossa within an osteofascial compartment (Rouviere & Delmas, 2005).

The infraspinatus fascia represents a very resistant structure that throughout its length – from the spine to the scapula – provides support to the infraspinatus, teres minor, and teres major muscles, adjoining its insertions (Rouviere & Delmas, 2005). It is firmly united to the medial and lateral borders of the scapula with strong and multidirectional fiber connections. The latissimus dorsi fascia is continuous with the fascia of the teres major muscle and is strengthened inferiorly by the deep layer of the axillar fascia. The fascia of the levator of the scapulae muscle is a thin sheet that accompanies the muscle throughout its length (Bochenek & Reicher, 1997).

The fascia of the subscapularis muscle covers the area of the subscapularis fossa separating the subscapularis and the serratus muscles. The rhomboid fascia is more robust in the lower end, where it is continuous with that of the trapezius and the latissimus dorsi muscles.

Brachial fascia

Anatomical attachments

From the shoulder complex and the axillar fossa, the fascial system enables effective integration transitioning into the brachial fascia, antebrachial fascia, and finally to the hand structures. The brachial fascia forms a strong layer that envelops, like a glove, the structures of the arm (Thiel, 2000). In the superior end (see Fig. 18.4) it is continuous with the pectoralis, the deltoid, the axillar, and the dorsal fascia. Then it continues with the thoracolumbar fascia (Testut & Latarjet, 2007; Rouviere & Delmas, 2005), thus linking the dynamics of the scapular girdle with the upper limb.

Morphological and biomechanical characteristics

Stecco et al. (2008) suggested that the presence of fascial expansions strengthens the anatomical design of the brachial fascia and places selective tension on it, which may increase the effectiveness of the arm's movement.

Brachial fascia compartments

The brachial fascia expands on its inner side into two fibrous, transversely oriented septa, thus forming the anterior/flexor and posterior/extensor compartments (Rouviere & Delmas, 2005). The anterior compartment involves biceps brachii, brachialis, and coracobrachialis muscles. The posterior compartment contains the triceps brachii and anconeus muscles.

Antebrachial fascia

Anatomical attachments

The antebrachial fascia arises as a direct continuity of the brachial fascia at its lower length and surrounds the forearm. In the dorsal aspect of the limb there is a direct link between the triceps muscle and the antebrachial fascia. One part of the triceps tendon is firmly inserted into the olecranon and the other continues into the antebrachial fascia. On the ventral surface, there is a direct continuity through to the bicipital fascia. The internal expansions of the antebrachial fascia wrap around the individual muscles of the forearm.

Morphological and biomechanical characteristics

The antebrachial fascia is denser at the back compared to the ventral surface and its density also decreases distally. On the ventral surface there is a very special connection between the brachial and the antebrachial fascia through the bicipital aponeurosis or lacertus fibrosus (Fig. 18.7). The fascial structure extends in a fan shape (Testut & Latarjet, 2007) from the lower tendon of the biceps brachii muscle and, crossing the joint line, is continuous with the antebrachial fascia at its proximal end. Then, it is inserted into the cubital region of the common mass of the

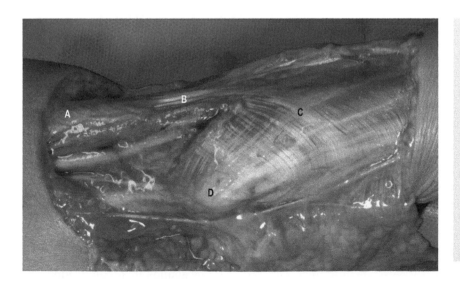

Figure 18.7
The elbow complex region of the left upper limb. **A** biceps brachii muscle; **B** biceps brachii tendon expansion to the lacertus fibrosus; **C** lacertus fibrosus (bicipital aponeurosis) expansion to the antebrachial fascia. Note the direction of the collagen fibers; **D** medial epicondyle

epitrochlear muscles (Blemker et al., 2005; Chew & Giuffrè, 2005). The lacertus fibrosus connection is perhaps one of the best examples of dynamic links, where the muscle contraction is transmitted directly from the fascia, to the fascia, reinforcing the bone–tendon connection.

Antebrachial fascia compartments

The forearm contains 17 muscles that cross the elbow joint. There are no 'intermuscular' septa per se; anyway every muscle is wrapped in its own envelope. These envelopes are mechanically inter-related via connections between the muscle epimysia. However, there are two recognizable compartments: the flexor compartment and the extensor compartment. The flexor compartment contains the following muscles: flexor carpi radialis, palmaris longus, flexor carpi ulnaris, pronator teres, flexor digitorum superficialis, flexor digitorum profundus, flexor pollicis longus, and pronator quadratus. The extensor compartment contains: brachioradialis, extensor carpi radialis longus, extensor carpi radialis brevis, extensor carpi ulnaris, anconeus, extensor digitorum, extensor digiti minimi, abductor pollicis longus, extensor pollicis brevis, extensor indicis, and supinator muscles.

Fascia of the hand

The palmar fascia extends as a fan and forms a direct continuance of the antebrachial fascia. It is firmly attached to the skin. It is a thick structure reinforced by the long palmar muscle. Laterally, it continues to the tenar and hypotenar eminences and manifests as a thin structure (Fig. 18.8). The deep fibers of the palmar aponeurosis relate to terminal branches of the median nerve and the superficial branch of the ulnar nerve. The dorsal fascia of the hand is continuous with that of the forearm. It covers the tendons of the extensor muscles and becomes thicker in the form of the extensor retinaculum over a transversal span of fibers. The main function of the retinaculum is to assist the extensors' tendons in accurate functional positioning, and also to avoid them becoming loose when contracted (Testut & Latarjet, 2007).

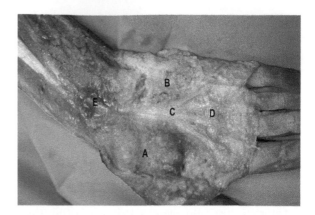

Figure 18.8
Palmar fascia. **A** thenar fascia; **B** hypothenar fascia; **C** palmar aponeurosis; **D** transverse fascicle of palmar aponeurosis; **E** tendon of palmaris longus

Anatomical considerations relating to the continuity of the fascial system of the lower extremity

Introduction

Analysis of the continuity of the fascial system in the lower extremities leads us to consider the anatomical links to the maintenance of body weight and the optimization of daily activities, in relation to the bipedal position and locomotion. The most important structure of this complex is the thoracolumbar fascia (TLF) (Fig. 18.9). Anatomically, the TLF fascia is the largest body aponeurotic structure and dynamic bridge connection between the trunk and limbs. At its superficial level it is connected to the latissimus dorsi and contralateral gluteus maximus muscles. This connection is expressed in the activities of locomotion and trunk stabilization (Carvalhais et al., 2013). Wood Jones (1944) considers that the topography and dynamics of fascia of the lower extremities is linked with the ectoskeletal function relating to the upright position of the human body. Therefore, the architectural orientation of the fascial system of the lower extremities is determined by its weight-bearing function.

Superficial fascia

The superficial fascia is firmly attached to the skin. It is characterized by abundant vascularization and

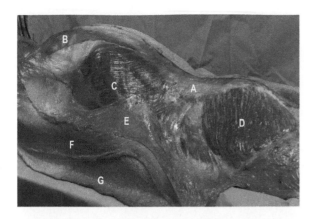

Figure 18.9

Thoracolumbar fascia. **A** thoracolumbar fascia; **B** trapezius **C** latissimus dorsi; **D** gluteus maximus; **E** deep fascia (inner view); **F** superficial fascia (inner view); **G** skin (inner view)

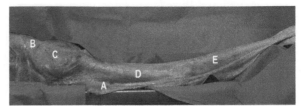

Figure 18.10

Deep fascia of the lower extremity. **A** skin with superficial fascia (inner view). Deep fascia continuity from the back region **(B)**, through to the gluteal fascia **(C)**, fascia lata **(D)**, and crural fascia **(E)** to the foot

innervation and also by a high fat content. Covering the thoracic and lumbar areas, it continues to the iliac crest. Subsequently it runs the length of the entire lower extremity up to the end of the foot structure. Anteriorly, it continues through the pectoral and abdominal region to the inguinal area. It then becomes the fascia of the thigh and leg and continues to the dorsum of the foot.

Deep fascia

The deep fascia manifests as a fibrous structure following a continuous path from the inguinal region and iliac crest to the foot structure without interruption. Throughout its length, depending on topography, it is named gluteal fascia, fascia lata, crural fascia, or fascia of the foot (Fig. 18.10).

Gluteal fascia

Anatomical attachments

As mentioned earlier, at the back, the superficial layer of the thoracolumbar fascia is continuous with the gluteal fascia, which covers the gluteus medius and gluteus maximus muscles. Proximally, it is attached to the iliac crest, sacrum, and coccyx and distally becomes fascia lata (Fig. 18.11).

Morphological and biomechanical characteristics

At the proximal portion, the gluteal fascia is a dense and fibrous structure covering the anterior part of the gluteus medius and the proximal part of the gluteus maximus muscles. The presence of loose connective tissue between both muscles facilitates the sliding process during movement (see Fig. 18.11).

Gluteal fascia compartments

The gluteus maximus muscle is surrounded by two sheets of gluteal fascia. The superficial sheet is thin, firmly attached to the muscle mass, and embedded by the fat nodules. It emits septa that penetrate muscle belly, creating spaces for their bundles. The deep sheet also emits fibrous septa that compartmentalize muscle belly. A third sheet is located at a deeper level and this covers the surface of the sacrotuberous ligament and also the piriformis, gemellus superior, obturator internus, gemellus inferior and quadratus femoris muscles (Fig. 18.12) (Testut & Latarjet, 2007; Bochenek & Reicher, 1997; Rouviere & Delmas, 2005).

Fascia lata

Anatomical attachments

The fascia lata surrounds the thigh. Anteriorly, it starts at the inguinal ligament and, continuing along the thigh, is inserted into the patella and tibia (Fig. 18.13). Posteriorly, it is continuous with the gluteal fascia (see Fig. 18.9). Laterally, at the iliotibial tract it forms a sheet

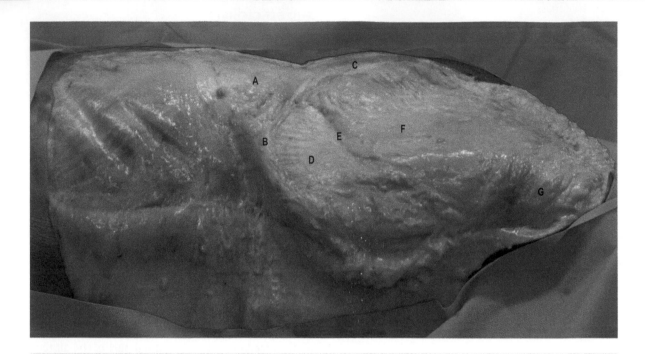

Figure 18.11

Continuity of deep fascia on the upper part of the lower extremity (close-up view). Note the fibrous appearance of the deep fascial tissue. **A** thoracolumbar fascia; **B** iliac crest; **C** sacrum; **D** gluteal fascia of the gluteus medius; **E** boundary between the gluteus medius and the gluteus maximus; **F** gluteal fascia of the gluteus maximus; **G** thigh region (fascia latae)

of greater thickness and resistance. It continues in the outer lip of the iliac crest and in the space between the tensor fascia latae and gluteus maximus muscles and above the gluteus medius muscle (continuing the path of the gluteal fascia). Then, laterally, it continues to the greater trochanter, bypassing the knee-joint level, and is inserted into the lateral border of the patella, the patellar ligament, and the lateral condyle of the tibia (Rouviere & Delmas, 2005).

Morphological and biomechanical characteristics

Fascia lata represents a thick fibrous sheet with aponeurotic appearance. The fact that the gluteus maximus and tensor fascia latae muscles are mainly inserted into the deep fascia rather than into the bone maximizes their mechanical efficiency (Benjamin, 2009).

Fascia lata compartments

From the deep surface of the fascia latae originate two intermuscular septa (lateral and medial), which continue toward the femur and, forming compartments, divide muscles and also the femoral vessels into groups along their longitudinal path. The lateral septum is inserted into the gluteal tuberosity and the lateral lip of the linea aspera. It is located between the vastus lateralis muscle and the short head of the biceps femoris muscles, thus defining the lateral compartment space. The lateral/gluteal compartment of the thigh contains: tensor fasciae latae, gluteus maximus, gluteus medius, gluteus minimis, piriformis, superior and inferior gemellus, and quadratus femoris muscles, and the obturator internus tendon. Posteriorly, it includes the continuity between the sacrotuberous ligament and the tendon of the long head of the biceps femoris muscle, as well as the path of the sciatic nerve. The medial intermuscular septum is

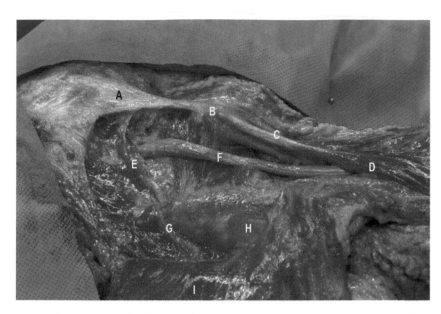

Figure 18.12
The gluteal fascia (deepest compartment).
A sacrotuberous ligament; **B** sciatic tuberosity; **C** biceps femoris (long head tendon); **D** biceps femoris. (long head belly); **E** piriformis; **F** sciatic nerve; **G** great trochanter; **H** iliotibial tract; **I** gluteus maximus (inner view)

inserted into the medial lip of the linea aspera of the femur and is located between the vastus medialis and medial thigh muscles, thus defining the anterior compartment space. The anterior/extensor compartment of the thigh contains the quadriceps femoris and the sartorius muscles. In some places these septum merge with ligaments (iliopsoas fascia with the inguinal ligament) or tendons (fascia of the tensor fascia latae with its tendinous sheet) (Benjamin, 2009).

Knee joint and popliteal fossa segment

At the level of the knee joint, the fibrous stabilizing structure of the patella forms a multilevel and multidirectional complex web. It relates mainly to the position

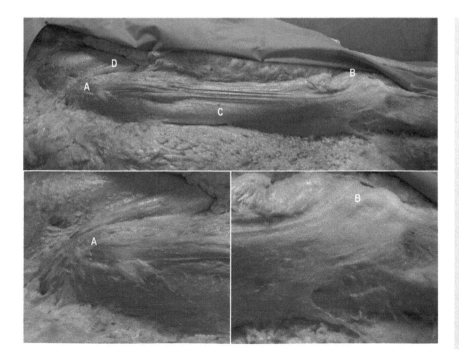

Figure 18.13
Top: lateral aspect of the thigh in an unembalmed cadaver dissection. Note the lines of tension on the iliotibial tract (an extremely strong, tough, and avascular fibrous structure). **A** anterior superior iliac spine; **B** patella; **C** iliotibial tract; **D** inguinal canal. Bottom left: close-up of proximal portion. **A** iliotibial tract: proximal insertion in the outer lip of the iliac crest. Bottom right: close-up of distal portion. **B** iliotibial tract: distal insertion

of the patella in between the quadriceps tendon, the infrapatellar ligament and the fascia latae. This system also assists in the control of lateral patella movements. Fascia creates – in the form of a roof – a system for protecting the nerves and vessels passing through the popliteal fossa. The most important of these is the tibial nerve, which is protected by an abundant layer of loose connective tissue containing a considerable amount of fat nodules (Benjamin, 2009).

Crural fascia

Anatomical attachments

The crural fascia forms a tubular investment of the leg, which incompletely surrounds its structures. It initiates through the dense insertion, into the anterior edge of the tibia, merging with its periosteum. It then surrounds the leg and ends at the posterior edge of the tibia. Thus it does not cover the anteromedial aspect of the tibia. In this zone, the deep fascia is missing and is covered only by the superficial fascial plane. At the proximal end, the crural fascia is continuous with the fascia lata, starting at the head of the fibula, patella, condyles, and tuberosity of tibia. It continues distally as the fascia of the foot (Bochenek & Reicher, 1997).

Morphological and biomechanical characteristics

The crural fascia is characterized by its fibrous appearance, being a multilevel and multidirectional construction of fibers. The fibers usually have a longitudinal path, intersecting with the oblique and transverse fibers. The arrangement of the collagen fibers gives the crural fascia its anisotropic characteristics, thus enabling the positioning of the foot. It also facilitates the protection of nerve structures, such as the superficial peroneal nerve (Fig. 18.14).

Crural fascia compartments

From the inner side of the fascia of the leg begins an intermuscular septa (anterior and posterior), which eventually is inserted into the fibula. Both septa, together with the interosseous membrane, form compartments that define and control the position of the leg muscles. The anterior septa are fixed at the anterior edge of the fibula and the posterior septa are fixed at the fibula's posterolateral edge. The third divisive structure, the interosseous membrane, links

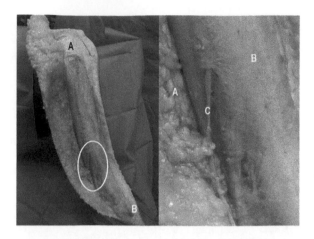

Figure 18.14
Anterolateral aspect of the crural fascia of the right leg from an unembalmed cadaver dissection. Left: **A** anterolateral aspect of the knee joint; **B** dorsal aspect of the foot. Right: close-up view. **A** superficial fascia with fat (inner view); **B** crural, deep fascia (note its fibrous structure); **C** superficial peroneal nerve

the tibia and fibula. Through these divisions three compartments are formed: anterior, lateral and posterior (divided into deep and superficial). The anterior compartment contains the following muscles: tibialis anterior, extensor hallucis longus, extensor digitorum longus and fibularis tertius. The lateral compartment contains the fibularis longus and fibularis brevis muscles. The deep posterior compartment contains the tibialis posterior, flexor hallucis longus, flexor digitorum longus, and popliteus muscles. Finally, the superficial posterior compartment contains the gastrocnemius, soleus, and plantaris muscles (Bochenek & Reicher, 1997).

Fascia of the foot

At its distal end, the crural fascia becomes the fascia of the foot. It forms the investment of the foot (Fig. 18.15). In the posterior aspect of the leg the fibrous aponeurotic expansion from the gastrocnemius muscles and the long path of the Achilles tendon with progressive densification of the fibers can be observed. In the dissection of the plantar fascia it seems that the Achilles tendon and the plantar fascia form an interrupted continuum,

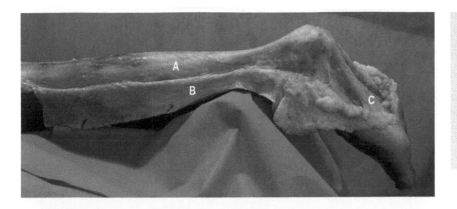

Figure 18.15
Crural and foot fascia from an unembalmed cadaver dissection. **A** posterior aspect of crural fascia; **B** superficial fascia and skin (inner view); **C** plantar fascia

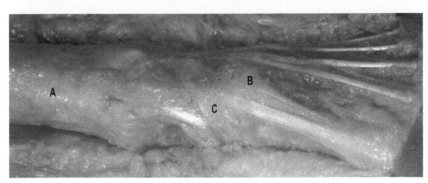

Figure 18.16
Dorsal aspect of the leg and dorsum of the foot in an unembalmed cadaver dissection. **A** crural fascia; **B** foot fascia; **C** inferior extensor retinaculum

by the periosteum of the calcaneus, with which both structures are merged. The fascia path ends at the sole, where it forms the plantar aponeurosis.

At the distal end of the crural fascia appear three groups of retinacula (flexors, extensors, and the peroneal) that fix the relationship of the muscles with the skeleton. Extensor (superior and inferior) retinaculum controls the position of the tibialis anterior, extensor hallucis longus, and extensor digitorum longus muscles (Fig. 18.16). The flexor retinaculum controls the position of the tibial posterior, flexor digitorum longuss, and flexor hallucis muscles. The peroneal retinaculum holds the long and short peroneal muscles.

References

Avelar J. 1989. Regional distribution and behavior of the subcutaneous tissue concerning selection and indication for liposuction. *Aesthet Plast Surg.* 13:155–162.

Benjamin M. 2009. The fascia of the limbs and back—a review. *J Anat.* 214(1):1–18.

Blemker S. S., Pinsky P. M., Delp S. L. 2005. A 3D model of muscle reveals the causes of nonuniform strains in the biceps brachii. *J Biomech.* 38:657–665.

Bochenek A., Reicher M. 1997. Anatomia czlowieka. PZWL: Warszawa.

Carvalhais V. O., Ocarino Jde M., Araújo V. L. et al. 2013. Myofascial force transmission between the latissimus dorsi and gluteus maximus muscles: an in vivo experiment. *J Biomech.* 46:1003–1007.

Chew M. L., Giuffrè B. 2005. Disorders of the distal biceps brachii tendon. *Radiographics.* 25:1227–1237.

Congdon E. D., Edson J., Yanitelli S. 1946. Gross structure of subcutaneous layer of anterior and lateral trunk in the male. *Am J Anatomy.* 79:399–429.

Fernández-de-las-Peñas C., Pilat A. 2012. Chapter 11.1 Soft tissue manipulation approaches to chronic pelvic pain (external). In: Chaitow L. Lovegrove Jones R. (eds) *Chronic Pelvic Pain and Dysfunction: Practical Physical Medicine.* Edinburgh: Elsevier.

Kapandji A. I. 2012. Le système conjonctif, grand unificateur de l'organisme. *Annales de Chirurgie Plastique Esthétique.* 57(5):507–514.

Markmann B., Barton F. E. 1987. Anatomy of the subcutaneous tissue of the trunk and lower extremity. *Plastic Reconst Surg.* 80:248–254.

Nakajima H., Imanishi N., Minabe T. et al. 2004. Anatomical study of subcutaneous adipofascial tissue: a concept of the protective adipofascial system (PAFS) and lubricant adipofascial system (LAFS). *Scand J Plast Reconstr Surg Hand Surg.* 38(5):261–266.

Pilat A. 2015. Chapter 63 Myofascial induction approaches. In: Fernández-de-las-Peñas C., Cleland J. A., Dommerholt J. (eds) *Manual Therapy for Musculoskeletal Pain Syndromes: An Evidence- and Clinical-Informed Approach*. London: Elsevier.

Rouviere H., Delmas A. 2005. *Anatomía humana.* Masson: Barcelona.

Stecco C., Porzionato A., Macchi V. et al. 2008. The expansions of the pectoral girdle muscles onto the brachial fascia: morphological aspects and spatial disposition. *Cells Tiss Organs.* 188:320–329.

Testut L., Latarjet A. 2007. *Compendio de anatomía descriptiva*. Masson, Madrid.

Thiel W. 2000. *Atlas fotográfico de anatomía práctica. Volumen I, abdomen y extremidad inferior.* Springer-Verlag Ibérica, Barcelona.

Wood Jones F. 1944. *Structure and Function as Seen in the Foot.* London: Baillière, Tindall and Cox.

FASCIAL ANATOMY OF THE VISCERA

Andrea Pasini, Antonio Stecco, Carla Stecco

Introduction

The word 'anatomy' comes from the Greek ανατομὴ, *anatomè*, meaning 'dissection', and is from ανά (*anà*) meaning 'between', and τέμνω (*tèmno*) meaning 'cut'. The study of anatomy and anatomy textbooks is the result of the author's ability to observe the human body, to represent it using drawings and models, and to give an interpretation of what he has seen. This is the reason why there are so many different interpretations in the literature. Anatomy textbooks focus on fascia as it relates to anatomy, different names are used for the same structures, and the same fascia has different names depending on the area and is described in different ways depending on the author, etc. This means it is impossible to identify the continuity of the visceral fascia as well as its precise organization. Fascial continuity will be the first key concept of this chapter. To understand the second key concept, we have to go back for a moment to the definition of 'anatomy', understood to mean a pure representation of dissections. The 'static' view of fascia, as tissue for filling and support, is inadequate today. This is verified by published studies and articles,[1] and the increasing recognition of the importance of fascial tissue in relation to motor coordination and proprioception.[2,3] To better organize and understand the continuity of this tissue it is necessary to link the practical (dissections) and theoretical (articles, studies) knowledge to the *function* of fascia. In this way, a new concept of 'functional anatomy of the fasciae' is born that includes not only images, but also the physiology of fasciae. Only by joining the concept of fascial continuity to the 'function' (from the Latin funcio + -onis, derived from fungi, meaning 'fulfill') is it possible to understand why some anatomical connections exist and what their role is.

The biomechanical model described in this chapter aims to provide the key to interpreting internal fasciae and, above all, to understanding their function.

Function and subdivision of internal fasciae

The proper functioning of each organ, be it viscera, a gland, or a vessel, is strictly connected to its own mobility and motility.[4] It is easy to imagine the concept of motility if you think about the intestinal tract: during the passage of food, the walls contract to ensure normal peristalsis, but the same thing happens, for example, to the glands as they secrete a hormone and contract to allow the squeezing of ducts. In contrast, an organ's mobility is the ability of the organ to move in the space within the cavity of the body, and the smaller glands, such as the prostate, have their own mobility.[5] There are several studies that demonstrate that in cases of pathology or dysfunction of an organ its mobility is altered,[6,7,8] and some studies also demonstrate that the fascia related to the organ is altered when there is a dysfunction.[9,10] Internal fasciae have the task of managing and coordinating these two functions (motility and mobility) but, as these are two completely different kinds of movement, fascia will change according to the function. Combining this hypothesis with what has been found in anatomical dissection, we can see that each organ has a thinner fascia that surrounds it, closely adherent; and another fascia that connects it to other organs or to the muscular fasciae of the trunk. Therefore, to simplify the anatomy we can say that internal fasciae can be divided into two types:

- Investing fasciae: adherent to the viscera (or vessels, or glands), closely related to the organ's wall.

- Insertional fasciae: connecting organs with other organs and with the fasciae of the trunk.

For example, the fascia that envelops the intestine is the peritoneum, and it is composed of two layers: the visceral and the parietal peritoneum (Fig. 19.1). The two layers are completely different from both the macroscopic and microscopic points of view. The visceral peritoneum is a layer of thin and elastic connective tissue, hardly separable from the organ. The parietal peritoneum, on the other hand, is a thick and resistant, fibrous lamina, easily separable from the internal organs and connected to the muscular fasciae at specific points. To better understand the internal fasciae we can compare them to the muscular fasciae. The visceral peritoneum (investing fascia) is similar to the epimysium (thin, more elastic, strictly adherent to the muscle and hardly separable), whereas the parietal peritoneum (insertional fascia) is similar to the aponeurotic fasciae (thicker, less elastic, easily separable from the muscle). The same example is true of the fasciae that envelop the lung:

there are the visceral pleura (investing fascia) and the parietal pleura (insertional fascia). The visceral pleura is closely connected to the organ's parenchyma, while the parietal pleura is free to move against the viscera and is closely related to the endothoracic fascia (muscular fascia). Thus, in the thorax we have a fusion between muscular and internal fasciae, but we don't have this in the abdomen, where the parietal peritoneum is divided from the fascia of transverse muscle by loose connective tissue.[4] The different relationship between internal and muscular fasciae in the thorax and in the abdomen reflects a different mechanical need. It is necessary to actively control the breathing, for example, during phonation, whereas intestinal mobility/motility has to be independent from the movement of the musculoskeletal system. Even in the renal region there is the same organization. The kidneys are enveloped by the renal capsule (investing fascia), a thin and elastic fascia that covers the organ and is barely separable from the parenchyma. More externally there is a thicker

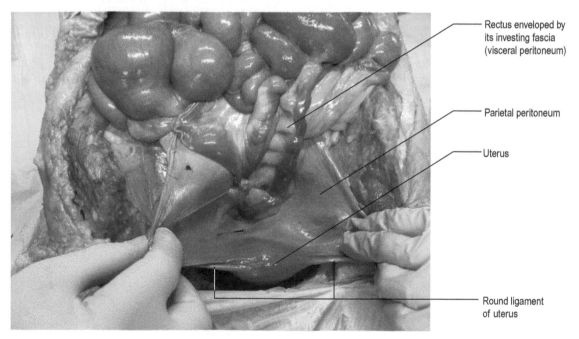

Rectus enveloped by its investing fascia (visceral peritoneum)

Parietal peritoneum

Uterus

Round ligament of uterus

Figure 19.1

Dissection of the abdomen and pelvis: anterior view. The parietal peritoneum (insertional fascia) is stretched to show its resistance and its fibrous aspect. It covers also the uterus and forms the round ligaments of the uterus. The rectus is enveloped by the visceral peritoneum (investing fascia)

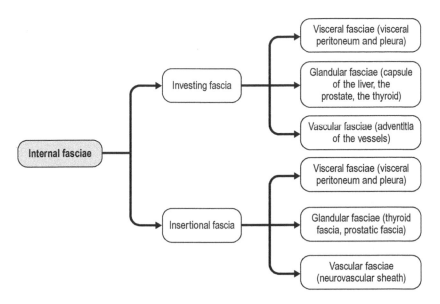

fascia, a whitish one, which creates a compartment all around the kidney: the renal fascia (insertional fascia). It extends to the vertebral column (prevertebral fascia) and continues with the insertional fascia of the aorta and vena cava, to reach the other kidney on the opposite side. Even for the aorta and vena cava, and in general for all the vessels, it can be noted how the adventitia has the same features as investing fascia, and in fact the vascular sheath connects the vessels to the organs (e.g., the continuity between aorta and renal fascia) or to the adjacent structures (e.g., aorta and pre-vertebral fascia). The renal fascia also has continuity with the iliac fascia (muscular fascia) and proximally with the diaphragmatic fascia. This is evidence that insertional fasciae are the ones that provide the connections between internal fasciae and muscular fascia, and between the different organs. The same pattern can be applied to the fasciae that surround the glands. For example, the capsule of the thyroid, which adheres to the gland and creates the dissepiments that enter the parenchyma, is its own investing fascia. Instead, the fascia of the thyroid gland, which forms the thyroid loggia and which is in continuity with the middle layer of the deep cervical fascia, is its own insertional fascia (Fig. 19.2).

Investing fascia

Investing fascia gives shape to the organ, it 'invests' it, and interacts closely with it. It is a very thin fascia (approximately 100 μm) and is rich in elastic fibers

so that it can adapt itself to the changing volume of the organ. As well as covering the organ, it also penetrates into the organ (viscera, or glands*), forming septa or lobes, and it organizes the structure of its own organ in the same way that the fascia of the epimysium arranges the structure and shape of the muscle. Investing fasciae don't have sensitive innervation, only autonomic innervation, so they are never responsible for the pain referred to an organ. Thanks to autonomic innervation, they have a key role in local coordination. Autonomic innervation in investing fasciae is very responsive to stretching.[11] Investing fasciae must be adaptable to every variation in the organ's volume to better interact with the neurons. In investing fasciae, the most important components of the autonomic nervous system are the intramural plexuses, among which the best known is Auerbach's plexus of the intestinal wall.[8] The autonomic plexuses within the investing fasciae form a neuronal net, sensitive to stretching and connected to the extramural ganglia. In anatomical literature, often the words ganglion and plexus are used in an interchangeable way, but by definition the plexus is

*The visceral (pulmonary) pleura adheres closely to the lung surface and follows the interlobar fissures, eventually ensheathing each pulmonary lobe.[4, p. 953]

'The esophagus adventitia is formed by dense, irregular connective tissue with a lot of elastic fibers. Its fibers penetrate also the deeper layers of the muscular tunica and surround them.'[4, p.1111]

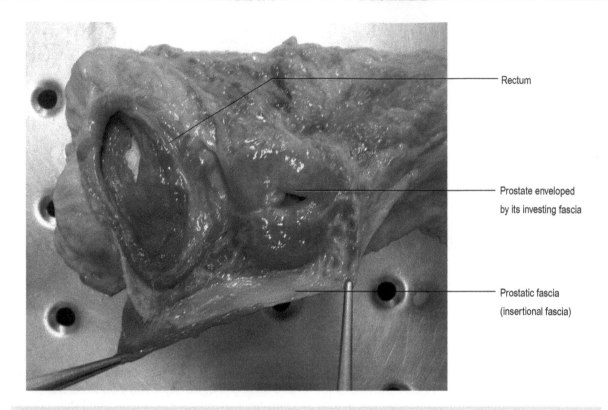

Rectum

Prostate enveloped
by its investing fascia

Prostatic fascia
(insertional fascia)

Figure 19.3
Fasciae of the prostate. The prostate is enveloped by investing fascia (corresponding to the capsule) and by insertional fascia (corresponding to the prostatic fascia). Note that the investing fascia is thin and strongly adherent to the organ, whilst the insertional fascia is a well-defined fibrous layer that creates a compartment around the prostate and the rectum

a set of dendrites and axons interwoven to form a local neuronal net; whereas the ganglia are clusters of neurons enveloped by a connective capsule placed along the course of the autonomic nerves, and they function as a 'relay' in nerve impulse transmission. Therefore, in the ganglion there is a 'reworking' of the information, while the plexus responds only to a precise mechanical stimulus, depending on the neuronal fibers' orientation.[12,13] We can take the intestinal wall as an example to better explain these concepts and the functioning of the enteric nervous system in relation to investing fascia. As the passage of food stretches the intestinal wall, the neuronal net (Auerbach's plexus) that is within the muscular tunica but strictly connected with the insertional fascia of the intestine (visceral peritoneum), feels the stretching and discharges. Intramural plexuses

(i.e., 'nets,') can respond to the stretching in every direction, but they are more sensitive in one precise direction[13] and they can discharge with different rhythms. It is likely that it is the organ's shape and, above all, the orientation of the fibers of the investing fascia (on which the intramural plexuses are implanted) that determine the direction in which these neuronal nets are more sensitive to stretching. According to their elasticity and composition, they determine also how much tension is necessary to produce the impulse. So everything suggests that an altered basal tension of the investing fascia assists peristalsis. From a 'segmental' point of view, the internal organs' motility is thus automatic and 'auto-maintained'. There is a stimulus that starts the circuit, and then the peristalsis continues in an autonomous way. In the digestive apparatus, the digestion starts with swallowing (voluntary in the first part, autonomous in the second part) and then continues in a completely autonomous manner according to the passage of the bolus/chyme along the various tracts. The passage stretches the intramural plexus, causing an inhibition downstream, a consequent relaxation of the wall, and a contraction of the wall upstream.[14] This way, the transit of the bolus/chyme is guaranteed to be in one direction. The article affirms that if an intestinal tract is cut, then turned 180 degrees, and in the end sutured, the transit of the material along the viscera's lumen is interrupted. This is further evidence that fascia is the perfect peripheral organization that assists peristalsis, without a central command. Certainly a central command can intervene and somehow change the rhythm of the internal organs, increasing or decreasing their activity, but even without a central command the peristalsis of viscera, glands, and vessels works properly.

Insertional fascia

Insertional fasciae appear as fibrous sheets, easily isolable from the internal organs (Fig. 19.3). They have the function of creating compartments and loggia, ensuring the vital space of the organs. They are very thick fasciae, richer in collagen fibers and not very elastic. In some specific points there is a connection between insertional and investing fasciae, as in the course along the mesentery (or the hilum in a gland), through which there is a passage of the vessels and nerves that reach the organ's parenchyma. Insertional fasciae also form all the ligaments of anchorage of the internal organ, for example, the round ligament of the liver, the pleural dome's ligaments, the broad ligament of the uterus, etc. Typical insertional fasciae are the parietal peritoneum and pleura, the renal fascia, and the thyroid fascia. Even the vascular sheaths can be considered insertional fasciae. In fact, they are fibrous laminae† that create the loggia for vessels and nerves.[15] It is important

to underline how insertional fasciae are connected to the muscular fasciae at specific points, ensuring in part the autonomy of the internal organs from the locomotor system, and in part the connection between them. Insertional fascia has, indeed, a dual role: to divide and to connect. Each organ has one or more very different functions and has to maintain its own autonomy from the locomotor system. It is easy to see how disastrous it would be if every movement of the body could affect, for example, normal intestinal peristalsis. Therefore, the function of insertional fasciae is to isolate viscera (glands or vessels) from the external environment and from other organs to create specific compartments. The degree of 'isolation' depends on the organ's function.[16] Thinking, for example, about the thoracic region, there are several important organs with great motility and mobility, but independent from one another: the respiratory rate and heart rate must be autonomous and must not influence one another. Intestinal peristalsis is continuous day and night, but it is not perceived by the individual, because otherwise it would be a disturbing feeling during normal daily activities. The peritoneum performs this function of isolation; it is no coincidence that between the peritoneum and in the muscular fasciae of the abdomen there is loose connective tissue, so as to have the least possible repercussion on the musculoskeletal system.[4] Here too we have further evidence of how 'functional' the architecture of the human body is.

The second function of insertional fasciae is connection, both between different organs, and with the muscular fasciae. We will focus more on the connections between internal and muscular fasciae in the next paragraph. Internal fascial continuity moves in two directions: longitudinal and transverse.[16] The longitudinal continuity between different organs that have the same function forms the apparatus. For example, the digestive apparatus is formed by the esophagus, the stomach, the small intestine, etc. They are all in continuity thanks to insertional fasciae and they have the same function, namely digestion. The respiratory apparatus is the same. The insertional fasciae of the larynx and trachea are in continuity with the parietal pleura to coordinate respiratory functions, like phonation. Therefore, a fascial dysfunction or an abnormal tension of some internal fasciae can

---

†The vascular sheath surrounds the vascular nervous bundle of the neck and with its secondary extensions envelops the singular element of the bundle itself. They are denser around the jugular vein and more loose around the carotid artery. The vascular sheath is connected to the middle layer of the cervical fascia.[15]

AQ2

be transmitted far away along the apparatus or all over the apparatus.[17] Transversal connections from insertional fasciae link organs within different apparatuses. The lesser omentum, for example, originates from the lesser curvature of the stomach and reaches the liver and the gallbladder, covering the pancreas, the vena cava, and the aorta. It has all the features of insertional fascia and it connects organs of different apparatuses. This connection is found where these organs work together to execute a function. In fact, during the digestive process, when the stomach has to empty itself, there is a need to secrete bile (gallbladder), and there is a need to produce and free enzymes (pancreas, liver), etc. The lesser omentum, with its anatomical connections, coordinates the different organs of the subdiaphragmatic region. It is our belief that this mechanical connection supports the hormonal and chemical digestive processes. It is not by chance that in every segment of the trunk where a connection/coordination between different organs is needed there is a particular insertional fascia, like the lesser omentum. In the cervical region there is the retropharyngeal fascia. In the thoracic segment (in which it is important to divide and coordinate the heart and respiratory rate, during a sudden increase in activity, for example) there is the bronchopericardial membrane. In the pelvic region there is the rectovesical membrane that connects the rectum to the seminal vesicles and to the bladder. Abnormal tension in this fascia can in some patients cause activation of the ganglia, making it difficult to control urination during defecation. Insertional fasciae are innervated by somatic nerves, therefore, they are able to register an alteration in the form of pain. The somatic nervous system enables the patient to describe in a precise way the region and features of the pain. Insertional fasciae have, in addition, an autonomic innervation. Specifically, the key element is represented by the extramural ganglia. The extramural ganglia receive the information from the intramural plexuses and they rework them, producing a response that can be distributed to the organs in the direction determined by the connections of the insertional fasciae.[18] Even in this case, the timing and the activation modalities are determined by the morphology of the fascia. Intramural plexuses immediately react to the stretching and, according to the intensity of the stimulus, they activate a

segmental motor response and transmit the signal to the extramural ganglia. They rework the inputs from different plexuses (working as little peripheral brains) and transmit a new message in the direction of the insertional fasciae. This illustrates the importance of the fascial structure: there are some extramural ganglia set in series (along the longitudinal continuity of the insertional fasciae), and others set in parallel (in the transversal connections). The extramural ganglia placed in series manage the continuity of the peristalsis from one organ to the another within one apparatus. For example, the impulses produced by the stretch of the stomach's investing fasciae, and so of the intramural plexuses, activate at a later time the extramural ganglia, which determine a massive contraction and the emptying of the stomach itself. To summarize, we can affirm that that the intramural plexuses are responsible for the segmental organ's peristalsis (or gland, or vessel). The extramural ganglia ensure a 'global' peristalsis, namely the apparatus continuity. The ganglia set in parallel ensure a 'more global' peristalsis. As mentioned earlier in this chapter, the lesser omentum connects and 'coordinates' the different components (visceral, vascular, glandular) that participate in digestion in the duodenal tract. Abnormal tension in the fasciae of this region can result in improper activation of the extramural ganglia set in parallel (hyper- or hypoactivation). Thus a patient may be affected by the same digestive disorder whether the problem is due to the visceral component (stomach, pylorus, etc.), the glandular component (pancreas), or the vascular component. This is because the correct functioning of all these structures as a whole produces correct physiological peristalsis.

It is our opinion that it is not always essential to understand which organ has a dysfunction, given that it is not easy to know that, but it is important to know which region of the body is affected and, consequently, which fascia is affected.

Internal fasciae and muscular fasciae

Internal fasciae and, more specifically, insertional fasciae, have several connections with muscular fasciae. If these are altered it may disturb normal internal peristalsis, and vice versa. Analyzing the abdominal and pelvic region, the peritoneum has few direct connections with the muscular fasciae and there are only some laciniae that maintain the position of the peritoneal sac (e.g., in the iliac crest).[18,19] The renal fascia is retroperitoneal and is connected with the prevertebral fascia and with the fasciae of the quadratus lumborum and the psoas.[18] The ureters are supported by the fascia of the iliopsoas. The type of connection always depends on the degree of 'isolation' that the organs need. The endoperitoneal organs need to move as autonomously as possible, as opposed to the musculoskeletal system. Nevertheless, some connections are necessary to maintain the organ's position. The abdominal wall is like a tarpaulin that covers these structures and ensures their vital space, together with the fascia of the obliques and transverse muscles.[20] It is important that this vital space is maintained, irrespective of the position and of the muscle's contractions. An anomalous tension of this covering can give a traction along the laciniae, but, above all, it can generate compression and modification of the 'organ's vital space'. The intramural plexuses within investing fasciae are really sensitive to a minimal stretch.[21] So if insertional fasciae are not able to ensure the space/autonomy around the viscera, the function of the intramural ganglia may be compromised, resulting in an alteration in the organs' function/motility. Then the aim of the fascial therapist[22] is to ensure the vital space around the organs, normalizing the tensions that the muscular fasciae can create in insertional fasciae. Therefore, in the clinic, the focus should be on the content rather than the container – the treatment should not be focused directly on the internal organs but on the muscular fascia, and on investigating and treating the densification areas.[16,18,19] The anatomical continuity of the muscular fasciae explains how a fascial peripheral densification can result, after some time, with an internal dysfunction. From this point of view, it is difficult to establish how much a disorder has a visceral or somatic origin because both fascial systems (muscular and internal) interact with each other and dysfunctions in both may result in a somatic problem or an internal problem.

References

1. Findley T. W., Shalwala M. Fascia Research Congress evidence from the 100 year perspective of Andrew Taylor Still. *J Bodyw Mov Ther.* 2013;17(3):356–364.

2. Stecco C., Macchi V., Porzionato A. et al. The ankle retinacula: morphological evidence of the proprioceptive role of the fascial system. *Cells Tissues Organs.* 2010;192(3):200–210.

3. van der Wal J. The architecture of the connective tissue in the musculoskeletal system – an often overlooked functional parameter as to proprioception in the locomotor apparatus. *Int J Ther Massage Bodywork.* 2009;2(4):9–23

4. Standring S. (ed). *Gray's Anatomy: The Anatomical Basis of Clinical Practice, 41st edn.* Elsevier, 2016.

5. Raptopoulos V., Touliopoulos P., Lei Q. F. et al. Medial border of the perirenal space: CT and anatomic correlation. *Radiology.* 1997;205(3):777–784.

6. Bassotti G., Stanghellini V., Chiarioni G., et al. Upper gastrointestinal motor activity in patients with slow-transit constipation. Further evidence for an enteric neuropathy. *Dig Dis Sci.* 1996;41:1999–2005.

7. Coyne K. S., Cash B., Kopp Z. et al. The prevalence of chronic constipation and fecal incontinence among men and women with symptoms of overactive bladder. *BJU Int.* 2011;107:254–261.

8. Furness J. B. *The Enteric Nervous System.* Oxford: Blackwell Publishing, 2006, pp. 1–160.

9. Barbarić Z., Renal fascia in urinary tract disease. *Radiology.* 1976;118(3):561–565.

10. Bechtold R. E., Dyer R. B., Zagoria R. J., Chen M. Y. (1996) The perirenal space: relationship of pathologic processes to normal retroperitoneal anatomy. *Radiographics.* 16(4):841–854.

11. Kandel E. R., Schwartz J. H., Jessell T. M. Principles of Neural Science. McGraw-Hill, 2000.

12. Furness J. B., Clerc N., Lomax A. E. et al. Shapes and projections of tertiary plexus neurons of the guinea-pig small intestine. *Cell Tissue Res.* 2000;300(3):383–387.

13. Kunze W. A., Clerc N., Furness J. B., Gola M.The soma and neurites of primary afferent neurons in the guinea-pig intestine respond differentially to deformation. *J Physiol.* 2000;526(Pt 2):375–385.

14. Hall J. E. *Guyton and Hall Textbook of Medical Physiology.* 13th edition Saunders Elsevier, 2015, pp. 797–816.

15. Testut L. *Trattato di anatomia topografica.* Firenze: UTET, 1987.

16. Stecco L., Stecco C. *Fascial Manipulation for Internal Dysfunctions*. Piccin Nuova Libraria, 2013.

17. Jiang Y., Bhargava V., Mittal R. K. Mechanism of stretch-activated excitatory and inhibitory responses in the lower esophageal sphincter. *Am J Physiol Gastrointest Liver Physiol*. 2009;297(2):G397–405.

18. Stecco L., Stecco C. *Manipolazione fasciale per le disfunzioni interne*. Parte Pratica. Piccin Nuova Libraria, 2014.

19. Stecco C., Hammer W. *Functional Atlas of the Human Fascial System*. Churchill Livingstone Elsevier, 2014.

20. Lancerotto L., Stecco C., Macchi V. et al. Layers of the abdominal wall: anatomical investigation of subcutaneous tissue and superficial fascia. *Surg Radiol Anat*. 2011;33(10):835–842.

21. Wladyka C. L., Diana L. Kunze D. L. KCNQ/M-currents contribute to the resting membrane potential in rat visceral sensory neurons. *J Physiol*. 2006;575(Pt 1):175–189.

22. Stecco C., Day J. A. (2010) The fascial manipulation technique and its biomechanical model: a guide to the human fascial system. *Int J Ther Massage Bodywork*. 2010;3(1):38–40.

THE DIAPHRAGM

Michel Puylaert

General considerations

The diaphragm is a broad, unpaired, and asymmetrical musculotendinous sheet.

It is dome-shaped and oriented transversely in a posterodorsal direction. It is broader laterally than in the anteroposterior dimension.

Apart from its main role as the primary muscle of respiration, the diaphragm fulfills a number of additional functions. For example, it comprises the most important intrathoracic buffer zone for mechanical stresses as conveyed by fascial structures.

Structurally, the diaphragm is described as consisting of four parts:

- *The central tendon* is a thin, central tendinous sheet. Muscular fibers attach to its circumference and it is anchored to a strong fascial structure, the pericardium.

- *The lumbar part* extends from the anterior longitudinal ligament of the lumbar spine to the central tendon. Furthermore, this part can be divided into left and right crus of the diaphragm, and attaches the diaphragm to the inferior thoracic outlet. The muscular slips of this part of the diaphragm constitute proximally the passageway of the esophagus. Distally, they are pierced by the major and minor splanchnic nerves. Both crurae are connected centrally by the median arcuate ligament, which lies directly anterior to the aorta.

- *The costal part* is attached to the inner aspect of the ribs. Anteriorly and laterally it attaches to ribs 6–12, and posteriorly to ribs 9–12. It also extends to the central tendon.

- *The sternal part* is attached to the posterior aspect of the xiphoid process and is comprised of two parts that extend to the central tendon.

While separating the thoracic and abdominal cavities, the diaphragm at the same time constitutes the main connecting structure between these cavities. Thus, the diaphragm can be looked upon as a transitional zone between the negative pressure of the thoracic cavity and the positive pressure of the abdominal cavity. The pleural cavity appears to attract the peritoneal structures, particularly the proximal abdominal organs, almost as if it were a magnet. Conversely, the weight of the abdominal organs exceeds an inferior pulling force transmitted by abdominal fascia. The pliability of the diaphragm allows for an elastic relationship between the two cavities.

As the primary muscle of respiration the diaphragm accounts for two-thirds of thoracic extension during deep inspiration. Ninety-five per cent of expiration is controlled eccentrically by the diaphragm. During inspiration the diaphragm shortens more posteriorly than anteriorly. During expiration, the diaphragm shifts from an anterior to a more posterior position.

Embryology

The diaphragm (Fig. 20.1) develops from the mesoblast. Its development starts on day 27 or 28. It derives from four primitive structures:

- Ventrally: the transverse septum between the pericardial cavity and the yolk stalk.

- Laterally: two parts from pleuroperitoneal folds.

- Dorsally: from the dorsal meso-oesophagus.

- Cranially: myoblasts of striated skeletal muscle that have migrated away from cervical myotomes.

Figure 20.1
The diaphragm

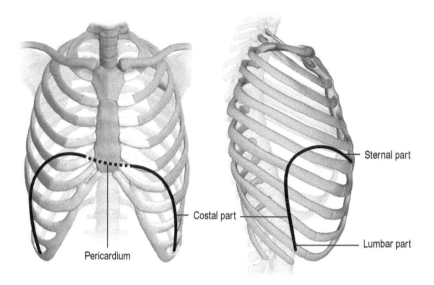

Sternal part

Costal part

Lumbar part

Pericardium

Connections

The diaphragm is connected to many other structures of the body. Important examples include:

- Fibers of the lumbar portion extend to the anterior aspects of vertebral bodies. They are connected to the intervertebral discs of L1–L2, L2–L3, and occasionally even L3–L4 on the right.

- At the level of L1, tendinous arches – the medial and lateral arcuate ligaments – connect the lateral aspects of the diaphragm to the transverse processes of L1, parts of the 12th ribs, and also to the psoas and quadratus lumborum muscles.

- In addition, the diaphragm is intimately related to the transversus abdominis muscle and the transverse abdominal fascia. It responds immediately to changes in the abdomen.

- The superior part of the diaphragm is connected to the pericardium by the phrenopericardial ligament. The endothoracic fascia and phrenicopleural fascia connect the pleura and the diaphragm.

- The inferior aspect is mainly covered by the peritoneum and is in contact with several organs: the liver and falciform ligament, the stomach and gastrophrenic ligament, the spleen, the left–right flexure of the colon, and the phrenicocolic ligament (right to left).

- By providing continual movement, the diaphragm contributes significantly to pressure ratios between and nutrient supply to abdominal organs.

- Posterior to the diaphragm lies the renal fascia, which covers the superior poles of the kidneys and the adrenal glands.

- Amongst others, the diaphragm is pierced by the inferior vena cava, the aorta, the thoracic duct, the esophagus, the sympathetic chains, and the phrenic nerves.

Muscular chains

The diaphragm has direct connections to the fasciae of the psoas muscles, quadratus lumborum, and the abdominal muscles. Thus, it forms a 'psoatico-(quadratico)-diaphragmatico-abdominal chain', which is closely connected to the central tendon. Diaphragmatic dysfunction (e.g., adhesions in the subdiaphragmatic recesses) often leads to an increased lumbar lordosis and a more kyphotic thoracic spine. There are about 20,000 respiratory cycles a day. Respiratory motion dominates any other repetitive motion of the body and can thus have an effect on all fascial or muscular chains of the body.

Innervation

The right and left phrenic nerves (C3–4) provide motor innervation to the diaphragm. Additionally, the sympathetic nervous system significantly influences its muscle tone. Apart from supplying the diaphragm, the phrenic nerves also innervate the pericardium; the superior and inferior vena cava; and the capsule of the liver. The phrenic nerves also form anastomoses with subclavian, hypoglossal, and vagus nerves, and cervical portions of the sympathetic nervous system. The phrenic nerves contain some sensory fibers, while the main sensory innervation of the diaphragm is, however, provided by the inferior six intercostal nerves. The right phrenic nerve is supplied directly by an anastomosis from the celiac ganglion.

Gastroesophageal junction

The gastroesophageal junction is a key area between the thoracic and abdominal systems. At the level of T10, the esophagus enters the abdominal cavity through the esophageal hiatus of the diaphragm. The distal end of the esophagus is anchored to the crurae of the diaphragm by the phrenoesophageal membrane. Embryologically, the membrane is of both thoracic and abdominal origin. The stability of the esophageal fascial fixation to the diaphragm differs individually and is age-dependent.

Examination

As direct contact with the diaphragm is not possible, both examination and treatment rely on indirect techniques. Testing and treatment often merge into each other and pure examination techniques thus remain limited.

Thoracic and diaphragmatic movements

Positioning: the patient is supine, with knees slightly bent. The practitioner stands next to the patient with his hands placed bilaterally on the patient's thorax, with fingers pointing laterally along the intercostal spaces and thumbs moving posteriorly behind the costal margins.

Technique:

Phase 1: the thoracic cage is moved alternatively left and right. The ease of this passive movement is judged using both fingers and thumbs.

Phase 2: during slightly deeper respiration, the diaphragm should descend and the intercostal spaces should widen.

Note: the right side may, due to the liver, feel slightly heavier. Otherwise, there should be no major differences. The movements should feel fluid.

Testing of the thorax

Positioning: the patient is supine, with knees slightly bent. The practitioner stands at the top end of the plinth near the patient's head, with hands resting on the anterolateral aspects of ribs 8, 9, and 10.

Technique: both hands follow the costal movements. At the end of both inspiration and expiration, an additional push is given with the hands.

Assessment: elasticity (amplitude), pain of thorax, or diaphragm are assessed.

Connective tissue zones

In diaphragmatic dysfunction, tender round areas of skin can be found on both sides of the xiphoid process.

Treatment
Domes of the diaphragm

Positioning: the patient is supine, with knees slightly bent. The practitioner stands at the level of the patient's pelvis and places his hands onto the anterolateral aspects of the lower ribs.

Technique: the practitioner applies pressure diagonally toward the sternum and in a posterior direction. Pressure is only increased by shifting the practitioner's weight toward the patient. The applied pressure is adapted to the resistance of the thorax. The fingertips can make firm contact with superficial fascia in order to minimize gliding movements. Pressure is sustained for one minute and then removed slowly. Repeat until the thorax feels elastic.

Diaphragmatic release
Muscular diaphragm techniques

Positioning: the patient is supine, with knees bent. The practitioner stands next to the patient, with his hands placed bilaterally on the patient's thorax, with the fingers pointing laterally along the lower ribs. The thumbs are placed onto the inner aspect of the costal margins and move as far craniolaterally as possible.

Technique: adhesions and fixations are released using stretch-and-glide movements and inhibition. Both sides of the thorax are treated.

Harmonizing diaphragm technique

Positioning: the patient is supine, with knees slightly bent. The practitioner stands on the right-hand side of the patient, with one hand on top of the costal margin and the other underneath, moving slightly craniolaterally.

Technique: the upper hand moves the costal margin caudally and medially, while the other hand increases the craniolateral pressure. The technique ends when a release is brought about, with movement directions changing according to fascial tension.

Lumbar parts and lumbocostal arch

Positioning: the patient sits on the edge of the plinth. The practitioner stands behind the patient, slightly off to one side. With one hand he holds the patient's trunk, while the fingertips of the other hand are placed directly lateral to the erector spinae muscle at the level of L1.

Technique: move the patient's trunk into ipsilateral side-bending and extension. Then, below rib 12 and lateral to the transverse process of L1, direct your fingertips anteromedially into the deeper tissues.

Phase 1: during inspiration, the practitioner allows the patient to push his fingers out slightly. During expiration, the fingers move in deeper and slide the tissues of the arcuate ligaments, the fascia of the quadratus lumborum and psoas, and the lumbar part of the diaphragm against each other.

Note: the renal fascia and Toldt's fascia can also be treated using this technique.

Phase 2: when the practitioner palpates a considerable change, he moves the patient into contralateral side-bending and possibly ipsilateral rotation, if needed. The fingers continue to move the tissues against each other.

Phase 3: a flexion and extension movement is conducted and the patient intensifies his breathing.

Phase 4: release slowly.

The patient feels that he can breathe more freely.

Fascial balancing of the diaphragm

Coordination of prevertebral fascia and dome of the diaphragm

Positioning: the patient is supine, with knees slightly bent. The practitioner stands at the level of the patient's shoulder girdle and places his more caudal hand on the anterolateral aspect of the lower ribs. His proximal hand is placed under the patient's thoracic spine.

Technique:

Phase 1: the distal hand induces a transversal movement and follows into the direction of ease.

Phase 2: the distal hand pushes cranially and follows the movement of the lower rib cage.

Phase 3: the distal hand continues to follow the movement of the lower rib cage until a movement of the upper thoracic spine can be felt. Both hands follow the movements of the upper thoracic spine and the thoracic cage, until the entire half of the thorax moves in a fascially harmonic fashion. The other side of the thorax is treated the same way.

Note: this technique can help with reflux in particular.

Esophageal hiatus

Specific fascial release

Positioning: the patient is supine, with knees slightly bent. The practitioner stands on the left-hand side of the patient at the level of the thorax. The pisiform bone of the proximal hand is placed onto the 5th intercostal space, just a finger's breadth lateral to the sternum. The distal hand is placed on top of the proximal hand to stabilize the contact.

Technique:

Phase 1: the practitioner applies posterior pressure until a clear resistance can be felt.

Phase 2: without releasing the backward pressure, the tissues are rotated in a clockwise or counter-clockwise direction. The technique can be used as a direct or indirect technique.

Generalized fascial release

Positioning: the patient is supine, with knees slightly bent. The practitioner stands at the level of the patient's pelvis. The proximal hand is lying flat on the epigastrium, directly distal to the xiphoid process. The distal hand is placed on top of the proximal hand to reinforce the contact.

Technique: the practitioner applies a mild pressure in a posterior direction, pulling the tissues caudally. The position is maintained until a release is effected.

Mobilization of the esophagus in relation to the diaphragm

Positioning: the patient is supine, with knees slightly bent. The practitioner places the thumb of his right hand lateral to the cardiac sphincter on the corpus of the stomach. The left hand wraps around the left costal margin to fix both diaphragm and ribs in a cranial position.

Technique: the practitioner moves the corpus of the stomach in a caudal direction while fixing ribs and diaphragm cranially. The stomach is mobilized either rhythmically or contrary to respiratory movements until the resistance of the tissues has eased off considerably.

Further reading

Finet, G., Williame C. (2000) *Treating Visceral Dysfunction: An Osteopathic Approach to Understanding and Treating the Abdominal Organs.* Stillness Press, Portland, Oregon.

Netter, F. H. (2003) *Atlas der Anatomie des Menschen.* 3. Aufl., Thieme, Stuttgart/New York.

Rohen, J. W. (2000) *Morphologie des menschlichen Organismus.* Freies Geistesleben, Stutgart.

Wancura-Kampik, I. (2009) *Segment-Anatomie.* 1. Aufl., Urban und Fischer, München.

ANATOMY OF THE DURA MATER

Torsten Liem

The dura mater represents the outermost of the three layers of the meninges, a thick and dense inelastic membrane that surrounds the brain and the spinal cord, and is impermeable to the cerebrospinal fluid (CSF). The cranial dura mater differs anatomically from the spinal dura mater in many aspects, hence it is necessary to describe them separately. However, the reader should note that both forms are part of one complete membrane, which is continuous at the foramen magnum.

In conjunction with the CSF, the dural system is responsible for the support and maintenance of brain functions, as well as serving as a form of protection in case of mechanical traumata. Mechanical forces directed to the skull are countered by shock-free absorption, due to the elasticity of the bones, the pillar construction of the skull, the nasal sinuses, and the attachment of the viscerocranium to the neurocranium (Drenkhahn & Zenker, 1994).

Cranial dura mater

The cranial dura mater lines the interior of the skull. It is composed of two layers, the outer endosteal layer and the inner meningeal layer. Both layers are closely connected, except when they form sinuses for the passage of venous blood. The cranial dura mater consists of white fibrous tissue and a specific layer of flattened fibroblastic cells without extracellular space and collagen, which can be found at the transition between the dura mater and the arachnoid mater (Haines et al., 1993). The outer surface of the dura mater adheres closely to the inner surfaces of the bones, with these adhesions being most prominent at the base of the skull and opposite the sutures. The outer surface of the dura is rough and fibrillated, whereas the inner surface is smooth and lined with endothelium.

The dura mater continues at the outer surface of the skull via the various foramina that exist at the base of the skull. Its fibrous layer forms sheaths for the nerves that exit the cranium, hence passing through these foramina. The dura is attached to the bone at the foramen magnum, and is continuous with the spinal dura mater.

The skin of the scalp and the dura are connected by emissary veins. The dura is particularly flat in the regions of the ethmoid bone cells, the tegmentum, and the sigmoid sinus. The inner meningeal layer of the dura is structurally weaker than the outer endosteal layer (Haines et al., 1993). The dura of an adult is able to resist greater force than the dura of a newborn (Dragoi, 1995). According to Arbuckle, a specific fiber structure enables the cranial and spinal dura to transmit different forces (Arbuckle, 1994). These so-called 'stress fibers' are structured in defined groups: horizontal, vertical, transverse, and circular. This direction of fibers in the cranial dura mater may be the result of mechanical forces during embryonic development, when collagenous fibers are brought into line by stress forces (Hamann et al., 1998).

As well as the venous blood sinuses, other important structures between the endosteal and meningeal layers of the dura are: the meningeal arteries, which are terminal branches of the carotid arteries; the endolymphatic bag, which is part of the ductus endolymphaticus, and which is located at the petrous bone between the two dural layers; the trigeminal cave (Meckel's cavity), which represents an outpouching of the dura for the ganglion of the fifth cranial nerve and which is located at the frontal side of the petrous part of the temporal bone above the foramen lacerum; and the passage of sympathetic nerve fibers between the dural layers of intracranial vascular walls.

Horizontal and vertical dural system

The cavity of the skull is divided into four compartments, which serve as protection for the different parts of the brain: falx cerebri, tentorium cerebelli, falx cerebelli, and diaphragma sellae. They are anatomically and functionally connected, hence they affect each other.

The **falx cerebri** is a small, sickle-shaped fold of the dura mater, which descends vertically into the longitudinal fissure between the cerebral hemispheres. At the front it is attached to the crista galli of the ethmoid, and at the back it is connected with the tentorium cerebelli. Its lower margin is free and concave, and contains the inferior saggital sinus, whereas the upper margin is attached to the inner surface of the skull in the midline, reaching back to the internal occipital protuberance (Jinkins, 2000; Herle, 2012; Standring, 2008).

The **tentorium cerebelli** is a dural fold that lies in the axial plane and divides the cranial cavity into supratentorial and infratentorial compartments. It covers the superior surface of the cerebellum, and supports the occipital lobes of the brain. Anteriorly, the deep tentorial notch, which allows communication between the supratentorial and infratentorial compartments, attaches to the clinoid processes and forms the lateral part of the cavernous sinus. Posteriorly, by its convex border it is attached to the inner surface of the occipital bones, and there encloses the transverse sinuses. Anteriorly, it attaches to the petrous parts of the temporal bones, enclosing the superior petrosal sinuses. The tentorium is also attached to the falx cerebri, with the straight sinus being placed at their junction (Singh, 2011; Standring, 2008).

The **falx cerebelli** is a small infolding of the dura over the floor of the posterior cranial fossa. It separates the two cerebellar hemispheres. Superiorly, the falx cerebelli is attached to the tentorium cerebelli, inferiorly it extends to the foramen magnum. Posteriorly, it attaches to the internal occipital crest of the occipital bone, containing the occipital sinus (Singh, 2011).

The diaphragma sellae is a small, circular horizontal fold, which covers the sella turcica and forms the roof of the hypophyseal fossa. It consists of two horizontal leaves of dura mater on the sphenoid bone.

The falx cerebri and falx cerebelli are made up of collagenous fibers and arcs in the anterior, intermediate, and posterior region, which cross each other perpendicularly. The fibers are able to organize themselves and move in different directions during the course of growth (Dragoi, 1995). This vertical system has the potential to tighten the cranial vault, in comparison with the horizontal system made up of the entorium cerebelli and diaphragma sellae, which may be able to act as a tightener of the cranial base (Newell, 1999).

Vascularization

The dural blood supply generally concerns the outer layer of the dura, as the inner layer does not require a large blood supply. The dura mater is supplied by numerous arteries. The anterior meningeal branches of the anterior and posterior ethmoidal and internal carotid, and a branch from the middle meningeal artery, are located in the anterior cranial fossa. The middle cranial fossa contains frontal and parietal branches of the middle meningeal artery, which enters the middle cranial fossa via the foramen spinosum; the accessory meningeal and pharyngeal arteries; and branches from the internal carotid artery. Those in the posterior cranial fossa are meningeal branches from the occipital artery, the posterior meningeal branch from the vertebral artery, occasional meningeal branches from the ascending pharyngeal artery, and a branch from the middle meningeal artery.

Venous drainage from the cranial dura mater occurs by anastomosis with the diploic veins, and ends in the various sinuses. The middle meningeal veins open into the pterygoid plexus, into the maxillary vein, or via the pterygoid plexus into the inferior ophthalmic vein and the cavernous sinus. Meningeal veins empty directly or indirectly into the jugular vein via the sinuses.

Innervation

The innervation of the upper part of the dura mater is primarily provided by meningeal branches of the trigeminus and vagus nerves, the lower part being innervated by the upper cervical spinal nerves. Nerve supply in the anterior cranial fossa is provided by the ophthalmic division of the trigeminal nerve; the naso-ciliary branch; and anterior and posterior ethmoidal nerves. The middle cranial fossa is innervated by meningeal branches of the ophthalmic, maxillary, and mandibular divisions of the trigeminal nerve. The innervation of the posterior cranial fossa is provided by the second and third cervical branches (C2, C3) and the meningeal branches of the vagus and hypoglossal nerves, with contributions from C1 and C2.

Spinal dura mater

The spinal dura mater (SDM) is a relatively inelastic tube of collagenous fiber, which forms a loose sheath around the medulla spinalis and follows closely the curvature of the vertebral canal. The dura is held under tension by the CSF, which depends on hydro-static, respiratory, and pulsatory factors (von Lanz, 1929). The dura extends from the foramen magnum of the occipital bone to the sacral canal, becoming invested with the filum terminale of the spinal cord at the level of S3, which blends with the periosteum of the coccyx.

The spinal dura mater is separated from the arachnoid mater by a potential cavity, the subdural space. However, both membranes are mostly in close contact with each other, except where they are separated by a minute quantity of CSF.

The dura mater is divided into three layers: an outer fibroelastic layer of flattened cells with thin and long cell extensions toward the epidural space; a middle fibrous layer; and the inner dural border cell layer with extracellular spaces, few cell junctions, and no extracellular collagen (Vandenabeele et al., 1996).

Within the dura, numerous elastic fibers are present, which indicate considerable flexibility and elasticity during movement and postural changes (Vandenabeele et al., 1996). Deforming forces applied to the spinal cord and the meninges are dispersed by the subarachnoid space and the fibroadipose tissue within the extradural space (Vandenabeele et al., 1996).

Two dural layers can be distinguished at the transition from the foramen magnum to the vertebral canal:

the outer, periostal layer that ceases at the foramen magnum, with its place being taken by the periosteum lining the vertebral canal, and the inner layer – the true SDM. These two layers are separated by the epidural space, which is not present inside the cranium, and which permits gliding movements between the dura and the spine. The posterior longitudinal ligament borders the epidural space anteriorly; the medial aspect of the pedicles and the intervertebral foramina are located laterally; and the anterior aspect of the laminae and the ligamentum flava border posteriorly (Westbrook, 2012). Superiorly, the dura blends with the periosteum of the foramen magnum.

The size of the dura mater is greater in the cervical and lumbar regions compared with the thoracic region.

Fascial relationships and attachments of the spinal dura mater are described in more detail below. These structures support the movement of the dural tube inside the spinal canal and prevent folding or other injury-causing mechanisms to the dura or the spinal cord.

Fascial relationships of the spinal dura mater

von Lanz originally described the **ligamentum craniale durae matris spinalis** (CDMS ligament) as fibrous strands extending from the dura mater to the occipital bone, the posterior longitudinal ligament, and the transverse ligament of the atlas (von Lanz, 1929). Posteriorly, the CDMS attaches to the arch of the atlas and axis, the periosteum of the occipital squama, and laterally to the atlanto-occipital and atlantoaxial joints (von Lanz, 1929). Further fibers were identified arising from the flaval ligaments between C1–C2 and C2–C3, and other fibers connecting to the dura were identified between the arch of C2 and C3 (Rutten et al., 1997). Rutten and colleagues suspect that parts of the CDMS ligament function as a tensioner of the upper cervical vertebral column during movement (Rutten et al., 1997).

The SDM is also associated with the **rectus capitis posterior minor** (RCPmi) muscle (Kahkeshani & Ward, 2012; Zumpano et al., 2006; Nash et al., 2005;

Humphreys et al., 2003; Hack et al., 1995; Hack & Hallgren, 2004), the **rectus capitis posterior major** (RCPma) muscle (Scali et al., 2011; Scali et al., 2013; Kahn et al., 1992), and the **obliquus capitis inferior** (OCI) muscle (Pontell et al., 2012; Pontell et al., 2013) via a connective tissue bridge (Fig. 21.1). The fibers of the connective tissue bridge between the RCPmi muscle and the dura are oriented primarily perpendicular to the dura (Hack et al., 1995).

The SDM is also connected to the posterior atlanto-occipital (PAO) membrane at the atlanto-occipital joint by connective tissue bands, which create a unit and is where the RCPmi can also be identified (Kahke-shani & Ward, 2012; Hack et al., 1995). The RCPmi may be able to directly affect the biomechanics of the SDM via the connection to the PAO membrane. The myodural connection between the RCPmi and the SDM may prevent the folding of the SDM toward the spinal canal, which tends to occur during neck and head extension (Hack et al., 1995; Adams & Logue, 1971; Tachibana et al., 1994; Hallgren et al., 1997;

Alix & Bates, 1999; von Lüdinghausen, 1967). The OCI is attached to the posterolateral part of the dura mater (Pontell et al., 2013), and the RCPma extends to the posterior dura mater via the atlantoaxial interspace (Scali et al., 2012).

The myodural bridge between the SDM and the suboccipital muscles exhibits considerable clinical significance, in that excessive tensions may be transmitted across the myodural bridge to the dura, which manifest as cervicogenic headache (Hack et al., 1995; Scali et al., 2011; Scali et al., 2013; Pontell et al., 2012; Pontell et al., 2013; Alix & Bates, 1999; Scali et al., 2012; Fernández-de-las-Peñas et al., 2007; Tagil et al., 2005).

Attachments between the posterior SDM and the **nuchal ligament** at the level of the first and second vertebrae have been identified, which is of importance in rotation movements of the head (Humphreys et al., 2003; Mitchell et al., 1998; Dean & Mitchell, 2002) (Fig. 21.2).

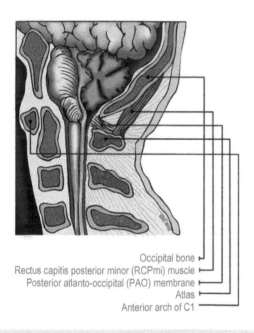

Occipital bone
Rectus capitis posterior minor (RCPmi) muscle
Posterior atlanto-occipital (PAO) membrane
Atlas
Anterior arch of C1

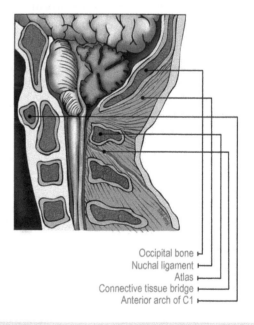

Occipital bone
Nuchal ligament
Atlas
Connective tissue bridge
Anterior arch of C1

Figure 21.1

Myodural connections with suboccipital muscles. © Stefanie Lenk (www.medicalartandgraphics.com)

Figure 21.2

Continuity of the nuchal ligament and SDM at the level of C1–C2. © Stefanie Lenk (www.medicalartandgraphics.com)

A connection between the **flaval ligament** and the SDM was identified in the upper and lower cervical spine at the level of the vertebral bodies (Rutten et al., 1997; Kubo et al., 1994. Other direct attachments at the level of C7/T1 have also been described (Hayashi et al., 1977). The posterior SDM is anchored to the flaval ligament via the posterior cervical epidural ligaments. In the absence or dysfunction of those ligaments, anterior displacement of the dura is suggested, which may lead to flexion myelopathy (Shinomiya et al., 1996).

The superficial layer of the **posterior longitudinal ligament** (PLL) is attached to the SDM (von Lanz, 1929). Likewise, Hofmann's ligaments are also located between the dura and the superficial layer of the PLL (von Lüdinghausen, 1967; Scali et al., 2012; Fernández-de-las-Peñas et al., 2007; Tagil et al., 2005) (Fig. 21.3). Sometimes, the superficial layer of the PLL is regarded more as a protective membrane for the soft structures inside the vertebral canal than as a conventional ligament (Hayashi et al., 1977;

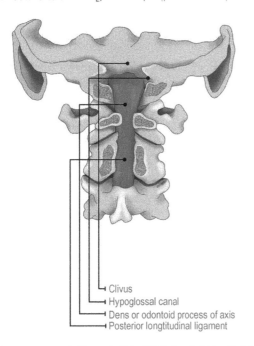

└ Clivus
├ Hypoglossal canal
├ Dens or odontoid process of axis
├ Posterior longtitudinal ligament

Figure 21.3

Posterior longitudinal ligament. © Stefanie Lenk (www.medicalartandgraphics.com)

Loughenbury et al., 2006). The ventromedian ligaments associated with the posterior longitudinal ligament (PLL) are sometimes called **Trolard's ligaments**. They are situated between the dura and the vertebral bodies and arc in the lower lumbar and sacral spine (Barbaix et al., 1996).

Soulié's ***trousseaux fibreux*** consists of a network of strong bundles supporting the anterior epidural venous plexus and connecting the dura mater with the posterior longitudinal ligament and the periosteum (Trolard, 1888).

The **denticulate ligaments** are fibrous structures that are located on either side of the spinal cord throughout its entire length, separating the ventral from the dorsal roots of the spinal nerves. The toothlike processes of these ligaments are attached to the dura mater. Extension and flexion of the spine is transmitted via the denticulate ligaments by the SDM to the pia mater, with the greater part of the forces being transmitted directly to the spinal cord via cranial and caudal attachments of the dura (Rossitti, 1993) (Fig. 21.4).

The rhomboid halter is a thin, diamond-shaped connective tissue plate that is attached to the dura mater via the upper toothlike processes of the denticulate ligaments (Rossitti, 1993; Key & Retzius, 1975). It has been suggested that the rhomboid halter keeps the cranial region of the spinal cord and the inferior medulla oblongata separated from the dens of the axis, the ligamentous apparatus, and the vertebral arteries during neck flexion (Lang, 1981; Breig, 1978).

The **opercula of Forestier** are located at the level of every intervertebral foramen, representing a connection between the dural coverage of the spinal nerves and the periosteum of the particular vertebra (Trolard, 1888; Forestier, 1922; Lazorthes, 1981). They are present at the inner and outer sides of the vertebral canal, enveloping the intervertebral foramina from both sides as well.

Vascularization

The course of the spinal cord arteries is highly variable. The SDM is supplied by the paired posterior spinal

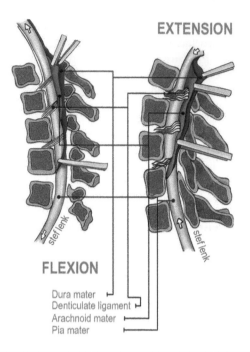

EXTENSION

FLEXION

Dura mater
Denticulate ligament
Arachnoid mater
Pia mater

Figure 21.4
Tensional changes in the denticulate ligament during flexion and extension of the vertebral column and their influence on the spinal cord. © Stefanie Lenk (www.medicalartandgraphics.com)

arteries and the anterior spinal artery. Venous drainage occurs via venous plexuses outside the vertebral column and segmental veins (Hu et al., 1995). These valveless plexus veins are of special physiological importance. They are able to communicate with the lumbar and intercostal veins, and with venous plexuses in the nuchal region, which enables multidirectional drainage of venous blood without congestion.

Innervation

Compared to the cranial dura mater, the SDM is sparingly innervated. In particular, the innervations are less dense dorsally than ventrally (Groen et al., 1988; Kumar et al., 1996). The dorsal dural nerves are derived from the ventral dural plexus, which is connected to the sinuverteral nerves, the nerve plexus of the posterior longitudinal ligament, and the nerve plexus of radicular branches of segmental arteries (Groen et al., 1988).

References

Adams C. B. T., Logue V. (1971) Studies in cervical spondylotic myelopathy. I. Movement of the cervical roots, dura and cord, and their relation to the course of the extrathecal roots. *Brain*. 94:557–568.

Alix M. E., Bates D. K. (1999) A proposed etiology of cervicogenic headache: the neurophysiologic basis and anatomic relationship between the dura mater and the rectus capitis posterior minor muscle. *J Manipulative Physiol Ther*. 22:534–539.

Arbuckle B. E.: (1994) The selected writings of Beryl E. Arbuckle. Indianapolis: American Academy of Osteopathy,. pp. 74–91.

Barbaix E., Girardin M. D., Hoppner J. P., Van Roy P., Clarijs J. P. (1996) Anterior sacrodural attachments – Trolard's ligaments revisited. *Man Ther*. Mar;1(2):88–91.

Breig A. (1978) *Adverse Mechanical Tension in the Central Nervous System: An Analysis of Cause and Effect: Relief by Functional Neurosurgery*. Stockholm: Almqvist and Wiksell.

Dean N. A., Mitchell B. S. (2002) Anatomic relation between the nuchal ligament (ligamentum nuchae) and the spinal dura mater in the craniocervical region. *Clin Anat*. 15:182–185.

Dragoi G. (1995) The mechanical properties of newborn dura mater. *J Leg Med*. 3(4):368–374.

Drenkhahn D., Zenker W. (Hrsg.) (1994) *Anatomie, Bd. 1*. 15. Aufl. München: Urban & Schwarzenberg, p. 489.

Fernández-de-las-Peñas C., Bueno A., Ferrando J., Elliot J. M., Cuadrado, M. L., Pareja J. A. (2007) Magnetic resonance imaging study of the morphometry of cervical extensor muscles in chronic tension type headache. *Cephalalgia*. 27:355–362.

Forestier J. (1922) In: Giradin M. Die caudale durale Insertion und das Ligamentum sacrodurale anterius (Trolard). *Naturheilpraxis*. 1996;4;528–536.

Groen G. J., Baljet B., Drukker J. (1988) The innervation of the spinal dura mater: anatomy and clinical implications. *Acta Neurochirurgica*. 92: 39–46.

Hack G. D., Hallgren R. C. (2004) Chronic headache relief after section of suboccipital muscle dural connections: a case report. *Headache*. 44:84–89.

Hack G. D., Koritzer R. T., Robinson W. L., Hallgren R. C., Greenman P. E. (1995) Anatomic relation between the rectus capitis posterior minor muscle and the dura mater. *Spine*. 20:2484–2486.

Haines D. E., Harkey H. L., al Mefty O.(1993) The "subdural" space: a new look at an outdated concept. *Neurosurgery*. 32(1):111–120.

Hallgren R. C., Hack G. D., Lipton J. A. (1997) Clinical implications of a cervical myodural bridge. *AAO J*. 7:30–34.

Hamann M. C., Sacks M. S., Malinin T. I. (1998) Quantification of the collagen fibre architecture of human cranial dura mater. *J Anat*. 192(Pt 1):99–106.

Hayashi K., Yabuki T., Kurokawa T., Seki H., Hogaki M., Minoura S. (1977) The anterior and the posterior longitudinal ligaments of the lower cervical spine. *J Anat*. 124:633–636.

Herle P. (2012) *Basic and Clinically Relevant Anatomy: A Guide for Students and House Surgeons*. Melbourne: Pradyumna Herle.

Hu J. W., Vernon H., Tatourian I. (1995) Changes in neck electromyography associated with meningeal noxious stimulation. *J Manipulative Physiol Ther*. 18:577–581.

Humphreys B. K. , Kenin S, Hubbard B. B., Cramer G. D. (2003) Investigation of connective tissue attachments to the cervical spinal dura mater. *Clin Anat*. 16:152–159.

Jinkins J. R. (2000) *Atlas of Neuroradiologic Embryology, Anatomy, and Variants*. Philadelphia: Lippincott Williams & Wilkins.

Kahkeshani K., Ward P. J. (2012) Connection between the spinal dura mater and suboccipital musculature: evidence for the myodural bridge and a route for its dissection – a review. *Clin Anat*. 25:415–422.

Kahn J. L., Sick H., Koritké J. G. (1992) Les espaces intervertébraux postérieurs de la jointure crânio-rachidienne. *Acta Anat Basel*. 144:65–70.

Key A., Retzius G. (1975) *Studien in der Anatomy des Nervensystems und des Bindegewebes*. Norstedt und Söner, Stockholm. Erste Halfte, pp. 88–89, 99, Tafel I (Figs 2,3,4).

Kubo Y., Waga S., Kojima T., Matsubara T., Kuga Y., Nakagawa Y. (1994) Microsurgical anatomy of the lower cervical spine and cord. *Neurosurgery*. 34:895-902.

Kumar R., Berger R. J., Dunkser S. B., Keller J. T. (1996) Innervation of the spinal dura: myth or reality? *Spine*. 21:18–25.

Lang J. (1981) *Klinische Anatomie des Kopfes*. Berlin: Springer, p. 436.

Lazorthes G. (1981) In: Giradin M: Die caudale durale Insertion und das Ligamentum sac-rodurale anterius (Trolard). *Naturheilpraxis*. 1996;4:528–536.

Loughenbury P. R., Wadhwani S., Soames R. W. (2006) The posterior longitudinal ligament and peridural (epidural) membrane. *Clin Anat*. 19:487–492

Mitchell B. S., Humphreys B. K., O'Sullivan E. (1998) Attachments of the ligamentum nuchae to cervical posterior spinal dura and the lateral part of the occipital bone. *J Manipulative Physiol Ther*. 21:145–148.

Nash L., Nicholson H., Lee A. S., Johnson G. M., Zhang M. (2005) Configuration of the connective tissue in the posterior altanto-occipital interspace: a sheet plastination and confocal microscopy study. *Spine*. 30:1359–1366.

Newell R. L. (1999) The spinal epidural space. *Clin Anat*. 12(5):375–379.

Pontell M. E., Scali F., Enix D., Battaglia P. J., Marshall E. (2013) Histological examination of the human obliquus capitis inferior myodural bridge. *Ann Anat*. 195:522–526.

Pontell M. E., Scali F., Marshall E., Enix D. (2012) The obliquus capitis inferior myodural bridge. *Clin Anat*. 26:450–454.

Rossitti S. (1993) Biomechanics of the pons-cord tract and its enveloping structures: an overview. *Acta Neurochirugica (Wien)*. 124:144–152.

Rutten H. P., Szpak K, van Mameren H., Ten Holter J., de Jong J. C. (1997) Anatomic relation between the rectus capitis posterior minor muscle and the dura mater (letter; comment). *Spine*. 22:924–926.

Scali F., Marsili E. S., Pontell M. E. (2011) Anatomical connection between the rectus capitis posterior major and the dura mater. *Spine*. 36:E1612–E1614.

Scali F., Pontell M. E., Enix D., Marshall E. (2013) Histological analysis of the rectus capitis posterior major's myodural bridge. *Spine J*. 13:558–563.

Scali F., Pontell M. E., Welk A. B., Malmstrom T. K., Marshall E. , Kettner N. W. (2012) Magnetic resonance imaging investigation of the atlanto-axial interspace. *Clin Anat*. 26:444–449.

Shinomiya K., Dawson J., Spengler D. M., Konrad P., Blumenkopf B. (1996) An analysis of the posterior epidural ligament role on the cervical spine cord. *Spine*. 21:2081–2088.

Singh I. (2011) *Textbook of Anatomy: Vol III*. Jaypee Brothers Medical Publishers.

Standring S. (2008) *Gray's Anatomy: The Anatomical Basis of Clinical Practice*. 40th edn. Elsevier.

Tachibana S., Kitahara Y., Iida H., Yada K. (1994) Spinal cord intramedullary pressure: a possible factor in syrinx growth. *Spine*. 19:2174–2178.

Tagil S. M. , Ozcakar L., Bozkurt M. C. (2005) Insight into understanding the anatomical and clinical aspects of supernumerary rectus capitis posterior muscles. *Clin Anat.* 18:373–375.

Trolard P. (1888, 1890) In: Giradin M. Die caudale durale Insertion und das Ligamentum sacrodurale anterius (Trolard). *Naturheilpraxis.* 1996;4:528–536.

Vandenabeele F., Creemers J., Lamprichts I. (1996) Ultrastructure of the human spinal arachnoid mater and dura mater. *J Anat.* 189:417–430.

von Lanz T. (1929) Über die Rückenmarkshäute. I. Die konstruktive Form der harten Haut des menschlichen Rückenmarkes und ihre Bänder. *Wilhelm Roux Arch Entwickl Mech Org.* 118: 252–307.

von Lüdinghausen M. (1967) Die Bänder und das Fettgewebe des Epiduralraumes. *Anat Anz.* 121:294–312.

Westbrook J. L. (2012) Anatomy of the epidural space. *Anaesthesia and Intensive Care Medicine.* 13:(11)551–554.

Zumpano M. P., Hartwell S., Jagos C. S. (2006) Soft tissue connection between rectus capitis posterior minor and the posterior atlanto-occipital membrane: a cadaveric study. *Clin Anat.* 19:522–527.

THE FASCIA OF THE PERIPHERAL NERVOUS SYSTEM

Michael Hamm

'All ... nerves go to and terminate in that great system, the fascia.'

A. T. Still

Clinicians working with the nerve–fascia interface depend on a clear understanding of the anatomical and physiological relationship of the two tissues. This chapter summarizes the structural and functional connections of peripheral nerves to fasciae, explores related findings from current fascia research, and suggests some ways that research findings may pertain to clinical practice.

Overview

A functioning peripheral nervous system (PNS) accomplishes the transmission of nerve signals and the maintenance of its cellular health despite significant potential disruption from mechanical stressors. Axons must pass from their cell bodies though heterogeneous fluid pressures, shifting interfaces, and rapidly tensioned limbs.

The structural strength, elastic recoil, and sliding capacity of the PNS are adaptations to these challenges, and are conferred primarily by fascial structures within and outside nerves. In addition, the reflexive actions of muscular and vascular elements to protect and supply neural structures are constrained and guided by the fascial architecture. Without such adaptations, the PNS is likely to suffer injury or dysfunction (Shacklock, 2005b; Topp & Boyd, 2006).

The clinical field of neurodynamics (Butler et al., 2000; Shacklock, 2005a) has explored in some detail the characteristic movements and physiologic changes that the main trunks of the PNS display in response to different stressors. Authors in this field have

emphasized the inadequacy of performing physical assessment of the PNS without a spatial understanding of its interface with surrounding structures.

Often this interface is schematized as a series of connective tissue tunnels through which a given nerve extends from midline to the innervated tissues. The nerves themselves are often shown as fully dissected from their fascial conduits. Simplifications such as these can be helpful for learning general principles, but the intact arrangement of fasciae is what determines the mechanical behavior of a living nerve (Topp & Boyd, 2006; Shacklock, 2005b).

Structural changes in the PNS may or may not be pathogenic, and likewise PNS pathology may or may not arise from changes in fascial architecture. Plausible mechanisms do not always correspond with clinical reality. Careful description of the nerve–fascia architecture is therefore necessary for clinical hypotheses to be made, tested, and refined.

The peripheral neurofascia

The fascia of the PNS can be classified as either *intrinsic* (comprising the nerves themselves) or *interfacing* (referring to fasciae that enclose, accompany, and confer force onto neural tissues).

Intrinsic fascia

Dissection of a nerve reveals it to be a nested arrangement of pressurized fascial tubes. Axons and Schwann cells are enclosed in *endoneurium* – a compartment containing interstitial fluid; longitudinal type I and

II collagen; and a basal lamina on the inner wall composed of type IV collagen, fibronectin, laminin, and heparin sulfate proteoglycan. Also inhabiting this environment are fibroblasts and somewhat rarer mast cells and macrophages. Not present within this axonal conveyance are blood vessels or lymphatics (Ombregt, 2013; Bove, 2008).

Endoneurial tubes are then tightly collected in multilaminar fascicles of *perineurium*, which have the capacity to slide and rearrange within the nerve in response to external forces. The number of separately mobile fascicles within a peripheral nerve varies widely along its length, and is generally correlated with the amount of bending or compression the nerve experiences during normal movement. In this way, transverse stressors can be taken up through the rearrangement of fascicles without requiring their deformation. Accordingly, fascicles within a nerve tend to multiply near joints and converge along diaphyses (Shacklock, 2005b).

Anchoring the fascicles is a loose mesh of *inner epineurium*, which connects to the dense *outer epineurium*. Each of these layers is a continuation of meningeal fasciae at midline (Ombregt, 2013; Bove, 2008).

Intraneural blood supply

Traversing the inner epineurium and perforating into the fascicles is a coiled vasculature (vasa nervorum) that delivers the metabolic resources for cellular repair, maintenance of membrane potential, and axoplasmic transport (Ombregt, 2013; Bove, 2008).

Blood vessels perforating into the outer epineurium are innervated by a perivascular plexus of serotoninergic, adrenergic, and peptidergic nerves. The arterioles contain only a small number of smooth muscle fibers, suggesting a limited capacity to modulate blood flow under changing conditions (Ombregt, 2013).

Blood–nerve barrier

Vessels inside the loose epineurium perforate and branch obliquely into the strata of the perineurium, terminating in large-diameter, longitudinal arterioles arrayed around the endoneurial tubes. Here the innermost layer of the perineurium forms a fluid barrier of collagen fibers enmeshed with interlocking

fibrocytes (Ombregt, 2013). Inflammatory processes can alter this barrier and allow a more direct interface between blood and endoneurium (Bove et al., 2003).

Intrinsic innervation of nerves

A population of small-diameter C and A∂ nerve fibers (nervi nervorum) travel along with the epi- and perineurium. These fascially-bound plexi have been characterized as *nocifensive* – regulating local inflammatory defense – and have been proposed as the key generator of nerve trunk pain (Fig. 22.1) (Bove, 2008).

Nerve injury and repair

Damage or lack of integrity in these intraneural fasciae has been suggested as a major cause of failure in the healing of peripheral nerves following injury. Given intact endoneurium (or a synthetic facsimile), glial cells can proliferate within the tube and release trophic factors guiding the regrowth of axons. A disrupted endoneurium may result in cessation of axon growth, or in the formation of a disorganized neuroma (MacKinnon, 2002).

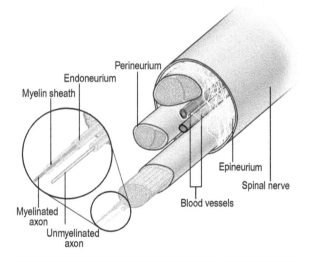

Figure 22.1
Intraneural fasciae shown in their nested arrangement. Each fascial layer is innervated, but vascular supply does not normally penetrate the endoneurial space

Fox & MacKinnon (2011) describe a six-stage model for assessing mechanical injuries to intraneural fasciae: axon/myelin disruption without endoneurial damage (stages 1–2), intact endoneurium with fibrous scarring (3–4), and some degree of fascial rupture within the nerve (5–6). Milder injuries show progressive improvement along the nerve's path in both manual and electrodiagnostic tests. More severe injuries exhibit a physiologic stasis and may require surgical repair for optimal recovery.

Interfacing fascia

While the integrity of nerves is conferred by intraneural compartments, their function within a moving body depends equally on the state of surrounding fascial tissues.

Mesoneurium and neurovascular bundle

Immediately outside the epineurium is a variably thick layer of loose connective tissue, commonly called *mesoneurium (*also *paraneurium)*, which enmeshes the attending vasculature and anchors the neurovascular bundle to surrounding tissues (Willard, 2012a).

Smaller blood vessels are observed to be coiled within loose strata along the nerve surface, whose layers telescope and take up vascular slack as the nerve slides. Branching nerves destined for neighboring fascial compartments also often take on coiled arrangements near sliding interfaces, presumably to allow for greater elongation without loss of function (Willard, 2012a).

Fibrous changes in the mesoneurium after surgery have been observed in human cadaver studies and ultrasonography by Millesi et al. (2007) to correlate with restrictions in the mobility of nerves, thus potentially diminishing their vascular supply and resistance to injury.

Epineurium is most directly attached to surrounding deep fasciae where it is perforated by blood vessels, and where the nerve branches. Nerves are also sometimes firmly attached to bony landmarks, such as the proximal fibula's anchoring of the common fibular nerve (Millesi et al., 2007).

Surrounding deep fasciae

The basic pattern of neurofascial interface is established in early embryologic development and then modified as tissues and compartments develop. The meningeal tube develops from paraxial mesoderm and (mostly) separates from the interior bony arches of the spinal canal. Meningeal sleeves gather around the filamentous connections of ectoderm from neural tube to skin, forming nerve roots. The major fascial compartments of the embryo are both perforated and circumnavigated by developing nerves (Franze, 2013; Willard, 2012a).

Two major compartments of deep fascia arise around neural midline: the axial (ventral) and hypaxial (dorsal) cylinders. At each neural segment, meningeal tubes perforate and follow these cylinders as ventral and dorsal rami. Ventral to the developing spinal column, the sympathethic trunk and rami communicantes traverse the prevertebral fascia and branch into visceral folds and neurovascular bundles. The vagus nerve develops within the mediastinum and branches toward local ganglia inside the capsules and suspensory folds of visceral fascia (Willard, 2012b).

Enclosure of major nerves in limbs

Willard (2012a) observes that both the brachial and lumbosacral plexi derive from nerve roots that perforate through an initial layer of prevertebral muscles, and then perform their exchange of fasicles within a narrow planar interface of deep fascia, whose branches follow along with nerves exiting the plexus.

The main neurovascular bundle is conveyed into the limbs by a dense, irregular septum or sheath that extends distally and continues to branch along with the neurovascular tree. This surrounding dense septum is most likely an extension of the prevertebral fascia at midline. It may serve to deflect and absorb forces of tension and compression in the vicinity of the bundle, and act as a diffusion barrier (Fig. 22.2).

Terminal interfaces

As peripheral nerves branch out from midline, the fascial continuity of meninges and epi-perineurium follows along with each nerve, until finally joining the collagen matrix of innervated compartments. The endoneurium follows along with the axon, joining with the architecture of its terminal receptor or effector (Ombregt, 2013).

Histologic studies of deep fascia by Stecco et al. (2008) and other teams reveal sparse but widespread investment of nerve fibers into collagen layers, with a

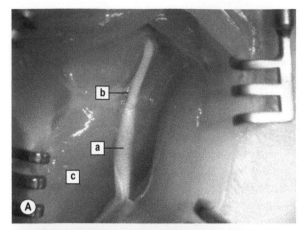

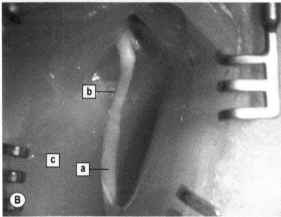

Figure 22.2

Sciatic nerve of a rat, shown with minimal dissection of surrounding fasciae. These structures change their conformation when, with the hip in resting position at 80° flexion (A), the knee is moved into extension (B). The nerve is drawn distally and narrows in diameter. A proximal branch point is drawn toward a fascial junction, and transverse 'bands of fontana' (British Medical Journal, 1972) seen in the epineurium at rest (A) disappear as the nerve approaches its elastic end range. **a** Nerve/outer epineurium; **b** mesoneurium; **c** adjacent deep (myo) fascia. Images courtesy of Dr Geoffrey Bove

The adhesion of neural structures to the surrounding extracellular matrix, combined with pressure and tension from the growth and migration of tissues, creates the fascial *pre-stress* seen in the adult human. The result is a nervous system with internal fluid pressure; intrinsic tensional forces; specific anchor points to midline and to target tissues; and a variety of fascial bindings along the sheaths of peripheral nerves. This environment is the baseline for cellular mechanotransduction, including mechanoreceptivity in nerve endings (Franze, 2013; Topp & Boyd, 2006).

Response to mechanical stress

A combination of direct force (compressive or tensile) and ischemia (mechanical or reflexive) can alter the function of nerves and their fasciae. If these factors are transient, the loss of function is quickly recovered. If prolonged or of sufficient magnitude, the cellular health and fascial architecture of a nerve may be chronically compromised.

Nerves in various experimental models display viscoelastic resistance and end-range stiffness before succumbing to damage. During the application of longitudinal stress, the nested fascial tubes and blood vessels elongate with progressively more resistance. Simultaneously the transverse diameter of the nerve decreases, meeting opposition from internal fluid pressure and thus increasing the overall stiffness of the nerve. (This relates to LaPlace's law regarding pressure–tension relationships within fluid chambers.) Progressively less structural stiffness is seen in the nerve as it is increasingly dissected away from surrounding tissues, suggesting that any dissective investigation involves a degree of departure from mechanical behavior in vivo.

Experiments on living nerves have shown a significant reduction in intraneural blood flow when the sliding of nerve meets its elastic end range. Blood flow is not impaired at 6% strain, is reduced by 50% at 11% strain, and is fully restricted at 16% strain (Topp & Boyd, 2006). These effects may be due to the ligation of perforating blood vessels or a lack of sufficient perfusion under higher pressure.

In cases of prolonged pressure or ischemia, nociceptors may respond by initiating a local dilation

volume fraction of about 1.2%. They are more numerous in the vicinity of blood vessels, and the majority terminate without specialized capsules.

of arterioles and a mechanical sensitization of the nerve (Shacklock, 2005c). In the short term, this may accomplish the restoration of blood supply and dissuade the larger organism from positions and actions that mechanically strain the nerve tissue.

Optimal pre-stress

As with all fascially bound structures, nerves are adapted for a level of mechanical stress, which depends for its maintenance on a regular, noninjurious amount of strain. Prolonged immobilization of a limb or tissue may expose nerves to levels of pre-stress below the physiological optimum, leading to adaptive changes such as decreased axon diameter and increased deposition of collagen, both of which may decrease the nerve's tolerance of mechanical stress when the tissue is re-mobilized (Ombregt, 2013).

Capacity for length change

Nerves appear to be physiologically tolerant of gradual length change over time. Studies of osteogenic bone-lengthening procedures have found that a rate of nerve lengthening by 0.5 mm to 1.0 mm per day does not significantly compromise local nerve function (Ombregt, 2013).

Defensive response

Experimentally induced inflammation, in addition to activating intraneural nociceptors, has been shown to cause the inward migration of immune cells into the peri- and endoneurium. Once inflammation is resolved, some immune cells have been observed to remain trapped, thus potentially leaving the tissue open to an amplified inflammatory response in the future (Bove et al., 2003).

Prolonged inflammation has also been theorized to interfere with axoplasmic transport, causing the deposition of transductive membrane proteins at the site of sensitization. Once embedded, these proteins respond readily to stimuli (thermal, mechanical, or chemical), and now may generate 'ectopic' action potentials, issuing bidirectionally from the site of generation. This ectopic impulse generation has been proposed, but not confirmed, as a noncentral mechanism in the maintenance of chronic pain (Bove, 2008).

Fibrosis

Repeated mechanical stress and immune-mediated degeneration have been observed to result in fibrous proliferation in the interior of nerves (MacKinnon, 2002; Ombregt, 2013).

Some surgical and cadaveric evidence suggests that fibrous thickenings can occur in the mesoneurium around nerves as well (Millesi et al., 2007; Willard, 2012a). The exact cause, or causes, of these fibrous changes in vivo have not been established. It is also unclear whether these fibrous changes are positively correlated with symptomatic pathology in patients. Indeed some authors (Bove, 2008) have cautioned against the existence of nerve 'tethering' as a generator of peripheral pathology.

Until more clarity emerges on the clinical significance of such thickenings, the clinician should keep in mind that fibrous change is not necessarily pathologic – though inflammatory sensitization is likely to increase the symptomatic effect of any local mechanical changes.

Clinical considerations

Elsewhere in this book, the reader will find a discussion of the sensory role of fascia per se, and the intrinsic functions of fascial structures. To the degree these findings relate to the peripheral nerve health of our patients, it can be helpful to incorporate some clinical model of nerve–fascia interaction into our treatment sessions.

Discussions of nerve entrapment have focused on places where nerves must perforate dense fascial structures or branch heavily into neighboring compartments. These interfaces are described as 'fulcrums' where the spatial movement of nerves is relatively constrained and thus more susceptible to entrapment.

Mechanical restriction may be a local phenomenon governed by fibrotic change, nerve irritation/edema, or myofascial contracture. Or it may involve more systemic factors, such as a summative restriction along the nerve bed, or the faulty engagement of an interfacing fascial plane during movement, or a centrally mediated inflammatory sensitization (Jänig, 2014). As more sophisticated models of fascial architecture and mechanics are developed, clinicians should strive to visualize the effects on the associated nerve anatomy.

During a seated slump test, for example, the head and spinal column are brought to a flexed position, passively drawing neural slack into the spinal canal. The fasciae innervated by the sciatic nerve are then carefully moved distally by flexing the hip, extending the knee, and dorsiflexing the foot. The combination of this central fixation and peripheral distraction is intended to increase the mechanical tension along the dura–epineurium, and accentuate any local stressors in the sliding interface. A provocation of familiar symptoms suggests to the clinician an increased neural sensitivity to deformation (Shacklock, 2005c).

Various modifications of the nerve–fascia interface during this test can help the clinician localize further the source of provocation:

- Shifting one joint position (e.g., inversion of the ankle) while the others remain stable may indicate which neural segments or branches are most sensitized.

- Changing the order of positioning (e.g., lifting the leg prior to flexing the spine) places different sections of dura–epineurium under stress from surrounding tunnels and turns, and thus often produces a different result.

- Tensioning or slackening of innervated skin along the axis of a cutaneous nerve (via manual engagement or taping) may indicate where the superficial fascia is involved.

- Careful palpation along the trunk of the nerve – using the interfacing tissues to engage with the dura–epineurium – may indicate where the neurovascular sheath is most restricted or sensitized.

(Note: Clinicians are advised to avoid prolonged stretch positioning of more than 30 seconds for the nervous system. Take breaks when testing.)

The literature on the physical health of the peripheral nervous system has seen an evolution in diagnostic and treatment models, from one primarily pathomechanical (tethered nerve) to one that takes into account concurrent changes in immune and central nervous system function (sensitized field) (Jänig, 2014; Butler et al., 2000; Shacklock, 2005a). It is a fast-evolving paradigm, still largely dependent on the discernment and skill of individual practitioners.

Clinical reports on nerve entrapment, such as those by Elkstrom & Holden (2002), Saratsiotis & Myriokefalitakis (2014), and Settergren (2013), exhibit some common themes. Emphasized is the importance of the nerve–fascia interface in diagnosis and pathogenesis. Both local and nonlocal factors contributing to dysfunction and recovery are taken into account. Manual fascial release methods are used in conjunction with neurodynamic tensioning to better mobilize the interfaces in and around the nerve. Most importantly, care is taken to treat the person and their total nervous system with respect, and not elicit a further sense of danger in the peripheral nerves.

Conclusion

When the health of a patient's peripheral nervous system is in question, the neurofascia – intrinsic and interfacing – are valuable objects of clinical inquiry. Practitioners who understand the adaptive responses of nerves and their fasciae will be better prepared to perform clear assessments, provide effective interventions, and interpret more skillfully the body's response to treatment. Perhaps most usefully, simple models of the nerve–fascia interface may be beneficially imparted to our patients, for the safety and self-care of their peripheral nervous systems.

References

Bove G., Ransil B., Lin H., Leem J. 2003. Inflammation induces ectopic mechanical sensitivity in axons of nociceptors innervating deep tissues. *Journal of Neurophysiology.* 90(3):1949–1955.

Bove G. 2008. Epi-perineurial anatomy, innervation, and nociceptive mechanisms. *Journal of Bodywork and Movement Therapies.* 12 (3):185–90.

Butler D. S., Matheson J., Boyaci A. 2000. *The Sensitive Nervous System.* Noigroup Publications. Chapters 1–2, 8.

British Medical Journal. 1972. Spiral nerve bands of fontana. [Editorial note]. (17 June) 671.

Elkstrom R., Holden K. 2002. Examination and intervention for a patient with chronic lateral elbow pain with signs of nerve entrapment. *Physical Therapy.* 82(11):1077–1086.

Fox I., MacKinnon S. 2011. Adult peripheral nerve disorders: nerve entrapment, repair, transfer, and brachial plexus disorders. *Plastic and Reconstructive Surgery.* 27(5):1–21.

Franze K. 2013. The mechanical control of nervous system development. *Development.* 140(15):3069–3077.

Jänig W. 2014. Sympathetic nervous system and inflammation: a conceptual overview. *Autonomic Neuroscience.* 182:4–14

MacKinnon S. E., 2002. Pathophysiology of nerve compression. *Hand Clin.*18 (2):231–241.

Millesi H., Hausner T., Schmidhammer R., Trattnig S., Tschabitscher M. 2007. Anatomical structures to provide passive motility of peripheral nerve trunks and fascicles. *Acta Neurochir Suppl.* 100:133–135.

Ombregt L. 2013. Pressure on nerves. In: *A System of Orthopaedic Medicine,* 3rd ed. Churchill Livingstone Elsevier. Chapter 2, pp. 21–27.

Settergren R. 2013. Conservative management of a saphenous nerve entrapment in a female ultramarathon runner. *Journal of Bodywork and Movement Therapies.* 17(3):297–301.

Saratsiotis J. Myriokefalitakis E. 2014. Diagnosis and treatment of posterior interosseous nerve syndrome using soft tissue manipulation therapy: a case study. *Journal of Bodywork and Movement Therapies.* 14(4):397–402.

Shacklock M. 2005a. *Clinical Neurodynamics.* Edinburgh: Elsevier Butterworth Heinemann, pp. xi–xii.

Shacklock M. 2005b. *Clinical Neurodynamics.* Edinburgh: Elsevier Butterworth Heinemann, pp. 12–15.

Shacklock M. 2005c. *Clinical Neurodynamics.* Edinburgh: Elsevier Butterworth Heinemann, pp. 20–25.

Stecco C., Porzionato A., Macchi V., Stecco A., Vigato E. 2008. Expansions of the pectoral girdle muscles into the brachial fascia: morphological aspects and spatial disposition. *Cells, Tissues, Organs.* 188(3):320–329.

Topp KS, Boyd BS. 2006. Structure and biomechanics of peripheral nerves: nerve responses to physical stresses and implications for physical therapist practice. *Physical Therapy.* 86:92–109.

Willard F. 2012a. Somatic fascia. In: R. Schleip, T. W. Findley, L. Chaitow and P. A. Huijing, eds., *Fascia: the Tensional Network of The Human Body.* London: Churchill Livingstone Elsevier, pp. 11–17.

Willard F. 2012b. Visceral fascia. In: R. Schleip, T. W. Findley, L. Chaitow and P. A. Huijing, eds., *Fascia: the Tensional Network of The Human Body.* London: Churchill Livingstone Elsevier, pp. 53–56.

Clinical aspects of fascia | 4

Therapeutic considerations | 4.1
Manual techniques | 4.2

4

INTRODUCTION

Anthony G. Chila, Paolo Tozzi

At first glance, this section might appear to be large, voluminous, and perhaps unwieldy to the reader. A bit of reflection will show that the overall content distributes easily into two major categories: Therapeutic Considerations and Manual Techniques. A comment or two about each category is in order. One of the difficulties encountered by clinical practitioners of various persuasions in manual bodywork is the issue of justification. It is perhaps for this reason that the series of Fascia Research Congresses I–IV has served an excellent purpose. Since the inception of the Congresses in 2007, the main theme has been to relate basic science implications to conventional and complementary health care. Meeting this standard has elevated the level of communication between and among these areas. In this light, the various mechanisms described are all part of an ongoing desire to improve fundamental understanding of experiential encounters with various manual interventions. By the same token, it is the experiential value of touch and manual intervention that seeks for and enables much greater appreciation of form, function, and motion. Across the spectrum of research and practice reflected throughout this text, the number and variety of authors contributes further to the expanding world of interest in fascia.

THE ABILITIES OF FASCIA

Rüdiger C. Goldenstein, Patrick Van Den Heede

Summary

The fascia represents a biological unit with distinct integrative and adaptive abilities. It mimics the shape and the image of the body (morphophenomonology). Entirely in line with the osteopathic principle of the interrelationship between structure and function, fascia is the organ of the body that embraces this principle.

During its development, it forms body cavities and generates the connection between the different compartments. The memory of this development is stored within the fascia and provides us with the tool for influencing 'body, spirit, and soul' through an osteopathic treatment in the sense of the founders of osteopathy. Therefore, the fascia clearly is more than a purely mechanical tool.

Introduction

There are still a lot of contrasting opinions over the abilities of the fascia, both with respect to its structure and regarding its function. The change in the use of the terminology of 'fascia' plays a considerable role; however, this has to be viewed critically since the newer definition describes what has been defined previously as the connective tissue part of the body.

At the Third International Fascia Research Congress in 2012, the term 'fascia' was used to mean the loose connective tissue that permeates the entire human body, providing an umbrella term for previously distinguished anatomical features, such as aponeuroses, tendons, ligaments, capsules, retinacula, epineurium, periosteum, and others.

On the other hand, a definition of fascia that is still valid in German-speaking countries describes it as 'slightly elastic, consisting of crossing-over collagen fibers and elastic networks, and covering single muscles and muscle groups.'[1]

Because of the aforementioned differences in definition, we would like to highlight that we will be using the definition originated by Frank H. Willard: an unorganized, loose connective tissue (mesenchyme).

Fascia in osteopathy and morphodynamics

Osteopaths generally tend to use the word fascia very arbitrarily to describe the tool through which they get into contact with the 'inside' of the body and the developmental story of its contents and exchange. A large number of osteopaths still have a very mechanical view with regard to the role of the fascia. A reason for this may well be that a large part of the research was carried out from a mechanical viewpoint with the aim of researching continuity and mechanical interaction.[2]

Some authors describe the connections of the fascia or the accompanying tension as the expression of a complex physiological interaction between different body systems, which serves to find a new balance point.[3] Nevertheless, only a few regard the fascia as an independently functioning organ. The main point is to understand whether fascia represents a continuum and can be defined as a histological unit.

Current views on fascia

Currently, fascia in general is regarded as a flexible and organized elaboration of loose, mobile and/or thick connective tissue, resulting in condensed, organized structures. These firmer structures function, for example, as tendons and insertions of muscles and bones, or extend the relations to, of, and between organs, both at a visceral and at a cranial level.

Often only the condensed, firmer and organized parts of the connective tissue are considered as a gateway to support osteopathic techniques. These parts are described as levers, bands, and cords that produce relations and fixations between structures in a highly organized, anatomical way. New to this approach is the justified call to match the description of the anatomy and dissecting anatomical specimens with the continuity of the tissue, in the sense that, for example, band structures could be viewed as a continuation of fascial tissue.[4]

Most of the time reference is made to classical anatomy books in which the osteopath can study the exact relation of these components in a reproducible way. The classic mechanical view tends to restrict comfortable access to the dynamic implications of more recent views. This in turn can contribute to restrictions on effective practice and teaching. On the other hand, there are contrasting and more innovative opinions on the actual function of fascia, where it is seen as an actual connection between body, spirit, and soul.[5] An obvious gap exists between those two views, which is yet to be filled through detailed research and which should explore what fascia really is, how it transmits its information into consciousness, and its role in autonomic and endocrine homoeostasis.

Development of the fascial concept in osteopathy

A. T. Still recognized the importance of the fascia more than 100 years ago and presented it as the highest communicating network, which is responsible for health and disease.[6]

A. T. Still repeatedly mentioned the mucous membranes, the mesenteria, the mesosystem, the omentum, and the connective tissue of the spine.[7] For Still, fascial relationships seemed to be significant based on many years of clinical experience and his own studies. From today's perspective, this is astonishing, since it took more than a century for the attention of modern science to be directed toward fascia.[8]

Still's understanding of fascia was as a matrix or system from which diseases develop and spread. Therapeutically, he dealt with the structural and functional components rather than the fascia directly. According to Stark, Still treated the fascia by seeking to improve the arterial, venous, and lymphatic circulation, as well as nerve function, usually through adjustments of bones. Still also treated the fascia by repositioning the viscera, for example, to influence mesenteric structures.[9] Based on the available literature, it is difficult to decide whether Still initially treated the supporting membrane to influence the position of the organs, or vice versa, or both.[9]

Concerning fascia as a therapeutic tool, an overview of the classical writings, concepts, and principles of American osteopaths can help define fascia as all-embracing scaffolding that integrates mechanical, metabolic, and immunological functions. The best-known early osteopaths who have taught on the subject of fascia and influenced our present concepts and understanding are A. T. Still, W. G. Sutherland,[10] R. E. Becker,[11,12] A. G. Cathie,[13] and J. G. Zink.[14] Their knowledge of the principles and basics is known to us through their writings.

Outstanding American descendants continue to pass on their knowledge, including V. M. Frymann, A. G. Chila,[15] and R. J. Hruby.[16]

Historically, what was taught about fascia?

1. Fascia is seen as an envelope of the body. It connects each structure and each anatomical part within the body. By guiding the essential structures like blood vessels, lymphatic ducts and nerves, it secures their function. Fascia can be described as a connecting tissue throughout the entire body.

2. A. G. Chila explained: 'If someone carries out a dissection and takes away all except fascia, we still remain with the form, size and basis for movement.'[17]

3. A. T. Still described fascia as the hunting grounds, being the basis of all techniques; and each supporting measure should start at the fascia.

4. The fascia of the body can be subdivided into three types: a superficial, a deep, and a visceral fascia.

There is the possibility of space formation between the superficial and the deep fascia. This space has the function of a gliding surface. It is this space in which clinical problems appear, due to imbalances in the fluids, metabolites, waste removal, and inflammation.

Fascia essentially maintains two characteristics:

- It secures the intactness and integrity of function and structure, and therefore organizes the body as a biomechanical unit.

- It directs the fluids and the electric field of the body.

Moreover, the fascia has two outstanding functions:

- A mechanical function, leading movement and mobility and supporting the body as a biomechanical unit: 'There is no muscle in the body that is not connected with the bone over connective tissue. The periosteum also has to be looked at as a connective tissue.'[17]

- A biomechanical function, possessing a conducting function for nerves and all types of pathways, which are integrated within it for appropriate fluid exchange and drainage

The visceral fascia also represents a fundamental part of the complete fascial body and does not possess any other distinguishable function. In the classic concept, there is no difference between a visceral function and a mechanical, supporting function: 'One cannot treat the visceral space as a separate unit. Even the cranial fasciae belong to the same organ system'.[17]

A. G. Cathie noticed that the dural membrane is a specialized form of connective tissue that supports and integrates the function of the other fasciae.

The ability of the fascia has been described as follows:[13]

- It contains sensory nerves.

- It is elastic and contracting.

- It provides attachments for muscles.

- It regulates the circulation (especially the venous–lymphatic exchange).

- It contributes to generating movement, to controlling it, and to influencing movement between body areas.

- It supports posture.

- It is the place of inflammation.

- It moves fluids and infectious processes through the entire body.

- The dura mater is a specialized connective tissue.

It seems evident that earlier osteopaths did not look at fascia as a solely mechanical tool. This is in contrast to what we often read, or possibly are taught, during our osteopathic studies.

Fascia from a morphodynamic view

The actual function of the fascia should, from our point of view, be derived from its pathway of development during embryogenesis and later organogenesis. During development, the fascia is situated between ectoderm and endoderm, and acts as a mediator of information between all tissues, in the same way as the intermediate mesoderm it has emerged from.

Fascial development

Fascia derives from embryological mesenchyme, which originates and develops its function during the first moments of gastrulation. According to Blechschmidt, the characteristic feature of mesoderm is its functioning as a zone of inner tissue situated between two different layers of limiting tissue.[18] The essential difference between a limiting tissue and inner tissue is the existence of intercellular matrix and space (see also Chapter 9).[19]

Mesenchymal cells proliferate and migrate throughout the embryo in order to fill unoccupied spaces and intercalate between the cells that later differentiate into organs (Fig. 23.1).

Gastrulation – the rise of intraembryonic mesoderm – occurs as early as the first epiblast cells proliferating and congregating along the midline to form the primitive streak and primitive node. They contribute toward the development of the notochord, the prechordal plate, and lateral plate mesoderm (Fig. 23.2).

Figure 23.1

Interplay between embryonic structures and mesenchymal tissue. ECF = extracellular fluid; EMT = epithelial-to-mesenchymal transformation; NCC = neural crest cells

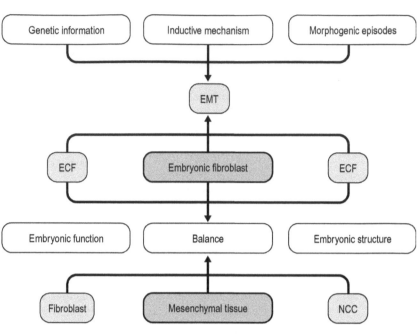

During the development of the notochord, these flat epithelial cells are influenced by a chemical field, which defines further cellular behavior through the effects of certain chemical gradients. Cells begin to migrate and transform during the epithelial-to-mesenchymal transformation. This process and the development of the primary mesenchyme both contribute to the formation and development of organs, and the development of body cavities. Organs, muscles,

and blood vessels all grow within the mesenchyme. The mesodermal formation is shown in Figure 23.3. All forms of stress (i.e., poor nutrition, mechanical stress, epigenetic factors, etc.) during embryological development influence the alignment of the original organization of the mesenchyme.

Fascia cannot be regarded as epithelium because it does not have a basement membrane. For this reason,

Figure 23.2

Origin of the axial (investing) fascia

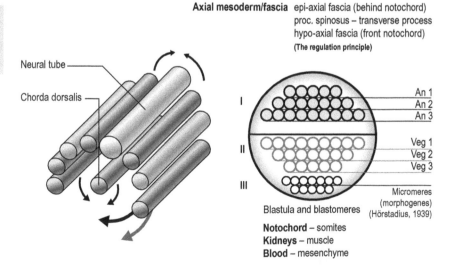

Axial mesoderm/fascia epi-axial fascia (behind notochord)
proc. spinosus – transverse process
hypo-axial fascia (front notochord)
(The regulation principle)

Neural tube

Chorda dorsalis

I
An 1
An 2
An 3

II
Veg 1
Veg 2
Veg 3

III
Micromeres
(morphogenes)
Blastula and blastomeres (Hörstadius, 1939)

Notochord – somites
Kidneys – muscle
Blood – mesenchyme

Splanchnopleura/somatopleura para-axial mesoderm

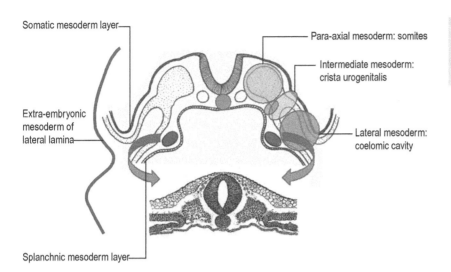

Somatic mesoderm layer

Extra-embryonic mesoderm of lateral lamina

Splanchnic mesoderm layer

Para-axial mesoderm: somites

Intermediate mesoderm: crista urogenitalis

Lateral mesoderm: coelomic cavity

Figure 23.3
Mesodermal differentiation

it can spread out into different directions and can unite different structures. At this time, it consists of stretched cells and appears as a loose, not particularly well-aligned tissue (Fig. 23.4).

Organs develop within the mesoderm. Muscles grow within the mesenchyme, which forms an investing fascia in and around the muscle. In fact, the whole somite develops as mesoderm and all of the related structures will develop within the mesenchyme:

- The dermatomes are essentially mesenchymal.

- At this stage the myotomes help initiate the development of the neural tube.[20]

- The sclerotome will give rise to hard tissue (bones and tendons), which also develop from mesenchyme.

Histomorphologic view

F. H. Willard mentions that fascia appears as a loose or firm, irregular connective tissue during histomorphologic studies.[21] It is not really an organized tissue. If a tissue has regularly aligned collagen fibers, it

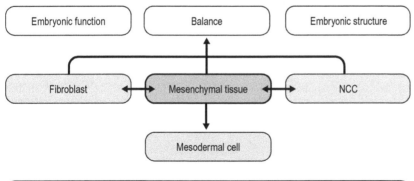

Figure 23.4
Organization of the mesenchyme

Embryonic function

Balance

Embryonic structure

Fibroblast   Mesenchymal tissue   NCC

Mesodermal cell

Embryonic mesenchyme: **primitive fascia**

Organization is loose

Always elongated cells

Stress lines in embryonic development set up lines of cell specialization and orientation

Stresses during embryological development reconstruct pathways of original organization

cannot be considered as fascia anymore and should be called an aponeurosis or a tendon.

As long as one finds irregularly laid-down collagen fibers, the tissue will:

- resist multi-directional forces
- serve as an investing tissue (enveloping, condensing, binding)
- fill the spaces between stable structures and other vulnerable components (e.g., blood vessels and others) so that these are not damaged.

Highly irregular patterning can also be found within the visceral fascia, in which the adventitia of the blood vessels blends with the surrounding tissue, blurring any clear boundaries.

Misnomers occur frequently with regard to the visceral fascia. Since it looks thicker in certain areas, many wrongly speak of ligaments, such as the Treitz fascia or the lateroconal fascia (paracolic gutter/ descending mesocolon). Histologically this is not correct, since these 'ligaments' show no regularity. However, for example, an aponeurosis should not be termed fascia because it appears as a spread-out, flat sheet of regular and firm connective tissue. According to the aforementioned description, this would not be classified as fascia. We must speak of aponeuroses instead of fasciae when we talk about the latissimus dorsi, the erector spinae, the plantar aponeurosis, the thoracolumbar aponeurosis, etc.

Fascial function from a morphodynamic view

In some respects, fascia serves as a transit (passage) zone between metabolic, mechanical, and histoimmunological driving forces. If the tissue suffers a tear or stress exertion (pressure/load), the fibroblasts can return to their stem-cell function. They are converted into protomyofibroblasts, which in turn can develop into myoblasts. The fibroblasts form the biomechanical center of the mesenchyme and can adapt their production of molecules by secreting cytokines in response to environmental changes (Fig. 23.5). In certain respects, they react in the same manner as the fibroblasts in the extracellular matrix (ECM).

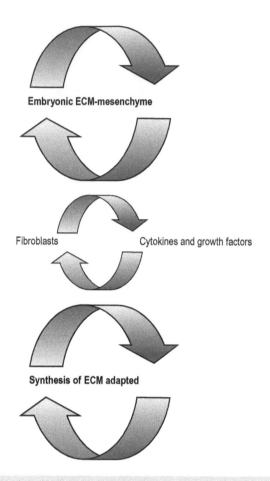

Embryonic ECM-mesenchyme

Fibroblasts   Cytokines and growth factors

Synthesis of ECM adapted

Figure 23.5
The embryological extracellular matrix: the mesenchyme

They can build up or destroy the matrix through metalloproteins or serine protease inhibitors (serpins) (Fig. 23.6). This is how the fibroblasts adopt an embryological pattern of function, protecting the tissue and its surroundings against further damage, for example, as in the case of the myocardium, by transitioning into a type of hibernation (Fig. 23.7).

Subdivision of the fascial system (according to F. H. Willard)

As mentioned above, F. H. Willard regards the original fascia as a loose, irregular connective tissue. He subdivides the fascial system into four main groups (Fig. 23.8):

- The paniculate fascia (superficial fascia)

- The axial fascia (described as the investing fascia), which lies beneath the dermis/subcutaneous tissue

- The meningeal fascia, which covers the entire cerebral nervous system.

- The visceral fascia, which connects organs and organizes the visceral cavity.

The axial or investing fascia can further be subdivided into:

- epiaxial fascia (develops behind the notochord)

- hypaxial fascia (develops in front of the notochord).

The axial fascia terminates at the base of the skull and only covers the part that derives from the somites. At the base of the skull, it is extended by the pretracheal fascia, which starts at the base of the heart where it originates embryologically from the covering of the Truncus arteriosus. Distally the end can be defined as being at the height of the division of the common iliac artery. The axial fascia forms a large covering sac in which most of the organs are contained.

Working on the fascia in these different compartments can be considered as accessing the trusted, most intimate 'workbench' of the body. On this 'workbench', most of the 'software' that ensures the homoeostatic adaptation of the body is developed. Additionally, the forwarding of substances to different zones in need of provision occurs in conjunction with physiological processes and according to specific times.

Conclusion

Fascia is a complete and purposeful organ. It develops from the mesenchymal 'workbench', which contains and controls the entire history of the embryogenetic, organogenetic, and developmental processes. Fascia represents an up-to-date function for receiving, conducting, exchanging, and storing information from different origins and for different destinations. In order to understand the function of the fascia,

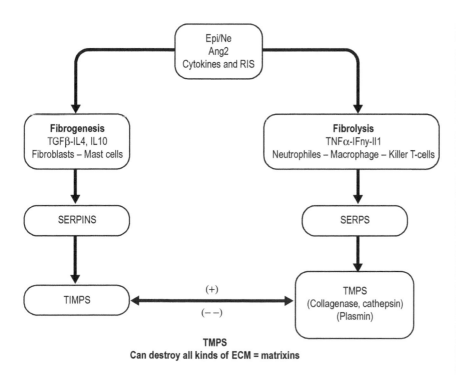

TMPS
Can destroy all kinds of ECM = matrixins

Figure 23.6
Regulation of inflammatory processes in the extracellular matrix. ECM = extracellular matrix; SERPINS = serine proteinase inhibitors; SERPS = serine proteinases; TIMPS = tissue inhibitory metalloproteinases; TMPS = tissue metalloproteinase. Reproduced with permission from Figure 1.9, p. 33, in H. Heine, *Lehrbuch der biologischen Medizin, Auflage 4*, Haug in MVS Medizinverlage, Stuttgart, 2015

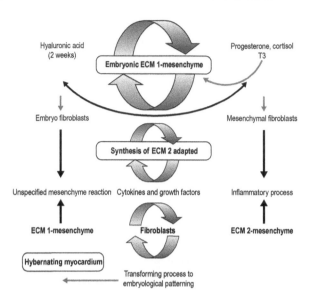

Figure 23.7
Hibernation of the myocardium

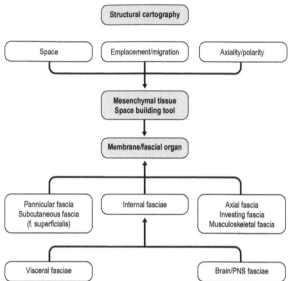

Figure 23.8
Groups of fascia according to localization.
PNS = peripheral nervous system

a detailed study of the function of the connective tissue is necessary. The exchange between extracellular matrix, fluids, and fibroblasts needs to be understood before one can participate in the great event of the body 'telling' us its most intimate stories of life. Through this it is easier to understand that movement and stillness have a most intimate relationship with all bodily functions and that the concept of A. T. Still on the trinity of body, mind, and soul is not a mere illusion.

References

1. *Pschyrembel Clinical Dictionary* (German Language). 252nd edition. Walter De Gruyter, Berlin, 1982.

2. A. Vleeming. 3rd Interdisciplinary World Congress on low back and pelvic pain. Vienna, Austria, November 19–21, 1998.

3. J. J. Debroux. Les fascias, du concept au traitement, pp. 163-170. Olivier Éditeur, 2002.

4. T. Dobler, M. Puylaert, J. van der Wal. Faszien. In: T. Liem, T. Dobler. *Leitfaden Osteopathie*. Elsevier, München, 2009.

5. J. McGovern & R. McGovern. *Your Healer Within*, pp. 86–90, Fenestra Books, 2003.

6. C. Ciranna-Raab. Das Tensegrity Modell. In: T. Liem, T. Dobler. *Leitfaden Osteopathie*. Elsevier, München, 2009.

7. A.T. Still. *Die Philosophie und die mechanischen Prinzipien der Osteopathie*. In: Das große Still-Kompendium, 2. Auflage, p.143f. Jolandos, Pähl, 2005 [dt. Übers. *The Philosophy and Mechanical Principles of Osteopathy* 1908].

8. See Chapter 2 'Nomenclature of fascia' in this book.

9. J. Stark. *Still's Fascia*, p. 156, Jolandos, Pähl, 2007.

10. W. G. Sutherland. *Teachings in the Science of Osteopathy*, pp. 5–6, 107, 218, Rudra Press, 1990.

11. R. E. Becker. *Life is Motion*, Stillness Press, 2001.

12. R. E. Becker. The Stillness of Life, Stillness Press, 2000.

13. A. G. Cathie. The fascia of the body in relation to function and manipulative therapy. *Yearbook American Academy of Osteopathy*, 1974.

14. G. J. Zink. Respiratory and circulatory care: the conceptual model. *Osteopathic Annals*, pp. 108–112, March 1977.

15. A. G. Chila. Conference on the fasciae, Namur, Belgium, Aug 4–6, 2001.

16. R. J. Hruby & P. Masters. The respiratory and circulatory model of Gordon Zink, Conference, Namur, Belgium, 1998.

17. A. G. Chila. Conference, Namur, Belgium, May 4–5, 2002.

18. E. Blechschmidt. Die ersten drei Wochen nach der Befruchtung. [The first three weeks after fertilization] Image Roche (Basel), 47:17–24, 1972.

19. J. van der Wal. Faszien. In: T. Liem, T. Dobler. *Leitfaden Osteopathie*. Elsevier, München, 2009.

20. M. S. Dias & M. Partington. Embryology of myelomeningocele and anencephaly, *Neurosurg Focus*, 16(2):E1, 2004.

21. F. H. Willard & G. Stevens. Skin and fascia. Conference, Limelette, Belgium, 2012.

FASCIA AND POSTURE: FROM THE BIOMECHANICAL MODEL TO THE NEUROMYOFASCIAL POSTURAL MODEL

Paolo Zavarella, Maurizio Zanardi, Christian Lunghi

The biomechanical postural model used in the osteopathic field

The concept of 'ideal posture' is historically related to the biomechanical, compressive, and structural models of the body and seems to be achievable by adequately activating the linear mechanisms of compression, tension, and balance.

Today it is understood that posture, like any other adaptive system, can no longer be interpreted as a static and reproducible state, but must be considered a dynamic 'strategy'. Therefore, the understanding of posture has evolved from mechanical efferent concepts of 'posturometry' to dynamic and afferent concepts of 'posturology'. The only form of balance possible in biological systems is the dynamic one, due to inertia, acceleration, and gravity: the parts have a rhythmical and reciprocal relationship between themselves and with the whole, and are constantly changing via internal and external homeostatic and allostatic mechanisms.

The research on the ability 'to keep a straight or a leaned posture against a blowing wind' (Bell, 1837), therefore on the relationship between posture and vision, oculomotricity, vestibular function, weight-bearing, and proprioception (Levinson, 2013; Housman et al., 2014) was focused on the idea that there was a system that was regulating balance in a complete, autonomous, and unique manner. Recently, due to the development of computer systems and stabilometry (Ranquet, 1953), it is known that balance, posture, and the fine postural system (FPS) are able to receive afferent information from several receptors that work with each other in a nonlinear way, coordinated by the central nervous system (CNS).

Looking at the historical definition of posture, one can understand the slow acquirement of the awareness of the complex, dynamic, and nonlinear phenomenon that is posture. Posture can be considered as the relationships between the whole body, its different parts, and the environment with which it is surrounded. This represents the whole accommodation to a certain environment and the correlation between somatic and mental aspects of the body (Tribastone, 1985; Caillet, 1977). Posture can be associated with behavioral embryology, which determines how the embryo behaves in its surrounding environment (Thelen & Adolph, 1992). A baby is thought to learn how to adapt and maintain a correct body position in space, to move its eyes in order to have control of its surrounding environment, to adequately regulate its heartbeat and breath to a specific situation, to be aware of its position in space, and to adopt a psychological well-being in every environmental situation (Guidetti, 1997).

Posture constitutes the combination of reflexes with polysensorial interactions that aim to achieve upright position (Gagey & Weber, 1997). The latter can be defined as the spatial relationships between body parts (Boccardi & Lissoni, 1998) achieved by the passive properties of ligaments and joints and the active properties of tonic muscles, in harmony with the gravitational forces (Caradonna, 1998) at a specific moment (Kandel et al., 2000).

For every individual, the best posture is achieved when body parts are confronted to minimum straining forces and have the maximum stability. Balance is a state, however, posture is a 'holistic strategy' that needs to be studied, analyzed, and used to better understand function, dysfunction, and the degree of adaptability in the structure-and-function relationship. The upright posture is unique to human beings and depends on the activity of coordinated mechanisms, which are responsible for its maintenance and stability. We believe that posture mirrors the adaptive neuromyofascial abilities of involuntary biological rhythms and of the allostatic load that constantly and dynamically changes balance.

The classical concept of 'ideal posture' (Charpentier, 1979; Gagey & Weber, 2010) has always been appealing, even though many authors point out its rarity in the clinical setting (Lunghi et al. 2016). It has been argued that an individual with adequate 'compensations', even should he be asymmetrical, can 'function' well (Kuchera, 2011). Passive muscular tonicity helps to maintain an orthostatic posture with a minimal increase in the body's energetic demand (+7% more than in supine position), often for a long period of time, due to polymorphic variations of the myofascial tone. Postural adaptations of the human body to the gravitational forces seemed to have developed due to the relationship between neurological evolutionary mechanisms and musculoskeletal tissue compensations aiming to reduce energetic waste (Zanardi, 1998; Zavarella et al., 2002).

In this chapter, the need for osteopathy to walk away from the 'ideal posture concept' will be described, although many clinicians still focus on correcting misaligned body structures in their clinical practice.

In the past few years, many authors have questioned whether the biomechanical postural model (BPM) was over-rated and stressed the urgent necessity of its renewal (O'Sullivan, 2010). To analyze these topics with criticality, *The Journal of Bodywork and Movement Therapy* invited five experts on manual medicine, osteopathy, chiropractic, and physiotherapy to confront their ideas on the topic (Chaitow, 2011), discussing whether the use of manual techniques to correct and rebalance the misaligned body parts is justifiable (Lederman, 2010). They concluded that unless the 'postural balance, mobility, energy and resistance' are re-established, the normal body function without pain might be hard to obtain using rehabilitation strategies. Therefore, it is necessary to consider holistic approaches, such as osteopathic manipulative treatment (OMT), aiming to integrate structure and function (Irvin, 1997; Chaitow, 2011).

The evolution of a postural concept

Clinical experience shows that in people with musculoskeletal symptoms, hypertonic areas at rest or hard surfaces, even with silent electromyographical signal, such as the superior trapezius in people who are affected by tension headaches or at the dorsolumbar erector spinae in people suffering with lumbar degenerative disc disease or ankylosing spondylitis can be palpated.

Research shows that human muscular tonicity at rest comes from viscoelastic tissue properties. The basic level of passive tension and the lengthening resilience contributes to maintaining postural stability in balanced positions and is defined as 'human resting myofascial tone or tension' (HRMT). HRMT is found within the kinematic body chains, independently of the CNS activity, and derives from molecular interactions between actin-myosin filaments within the sarcomere and within the myofibroblasts (Masi et al., 2008). On the contrary, the cocontraction of muscular groups is the effect of an active neuromotor control, which allows greater levels of stability associated with major energetic waste. Functionally, HRMT has relationships either with passive tensional fascial webs and ligamentous tendinous structures to build up a biotensegrity system that gives a stable support to maintain balanced posture. Significant reduction or excess of postural HRMT can cause musculoskeletal or pathological disturbance (Masi et al., 2010). Taking into account the evolution of the idea of posture and integrating the observations made on the importance of HRMT, one can immediately understand its different aspects, each of them being significant for the end results.

Postural control classically implies the control of the body position and its different parts, statically and dynamically. It is made up of:

- postural reflexes

- postural tone (the relationship between muscular tonicity and HRMT).

Therefore, there is not 'one posture,' but an indefinite number of 'postures' related to:

- any position assumed by the body or one of its parts that maintains:
  - a state of balance
  - a state of unbalance.

A dysfunctional memory, such as a somatic dysfunction (SD), is maintained by an increase in fibrous tissue and several links between collagen fibers in nodal points within fascial bands, with a progressive loss of the tissue's elastic properties. These myofascial tissue changes may alter the abilities of higher centers responsible for proprioceptive and interoceptive sensorial integration, as well as centers coordinating motor control and posture (Schabrun et al., 2013; Tsao et al., 2008; Tozzi, 2014).

A new concept of posture has emerged; indeed, today in theoretical scientific terms, it no longer exclusively relates to compressive, static, and linear concepts. A more recent definition of posture is based on the multiple strategies continuously used by the neuromyofascial system to adapt to gravitational forces and interoceptive, proprioceptive, and biopsychosocial stresses.

Should we then walk away from the concept of 'ideal posture'?

Renewing the biomechanical postural model: the neuromyofascial postural model

As we are debating posture in the field of fascia in osteopathy in this chapters, we will discuss:

- the historical concept of posture
- Lederman's criticism of BPM
- our own considerations on the debate surrounding the 'BPM crisis'.

We will propose a model that is coherent with the multifactorial nature of biomechanical, homeostatic, and allostatic adaptations: the neuromyofascial postural model (NMPM).

'Adaptations' are homeostatic (close to balance) and allostatic (away from balance) mechanisms. Allostasis (a metasystem of changes that maintains the systems essential to life) is the coherent answer of the system to stressors (Selye, 1956; Schulkin, 2003) and has been revealed as a 'syntropic' phenomenon rather than an 'entropic' one (Fantappié, 2011).

Adaptation is the main element of the stress response; it is a biological mechanism that is useful in restoring balance and minimizing internal effects, thus maintaining the interdependency between structure and function.

To conclude, 'posture' is the strategy used by the neuromyofascial and skeletal systems in response to gravitational forces and the accelerations (static or dynamic) ready to be used, when needed:

- in the most economical way (with the least energetic costs and myofascial tonic–phasic activity)
- with maximal stability (maximal 'dynamic balance')
- with maximal comfort (minimal stress on the osteoligamentous and myofascial structures);
- with no pain.

We believe that an evolution is necessary to keep the NMPM alive, and this evolution should take into account the multifactorial nature of the complex systems within posture and lead the osteopath toward a global approach. The NMPM considers:

- Integration between structures of an area and their function, to observe how much not only this relationship has an effect on the individual allostatic load, but also its reflection on posture.
- Neuromyofascial aspects in response to internal and external stimuli and the integration in the body of interoceptive and proprioceptive mechanisms.
- Biopsychosocial aspects, with the psychoemotional load that makes the individual unique, that allow an adaptive answer to be particular and individualistic (Laborit, 1979).

Consequently, the complexity of the expression of this process emerges, which progresses neither in a linear nor in a predictable way but in an observable and modifiable manner.

From molecules to cells, to tissues, and organs – each level is connected in a hierarchical organization able to integrate tensional stimuli of biomechanical forces in order for them not to be dissipated into the biotensegrity structure of the body. These stimuli are therefore converted into biochemical intercellular signals aiming to maintain structural integrity (Swanson, 2013).

The complex relationship between input (receptor afferents – visual–acoustic, podalic, somatoemotional, and occlusional/cranio-cervical mandibular) and output (compensations, postural adaptation) is possible with HRMT, in constant search of a new dynamic balance. This concept helps us to realize how the energies applied by an osteopath on the skin can have an effect at the cellular level by changing gene expression (Maas & Sandercock, 2010) and postural adaptations (Cao et al., 2013).

The new NMPM described in this chapter considers the posture to be an epiphenomenon and an efferent result (musculoskeletal) of an underlying afferent complexity (neuromyofascial): this concept can be read and interpreted and not judged or corrected.

For example, the information deriving from a scar or from traumatized ankle tissues returning to mobility via an efferent system causes global postural adjustments. A symptom can emerge in an area less capable of 'compliance' (Bordoni & Zanier, 2013) involving even the sympathetic nervous system and causing local vasoconstriction (Macefield, 2005; Mouchnino & Blouin, 2013), which allows a dysfunction to happen. A patient may suffer from pain, even if the scar is small and looks aesthetically good, due to the adhesions that can 'trap' the peroneal nerve not only mechanically, but also in response to afferent stimuli that lead the FPS to develop involuntary, local, and segmental contractures (Gilbey, 2007; Raju et al., 2012; Charpentier, 1979; Gagey & Weber, 2010). As a result of constant painful stimuli, the central and peripheral nervous systems adapt themselves, changing function and structure (allodynia and hyperalgesia) and creating a domino effect (Zwerver et al., 2013; Day et al., 2012). The nociceptive visceral, interoceptive, protopathic, unconscious stimuli create the same effect, as the central sensitization builds up at a subcortical level (in encephalon and/or in marrow). It interests dorsal horn activity without involving the conscious level (Jänig, 2013).

Changes in walking, chewing, weight distribution, and cervical and lumbar aches can be maintained by scars and adhesions only in areas apparently far from the lesion (Rowe et al., 2005; Skraba & Greenwald, 1984; Harrison et al., 2005; Leijnse & Rietveld, 2013; Stecco, 2009a; Stecco, 2009b).

The recommended osteopathic treatment in the NMPM aims not to elicit the efferent (motor) but the afferent (sensorial) stimulation, leading to:

* focus (to question)
* integration
* treatment (to normalize).

The information (SD) related to postural alteration, to be interpreted as 'dysfunctional attractor' (DM) of complex systems (Zavarella et al., 2002), that follows the same mechanism of afferent alterations coming from a scar, is able to create the foundations for more difficult postural disturbances (Gary, 2011).

The fascia, the ectoskeleton, and postural patterns

One can hypothesize that a vertebral dysfunction gives pain due to a muscular imbalance and an alteration of the weight distribution (postural imbalance), giving an autonomic-efferent response, affected by electrical and biochemical afferents (Brumagne et al., 2008; Shirzadi et al., 2013). The afferent stimuli able to elicit physiopathological reflexes can modify the posture (a complex and instantaneous strategy that links structure with function) and they originate from the neuromyofascial tissue: derma, fascia, dura mater, tendons, and supertendons (Kumka & Bonar, 2012; Benjamin, 2009).

When the fascia is not in its physiological condition, receptors such as the free nerve endings (Kumka & Bonar, 2012) can behave as nociceptors and lead to the development of a complex symptomatology (Stecco, 2009a; Benjamin, 2009; Kumka & Bonar, 2012). The fascial system of the limbs communicates with the whole body, in particular via the thoracolumbar fascia, which is one of the structures that is often a cause of low back pain or arthrokinematic anomalies of the shoulders (Willard et al., 2012).

Consequently, Benjamin has introduced the concept of 'supertendon', revealing how the tendons and fascia webs (articular capsules, tendons, retinacula, bursae), in particular of the hand and foot (von Schroeder & Botte, 1997), constitute the soft tissue for muscle insertions. A similar ectoskeleton is found in invertebrates

(Wood Jones, 1944a; 1944b) and its entire function is superior to the function of the individual limbs (Benjamin et al., 2008). It is a functional network that performs a non-neural 'somatic logic' brain–body coevolution and neuromuscular control (Valero-Cuevas et al., 2007) to guarantee the functioning of the cellular webs within the motor systems.

In the field of osteopathy, since the 1920s, techniques defined by Neidner as 'fascial twist' have been used. These techniques using torsional forces on the supertendons (palmar fascia, plantar fascia, fascia lata) of the extremities aim to find fascial balance and symmetry in transitional areas of the spinal junctions (De Stefano, 2011).

By using the NMPM, the osteopath examines the patient considering 'the body as a unit' and describes the adaptations within a biotensegrity system in which a minimal change in a region can cause biomechanical, tensional, and ergonomic changes from the original structural components to the neurological, respiratory-circulatory, metabolic, and behavioral functions. Fascia represents the *trait d'union* among these elements, integrating the whole-body mechanical forces (Tozzi, 2012). If the existence of this 'meta-system' were proved this would greatly modify our traditional understanding of physiology (Langevin, 2006).

In osteopathy postural patterns are used: the condition of general fascial adaptation to stresses, determined via palpatory tests, can indicate the degree of allostatic load (Zink & Lawson, 1979). It is known that 'postural compensation' represents a useful and functional response to genetic potential, structural asymmetries, allostatic overload, etc.

'Postural imbalance' highlights that the results of adaptations are dysfunctional and symptomatic when the person is manifesting a reduction of homeostatic mechanisms. According to Zink, by exploring the postural patterns it is possible to see signs of function and dysfunction anatomically, physiologically, and psychosocially.

When applying the NMPM, the osteopath 'prepares' the autonomic-connective system so that it can respond to the postural realignment

(Dunnington, 1964). 'Postural misalignment' indicates 'a loss' of individual energies compared to those of gravity and of allostatic loads. A primary role, in the regional compensatory patterns and in the creation of the groups of curvatures in the spine, is played by the anatomical 'transitional areas' (plantar fascia, lumbopelvic, thoracolumbar, cervicothoracic, occipitalatlanto, and craniocervical mandibular), both during adolescence and throughout adult life. The right posture for an individual in a determined period of time will be the best attempt the body will make via the integration of sensorial information and the distribution of body weight, reducing energy waste and harmonizing compression forces using the minimal ligamentous tension. If any asymmetry shows, pain and restrictions will be noticed, 'postural misalignment' will arise (such as the stresses caused by soft tissues sensitive to pain, anomalies, and/or structural restrictions/SD) and may facilitate pathophysiology from gravity strain (PGS) with symptoms such as fatigue, low back pain, and headache (Irvine, 1973).

The concept in which emotions, psyche, body perception and environment influence the posture (Irvine 1973) is integrated in the new NMPM. Individuals affected by psychological problems, such as depression, aggressive behavior, etc., show rigid and misaligned postural patterns, compared to healthy individuals who present good posture and flexibility.

The biomechanical model leads the osteopath to value the local adaptations to stressors (SD) (Lunghi et al. 2016): the neuromyofascial reinformation at the dysfunctional segment. OMT allows the individual to restore structural, vascular, neurological, metabolic, and behavioral functions. The aim of OMT is to optimize the patient's potential, restore functional and structural integrity, and improve dysfunctional postural patterns (LeBauer et al., 2008; Brooks et al., 2009; Posadzki et al., 2013).

Fascia, water, and the postural memory

At this point it is necessary to highlight the afferent aspects of an SD or of the degree of global misalignment. The analogy of water molecules and their behavior in living tissue can be used to describe the ability of fascia to store memory. Water molecules oscillate together, trapped in electromagnetic fields (Del Giudice & Tedeschi, 2009). Oscillations produce free electrons, able to gain electricity, from the background noise, and transform it into 'coherent energy of high quality' in the form of an electron vortex that can activate biomolecules which are resonant with water molecules. Therefore, material, energy, information, and knowledge or memory can be distributed and memorized due to an autotransport mechanism (Del Giudice et al., 2010). A dysfunction corresponds to the expression of altered neural information transmission within which electromagnetic and electro mechanic forces interact. Using palpation, the osteopath may perceive an alteration of the tissue quality, the vitality of the body fluids defined as 'present movement,' which represents the spontaneous motion of the particles that make up the human body (Del Giudice, 2011).

Osteopathy uses techniques based on the quantum physics principle known as the 'principle of the minimal stimulus'. If a proprioceptive, exteroceptive, interoceptive stimulus of very minimal energy is applied, the result is not a direct efferent response, but a neuromyofascial rebuilding/reorganization; the smaller the stimulus, the greater the response.

Osteopaths can achieve therapeutic results by freeing the tissue's memories held in the aqueous body, resulting in health and improved postural patterns. Research demonstrates that alterations in the interaction between calcium and free particles of water can increase after fascial osteopathic treatment aiming to promote motion of the interstitial fluid (Tozzi, 2014).

Procedures for the application of the NMPM

The evaluation process of the NMPM consists of deciding whether the patient will positively respond to a postural treatment considering the time, costs, and efficacy and whether the individual's posture:

1. plays a role in the current complaint (Lunghi et al. 2016)

2. represents a significant risk factor for pain, dysfunction, or future pathology

3. is the best possible adaptation to neurofascial disorders (Lunghi et al. 2016)

4. is the manifestation of local, segmental and/or global disharmony of the interdependent relationship between structure and function (Lunghi et al. 2016)

5. is being conditioned by an area of SD (the osteopath will then operate with a minimalistic approach)

6. has functions (linked to posture) that are influencing local structures causing SD (the osteopath will operate with a maximalistic approach).

The osteopathic evaluation process (Lunghi et al. 2016) (Fig. 24.1) consists of the following:

- Global tests on the general adaptation ability of an individual (allostatic load).

- Local tests on the ability of local adaptation (somatic dysfunction).

- Test of the interdependent relationship between structure and function, which, in the case of the NMPM, aims to evaluate when the SDs are clinically relevant to the postural adaptations.

The postural approach in the osteopathic field heralds the implementation of classical evaluation procedures with those emerging from the integrative postural analysis protocol (IPA) (Box 24.1).

Enrolment of an individual to OMT

Throughout a differential and objective evaluation, the osteopath proceeds to the treatment or to the referral of the patient to his general practitioner (GP) (Lunghi et al. 2016).

Global tests

These tests are to confirm the presence of a postural imbalance and indicate the adaptation capacity of an individual (Irvin, 1998; Zink & Lawson, 1979). The IPA protocol recommends carrying out this test with the help of a scoliometer (Parker et al., 2008), using observation and tissue palpation in transitory areas of the body. In accordance with Zink, transitional areas correspond to neuromyofascial transversal structures and kinematic chains demonstrating a 'fascial twist' in between articular segments.

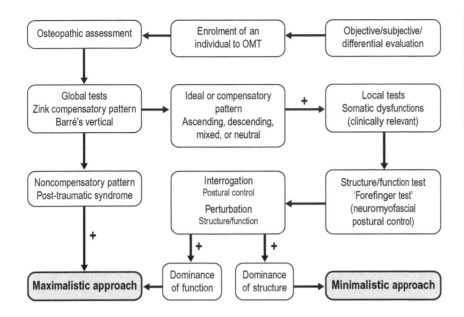

Figure 24.1
The evaluation process of the neuromyofascial postural model (NMPM)

Box 24.1

Protocol for Integrative Postural Analysis (IPA)

The IPA protocol is a method used to analyze the relationship between posture and the neuromyofascial system. It is made up of a series of clinical tests undertaken in a neutral position, after the examination and perturbation phases to test afferent stimuli, which communicate with the whole system via a neuromyofascial network. Comparing the results has shown an internal hierarchy of structure–function relationships. This clarifies whether the postural system is 'suitable' for the allostatic load or whether it has left intact or worsened its own dysfunctional components. Some of the IPA concepts explained below are used in the NMPM.

Base phase

The nine tests may be performed using tools, if required. The tests will highlight specific information to enable you to complete the prognosis, establish the primary area to be treated, and identify the dysfunctional attractors.

1. **Prognosis** (disharmony/dysfunction of the neuromyofascial FPS)

   a. **Postural Romberg test** (reveals the integration rate of the neurological oculocephalic reflexes with static otholithic vestibular reflexes)

   b. **Test of harmonic postural tone** (reveals the rate of integration between myofascial chains, of the diaphragm and of the transitional areas)

   c. **Fukuda–Utenberg test** (reveals the general rate of integration in the dynamic and bilateral distribution of the muscular and antigravitational tone elicited by the cervicospinal reflex)

2. **Primary area** (primary origin of active dysfunctional vectors and the hierarchy between SD)

IMPORTANT: You should look for the primary vector of SD, but if the dysfunctional (disharmonic) posture is present it is not easily assessable.

a. **Barré's posteroanterior vertical test** (studies the static distribution of body parts showing an ascendant or descendent, mixed or neutral, post-traumatic vector)

b. **Test of the external rotators of the hip** (Bernard Autet's test – studies the dynamic response of the neuromyofascial tone of the lower extremity external rotators showing an ascendant or descendent, mixed or neutral, post-traumatic vector)

3. **Dysfunctional attractors (DAs)** (structural and/or functional area where it is very easy to find SD)

a. **The forefinger test** (derived from De Cyon's test – shows the presence of SD in a specific area, by checking the variation in neuromyofascial tone before and after the examination phase)

b. **Podalic weight-bearing test and Barré's lateral vertical test** (show the correlation between dysfunctional attractors during weight-bearing of the hind foot, the angle of flexion/extension for the lower extremity, sacrum, weight-bearing of the head, craniocervical mandibular relationships, and temporomandibular joint (TMJ))

c. **Oculomotor test** (studies the correlation between oculomotor muscles, semicircular canals, cranial innervation, and presence of SD)

Examination phase

The examination phase measures *internal* stress caused by tension and/or perceptive contact and/or lever closure of a single element in the FPS. It allows us to verify, by an efferent reflex arc, the degree of integration, adaptation, and homeostasis of the entire system, highlighting the dysfunctional attractors that correspond to the palpable SD.

The examination phase happens exclusively on the afferent arc while the response happens on the efferent arc. The rational base is made up of the postural reflexes of oculomotor and vestibular origin.

Any of the tests in the IPA Protocol are effective after the examination phase for comparing the answers. If the adaptations are pertinent (the examination allows the elicitation) we will know that neuromyofascial DAs are not present in the area where the examination took place. If the adaptations are not adequately expressed (the examination inhibits or inverts the elicitation), you will find a system, which will correspond to the neuromyofascial system, and you will probably find SD.

Perturbation phase

Perturbation measures *external* stress, modified by the direct or indirect stimulation of a singular element used in the FPS. This allows us to verify, via an efferent reflex arc response ('perturbation' test), the significance of the DA tested compared to its integration and homeostatic approach on the entire system, adding precious information on the nonlinear parameters: primacy, coprimacy, priority, potency, and hierarchy.

Perturbations should have an aim and a specific direction, as they tend to invert (direct approach) or to worsen (indirect approach) the dysfunctional parameters. Therefore, they necessitate an evaluation by the operator to create (in the functional/ structural area with DA) a functional diagnosis. Furthermore, they have to be 'transitory' as they can be deleted from the FPS memory if they cannot reach the aims, to be able to introduce a new perturbation (short-term memory).

Characteristics of the perturbation:

- **Pinpoint**: Works only on a single afferent system

- **Oriented**: Inverts (direct) or worsens (indirect) dysfunctional parameters

- **Transitory**: Refers to the 'neuromyofascial postural' short-term memory

After having used the single perturbation on the primary dysfunctional attractor (PDA), the principal tests (i.e., the base phase test and the examination test) are used again. If the decompensated patterns disappear and/or primacy is deleted, you can find the PDA and you can proceed with a minimalistic approach.

On the other hand, if:

1. The active neuromyofascial element has not been found as PDA – continue focusing on another neuromyofascial element, which is likely to be PDA.

2. The active neuromyofascial element is found as PDA, but it has a coprimacy or a priority, which does not allow the FPS to reach harmony – continue with tests looking for the next active receptor as Coprimary Dysfunctional Attractor (CoPDA).

(Zavarella et al. 2002)

Zink and Lawson believe that it is possible to classify these patterns in a useful, clinical way:

1. Ideal patterns (minimal adaptation loads transferred throughout the regions).

2. Compensatory patterns, which alternate in direction from one area to another and that indicate a good adaptation (e.g., atlanto-occipital/cervicothoracic/thoracolumbar/lumbosacral, which are demonstrated in contralateral rotation and side-bending). In the IPA protocol, in accordance with Irvin's 'boundaries' concept (Irvin, 1998), the plantar arch is considered as another area of transition, which in this case represents a tissue preference ipsilateral to the lumbosacral area (if the plantar arch is in harmony with the ipsilateral lumbosacral area, the lower extremity will not present any dysfunction).

3. Noncompensatory patterns (ipsilateral) are normally activated by a stimulus/trauma or microstimulus/repetitive microtrauma (i.e., atlanto-occipital, cervicothoracic, thoracolumbar, lumbosacral present with ipsilateral rotation and side-bending). In this condition the plantar arch inverts its tissue preference in relation to the lumbosacral area (Zink & Lawson, 1979).

In his description of gravitational stressors, Kuchera maintains that signs and symptoms of physiopathology from gravitational efforts are only manifested after compensatory mechanisms become activated (Kuchera, 1995). Therefore, if a compensatory pattern is observed, the osteopath proceeds using a maximalistic treatment approach (Parsons & Marcer, 2006), walking away from using direct approaches considered in this case as further stressors for an already compromised system (Chaitow, 2002).

Global test of the neuromyofascial tone (i.e., Barré's vertical test)

This test verifies the presence of an SD that alters the relationship between structure and function and affects the postural pattern of an individual (distribution and control of the neuromyofascial tone). In the evaluation of areas of SD in the IPA protocol, the Barré posteroanterior vertical test can be used to evaluate the distribution of postural tone, which indicates the palpable and observable expression of HRMT (Masi et al., 2008), defining a descendent, ascendant, mixed, post-traumatic, or even neutral primary vector (Zanardi, 1998; Zavarella et al., 2002).

The individual is examined statically with a scoliometer, centered using a plumb line, with a reproducible and standard stance (heels at the same height, distance 6–8 cm apart, forefeet rotated 30 degrees external to the heels). The plumb line must pass through the center of the medial malleoli.

The test evaluates the distribution of landmarks correlated with transitional areas (gluteal line, spinous process of C7, vertex) compared to the plumb line, against which a dysfunctional primary vector causing the individual's altered posture can be observed.

Ascending

Possible (neuromyofascial) SD localized below C1–C2 (somatosomatic reflex). The afferent information is transmitted through the fasciculi cuneatus and gracilis in the spinal cord with a high percentage of decussation (for afferent information coming from proximal and axial motor systems).

Descending

Possible (neuromyofascial) SD localized above C1–C2 (somatosomatic reflex), with possible extension down to T4. Afferent information is transmitted by the trigeminal lemniscus, which is formed and runs into the brainstem with a low percentage of decussation.

Mixed

Possible (neuromyofascial) SD localized above and below C1–C2 (viscerosomatic, fascial, neurovegetative reflexes). Afferent visceral information and/or interoceptive information is transmitted by the somatic–visceral–medullary interactions and by the vagal visceral afferents (Jänig, 2013; Jänig et al., 2000).

Neutral

Absence of clinically relevant (neuromyofascial) SD can highlight (somatoemotional) dysfunctions in an individual with high activity of control (borderline personality disorder).

Post-traumatic

Possible (neuromyofascial) SD localized at the level of the cranial and spinal dura mater (alteration of the PRM), generally of traumatic origin. Afferent information is transmitted via the trigeminal, glossopharyngeal, vagus nerve, and recurrent branches of the spinal nerves.

Local tests: evaluation of SD

The osteopath proceeds to the application and verification of biomechanical laws and biotensegrity that rule the stress adaptations of:

- vertebral, thoracic, cranial, and appendicular joints (Fryette, 1917; Gibbons & Tehan, 2001; Bogduk & Mercer, 2000; Herzog, 2000; McCarthy, 2001; Beal; 1987; Cummings, 1994; Fraix et al., 2013)

- soft tissues; fascia; and visceral, vascular, and neural structures (Swanson, 2013; Findley & Shalwala, 2013; Bordoni & Zanier, 2013; Tozzi, 2012).

The palpatory procedure used by the osteopath utilizes some of the palpatory tests that have been demonstrated to be useful to find SD (Degenhardt et al., 2005; Degenhardt et al., 2010).

Test of structure and function interdependence

The inhibition test (Chauffour, 2002) is used to evaluate:

- the influence of structure (SD) on function (postural control: muscular tone, HRMT, reflexes) influencing health.

- the influence of function on structure influencing health.

The forefinger test (Box 24.2) uses the variation in the distribution of muscular tone of extensor muscles in the upper extremities introduced by internal variations to evaluate the relationship between neuromyofascial functions and body biomechanics.

There are three steps to follow: 1) base phase, 2) examination phase, and 3) perturbation phase (see Box 24.1 and 24.2).

1. The base phase measures the neuromyofascial tone.

2. The examination phase measures the grade of postural control: the relationship between muscle tone, HRMT, and myofascial vestibulo–occulo–cervical and viscerosomatic reflexes. It evaluates whether a manually applied stimulus is able to modify (or not) the neuromyofascial tone compared to the one evoked in the base phase. If an examination is able to elicit a postural reflex, it has modified the HRMT in the efferent motor reflex arc, and the function does not indicate overload of the individual's postural control. If, on the contrary, an examination is not able to elicit a postural reflex, there is a dysfunctional relationship between the function and the postural control in the HRMT.

3. The perturbation phase measures the degree of influence in the structure/function. In this phase, the test can be repeated after the tissue-articular barrier of a SD area has been stimulated with specific direct or indirect vectorial parameters

BOX 24.2

The forefinger test

The forefinger test is a neurophysiological test using variation in the symmetry of the tone of the extensor muscles in the upper extremity introduced by internal variants (examination phase). To carry out the test, extend the upper extremities of an individual in a static position, with the forefingers forward, with a neutral gaze, with the jaw relaxed, with teeth not in contact, and with feet aligned.

Base phase

During the base phase the practitioner considers certain physiological functions in the patient, observing at each step whether either of the upper limbs is positioned more posteriorly at the end of the movement of elevation. If this is the case, a degree of hypertonia of the corresponding limb extensor muscles can be detected. The degree to which the limb is positioned posteriorly and the degree of extensor hypertonia can be defined as low, medium, or high.

Examination phase

Perform the test while other body areas fulfill their function (e.g., walking, chewing, swallowing). Some functions and postures elicit oculocephalic or vestibular reflexes that modify the muscular tone. The following are some examples of examination test:

Walking: The patient weight-bears first on one leg, then on the other, without losing contact with the surface and the other foot. You can perform the test and the examination without allowing the patient to change the HRMT tone. If the base phase is different, overload of postural function is found in correlation to the lower extremity, which is weight bearing.

Craniocervical thoracic brachial mobility:

- *Rotation of the head:* The patient rotates the head to the right and then to the left side, without moving the eyes. When you perform the forefinger test the examination has to change the muscular tone by increasing the ipsilateral tone of the extensor muscles and the posteriority of the extremity. If the base phase test results do not change, there is an overload of the postural function related to the cervical spine (C0–C3) and/or the cervical spine muscles and/or the scapular muscles.

- *Side-bending of the head:* The patient side-bends the head to the right and then to the left side very slowly, so that there is no activation of the semicircular canals. When you perform the forefinger test the examination should not allow any change in the muscular tone.

- *Head extension and flexion:* The patient extends and then flexes the head slowly so that there is no activation of the semicircular canals. When you perform the forefinger test the examination should not allow any change to the muscular tone. If the base phase test is modified, there will be an overload of the postural function related to the lower cervical spine (C3–C7) and/or cervical spine muscles. The examination with hyperextended head is used in forensic medicine for its precision in finding (on the stabilometric platform) postural alterations (and balance alterations) following trauma.

Oculomotricity: The patient changes gaze orientation toward the right and then the left, slowly, without rotating the head. The forefinger test is done and the examination phase should change the tone, increasing the tone of the contralateral extensors, and the posteriority of the extremity. If the base phase test results do not change, you may find an overload of the postural function related to the oculomotor muscles.

Occlusion: The patient opens and then closes the jaw. When you perform the test the examination should not change the muscular tone. Conversely, if the practitioner finds an increased muscle tone and a posteriority of the extremity, there will be an overload of the postural function related to the TMJ, to the opening muscles and/or to the jaw, hyoid bone, and the swallowing muscles.

Swallowing: The patient opens the jaw and pushes the tongue out toward the right and then the left. The examination should not change the muscular tone. If the osteopath finds increased muscle tone and a posteriority of the extremity, there will be an overload of the postural function related to the hyoid bone, i.e., to the stomatognathic functions (sound, mastication, and respiration).

(Zavarella et al., 2002)

verifying the answer on a neuromyofascial component related to the overload function that was evoked in the examination phase.

If the test is repeated after the perturbation focused on the SD and is able to elicit a postural reflex, this will be the confirmation that the structure governs the function: the previous SD significantly influences function. The osteopath can now proceed with a minimalistic approach (Parsons & Marcer, 2006) (Fig. 24.2). If the perturbation focused on the SD has given a finding with a direct perturbation, the osteopath will choose direct techniques (i.e., specific adjustment technique – SAT), otherwise in the case of an indirect perturbation (i.e., balanced ligamentous tension technique – BLT).

If the test is repeated after the perturbation focused on the SD and the osteopath is not able to elicit a postural reflex, this will be sign of function governing structure and influencing health. A maximalistic approach (Fig. 24.3) is therefore advised, aiming:

• to normalize the dominant function using homeostatic techniques. For example, the 'occlusion function' indicates balance of the membranous and ligamentous tensions in the cranial area (Cuccia et al., 2011) associated with Galbreath's mandibular drainage techniques (AACOM, 2009) and/or an osteopathic approach to fluids and involuntary movements in the biodynamic cranial field (McPartland et al., 2005). In the case of a dominant 'oculomotor function', the osteopath can proceed with a general routine treatment of the orbit, the

ocular bulb, and its vascular component using Ruddy's technique (Ruddy, 1962).

• to integrate the ectoskeleton and exoskeleton using, for example, the general osteopathic treatment (Parsons & Marcer, 2006) to encourage the coordination and correlation of somatic dysfunctions with the rest of the body, using a rhythmic and oscillatory routine with long levers.

Final considerations

The most important problem in the postural approach to fascia in osteopathy 'is the Question, our main focus, is the Question that has led us here ...' (from *The Matrix*, Lana and Andy Wachowski).

The input of the neuromyofascial afferents governs posture. The osteopath should focus and work on the afferent input (the question), not on the biomechanical efferent input.

The biomechanical is the epiphenomenon of a strong world, made up of *information* transmitted by fascia, tendons, supertendons, ligaments, aponeuroses, and myofibroblasts: neuromyofascial tissues distributed and correlated to each other (Lunghi et al. 2016).

The minimal stimuli law, the examination and perturbations of the afferent input, the distribution of the HRMT, the presence of SD, the complexity of the postural efferent response ... the implications of all of these are described in this chapter, pushing the osteopath toward a critical re-evaluation of the NMPM, aiming for a new neuromyofascial postural model.

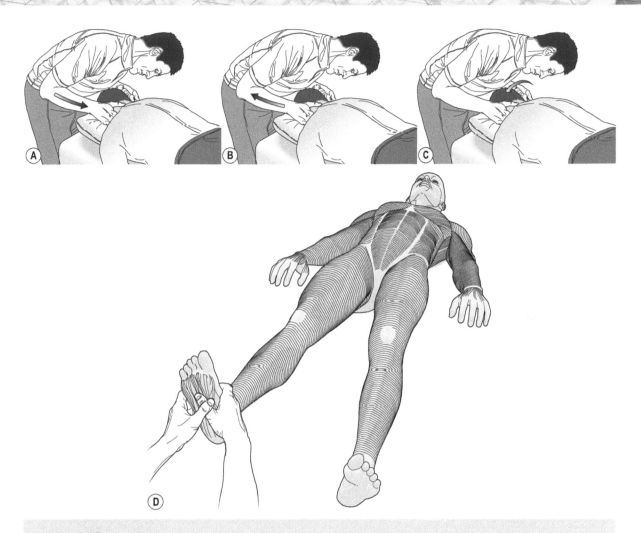

Figure 24.2

Minimalistic approach. The postural governance of structure on function leads the osteopath toward a minimalistic approach with:

- Direct techniques such as specific adjustment technique (SAT) applied to the somatic dysfunction discovered by using palpation. The osteopath approaches the high cervical area using SAT (A, B, C) with harmonic oscillations (A) aiming to find out the vector where all the tensions are neutralized. The operator proceeds with a thrust or a toggle at high velocity and minimal input (B, C) toward the neutral vectors, aiming to improve the tensions memorized in the tissue. Knowledge of the patient's clinical condition is essential before starting any manipulative treatment, especially when the osteopath decides to use SAT (Cicconi et al., 2014).

- Indirect techniques such as balanced ligamentous tension (BLT) technique (D). This indirect technique requires an initial disengagement of the tensioned tissue by using a compressive force (in this example) on the plantar fascia. This phase is often followed by an exaggeration of the vectors used, by engaging a distractive force until a neutral point of tension within the elastic barriers is achieved. Inherent movements of tissue remodeling are reached, such as the vasomotion while the tensional and neurological information is processed. This process goes on until capsule-ligamentous tension is released and the somatic dysfunction normalizes.

Drawings by Mariantonietta Alò

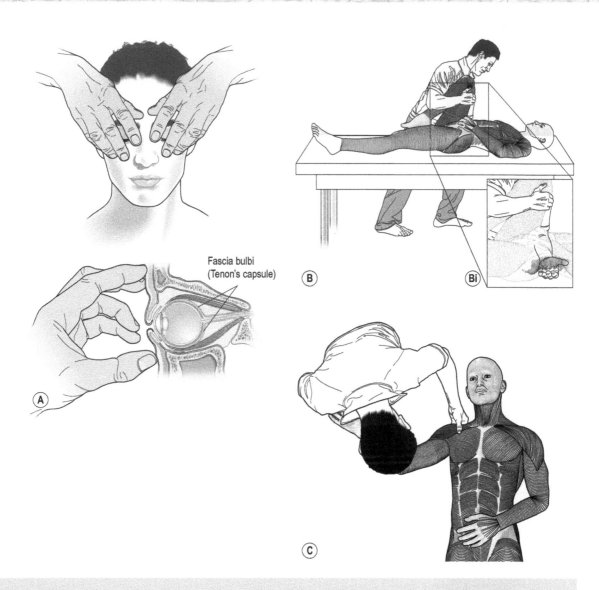

Fascia bulbi
(Tenon's capsule)

Figure 24.3

Maximalistic approach. Postural governance of function on structure leads the osteopath toward a maximalistic approach. In this example one can hypothesize that the evaluation test of the interdependency of structure and function highlights that the oculomotricity and the visual overload are centrally located due to the individual postural function. The operator can then proceed with:

- Treatment of the ocular globe (A) with techniques classically used in case of abnormal tension of the ocular muscles, aiming to improve the eye blood supply working at the capsule of Tenon. After Liem T., 2004. *Cranial Osteopathy: Principles and Practice*, Elsevier Health Sciences, pp. 565–567.

- General osteopathic treatment (B, C). The operator proceeds with a long lever, rhythmic, oscillatory routine to coordinate the kinematics between the lower extremity, the thoracolumbar fascia, and the upper extremity.

Drawings by Mariantonietta Alò

References

AACOM (American Association of Colleges of Osteopathic Medicine), 2009. Glossary of Osteopathic Terminology. Available at: https://www.aacom.org/docs/default-source/insideome/got2011ed.pdf?sfvrsn=2 [accessed March 20, 2016].

Beal M. C. 1987. Biomechanics: a foundation for osteopathic theory and practice. In: Northup G. W. ed. *Osteopathic Research: Growth and Development*. Chicago IL: American Osteopathic Association, pp. 37–58.

Bell Ch. 1837. *The hand: Its Mechanism and Vital Environment*. 4th ed. London: V. Pickering, pp. 234–235.

Benjamin M. 2009. The fascia of the limbs and back – a review. *J Anat* 214:1–18.

Benjamin M., Kaiser E., Milz S. 2008. Structure–function relationships in tendons: a review. *J Anat* 212:211–228.

Boccardi S., Lissoni A. 1998. *Chinesiologia, vol. I.* Roma: Società Editrice Universo.

Bogduk, N., Mercer S. 2000. Biomechanics of the cervical spine. I: Normal kinematics. *Clin Biomech* 15:633–648.

Bordoni B., Zanier E. 2013. Anatomic connections of the diaphragm: influence of respiration on the body system. *J Multidiscip Healthc* 6:281–291.

Brooks W. J., Krupinski E. A., Hawes E. A. 2009. Reversal of childhood idiopathic scoliosis in an adult, without surgery: a case report and literature review. *Scoliosis* 4:27.

Brumagne S., Janssens L., Knapen S. et al. 2008. Persons with recurrent low back pain exhibit a rigid postural control strategy. *Eur Spine J* 17:1177–1184.

Caillet R. 1977. *Il dolore lombo-sacrale*. Roma: Ed. Lombardo.

Cao T. V., Hicks M. R., Campbell D. et al. 2013 Dosed myofascial release in three-dimensional bioengineered tendons: effects on human fibroblast hyperplasia, hypertrophy, and cytokine secretion. *J Manipulative Physiol Ther* 36:513–521.

Caradonna D. 1998. Argomenti di posturologia. Atti del II Congresso Mondiale di Posturologia – Fiuggi. Bologna: GSC Editrice.

Chaitow L. 2002. *Positional Release Techniques*, 3rd ed. Churchill Livingstone, Elsevier.

Chaitow L. 2011 Is postural–structural–biomechanical model within manual therapies, viable? A JBMT debate. *J Bodyw Mov Ther* 15:130–152.

Charpentier A. 1979. Postural tonic activity: discussion by doctors Baron, Nasse and Gagey. *J Belge Med Phys Rehabi* 2:13–29.

Chauffour P., Prat E. 2002. *Mechanical Link: Fundamental Principles, Theory, and Practice Following an Osteopathic Approach*. Berkeley, CA: North Atlantic Books, pp. 15–18.

Cicconi M., Mangiulli T., Bolino G. 2014. Onset of complications following cervical manipulation due to malpractice in osteopathic treatment: a case report. *Med Sci Law* 54:230–233.

Cuccia A. M., Caradonna C., Caradonna D. 2011. *Manual Therapy of the Mandibular Accessory Ligaments for the Management of Temporomandibular Joint Disorders. J Am Osteopath Assoc* 111:102–112.

Cummings C. H. 1994. A tensegrity model for osteopathy in the cranial field. *Am Acad Osteopath J* 49–13, 24–27.

Day J. A., Copetti L., Rucli G. 2012. From clinical experience to a model for the human fascial system. *J Bodyw Mov Ther* 16:372–380.

Degenhardt B. F, Johnson J. C., Snider K. T. et al. 2010. Maintenance and improvement of interobserver reliability of osteopathic palpatory tests over a 4-month period. *J Am Osteopath Assoc* 110:579–586.

Degenhardt B. F, Snider K. T., Snider E. J. et al. 2005. Interobserver reliability of osteopathic palpatory diagnostic tests of the lumbar spine: improvements from consensus training. *J Am Osteopath Assoc* 105:465–473.

Del Giudice E., Tedeschi A. 2009. Water and autocatalysis in living matter. *Electromagn Biol Med* 28:46–52.

Del Giudice E., Spinetti P. R., Tedeschi A. 2010. Water dynamics at the root of metamorphosis in living organisms. *Water* 2:566–586

De Stefano L. A. 2011. *Greenman's Principles of Manual Medicine*. 4th ed. Baltimore, PD: Williams & Wilkins, p. 155.

Dunnington W. P. 1964. A musculoskeletal stress pattern: observations from over 50 years' clinical experience. *J Am Osteopath Assoc* 64:366–371.

Fantappié L. 2011. *Che cos'è la sintropia. principi di una teoria unitaria del mondo fisico e biologico e conferenze scelte*. Roma: Di Renzo Editore.

Findley T. W., Shalwala M. 2013. Fascia Research Congress evidence from the 100 year perspective of Andrew Taylor Still. *J Bodyw Mov Ther* 17:356–364.

Fraix M., Gordon A., Graham V. et al. 2013. Use of the SMART Balance Master to quantify the effects of osteopathic manipulative treatment in patients with dizziness. *J Am Osteopath Assoc* 113:394–403.

Fryette H. H. 1917. Physiologic movements of the spine. *J Am Osteopath Assoc* 18:1–2.

Gagey P. M., Weber B. 1997. *Posturologia: regolazione e perturbazioni della stazione eretta.* Ed. Marrapese.

Gagey P. M., Weber B. 2010. Study of intra-subject random variations of stabilometric parameters. *Med Biol Eng Comput* 48:833–835.

Gary B. C. 2011. Building a rationale for evidence-based prolotherapy in an ortho pedic medicine practice. Part 1: A short history of logical medical decision making. *Journal of Prolotherapy* 2(4).

Gibbons, P., Tehan P. 2001. Patient positioning and spinal locking for lumbar spine rotation manipulation. *Man Ther* 6:130–138.

Gilbey M. P. 2007. Sympathetic rhythms and nervous integration. *Clin Exp Pharmacol Physiol* 34:356–361.

Guidetti G. 1997. *Diagnosi e terapia dei disturbi dell'equilibrio.* Editore Marrapese.

Harrison J. W., Siddique I, Powell E. S. et al. 2005. Does the orientation of the distal radioulnar joint influence the force in the joint and the tension in the interosseous membrane? *Clin Biomech* 20:57–62.

Herzog, W. 2000. *Clinical Biomechanics of Spinal Manipulation.* Philadelphia: Churchill Livingstone.

Housman B., Bellary S. S., Walters A. et al. 2014. Moritz Heinrich Romberg (1795–1873): early founder of neurology. *Clin Anat* 27:147–149.

Irvin, R. E. 1998. The origin and relief of common pain. *J Back Musculoskelet Rehabil.* 11:89–130.

Irvine W. G. 1973. New concepts in the body expression of stress. *Can Fam Physician* 19:38–42.

Jänig W. 2013. Functional plasticity of dorsal horn neurons. *Pain* 154:1902–1903.

Jänig W., Khasar S. G., Levine J. D. et al. 2000. The role of vagal visceral afferents in the control of nociception. *Prog Brain Res* 122:273–287.

Kandel E. R., Schwartz J. H., Jessell T. M. 2000. *Principles of Neural Science, 4th ed.* New York: McGraw-Hill.

Kuchera M. 1995. Gravitational stress, musculoligamentous strain, and postural alignment. *Spine: State of the Art Reviews* 9:463–489.

Kuchera M. L. 2011. Postural consideration in osteopathic diagnosis and treatment. In: Chila

A. (ed.) *Foundations of Osteopathic Medicine.* Philadelphia: Lippincott Williams and Wilkins, p. 437.

Kumka M., Bonar J. 2012. Fascia: a morphological description and classification system based on a literature review. *J Can Chiropr Assoc* 56:179–191.

Laborit H. 1979. *L'inhibition de l'action: biologie, physiologie, psychologie, sociologie.* Paris, New York: Masson.

Langevin, H. M. 2006. Connective tissue: a body-wide signaling network? *Med Hypothese* 66:1074–1077.

LeBauer A., Brtalik R., Stowe K. 2008. The effect of myofascial release (MFR) on an adult with idiopathic scoliosis. *J Bodyw Mov Ther* 12:356–363.

Lederman E. 2011. The fall of the postural–structural–biomechanical model in manual and physical therapies: exemplified by lower back pain. *J Bodyw Mov Ther* 15:131–138.

Leijnse J. N., Rietveld A. B. 2013. Left shoulder pain in a violinist, related to extensor tendon adhesions in a small scar on the back of the wrist. *Clin Rheumatol* 32:501–506.

Levinson S. 2013. Return of the living dead: Re-reading Pierre Flourens' contributions to neurophysiology and literature. *Prog Brain Res* 205:149–172.

Liem T. 2004, *Cranial Osteopathy: Principles and Practice.* Elsevier, pp. 564, 573.

Lunghi C., Tozzi P., Fusco C. 2016 The biomechanical model in manual therapy: Is there an ongoing crisis or just the need to revise the underlying concept and application? *J Bodyw Mov Ther* [In press]

Macefield V. G. 2005. Physiological characteristics of low-threshold mechanoreceptors in joints, muscle and skin in human subjects. *Clin Exp Pharmacol Physiol* 32:135–144.

McCarthy C. J. 2001. Spinal manipulative thrust technique using combined movement theory. *Man Ther* 6:197–204.

McPartland J. M., Skinner E. 2005. Biodynamic model of osteopathy. *EXPLORE (NY)* 1:21–32.

Maas H., Sandercock T. G. 2010. Force transmission between synergistic skeletal muscles through connective tissue linkages. *J Biomed Biotechnol* Vol. 2010. Article ID: 575672.

Masi A. T., Hannon J. C. 2008. Human resting muscle tone (HRMT): narrative introduction and modern concepts. *J Bodyw Mov Ther* 12: 320–332.

Masi A. T., Nair K., Evans T. et al. 2010. Clinical, biomechanical, and physiological translational interpretations of human resting myofascial tone or tension. *Int J Ther Massage Bodywork* 3:16–28.

Mouchnino L., Blouin J. 2013. When standing on a moving support, cutaneous inputs provide sufficient information to plan the anticipatory postural adjustments for gait initiation. *PLoS One.* 8:e55081.

O'Sullivan P. 2010. Diagnosis and classification of chronic low back disorders. Proceedings Book, 7th Interdisciplinary World Congress on Low Back and Pelvic Pain, pp. 160–177.

Parker N., Greenhalgh A., Chockalingam N. et al. 2008. Positional relationship between leg rotation and lumbar spine during quiet standing. *Stud Health Technol Inform* 140:231–239.

Parsons J., Marcer N. 2006. *Osteopathy: Models for Diagnosis, Treatment and Practice.* Edinburgh: Elsevier Churchill Livingstone.

Posadzki P., Lee M. S., Ernst E. 2013. Osteopathic manipulative treatment for pediatric conditions: a systematic review. *Pediatrics* 132:140–152.

Raju S., Sanford P., Herman S. et al. 2012. Postural and ambulatory changes in regional flow and skin perfusion. *Eur J Vasc Endovasc Surg* 43:567–572.

Ranquet J. 1953. Essai d'objectivation de l'équilibre normal et pathologique. Thèse Médecine (Paris).

Rowe M. J., Tracey D. J., Mahns D. A. et al. 2005. Mechanosensory perception: are there contributions from bone-associated receptors? *Clin Exp Pharmacol Physiol* 32:100–108.

Ruddy T. J. 1962. Osteopathic manipulation in eye, ear, nose and throat disease. *Academy of Applied Osteopathy Yearbook.* 133–140.

Schabrun S. M., Jones E., Kloster J., Hodges P. W. 2013. Temporal association between changes in primary sensory cortex and corticomotor output during muscle pain. *Neuroscience* 235:159–164.

Schulkin J. 2003. *Rethinking Homeostasis: Allostatic Regulation in Physiology and Pathophysiology.* Cambridge MA: MIT Press.

Selye H. 1956. *The Stress of Life.* New York: McGraw-Hill.

Shirzadi A., Drazin D., Jeswani S. et al. 2013. Atypical presentation of thoracic disc herniation: case series and review of the literature. *Case Rep Orthop* Vol. 2015. Article ID: 621476.

Skraba J. S., Greenwald A. S. 1984. The role of the interosseous membrane on tibiofibular weightbearing. *Foot Ankle* 4:301–304.

Stecco A., Masiero S., Macchi V. et al. 2009a. The pectoral fascia: anatomical and histological study. *J Bodyw Mov Ther* 13:255–261.

Stecco A., Macchi V., Masiero S. et al. 2009b. Pectoral and femoral fasciae: common aspects and regional specializations. *Surg Radiol Anat.* 31:35–42.

Swanson R. L. 2013. Biotensegrity: a unifying theory of biological architecture with applications to osteopathic practice, education, and research—a review and analysis. *J Am Osteopath Assoc* 113:34–52.

Thelen E., Adolph K. E. 1992. Arnold L. Gesell: The paradox of nature and nurture. *Dev Psychol* 28:368–380.

Tozzi P. 2012. Selected fascial aspects of osteopathic practice. *J Bodyw Mov Ther* 16:503–519.

Tozzi P. 2014. Does fascia hold memories? *J Bodyw Mov Ther* 18:259–265.

Tribastone F. 1985. *Compendio di ginnastica correttiva.* Roma: SSS.

Tsao H., Galea M. P., Hodges P. W. 2008. Reorganization of the motor cortex is associated with postural control deficits in recurrent low back pain. *Brain* 131:2161–2171.

Valero-Cuevas F. J., Yi J. W., Brown D., McNamara R. V. et al. 2007. The tendon network of the fingers performs anatomical computation at a macroscopic scale. *IEEE Trans Biomed Eng* 54:1161–1166.

von Schroeder H. P., Botte M. J. 1997. Functional anatomy of the extensor tendons of the digits. *Hand Clin* 13:51–62.

Willard F. H., Vleeming A., Schuenke M. D. et al. 2012. The thoracolumbar fascia: anatomy, function and clinical considerations. *J Anat* 221:507–536.

Wood Jones F. 1944a *The Principles of Anatomy as Seen in the Hand.* London: Ballière, Tindall and Cox.

Wood Jones F. 1944b *Structure and Function as Seen in the Foot.* London: Baillière, Tindall and Cox.

Zanardi M. 1998. *Posturologia clinica osteopatica: prontuario tecnico pratico.* Roma: Editore Marrapese.

Zavarella P., Asmone C., Zanardi M. 2002. *Le asimmetrie occluso-posturali.* Volume 2. GLM Editore.

Zink J. G., Lawson W. B. 1979. An osteopathic structural examination and functional interpretation of the soma. *Osteopath Ann* 7:12–19.

Zwerver J., Konopka K. H., Keizer D. et al. 2013. Does sensitisation play a role in the pain of patients with chronic patellar tendinopathy? *Br J Sports Med* 47:e2.

FASCIA AS A SENSORY ORGAN: CLINICAL APPLICATIONS

Robert Schleip

Basic orientation

In line with Chapter 7, the following descriptions provide examples of how specific techniques can be utilized in order to optimize an intended stimulation of specific mechanoreceptors in fascial tissue.

Stimulation of muscle spindles

Of the five traditional elements of Swedish massage it is the 'petrissage' – a form of deep, rhythmical kneading – that can be best applied for this purpose. In order to use the myotatic reflex arc in a muscular relaxation direction, the practitioner uses both hands to grab hold of two larger muscular tissue portions and moves them towards each other in a compressional manner. Using a more rhythmical style the practitioner attempts to quickly decrease the length of the muscle spindles in the zone between the two hands. A different version of this basic technique is sometimes used in sports massage for the purpose of increasing muscle tone before an athletic performance. In this case the two hands move away from each other in a rhythmic fashion, thereby inducing a stretching effect – rather than compression – in order to ignite the well-known myotatic reflex in a way that stretches muscle spindles and thereby exerts a stimulatory effect on the active muscular tonus regulation. In contrast, in the style described here, the two hands attempt to create a rapid tonus decrease within the spindle fibers, which is expected to induce a tonus-decreasing effect on alpha motor tonus activity.

Stimulation of Golgi receptors

In myofascial therapeutic mobilization it is typical that slower tissue deformations are created, and, in contrast to some forms of sports massage, the focus is usually on relaxation rather than on tonus augmentation. The Golgi receptors are a good target for such an approach, since stimulation of these neural receptors tends to induce muscular relaxation in those muscle fibers that are mechanically linked with the area of stimulation. However, as outlined in Chapter 7, when applying stretch in tissue areas that are serially arranged with soft and compliant muscle fibers, all stretch is 'swallowed' by the softer myofibers (instead of the more rigid collagen fibers) and the Golgi receptors within the collagenous fibers are not sufficiently lengthened.

One way to prevent this seems to be a cross-fiber mobilization across the muscle belly area (rather than the muscular attachments) in order to lower the described spreading effect towards the compliant muscle fibers. A common technique often taught as part of the Bowen method involves cross-friction across the muscle bellies, which might in fact induce at least a temporary regional muscular relaxation via stimulation of related Golgi receptors.

If one wants to work within the more tendinous areas, another approach is advocated. Here the patient is asked to activate the related myofibers against external resistance, while the practitioner applies moderate to strong stimulation (usually $10–50\,\text{N/cm}^2$) to the tendinous collagenous tissues that are tensed by the respective muscular contraction. One way of achieving this seems to be by using the postisometric relaxation technique, as frequently taught within the proprioceptive neuromuscular facilitation or PNF concept in manual therapy. Here the patient is usually instructed to contract a joint musculature against the handheld resistance of the practitioner for a period of between 60 and 90 seconds and a 'tissue release' is often observed during the subsequent relaxation. Sometimes there is also a brief antagonistic contraction included immediately before the final relaxation.

A more advanced – and proprioceptively stimulating – approach was taught as 'pandiculations' by Thomas Hanna (1998). Here too the practitioner provides external resistance to the actively moving body part of the patient, however, patient and practitioner cooperate in such a way that the patient is instructed to move against the resisting hand of the therapist in a super-slow continuous fashion. Subsequently the respective limb is pulled back towards the body, again against a moderated resistance of the therapist; and this movement is also performed in a smooth and super-slow fashion. Patient and practitioner direct most of their mindful attention toward achieving a nonerratic movement quality (i.e., without any perceived 'stop and go' interruptions). As soon as such an erratic moment is detected, the patient is instructed to return to the position immediately before it happened, and then try to repeat the movement at an even slower speed and, hopefully, with less bumpy movement orchestration. This active resistance phase – with the patient participating in both concentric as well as eccentric activation – is usually practiced for between 60 and 90 seconds and – as in the respective PNF technique – is then followed by a brief moment of isometric contraction of the respective antagonistic muscles. In addition, the practitioner provides a strong myofascial stimulation (yet not beyond the comfort zone of the pressure–pain tolerance of the patient) to the fascial tissue area within the tendinous portions of the related musculature.

For example, when sitting, a patient may be instructed to slowly raise her right shoulder against the external resistance of the practitioner. Then she is asked to gradually lower her muscular activation in order to allow the downward pushing force of the practitioner to gradually lower the shoulder to the starting position. Each of these two movements should occur in a smooth, uninterrupted, continuous manner, lasting at least five seconds each. Whenever a tiny 'jerk' is detected by either the patient or practitioner, the movement is repeated with increased mindfulness from the position shortly before it occurred. During all of this the practitioner works with a deep stretching myofascial release approach on the aponeurotic insertions of the upper trapezius on the superior nuchal line of the cranium. After approximately 60 to 90 seconds the myofascial hands-on work is finished and the patient is asked to perform a downward active shoulder movement for one or two seconds only, with her elbow pressing isometrically against the resisting hand of the practitioner. Finally, the patient is asked to relax and to subjectively compare the perceived height and sensation of the treated shoulder with the other shoulder.

Stimulation of Pacini corpuscles

The following example is for the stimulation of spinal joint receptors in the cervicothoracic region. The patient is asked to lie comfortably on her right side with the practitioner sitting behind the patient's back. The practitioner starts with a prominent spinal process, for example, from C6, C7, or T1, and lifts this process a few millimeters away from the table toward the ceiling. It is then wiggled two to four times in a random manner before it is lowered again to the starting position. This is repeated in slightly different lifting directions, varying between slightly more cranial and more caudal lateral directions. The lifting amplitude is calibrated so that the maximal delay occurs between the movement of the manipulated vertebrae and its two adjacent neighbors. The intention of the practitioner is to show the central nervous system of the patient that the spine in this region is not a rigid column but rather a series of mobile elements that are arranged like a string of pearls. If successful, this may support a related reformation of the respective cortical mapping of what is called 'body schema' representation in the brain.

One or two minutes are spent in this way on each vertebra before the neighboring vertebra is approached in a similar manner. The natural breathing movements of the patient are carefully observed. Sometimes during a slow lifting movement of a thoracic spinous process a normal inhalation movement is slightly increased in time and amplitude (maybe 10% more than usual). If this happens, the practitioner may play with the concept of 'taking a ride' on this extended inhalation and lifting the vertebra a tiny bit more (and for a second longer) at the apex of the inhalation movement. If successful this may result in a release-like response around the costovertebral joints of the respective vertebrae on the side on which the lifting movement causes a temporary decompression.

Note that it may take 10 minutes to apply this technique to the spinous processes of, for example, C6 to T5. In most cases the technique does not need to be repeated for the opposite side-lying position – at least not in those cases for which the main intention is to produce a more refined representation of this spinal area in the patient's body schema in terms of a more mobile rather than rigid body portion.

Stimulation of Ruffini corpuscles

Here a slow but firm touch is provided that exerts a lateral tangential shearing motion to the skin, as well as to fascial membranes below the subcutaneous loose connective tissue. Once the pressure achieves a slow gliding of the practitioner's hand in relation to the skin of the patient, the speed of this gliding motion is calibrated toward the slowest possible continuous speed. For a beginner this may be a speed of 5 cm per second, while for a more experienced practitioner much slower gliding motions of around 1 cm per second or less are possible. If possible the patient can be instructed to assist this technique by conducting a slow active movement participation that provides an expansional stretch to the working area (Fig. 25.1).

During the gliding motion the practitioner feels for the optimal vectorial direction of his hands – whether slightly more vertical/horizontal, more distal/proximal, or more medial/lateral, etc. – at which the local tissue relaxation response spreads out most readily toward a larger, more spacious tissue response. The analogy of a school of fish can be employed to foster the related empathic palpatory sensitivity of the practitioner (Fig. 25.2).

Stimulation of free nerve endings

The recent discovery of the tactile C-afferents in the dermis of the hairy skin of humans (and other mammals) has led to an increase in research on 'affective touch'. Based on this, therapeutic meth-

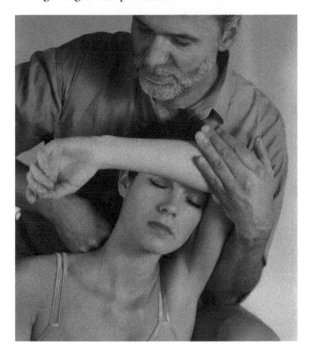

Figure 25.1
Example of the use of AMPs (active movement participation) with the patient during a Ruffini-oriented release technique. While deeply melting with one hand into the tissue and specific joints of the upper thorax, the practitioner guides the patient to support his myofascial work with subtle and random slow-motion participations. Here the patient performs a lateral bending movement of the thorax combined with a cranially directed extension (following the elbow) in order to increase an opening of the thoracic vertebral joints

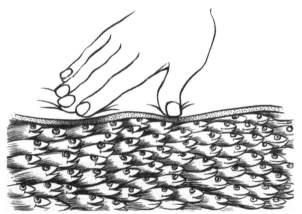

Figure 25.2
Myofascial tissue illustrated as a school of fish. A practitioner working with myofascial tissue may feel several of the motor units responding to the touch. If the practitioner then responds supportively to their new behavior, the working hand will feel other fish joining this release, and so on

ods – usually involving gentle and slow stroking – are explored, and these provide the cortical insula with a sensation of nurturing touch, also called 'social touch', which can induce a general sense of well-being and relaxation in the patient. The depth of responses can involve profound shifts in immunological, psychosocial, and neurophysiological parameters (McGlone et al., 2014). For related instruction on this intriguing aspect of therapeutic touch the reader is referred to the new literature on this subject, for example, Lloyd et al. (2015) and McGlone et al. (2014).

Another method for stimulation of C-fibers or A-delta fibers (both terminating in free nerve endings) targets the high density of their related nerve endings in the periosteum (i.e., the fascial envelope around bones). This approach is inspired by the ancient *Chua K'a* method, as taught by Oscar Ichazo (Hertling & Kessler, 2006). Here strong pressure is applied to bony surfaces until a slight sympathetic activation is observed in the patient. This response may involve a slight dilation of the pupil, an increased and elongated inhalation, an increased circulation in the face, and/or a turning of head and eyes toward the respective body part. It should be an expression of the so-called 'orienting response' in behavioral biology, during which an animal responds to a new challenging stimulus by straightening its neck upwards toward the perceived place of stimulation in a general state of alertness. Care should be taken that an avoidance-and-withdrawal response is avoided, which expresses itself in very different behavior involving a flexion movement of the trunk and limbs, a turning away from the perceived stimulus location, a shortening of the neck, and either a halt in breathing or an augmented breathing speed. The patient may be instructed to participate with an active movement that intensifies the perceived pressure with an assertive gesture, such as arm abduction and pushing the elbow into the working stimulus of the practitioner. The use of tools – such as in instrument-assisted manual therapies – could be used to work with more precision (Fig. 25.3).

Once a slight sympathetic orienting response is achieved, a moment of rest – without any touch – is added, during which the practitioner waits for at

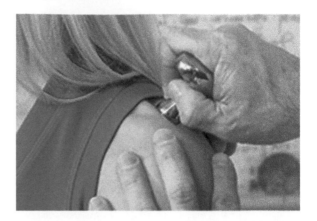

Figure 25.3

Use of a stainless steel tool (a third thumb) for stimulation of periosteal free nerve endings

least three to five of the patient's breathing cycles until a parasympathetic shift (or general relaxation) is observed. Subsequently a spot on the periosteum in very close proximity to the first spot is treated in a similar manner. If there is a hyperalgesic zone, the treatment starts first in the nearest area with a normal pressure sensitivity. Once a relaxation response is achieved there, gradually periosteum zones nearer to the hyperalgesic spot are treated. The goal is a gradual desensitization process leading to increased resilience to pain. Most likely this process will involve an activation of cortical descending modulatory pathways (Bingel & Tracey, 2008).

In a nutshell (see Table 25.1):

- Stimulation of spindle receptors can be facilitated by quick compressional impulses to the muscle bellies.

- Golgi receptors can be stimulated by techniques that require temporary resistance by the patient.

- Ruffini techniques attempt to apply slow shear sensations while finding the respective optimal vectorial direction.

- Pacini corpuscles require constantly changing novel sensations.

- Free nerve endings can be stimulated by work on the periosteum.

Receptor	Triggered response	Potential usage in manual therapy
\n\n**Muscle spindle**	• Tonus decrease in related myofibers	• Petrissage element of Swedish massage: compressional moves toward muscle belly
\n\n**Golgi receptor**	• Tonus decrease in related myofibers	• Cross-fiber techniques at muscle belly • Postisometric relaxation techniques • Hanna's pandiculation
\n\n**Pacini corpuscle**	• Enhancement of local proprioception, plus – hopefully – improvement in local neuromuscular self-regulation	• High-velocity manipulations • Recoil technique • Harmonic technique • Trager work
\n\n**Ruffini endings**	• Inhibition of sympathetic activity	• Classical myofascial 'melting' work (e.g., Rolfing)
\n\n**Interstitial free nerve endings**	• Tactile C-afferents: affiliation, well-being, pain-inhibition • Threatening pain: withdrawal response and pain sensitization • 'Relieving pain': orienting response, pain desensitization	• Slow skin-stroking techniques • Periosteum stimulation: induction of novel nociceptive stimulation within same fasciatome

Table 25.1
Overview of the different sensory receptors in myofascial tissue, the responses triggered by their stimulation, and the manual techniques that can evoke those responses

References

Bingel, U., Tracey, I. 2008. Imaging CNS modulation of pain in humans. *Physiology.* 23:371-380.

Hanna, T., 1998. *Somatics: Reawakening the Mind's Control of Movement, Flexibility, and Health.* Da Capo Press, Cambridge MA, USA.

Hertling, D, Kessler, R. M 2006. *Management of Common Musculoskeletal Disorders.* Lippincott Williams & Wilkins, Philadelphia, p. 170.

Lloyd, D. M., McGlone, F. P., Yosipovitch, G. 2015. Somatosensory pleasure circuit: from skin to brain and back. *Experimental Dermatology.* 24(5):321–324.

McGlone, F., Wessberg, J., Olausson, H. 2014. Discriminative and affective touch: sensing and feeling. *Neuron.* 82(4):737–755.

TOUCH RELATED TO FASCIA

Maurice César

Warning

A text, more than pictures or drawings, requires you to read carefully and can also give birth to an emotion, a feeling, a soul, a sensitive experience. The mental image of the different tissue structures in three dimensions thoroughly describes the reality of the area in question.

Words, much more permissive and less directive than an image or a drawing, force you to search, discover, and feel. If the touch is professional, the resulting feeling is even more personal. It shapes the tone of the contact and the corrective movement. It defines your specific qualities as a therapist.

I could write an entire book on this topic but, having only one chapter at my disposal, I will only make a high-level analysis. Rest assured all the important and relevant principles will be present in this chapter. The osteopath, who is a tactile practitioner, will waste no time in putting theory into practice.

Even though the content of this chapter has a direct impact on practice, it is essentially theoretical. Please do not expect any techniques; there will not be any. I could have called this chapter 'back to the roots', in other words, back to the philosophy of osteopathy, or its essence, as the things I describe here seem so basic to me. However, I see too many practitioners learning more and more sophisticated techniques, but neglecting what are, to my mind, three essential and primordial elements:

- Firstly, the power of touch, for the indispensable precision it brings to the investigating or corrective movement.
- Secondly, the importance of anatomical knowledge. Touch is nothing without it.

- Thirdly, the intelligence and the ability of our interlocutor – the tissue. We call it 'fascia' and without it healing is impossible.

Introduction

It is common knowledge that the function defines the organ. It has allowed the evolution of humans and other species as well as the perpetual search for a more effective, energy-efficient, and comfortable inner life. All of that is only possible because around and inside this organ there is a structure that allows the idea itself of performance or willingness to perform that function. That structure is called 'fascia'. It has a rich and exciting life of its own. It has its own laws and codes. It deserves our respect and support when needed. In this chapter, I will describe a small but very significant part of that supportive relationship.

It is also established that in osteopathy we only see one symptom, one disease: lack of mobility. It cannot be detected by doing a blood test, in an ultrasound, in an X-ray, or by any other classical medical investigation. Nor can it be deducted or concluded from the patient's complaints or descriptions. Neither can it be seen. It is not redness, paleness, an angulation, a spasm, a swelling, or a tight spot. No, in order to find it we need to touch. It is in the tissue. The only tools we have are our hands. As our hands only allow us to get in touch with a few square millimeters, we are obliged to optimize as much as we can the impact on this surface. In the next couple of sentences, I will provide you with some important details that will enable you to make the relationship that you have with the tissue as relevant and effective as possible, through your touch.

Touching is a tool as old as life. It is archaic, and therefore puts our profession, manual therapy, in a rather nonelitist position compared to 'high-tech' medical practice. However, it gives me the opportunity to proudly call myself a 'medical artisan'. Thanks to that touch, a true therapeutic act, we help our fellow human beings to improve their performance and internal comfort.

In this chapter, I will provide you with a few simple and elementary rules to help define whether the touch is diagnostic or therapeutic. I will also take a closer look at the qualitative and quantitative aspects of the pressure of our contact and will describe the different kinds of touch:

- The cutaneous touch defines a situation and a location.

- The anatomical touch identifies a structure and determines a configuration.

- The histological touch shows tissue composition and constitution.

- The physiological touch reveals the move that we want to normalize.

I will try to describe with words, step by step, our conversation with the fascia, or even the life that inhabits it. Its main specificity is its incredible will to survive. We can feel that will in our first contact, and it will never fade. That profession, that I refuse to call 'work', is a daily lesson in optimism and persistence.

Happy reading.

The cutaneous touch

For the tissue, eager to live, everything has a value for information, indication, and reaction. No contact point is insignificant for the fascia. Sometimes the latter has difficulty in distinguishing informative touch from technical touch when it is subject to three or four points of contact, especially if the first contact is imprecise or perhaps weaker than the second contact. The more the information is isolated, the clearer the language, hence the more prompt and complete the desired response will be. The one thing the tissue is looking for is to normalize itself. Give it an opportunity and it will not hesitate to grasp it.

The skin is the first selective barrier. It is up to us to use that feature to our advantage. But, first things

first: let's limit the information as much as possible. The main thing that we want to accomplish with every new touch is to create an overview of these new points of contact. We should never touch the body where unnecessary. If the applied technique requires only three fingers, we should only touch with three fingers and nothing more. We should avoid any unnecessary contact. We should even be vigilant that our clothes do not touch the patient in any way. Let's refrain from any contact that is not directive or active.

In my book *L'action Ostéopathique: Une Intrusion Autorisée dans le Conscient Tissulaire*, I have described in detail all the precautions to take in order to help reassure, relax, and disconnect the patient in order to ease and optimize the contact with their tissue, of which they are totally unaware (César, 2007). At this level the challenge remains the same. As far as we can, we should not distract the tissue with useless information.

A certain amount of nonoperative contact is, however, necessary and essential. It assists with support, posture, fixation, or counterpressure. It should be strictly limited according to necessity and should be clearly identified. Gravitating touch is only there to help. Nonoperative contact should be as wide and multistructural as possible. It is therefore particularly inaccurate in relation to the underlying anatomical structures. It consciously covers several internal structures, without any anatomical or functional correlation, or therapeutic consistency with the zone of treatment. The pressure on the whole surface of contact will be highly uniform and always lighter than the pressure coming from any corrective touch. Nonoperative contact must remain vague, cutaneous, and without any message attached. It would not make sense during a technique of abdominal normalization with long lever for the hand that encloses the ankle and mobilizes the lower limb to apply more pressure at the level of the limb than the guiding hand working in the abdomen. That would distract the sensitivity of the tissue from the primary purpose. The weakness of the counterpressure will automatically be compensated for by an increase in the counterpressure surface. Nonoperative contact must be of a secondary and complementary nature, and be perceived as such by the tissue. We should also focus on limiting as much as possible any change in position. Each new piece of information is a new development for the tissue, and, therefore, can only distract it from its normalization task.

Being careful and precautionary is really meaningful for the tissue. It indirectly contributes to it focusing its proprioceptive attention on the treated area. By limiting and depolluting the given information, we will help the tissue in its task.

By contrast, the corrective touch will be striking with precision. More than anything else it will be transcutaneous and transdermal. Increasing the pressure by even one gradient will be a strong indicator for the tissue but must not saturate the receivers under any circumstances with too much pressure or stretching. That would make the therapeutic move useless and this area impossible to treat for a short time. We would have to wait for complete relief of the cutaneous tissue. The recovery time for sensitivity to normalize can vary a lot. Moreover, you have to awaken the patient's attention. It won't always be easy to get relaxation and trust back. We must simply materialize the difference between what is more and less important. The pressure disparity between different points of contact is clear information for the tissue. You show your willingness to communicate with the underlying structures by crossing the skin border. As I have already mentioned, that touch should be as precise as possible. It will identify an area to work on and target one underlying structure by fine contact points. Please never forget that your touch will have more impact when limited in its surface. Pressure will of course be uniform on all contact points if the touch needs to be double or multiple. We will define an area, a site that will be almost a single structure. The tissue will understand that all the action will take place there. It must be able to recognize, localize, and identify the officiating and monitoring hand from its associate. It must know where you work, where you want to help, what you are treating. Your touch must bear a message.

These are all essential components for the tissue that will be selective and will identify the corrective touch. Only one range of information must reach the medullary and superior centers. Only one must attain consciousness and raise awareness from the tissue.

Be careful with the duration of contact as it could be perceived as aggression if too quickly established. You should also respect all the different tissue layers. Contact will only create doubt and surprise if it is too furtive or too quickly broken.

I would like to bring to your attention that skin sensitivity varies depending on the location. Contact points that are too close might be understood as one and therefore be perceived as puncturing. Waking up the skin sensitivity equals waking up the patient and de facto closing all communication with the tissue. However, as soon as the skin obstacle is overcome, the delight is absolute; the relationship is real and complete; we enter the third dimension.

This is a close encounter of the third kind with a bubbling life, even in time of 'peace' for the tissue. The patient is not aware of that life. It takes form and becomes conscious only in discomfort. For the patient, good health is the absence of feeling, the ignorance of the inside.

The patient will soon realize that they are not part of that relationship. Generally, convinced that they made the right choice by delegating the problem-solving to you, they will 'go to sleep' pretty easily, thanks to the trust they put in your cutaneous contact and the precision of the actions on the tissue. Your touch will quickly determine the level of trust that they will place in your therapeutic approach. Contact comes long before the corrective action. It must be absolutely meaningful from the very beginning, as much for the patient as for the body.

The diagnostic touch – therapeutic touch

Before we get into the subject, let's set the scene: the fascia is the star and it has the leading role. Getting in contact with it means being side by side with a life that dates back 540 million years, when single-celled organisms that appeared a long time before that (about 3.8 billion years ago) have joined together around one unifying element: the collagen, the fascia (600 million years). Other convening elements will appear soon: blood and its constituents (hormones, nutrients, etc.) and the nervous system. Because of their ubiquitous nature (and in reverse order to the one I have just used), those three elements fostered A. T. Still's reflections. They inspired and influenced his philosophical path throughout his life.

So we are in the presence of an organism, a structure, where all components are driven by one basic (archaic) program: to improve its internal environment in order to live one moment more and, if possible, in a better way. That pursuit is continuing, always looking for the absolute goal, which is clinical and functional silence for minimal effort. It is constantly searching for the absence of pain, for comfort, for a situation of balance, effective and energy efficient. Only the fascia knows its history, its trials, its mistakes, its successes. And it is also the only one knowing its basic initial structure, its specific and personal imbalance; in a nutshell, its optimal norm.

So we are in a situation where only the leading actor knows the script. We only know the bits and pieces that it selects for us. Remember that we are not repositioning. If there is repositioning, it will be because of the tissue's work, following our treatment, using any technique. The touch will not be insignificant, thanks to that knowledge, that logistical support, and its speed of action. This is already a technique. The fascia will use it as a springboard to normalize itself. Therefore, there is no need to use strength. Precision is enough. And it provides us with a good dose of optimism because from now on we are not alone anymore in this pursuit of well-being. We have a strong ally: the tissue, the fascia.

Three lessons can be learned from this.

First of all, as only the fascia knows its own history, we need to work as closely as possible to the structure of the fascia. Whether the touch is diagnostic or therapeutic, all the information that goes through the fascia, and only through it, will only result in a vague and imprecise idea of the problem if the touch is vague and imprecise. The contact must be carefully exercised before it can properly treat.

Secondly, because the fascia shows a tenacious will and is prompt to react, the diagnostic touch will be as furtive as possible. However, it will be precise, as light as possible, even tactile and subtle. A too-long contact

would only disturb your judgment. The tissue is constantly looking for balance and self-management. So please do not give it the opportunity to normalize itself at this stage. It is too soon!

In this therapeutic phase, I also need to insist on the notion of pressure, as much on the qualitative aspect as on the quantitative one. Please respect the different levels of pressure in your points of contact. Start lightly, and progress slowly. Evolve from not intervening to intervening by feeling the tissue. The latter will lead you, guide you. A therapeutic contact that is too strong from the beginning would overfill the sensitive sensors and would therefore nullify any lighter or superficial subsequent movement. Work toward a crescendo. Let the tissue get used to this increase of pressure. The tissue does not like to be forced into anything. The same applies to points of contact that would be too strong, too 'perforating', too close to each other, or too repetitive in one location. Once again, the tissue does not like to be compelled. The location is by far more important than the strength used. The optimal booster is never the maximum one. We understood that a long time ago.

Finally, the therapeutic touch will take time. It will be divided into two phases: a passive and an active one. As always, the first question will be: 'What will the tissue do under or with my fingers?' And only then: 'What should I do to the tissue to help it?' Even though they will both examine the same structures, the major difference between diagnostic and therapeutic contact is the duration. Diagnostic contact is characterized by speed and lightness. Conversely, with therapeutic contact we will take as long as we need, and we will help, accompany, and live with the tissue.

The anatomical touch

Through the skin, we will use our fingers as a scalpel. We will break down the structure and separate it from its direct environment, isolating the tissue or the tension. We will delimit the area to work on as precisely as possible, with the sole aim of locating our target area. The tissue will answer with as much force, power, and swiftness as the precision of the movement. The word 'anatomy' derives from Greek, meaning 'section through'. We need to penetrate deeply and break through the layers (the tissue strata). To reach the target area, we need to use respect and consideration for each of the layers. We must target that specific area and seize the tissue's attention there. But please do not forget to pause as you progress in depth. The tissue does not like to be rushed and neither does the patient.

It is also crucial to delimit the entire structure or organ. Even if your therapeutic approach is only looking at a fraction of the structure, take it first as a whole and then select a part of it. Do your best to respect its outlines, position in space, direction, thickness, form, roundness, and flatness before you penetrate more deeply.

As you know, here lies all the art of the 'probe', the 'toucher' that the osteopath is. It is the control of the knowledge of topographic anatomy, as well as the ability and the capacity to perceive and recognize normal trophicity, tonicity, and hydration in the tissue or, in short, normality in abnormality. The osteopath is therefore a geologist of touch, who works relentlessly on his or her knowledge of anatomy. The real foundation of the osteopath's art, its very essence, lies in not seeing anatomy only as adjacent parts with static relations between them, or the position of pieces compared to one another, but seeing it as interactions of movement, each contact between structures being an articulation, as A. T. Still pointed out. Mobility of all parts comes first, long before location.

Your touch needs to be as flexible and light as possible, even as you progress through the different layers, and as you go deeper and deeper into the structure. It has to be 'fluid'. We like that word! All of the constituents of our body and also our patient's body live in liquid. Our fascia is only a flexible container. Let's not forget that the level of intensity of a lesion on a site can be qualified in terms of liquidity, fluidity, impregnation, and water absorption. Water remains our main constituent, our primary fascia. It is what we are and what we have the most of in our bodies. There is no life without water. There is no structure without water in the body. Even the reaction of tissue to any constraint will only be a reinforcement of its most resistant constituents (collagen) at the expense of its liquid component.

The osteopath can appreciate the disparity of water and collagen with their touch. Let's be more fluid and 'liquid' than the tissue itself. You will then appreciate the intensity of the lesion even more. Pressure is not necessary. The location, the coverage, and the direction of your fingers on the skin are efficient by themselves. There is no perfect topographic overlapping inside the body. No structure is positioned perfectly on top of another. Even on a deep and nonpalpable structure, curative action will only be perceived as such if the topography is well limited. Thanks to your fingers, the tiniest part of the body, as small as it is, can be 'peeled' or 'shelled' for diagnostic or therapeutic purposes. The structures, local or in transit, being veins, arteries, nerves, muscles, ligaments, sheaths, or bones, will be treated successively and individually, as indicated by the lesional processes, in a real 'scuffling'. All of these structures contain connective tissue and will respond to techniques of listening, myotensive mobilization, stretching, longitudinality, general positioning, recoils, motility reharmonization, or lemniscate activity, tonicity, or trophicity. And as we are talking about anatomically delimiting a structure, I would like to draw the reader's attention to a topic that is particularly close to my heart, namely phylogenesis, which is part of the therapeutic strategy, and will be discussed later in this chapter.

Earlier I used the word 'geologist' in relation to touch and tissue. To this I will add another phrase: 'archeologist of the structures'.

Phylogenetics – the comparative anatomical study of living beings, animals, and humans – shows us that many of our common ancestral characteristics have diversified in the course of evolution. They have persisted for tens of millions of years only to modify themselves for maybe a few millions or thousands of years. Inside these structures remains a synergy of life, of action, and of feeling that forces us to consider them as united. Treating those structures as a whole during my contact, and associating them with the techniques I use, has proved to me that I am right. I have seen the results and how quickly they have been achieved. That association, considered as functional anatomy, is the memory of our formation and evolution. This evolution, more than anything else, helps us to understand some of the processes that govern our inner life. Here are a few examples amongst many.

The pectoralis minor muscle and the coracohumeral ligament used to be one single structure. That ligament is none other than the former tendon of the pectoralis minor muscle that used to attach itself to the humerus, as is still the case in many mammals. If you wish to cure one, please do not forget the other. Include it in your touch and in your technique. Similarly, we can see the same connection between the subclavius muscle and its former tendon, the trapezoid ligament. The sacrotuberous ligament is nothing more than the former biceps femoris tendon from which it is still inseparable. In the case of horses and monkeys, this muscle is still inserted in the sacrum. We will leave this subject now as the list would otherwise be too long.

The bonds that link us to animals and to our own past are undeniable. Our body is a compilation of these successive transformations, which are souvenirs of previous evolutions, but still so vivid.

This is our history and we cannot deny it.

The histological touch

The histological touch is the anatomical touch, transposed to a microscopic dimension, at the cell level. If the anatomical touch selects a structure, the histological touch selects one of its constituent tissues. Also, in this situation it will be defined by the quality of the pressure, sense, and direction of the touch of your fingers. It will also adjust the preparation and the type of corrective movement. That precision of contact will be directive for the tissue, and the latter will understand your intentions. It knows.

If anatomy is the support of the movement, it is histology that determines its achievement criteria: sense, direction, and amplitude.

The division of one structure in different tissue layers or directions is there for a reason. It is a sharing of functions, a distribution of tasks and constraints.

Is it the direction or the layering of collagen fibers, according to a clearly defined plan, that determines the authorized direction of the action, or the latter

that modulates the tissue as it goes? No one can say. It is probably both. You will determine the layer you want to work on using the pressure of your hands to select the tissue layers from one single structure.

Between the tissue and therapists there is only one language: touch. The more this touch is pertinent, the more clear and close the understanding will be, and the more prompt and complete the reaction. Let's not forget that the tissue has only one desire: to heal, to improve its quality of life, and its performances. What it cannot heal, it will compensate for, bury into the mass by tissue sharing. What it cannot compensate for, it will express loud and clear. The ultimate permanent goal is to reach clinical and functional silence. In the course of the therapeutic adventure, tissue is our partner, our ally. It plays the leading role in this search for well-being. We are only supporting actors. Only it knows its history, its trials, its mistakes, and how to normalize itself. Our hands will only help it in its perpetual pursuit of well-being.

We could give a number of examples, but the length of this chapter does not allow us to do this. So, let's choose one amongst many: the medial collateral ligament in the knee.

This flattened and banded ligament inserts itself at the top of the tuberosity of the medial condyle just under the tuber of the adductor magnus. Then it goes downward and a little bit anterior and ends on the highest part of the anterointernal face of the tibia. Rather narrow at its upper end, it gets wider lower down, reaching its maximum width at the level of the meniscus, then it narrows gradually up to the tibial insertion. Thus it takes as a whole the form of a triangle, with the base represented by the anterior edge. It can be up to 9–10 cm long and is between 20–25 mm wide at its middle part, at the level of the joint gap.

It consists of three orders of fibers:

1. Vertical fibers that go downward directly from the femur to the tibia, and are the anterior edge of the ligament.

2. Descending oblique fibers that, coming from the femur, run backward and spread to end both on the capsule and on the meniscus.

3. Ascending oblique fibers that, from the tibia, move backward to the capsule and to the meniscus.

Therefore, that ligament gives us the opportunity to consider three different types of fibers. Determining which parts are damaged and applying tissue techniques on each of those parts, and only on those parts, means working at the heart of the tissue and increasing our effectiveness.

The physiological touch

We are only in the infancy of our knowledge of movement of tissue and its operating mode. We would like to share this life for a moment, to capture and take ownership of it, to endorse it, before correcting it with a normalizing motion. First things first: please do not impose yourself. We can only know someone if we live with them. Let's do the same with the tissue. Its life, its activity, is relentless, 24/7. It hardly decreases at night. The fascia is really hyperactive. Thus refrain from any action before you appropriate its rules, its rhythms, its mood swings, and its defects.

The physiological touch is the movement touch, the contact with life, the real one, the ancestral one. The touch that does not do anything in vain. It works in an energy-efficient way. It is compellingly consistent and logical. We are working here with total rationality.

Anatomy without the physiological touch, without movement, is a science for corpses.

The physiological touch is the science of movement. No function can take place without movement: no movement, no life. If you restrict it, you limit life, you amputate its life-capital. In a corpse and in a living body, anatomy and histology do not change, but in a corpse that indefinable spark that is life has disappeared. Therefore, inside the organ, the structure, or the chosen tissue, you will have to select the movement to normalize through mobility or primary cranial movement, lemniscate activity, blood wave, breathing, etc. Each one has its own rules, and it is important to share, if only for a brief instant, its way of living, even pathologically, before you make any correction.

Learn how to live with this tissue before you impose your own rules, your help.

The physiological touch is the dynamic touch. We move.

As soon as you make contact with a structure, follow it right away: it lives and so it moves. It is permanent. Every contact will only alter its quality of life, its well-being, and it will be 'fixating', which does not make any sense when the aim is to free it.

If you immobilize the structure with your touch, it will immediately try to defeat you, to restore its balance as much as possible, meaning additional work for it and disruption for the therapist. So, as soon as you are touching, you should live at its pace. Wait a while before you choose the corrective movement. Let the tissue express itself and it will lead you where it wants. And where it wants is exactly where you should be.

Please do not forget that we do not know anything about its history. Let's not impose ourselves in a world of which we are ignorant. Let's trust the life of the tissue that has evolved over 540 million years.

Conclusion

It is surprising to see human beings dedicating billions to probe space to look for another form of life, while on Earth many animal species disappear every day almost without being noticed. And also inside our bodies, in our own tissues, there is a life that palpitates with so many unexplored and unknown facets. Only little attention has been paid to the life of the tissue in its gestural expression. This is precisely why we want to pay tribute to that life, via the touch, and describe how we can, with the help of our hands, bring support to the tissue in its fight to defend itself and its fulfillment, without being presumptuous. The tissue lives by its own rules and codification. It also has a syntax of its own and is defined by the precision of contact, the finesse of touch, the respect of its constituents and their own particular rhythm, but above all a total absence of the will to impose. All qualities that we tried to describe in the most exact way.

We interact on a daily basis with that primary life, meaning 'original' but far from primitive in the sense of 'basic', and the delight is as absolute as in the early days. After so many years of companionship, we are still amazed to see what a hand can do helped only by heart, sensitivity, emotion, and a genuine will to help.

Unfortunately, everything comes to an end. This chapter is only a part of the osteopathic adventure, some selected pieces, some sequences from a feature film, of which you have only heard the soundtrack, a conversation, or, even better, an intimate dialogue between the osteopath and the fascia. By reading this, the reader/viewer will be able to imagine the overall spirit of the movie.

We are aware that this chapter, because of its apparent simplicity, in an elitist and high-tech society such as ours, could be seen as counter-speech. However, we ignore that fact and claim the genuineness of our relationship with the tissue. We enjoy it too much.

Put all discussions aside and stop intellectualizing. Let's close this chapter. Let's roll up our sleeves and touch. Therein lies our real secret. Thank you for reading.

Dedication

To Christiane, Carole, Cécile, Line, Julien, Lars, Nils, Joséphine, Nanuq, and Stig. My flesh, my blood, and so much more ...

Reference

César, M. 2007. *L'Action Ostéopathique. Une Intrusion Autorisée dans le Conscient Tissulaire.* Paris: Publibook, 2007. Translated from French by Hinz, K. 2009. *Osteopathisches Handeln*, München: Noëma Verlag.

MYOFASCIAL TRIGGER POINTS, SENSITIZATION, AND CHRONIC PAIN: EVALUATION AND TREATMENT

Jay P. Shah, Nikki Thaker

Introduction

Myofascial pain is the most common component of musculoskeletal pain conditions. As a form of muscle pain, myofascial pain can often be described as aching, cramping, deep, and difficult to localize. Muscle pain is distinguished from cutaneous pain in that muscle pain involves nociceptive-specific neurons in the brainstem and spinal cord.[1,2] In addition, muscle pain activates unique cortical areas that are associated with affective or emotional components of pain.[3] Although muscle nociception is inhibited more intensely by descending pain-modulating pathways,[4,5] persistent muscle nociception is more effective than cutaneous nociception at inducing maladaptive neuroplastic changes within the dorsal horn.[6] Such neuroplastic changes underlie the clinical observation that muscle pain is often persistent and difficult to resolve.

Myofascial pain syndrome (MPS) is a term used to describe a pain condition that can be acute (less than three months in duration) or, more commonly, chronic and that stems from the muscle and its surrounding connective tissue (e.g., fascia). Although the specific pathophysiological basis of myofascial trigger point (MTrP) development and symptomatology is unknown, several promising lines of scientific study (e.g., biochemical, tissue imaging, and somatosensory testing) as well as a recent systematic and comprehensive evaluative approach (including measures of range of motion, strength, and self-reports of pain, fatigue, mood, and health status) have revealed objective abnormalities.

For many clinicians and investigators, the finding of one or more MTrPs is required to assure the diagnosis of MPS. An MTrP is a discrete hyperirritable nodule in a taut band of skeletal muscle, which is palpable during physical examination (Fig. 27.1). The pain of MPS is associated with, but may not be caused by, an active MTrP. An active MTrP is clinically associated with spontaneous pain in the immediate surrounding tissue and/or to distant sites in specific referred pain patterns. Strong digital pressure

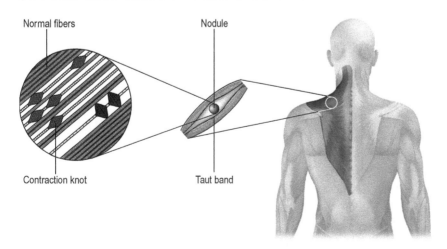

Normal fibers

Nodule

Contraction knot

Taut band

Figure 27.1
Schematic of a trigger point complex. A trigger point complex in a taut band of muscle is composed of multiple contraction knots

on the active MTrP exacerbates the patient's spontaneous pain complaint and mimics the patient's familiar pain experience. MTrPs can also be classified as latent, in which case the MTrP is physically present but not associated with a spontaneous pain complaint. However, pressure on the latent MTrP elicits local pain at the site of the nodule. Both latent and active MTrPs can be associated with muscle dysfunction, muscle weakness, and limited range of motion. Although pain of muscle origin does display unique clinical characteristics compared to cutaneous and neuropathic pain, the nature of the symptoms is highly dependent upon the individual's perception of its intensity, distribution, and duration. The way in which individuals report their symptoms presents a challenge for standardization and validation if these are to be used as diagnostic criteria, outcomes, measures of improvement, and/or in clinical trials. Characteristics like the quality of the pain, its distribution, and whether it radiates, have never been required for the diagnosis of MPS.

Origins and history of the approach

Although the clinical study of muscle pain and its associated myofascial trigger points (MTrPs) has proliferated over the past two centuries, the scientific literature often seems disjointed and confusing. Much of the terminology, theories, concepts, and diagnostic criteria are inconsistent, incomplete, or controversial.

The term 'myofascial' has evolved from the view that both muscle and fascia are likely to be contributors to the symptoms. Nomenclature from the past included 'fibrositis', which meant inflammation of the connective tissue lining muscle, along with chronic muscle pain. These terms have been replaced by the term 'myofascial pain'.

Guillaume de Baillou (1538–1616) of France was one of the first to write in detail about muscle pain disorders. In 1816, the British physician Balfour associated 'thickenings' and 'nodular tumors' in muscle with local and regional muscle pain.[7] Various other publications contained different descriptions and terminology, which reflects the slow evolution in the understanding of MTrPs. For example, Froriep in 1843 coined the term 'muskelshwiele' (muscle calluses) to describe what he believed was a 'callus' of deposited connective tissue in patients with rheumatic disorders.[8] Subsequently in 1904, Gowers suggested that inflammation of fibrous tissue (i.e., 'fibrositis') created the hard nodules.[9] However, the term fibrositis became discredited as biopsy data did not substantiate an inflammatory pathology. Schade (1919) later proposed that the nodules, which he called 'myogeloses', were high-viscosity muscle colloids.[10,11] In the mid-1900s, important work was conducted independently by Michael Gutstein in Germany, Michael Kelly in Australia, and J. H. Kellgren in Britain. By injecting hypertonic saline into various anatomical structures such as fascia, tendon, and muscle in healthy volunteers, Kellgren was able to chart zones of referred pain in neighboring and distant tissue. Among others, his work influenced the US physician Janet Travell, whose work on myofascial pain, dysfunction, and trigger points is arguably the most comprehensive to date. Travell and Rinzler coined the term 'myofascial trigger point' in the 1950s, reflecting their finding that the nodules can be present and refer pain to both muscle and overlying fascia.[12] The two-volume book *Myofascial Pain and Dysfunction: The Trigger Point Manual*, which Travell co-authored with her colleague, David Simons, represents decades of keen observation and study of myofascial pain and MTrPs.

The manual, together with more than 40 papers Travell published on the subject, was and remains instrumental in defining and popularizing the diagnosis and treatment of MPS and MTrPs among the health care community, including physical therapists, allopathic and osteopathic physicians, chiropractors, dentists, pain specialists, massage therapists, and myofascial trigger point therapists. Among the various allopathic medical specialties, physiatrists currently have the most comprehensive working understanding of MTrPs. This is, in part, because physiatrists see MPS and the MTrP as related to muscle and musculoskeletal dysfunction. Many physiatrists place a special emphasis on muscle, an 'orphan organ' few other specialties seriously consider. There are signs, however, that Simons' comments along with Travell's myofascial pain concepts are gaining ground in mainstream medicine.

The contemporary use of the term 'MPS' implies a specific condition that is distinguished from other soft tissue pain disorders such as fibromyalgia, tendonitis, or bursitis.[13] It presents as regional pain, sometimes with referred pain, often accompanied by increased tension and decreased flexibility. It has been reported to coincide with other diseases and syndromes associated with pain, for example, rheumatic diseases and fibromyalgia.[14] MPS has also been associated with other pain conditions including radiculopathies, joint dysfunction, disk pathology, tendonitis, craniomandibular dysfunction, migraines, tension-type headaches, carpal tunnel syndrome, computer-related disorders, whiplash-associated disorders, spinal dysfunction, pelvic pain and other urologic syndromes, post-herpetic neuralgia, and complex regional pain syndrome.[14] In addition, MTrPs have been associated clinically with a variety of medical conditions including those of metabolic, visceral, endocrine, infectious, and psychological origin.[15] However, MPS has generally been characterized by a physical finding and symptom cluster without demonstrable pathology, and it attracted little research attention until recently.

A definitive relationship between MPS and MTrPs is elusive. Although MTrPs are frequently associated with musculoskeletal pain, clinicians may also encounter painless nodules upon palpation. Unlike fibromyalgia, which is widespread, symmetrically distributed, and which frequently affects sleep and mood, the pain of MPS is usually local or regional, distributed in a limited number of select quadrants of the body, and has traditionally been thought to present independently of mood or sleep abnormalities. The definition and pathogenesis of MPS is still not fully understood, and there is not yet universal agreement about whether MPS is a disease or process rather than a syndrome. For many clinicians and investigators, the finding of one or more MTrPs is required to assure the diagnosis of MPS.

Aims and objectives

- To gain deeper understanding of the mechanisms of central and peripheral sensitization, and investigate the critical role of these neuroplastic changes in perpetuating chronic musculoskeletal pain.

- To summarize the reproducible physical manifestations of spinal segmental sensitization (SSS) associated with chronic musculoskeletal pain.

- To review how improved quantitative and objective diagnostic techniques are used to determine the spinal segments involved in SSS (including dermatomes, myotomes, and sclerotomes), and how such investigations are applicable in the diagnosis and treatment of chronic musculoskeletal pain.

- To discuss and demonstrate modalities and needling techniques used to desensitize the involved segments, eliminate chronic myofascial trigger points, and alleviate chronic *neuro*-musculoskeletal pain.

Background on sensitization

Sensitization is the lowering of activation threshold for nociceptors, which then increases neuronal activity in the central nervous system. Through sensitization, chronic pain syndromes, such as MPS, exhibit profound neuroplastic changes, altering neuronal excitability in the pain pathway (e.g., the spinal cord, thalamic nuclei, cortical areas, amygdala, and periaqueductal gray area). This dynamic process can fundamentally alter pain threshold, pain intensity, and emotional affect.[16] Common manifestations of sensitization are hyperalgesia (increased pain to a normally painful stimulus) and allodynia (pain to a normally nonpainful stimulus).

Signaling in the pain matrix may begin with activation of polymodal nociceptors, structures that can be sensitized by substances released from damaged tissue and the nociceptor terminals themselves. Peripheral tissue damage arising from muscle trauma and tissue inflammation triggers the release of numerous substances from damaged muscle, such as adenosine triphosphate (ATP), bradykinin (BK), serotonin (5-HT), prostaglandins, protons, and potassium. This inflammatory pool of biochemicals sensitizes and/or activates local nociceptors, an event known as peripheral sensitization. Continual bombardment of primary afferent activity over time leads to abnormal functional and structural changes in the dorsal root ganglia and dorsal horn, a process known as central sensitization. For example, a continuous barrage of noxious input into the dorsal horn (a process termed afferent bombardment) results in the co-release of L-glutamate and substance P (SP). Released together, these two substances can lower thresholds for synaptic activation and open previously ineffective synaptic connections in wide dynamic range (WDR) neurons, thus inducing central sensitization.[17,18]

The bombardment of nociceptive stimuli into the dorsal horn will lead to spinal facilitation, an increase in spinal cord neuronal activity.[19] Under normal circumstances, activation of primary afferent nociceptors in the dorsal horn is modulated by inhibitory mechanisms either locally or via descending pathways from the cerebral cortex or brainstem. However, persistent nociceptive afferent input may result in inhibitory neuronal cell death and wind-up, and sensitization of secondary order neurons in the dorsal horn. Circuits in the spinal cord (i.e., dorsal horn, ventral horn, and lateral horn) may develop lowered thresholds of activation, causing them to be more easily activated by minimal or no input at all.

The ensuing spinal facilitation is characterized by:

1. Increased ventral horn outflow that stimulates anterior motor horn cells, resulting in increased muscle tone in the myotome corresponding to its segmental level of afferent barrage.

2. Increased lateral horn outflow that results in autonomic reflexes that enhance nociceptive activity.

3. Increased dorsal horn outflow that causes antidromic electrical activity along a sensory nerve (also known as dorsal root reflexes).

Dorsal root reflexes activate dorsal root ganglion cell bodies to increase production and release of vasoactive neuropeptides (e.g., SP, CGRP, and somatostatin) both centrally and peripherally. These neuropeptides have been shown to cause leaky blood vessels and trigger the liberation of inflammatory mediators into the tissue, causing inflammation de novo, a condition known as neurogenic inflammation.[17] However, if inflammation is already present, the release of vasoactive neuropeptides will further exacerbate the condition. As a result, local tissue tenderness and mechanical hyperalgesia often ensue (or worsen, if already present), which may underlie the clinical findings of active MTrPs.

An understanding of segmental distribution of sensory nerve fibers is a vital component in proper pain management.[20] Innervation patterns of the skin, muscles, and deep structures occur at an early stage of human fetal development and little variability exists among individuals.[14] Accordingly, each spinal cord segment has a consistent segmental relationship to its spinal nerves. This allows clinicians to attribute the pattern of dermatomal, myotomal, and sclerotomal hyperalgesia to dysfunction in its corresponding spinal segment.[20,21]

Spinal segmental sensitization (SSS) is a hyperactive state of the dorsal horn caused by bombardment of nociceptive impulses from sensitized and/or damaged tissue (e.g., somatic structures such as active MTrPs or visceral structures such as the gall bladder). Manifestations in the sensitized spinal segment include dermatomal allodynia, in addition to sclerotomal tenderness and MTrPs within the involved myotomes.[20,22] Hyperalgesia of central origin is so prevalent that in one study it was found to be present in 61% of patients suffering from arthrosis-related pain. This suggests that both central and peripheral mechanisms are responsible for maintaining a chronic pain state in these individuals. Initially, hypersensitivity occurs at a local, affected site, but it is possible for central mechanisms to begin and persist separately from the peripheral process.[23] Further, segmental sensitization occurs through neuron hypertrophy as well as upregulation of excitatory neurons, prohyperalgesic peptides, and neurotransmitters at the dorsal horn. As a result, pain and inflammation occur as independent events; one condition is not indicative of the other.

Peripheral to central sensitization in muscle pain

Sensitization of primary afferents is responsible for the transition from normal to aberrant pain perception in the central nervous system that outlasts the noxious peripheral stimulus. A possible explanation for expanded referral pain patterns is increased synaptic efficiency through activation of previously silent (ineffective) synapses at the dorsal horn. This concept of opening previously ineffective connections was demonstrated in a rat myositis model. Experimentally induced inflammation unmasked receptive fields remote from the original receptive field, indicating that dorsal horn connectivity expanded beyond the original neurons involved in nociceptive transmission.[24] In this study, nociceptive input resulted in central hyperexcitability. This finding helps to explain referred pain patterns common to myofascial pain syndrome.

Central sensitization may also facilitate additional responses from other receptive fields as a result of con-

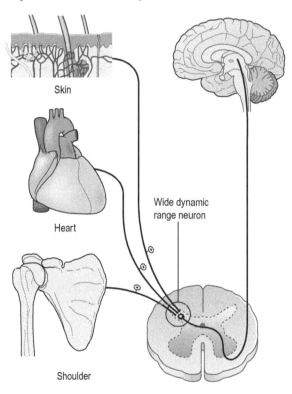

Figure 27.2
Wide dynamic range (WDR) neuron. A WDR neuron receives convergent input from cutaneous, visceral, and deep somatic afferents and subsequently sends signals to the thalamus. As such, the WDR neuron and higher-level brain centers can be driven by various inputs. Accordingly, central sensitization may facilitate responses from other structures (e.g., the shoulder, heart, and skin) that share convergent input

vergent somatic and visceral input at the dorsal horn[25] via WDR neurons (Fig. 27.2). Furthe more, afferent fibers have the ability to sprout new spinal terminals that broaden synaptic contacts at the dorsal horn and may also contribute to expanded pain receptive fields.[26] This change in functional connectivity may occur within a few hours, even before metabolic and genetic alterations occur in dorsal horn neurons.[27]

The role of the limbic system

After activating WDR neurons, afferent input from active MTrPs then ascends the spinothalamic tract to reach higher brain centers. In addition to activating the thalamus, muscle afferent input preferentially activates the limbic system (i.e., the anterior cingulate gyrus, insula, and amygdala), which plays a critical role in modulating muscle pain and the emotional or affective component of persistent pain.[28] Increased activity in the limbic system leads to greater fear, anxiety, and stress. Furthermore, Niddam et al. demonstrated increased anterior insula activity in patients with upper trapezius myofascial pain syndrome.[17]

The limbic forebrain and/or hypothalamus likely play a role in the sequence of top-down events leading to myofascial pain. These areas are influenced by emotions and hormonal fluctuations, which then modulate the periaqueductal gray (PAG) in the midbrain. The rostral ventral medulla (RVM) is a relay area between the PAG and the spinal dorsal horn. The RVM contains a population of ON cells, which can increase pain, and OFF cells, which can decrease pain. The ON/OFF cells are part of the descending inhibitory pain system that controls pain through projections that modulate activity in the dorsal horn. Following initial tissue injury, the ON cells serve a useful and protective purpose designed to prevent further damage. Under ordinary circumstances, tissue healing would lead to a decrease in ON cell activity and an increase in OFF cell activity.[17] However, in chronic musculoskeletal pain conditions, there appears to be an overall shift to a decrease in inhibition, presumably due to an imbalance of ON cell and OFF cell activity.[29] Thus, over time, maladaptive neuroplastic changes may develop, resulting in disinhibition in the spinal dorsal horn. As a result, dorsal root reflexes can create neurogenic inflammation, which then leads to local tissue tenderness, even in the absence of ongoing tissue injury or nociception. Negative emotions and stress as well as hormonal fluctuations may influence not only the perception of pain, but may actually create allodynia and mechanical hyperalgesia, the characteristic clinical findings of myofascial pain.

Evaluation of the MTrP and sensitized segments

The requisite examination skills are easy to learn and of fundamental importance to the evaluation and management of a chronic pain complaint. Furthermore, their application before and after treatment, aimed at desensitizing the involved spinal segment, provides the clinician and patient with meaningful, objective, and reproducible physical findings to guide treatment outcomes. In order to perform a comprehensive evaluation of MPS, the patient must be assessed not only for MTrPs but for sensitized spinal segments as well.

Palpation of the skeletal muscle for the objective physical findings of active and possibly latent MTrPs is the gold standard for diagnosis of myofascial pain. Identifying and adequately treating active and even latent MTrPs may have very important implications for complete resolution of a patient's pain complaint. Active MTrPs are a very common source of peripheral nociceptive bombardment, which may lead to central sensitization and perpetuation of the pain complaint. If left unresolved, active MTrPs (or other peripheral pain generators) will resensitize the dorsal horn, resulting in the re-emergence of segmental findings (e.g., allodynia and hyperalgesia) and the reproduction of the same pain complaint even after paraspinous needling treatment. It is also important to identify latent MTrPs because, under specific conditions, they can become active MTrPs. Latent MTrPs send excitatory, subthreshold potentials to the dorsal horn. Sensitization of the dorsal horn opens previously ineffective synapses to distant muscle sites. As a result of sensitization, normally non-noxious palpation of the latent MTrP induces pain locally, and upon opening of previously ineffective synapses, pain will also occur in remote areas. Thus, upon muscle palpation, pain is experienced at the site of the palpated latent MTrP and in distant, seemingly unrelated muscle.[30]

Excitatory subthreshold potentials from latent MTrPs can summate with subthreshold potentials from active MTrPs to surpass the threshold necessary for SSS to occur. Once the myotome is sensitized, all MTrPs in that myotome may become active.

If pain persists even after deactivating the trigger point(s), it may be because the related spinal segments are severely sensitized, and, accordingly, such segments should be assessed at the dermatomal, myotomal, and sclerotomal levels for MPS.

Adjacent dermatomal levels are examined paraspinally by checking for hyperalgesia and allodynia. Hyperalgesia is assessed by scratching the skin with the sharp edge of a paper clip or Wartenberg pinwheel. This noxious stimulus is applied across dermatomal borders and the patient is instructed to simultaneously report any sharpening or dulling in the sensation of pain during the procedure. An increased painful response is indicative of hyperalgesia. Allodynia is assessed by picking up the skin between the thumb and forefinger and rolling the tissue underneath, also known as a pinch-and-roll test (Fig. 27.3). This non-noxious stimulus is applied across dermatomal borders and the patient is instructed to simultaneously report any sensation of pain. The sensation of pain is indicative of allodynia, a finding that is the most sensitive indicator for the diagnosis of sensitization.

Adjacent myotomal levels are examined by palpating segmentally related musculature for tender spots, taut bands, and MTrPs and applying a pressure algometer to measure the local tenderness along the myotome.

Adjacent sclerotomal levels are examined by palpating segmentally related tendons (e.g., tendonitis), entheses (e.g., enthesitis), bursae (e.g., bursitis), and ligaments (e.g., supraspinous ligament sprain), and applying a pressure algometer to measure the pain pressure threshold (PPT) along these sclerotomal structures. (Note: PPT is the minimum pressure that elicits pain and is considered abnormal if it is at least $2 \, kg/cm^2$ lower than a normosensitive control point.)

These objective and quantitative findings help the clinician to identify the tissues and likely pain mechanisms involved in their patients' chronic pain. These segmental findings are not only reproducible, but they are often indicative of the severity of the sensitized

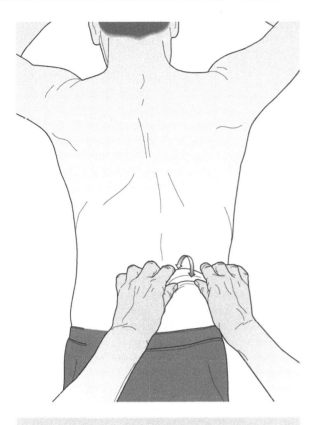

Figure 27.3
Pinch-and-roll test. The skin and subcutaneous tissue is gently pinched between the thumb and forefinger and rolled vertically across dermatomal borders. Elicitation of a painful response is indicative of allodynia

state and provide important clues about the underlying pathogenesis of the pain syndrome.

Principles and methods of treatment

While the etiology of MPS and the pathophysiology of MTrPs are not yet fully understood, some investigators recommend that treatments focus not only on the MTrP but also on the surrounding environment or fascia. The roles of muscle, fascia, and their cellular components are important contributors to both MPS and the formation of the MTrP. Thus, the evolution of thinking has led clinicians to try to reduce the size of the MTrP, correct underlying contributors to

the pain, and restore the normal working relationship between the muscles of the affected functional units. According to Dommerholt, all treatments fall into one or both of two categories: a pain-control phase and a deep conditioning phase. During the pain-control phase, trigger points are deactivated, improving circulation, decreasing pathological nociceptive activity, and eliminating the abnormal biomechanical force patterns. During the conditioning phase, the intra- and inter-tissue mobility of the functional unit is improved, which may include specific muscle stretches, neurodynamic mobilizations, joint mobilizations, orthotics, and muscle-strengthening exercises.[31]

Current approaches for management of MPS include pharmacological and nonpharmacological interventions. Among the pharmacological approaches are anti-inflammatory, analgesic, and narcotic medications: topical creams; and trigger point injections, which are now safer and more effective. Nonpharmacological interventions include manual therapies, including postisometric relaxation, counterstrain method,[32] trigger point compression, muscle energy techniques, and myotherapy,[33] along with other treatments like laser therapy,[34] dry needling, and massage.[35,36]

Stretching and strengthening of the affected muscles is important for any treatment. All forms of manual therapy include some form of mechanical pressure, and the underlying theory as to why they are effective continues to evolve with further study. Modalities and manual treatments are often clinically effective for deactivating active MTrPs and desensitizing sensitized spinal segments, and are commonly employed as a first line of treatment before attempting more invasive therapies.

Among the invasive therapies, scientific articles report mixed results. Generally, dry needling (Fig. 27.4), and injection of anesthetic, steroids, and botulinum toxin-A (BTA) into the MTrP have all been shown to provide pain relief. Regardless of the method used, there is considerable agreement that elicitation of an LTR produces more immediate and long-lasting pain relief than no elicitation of an LTR,[38–43] although some still believe that eliciting an LTR is not necessary for improvement. Nevertheless, within minutes of a single induced LTR, Shah et al. found that the initially elevated levels of SP and CGRP within the active MTrP in the upper trapezius muscle decreased to levels approaching that of normal, uninvolved muscle tissue. Though the mechanism of an LTR is unknown, the reduction of these biochemicals in the local muscle area may be due to a small, localized increase in blood flow and/or nociceptor and mechanistic changes associated with an augmented inflammatory response.[17,44]

In addition to studying application methods, researchers are also discovering better ways of categorizing and analyzing the clinical data they collect and determining if a treatment is effective. For example, researchers have begun to utilize classifications such as latent, 'nonpainful palpable', and 'painful, but no nodule' to categorize MPS. Gerber et al. have also begun to assess the effect of treatment on other important aspects in addition to pain, such as quality of life and function, disability, sleep, mood, and range of motion.[45] Clinicians are shifting the focus to improving the patient's quality of life as well as obtaining pain relief and increasing function.

Though many practitioners can attest to improvement in pain associated with MPS, improvement is typically measured using self-reports of pain levels pre- and post-treatment. To date, the number of randomized, placebo-controlled trials is few, and most of them have small numbers of participants. Additionally, because they have relied exclusively on self-reports, uncertainty remains about the validity of the findings. Thus, while a variety of pharmacological and nonpharmacological treatments have shown efficacy, studies of proper size and quantitative outcome measures need to be performed.

However, sometimes treating active MTrPs is insufficient. For example, manual therapy and trigger point injection procedures may only temporarily deactivate the MTrP(s) and the pain may therefore reoccur. In these situations, segmental dysfunction may be overlooked, and treatments need to target the SSS. While a number of recent reviews and meta-analyses have focused on needling, the effectiveness of manual therapy should not be overlooked and may be just as effective as needling.[37] For example, various forms of electrical stimulation including microcurrent, transcutaneous electrical nerve stimulation (TENS), percutaneous electrical nerve stimulation (PENS), manual therapies, such as osteopathic manipulative medicine, and spray and stretch are commonly used to treat myofascial pain and SSS. Researchers continue

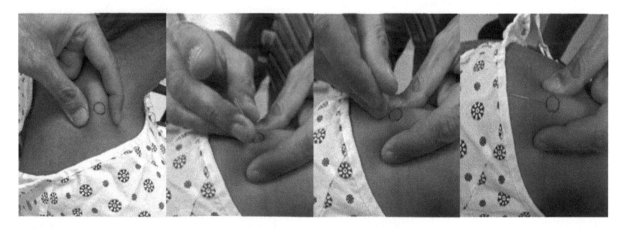

Figure 27.4

Dry needling. A series of images are shown in which the MTrP is identified and the needled is inserted in the MTrP using a swift tap. The muscle and surrounding fascia are probed with an up-and-down motion of the needle in a clockwise direction, and the needle is left in place for 1–2 minutes for full therapeutic benefit

to debate the effectiveness of laser and ultrasound for the deactivation of MTrPs but generally agree that these technologies are effective for pain management. Biofeedback and other relaxation techniques, like hypnotherapy, are also available to help patients with pain management by training them to regain control of their pain condition. Other effective but more invasive treatments for SSS include paraspinous injection block techniques and paraspinous needling, as discussed below. SSS is determined by findings of allodynia, hyperalgesia, and measurable pressure pain sensitivity over the sensory, motor, and skeletal areas along with viscera supplied by a particular spinal segment (i.e., the dermatome, myotome, sclerotome, and viscerotome, respectively).

The paraspinous injection block technique and paraspinous needling should be used particularly in chronic cases in which physical examination reveals severe and persistent allodynia and hyperalgesia, suggesting dense dermatomal, myotomal, and sclerotomal manifestations of SSS (Fig. 27.5). Often, dermatomal, myotomal, and sclerotomal segmental findings coincide, making diagnosis and treatment of the sensitized segmental level relatively straightforward. However, when they do not, or if pain relief is only partial/persists after treatment with modalities and manual treatments, affected segmental levels most closely corresponding to the principal pain complaint should be treated first with paraspinous needling, a technique that addresses the centrally sensitized component of pain.

If the patient experiences little or no pain relief, adjacent segmental levels may be needled paraspinally until the patient reports a decrease in pain. This subjective decrease in pain is typically accompanied by an objective improvement in segmental findings. However, effective management involves identification and treatment of both the peripheral and central components of sensitization. For example, as mentioned above, if active MTrPs are not treated, they will re-sensitize the dorsal horn, resulting in the re-emergence of segmental findings (i.e., allodynia and hyperalgesia) and reproduction of the same pain complaint. Accordingly, the clinician should identify and eradicate all foci of nociceptive bombardment responsible for initiating and/or perpetuating the centrally sensitized segmental findings.

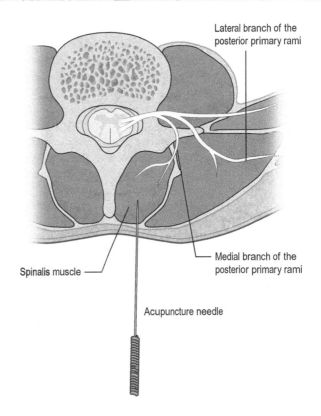

Lateral branch of the posterior primary rami

Medial branch of the posterior primary rami

Spinalis muscle

Acupuncture needle

Figure 27.5
Paraspinal needling. An acupuncture needle is inserted sagittally into the spinalis muscle and is then manipulated as described. Multiple acupuncture needles may be inserted to create a paraspinous block at each affected segmental level

So far, we have discussed how paraspinal muscles can be facilitated by active MTrPs elsewhere in the body. However, paraspinal muscles themselves, may have MTrPs, which act as a primary source of peripheral nociceptive input into the dorsal horn, further sensitizing the paraspinal muscles. In order to desensitize the muscles along a specific segment, Fischer et al. (2002) developed a paraspinous injection block technique that traditionally utilizes a 1% lidocaine injection. A 25-gauge needle, of sufficient length to reach the deep layers up to the vertebral lamina, is inserted in the sagittal plane. Injection is performed between the levels of the spinous processes corresponding to the affected segmental levels of sensitization as identified on physical examination. The needle is inserted through the paraspinal muscle to a maximal depth but without contacting the vertebral lamina. The needle is aspirated (in order to avoid blood vessels), and then approximately 0.1 mL of anesthetic is injected. The needle is then withdrawn to a subcutaneous level and redirected in the caudal direction, ending about 5 mm from the previous deposit of anesthetic solution. One continues this procedure, going as far as the needle reaches. The same procedures are repeated going in the cephalad direction. The result of this technique is multisegmental desensitization, which effectively blocks the medial branch of the posterior primary rami at affected segmental levels.[46]

Though many practitioners can attest to improvement in pain levels as a result of paraspinous block and paraspinous dry needling, these merely arise from clinical observation. Randomized, double-blinded, placebo-controlled clinical trials examining the effects of paraspinous block and paraspinous dry needling need to be conducted to demonstrate its efficacy.

Perpetuating factors of MPS

There are many conditions that may act as perpetuating factors of chronic MPS, including nutritional deficiency states such as iron insufficiency and vitamin B12 deficiency, hormonal disorders such as hypothyroidism, and trauma such as cervical strain injury. There are also mechanical causes of chronic MPS including structural, postural, and ergonomic problems. For example, Vitamin D deficiency is associated with musculoskeletal pain, loss of type II muscle fibers, and proximal muscle atrophy. One study found that 89% of subjects with chronic musculoskeletal pain were deficient in Vitamin D. The deficiency state can be reversed easily, but requires up to six months for restoration to normal Vitamin D levels. Another example is iron deficiency in the muscle, which creates an energy crisis by limiting an energy-producing reaction. As a result, iron deficiency may also play a role in the development or maintenance of MTrPs. Hypothyroidism is also considered a perpetuating factor because it produces a hypometabolic state, which may augment MTrP formation. Perpetuating factors may be structural, postural, or ergonomic if comorbid conditions such as scoliosis, leg length discrepancy, pelvic torsion, and/or hypomobility or hypermobility

of joints, among others, are present. Comorbid conditions, whether of medical or mechanical nature, may initiate or interfere with the treatment or recovery process. Thus, in cases of chronic myalgia, it is important to identify them through a thorough history and physical examination as well as a laboratory exam.[47]

Possible physiological mechanisms

Until recently, researchers have largely relied upon Simons' Integrated Trigger Point hypothesis, introduced in 1999, to explain the role of peripheral and central sensitization. According to the hypothesis, the presence of abnormal endplate activity is what augments the series of events leading to MTrP development. As hypothesized by Simons, during abnormal endplate activity, high levels of acetylcholine (Ach) are released, which travel down the sacroplasmic reticulum and open calcium channels. When calcium binds to troponin on the muscle fibers, the muscle fibers contract. In order to release the contraction, adenosine triphosphate (ATP) is needed to cause the conformational change of the muscle fibers and actively pump calcium back into the sacroplasmic reticulum. Thus, a lack of ATP perpetuates the sustained contracture near an abnormal endplate. This leads to increased metabolic demands, compressed capillary circulation (which reduces blood flow, forming local hypoxic conditions), and a polarized membrane potential. The increased demand for and reduced supply of ATP forms the energy crisis, which may evoke the release of neuroreactive substances and metabolic byproducts (i.e., BK, SP, 5-HT) that could sensitize peripheral nociceptors.[48] While Simons' hypothesis explains how sensitizing neuroactive substances are responsible for the pain associated with active MTrPs and is the most credible theory to date, it remains conjectural. Remarkably, key tenets of Simons' Integrated Trigger Point hypothesis overlap with the self-sustaining cycle suggested by the Cinderella hypothesis.

The Cinderella hypothesis[49] provides a possible explanation for the role of muscle in MTrP development. This hypothesis describes how musculoskeletal disorder symptoms may arise from muscle recruitment patterns during submaximal level exertions with moderate or low physical load. These types of exertions are typically utilized by occupational groups such as office workers, musicians, and dentists, in which myalgia and MTrPs have been commonly reported.[50] According to Henneman's size principle, smaller type I muscle fibers are recruited first and derecruited last during static muscle exertions. As a result, these 'Cinderella' fibers are continuously activated and metabolically overloaded, in contrast to larger motor muscle fibers that spend less time being activated and do not work as hard. This property makes the 'Cinderella' fibers more susceptible to muscle damage and calcium dysregulation, key factors in the formation of MTrPs.[51] A study by Treaster et al. supports the Cinderella hypothesis by demonstrating that low-level static continuous muscle contractions in office working during 30 minutes of typing induced the formation of MTrPs.[52]

MTrPs can also develop as a result of muscle overuse in cervical and postural muscles during the performance of low-intensity activities of daily living and sedentary work.[50,52] An intriguing possible mechanism involves sustained low-level muscle contractions routinely used in tasks requiring precision and postural stability of the cervical spine and shoulder. As a result of sustained low-level contractions, a decrease in intramuscular perfusion has been postulated. Thus, it is conceivable that ischemia, hypoxia, and insufficient ATP synthesis in type I motor unit fibers may occur and are responsible for increasing acidity, Ca^{2+} accumulation, and subsequent sarcomere contracture. This vicious cycle leads to increased sarcomere contracture, decreased intramuscular perfusion, and increased ischemia and hypoxia. As a result, several sensitizing substances may be released, leading to local and referred pain and muscle tenderness, which are clinical hallmarks of MPS. Shah et al. demonstrated and confirmed that active MTrPs have elevated levels of inflammatory mediators, neuropeptides, catecholamines, and cytokines, biochemicals known to be associated with inflammation, pain, sensitization, and intercellular signaling.[18,23,44]

Other researchers emphasize the 'neighborhood' of the MTrP (i.e., surrounding fascia) in order to explain the symptom complex and physical findings associated with MPS. Specifically, Stecco focuses on three anatomical layers: the deep fascia, the layer of loose connective tissue (which houses the highest concentration of hyaluronic acid), and the layer of epimysium below it. An important molecule in this system is hyaluronic acid (HA), an anionic, nonsulfated glycosaminoglycan distributed widely throughout various tissues, and one of the chief components of the extracellular matrix. Normally, HA functions as a lubricant that helps muscle fibers glide alongside one another without friction. However, Stecco theorizes that, as a result of muscle overuse or traumatic injury, the sliding layers start to produce immense amounts of HA, which then aggregate into supermolecular structures, changing both its configuration, viscoelasticity, and viscosity. Due to its increased viscosity, HA can no longer function as an effective lubricant, which increases resistance in the sliding layers and leads to densification of fascia, or abnormal sliding in muscle fibers. Interference with sliding can impact range of motion and cause difficulty with movement including quality of movement and stiffness. In addition, under abnormal conditions, the friction results in increased neural hyperstimulation (irritation), which then hypersensitizes mechanoreceptors and nociceptors embedded within densified fascia. This hypersensitization correlates with a patient's experience of pain, allodynia, paresthesia, abnormal proprioception, and altered movement. The fact that very few objective, repeatable studies have been conducted to elucidate these concepts demonstrates the constraints of our knowledge regarding the pathophysiology of MPS. Further research is needed to determine not only the role of the MTrP, but also its surrounding fascia.[53]

Case study

Nora is a 50-year old woman with a complex medical history, who develops a new onset of right upper quadrant pain. She is perplexed because this episode is identical to her previous experience with gall bladder pain, despite having undergone a cholecystectomy 20 years ago. Nora's new onset of 'gall bladder pain' is one of the many pain complaints she has developed over the years. However, alarmed that the pain appears to be coming from an organ that is no longer there, Nora decides to see an osteopathic physician.

Upon her first visit, her doctor collects a detailed medical history. She begins by telling him that in her teenage years, she was an elite soccer player. However, she sustained a serious sports injury during a game when an overaggressive opponent kicked the front of her right thigh, causing a noticeable limp. Nora complained of an achy, cramping pain deep in her right knee joint that also caused the knee to occasionally buckle. Due to the pain, Nora often had trouble sleeping at night. Since the injury, Nora also has a mild form of patellar tracking dysfunction, in which she experiences a painful popping or grinding of the kneecap as the knee is flexed or extended. After five years of massage and other manual therapies, her knee joint pain completely resolved, but she was unable to return to her previous level of physical activity due to continued muscle dysfunction, weakness, and a limited range of motion in her knee joint.

Over the years, doctors ruled out patellofemoral dysfunction and tendinitis of the quadriceps or patellar tendons as an explanation for her knee dysfunction. Nora was told that there were no abnormal findings in her right knee and thigh.

Coincidentally, around this time, Nora also developed lower back pain and pelvic pain, which continues to persist today. She obtains temporary relief from pain relievers and therapeutic massages, but has accepted that she is going to have to live with debilitating pain in her knee.

At age 35, she started to feel immense pain radiating from her gall bladder. She found out she had developed acute cholecystitis (gallbladder inflammation) for which she underwent a cholecystectomy. While the surgery relieved her original gall bladder pain, now at the age of 50, she feels the same pain has returned. *How is this possible?*

After carefully listening to Nora's medical history, her new physician suspected that no one had previously examined the muscles surrounding her knee joint and pelvic area for MTrPs. He conducted a thorough physical examination, palpating the soft tissue and muscles surrounding her knee and pelvic area. He found multiple latent MTrPs in her right vastus lateralis (knee extensor muscle) and active and latent MTrPs in her lower back and pelvic area. Nora's doctor suspected that the latent MTrPs could be responsible for her knee dysfunction, and her sports injury could have led to her other pain complaints. He went on to explain that her chronic knee pain could have triggered her other pain complaints as a result of

peripheral and central sensitization. However, there are still many unanswered questions. *Are Nora's pain complaints all related to one another? Are there other factors that are exacerbating her pain complaints? Lastly, could her pain symptoms be reversed or relieved?*

In order to find an effective treatment for Nora, it was important to make detailed notes of her medical history, including any emotional aspects, and to conduct a thorough physical examination. By doing so, Nora's osteopathic physician was not only able to organize her complex 50-year medical history into a coherent web of interconnected pain conditions, but was also able to attribute possible explanations as to their origins. Throughout her lifetime, Nora had experienced knee, pelvic, lower back, gall bladder, and phantom pain conditions along with patellar tracking dysfunction. All of her pain conditions started after her soccer injury. Her physician concluded that the kick to her right thigh during her soccer injury activated MTrPs in Nora's vastus medialis and led to her initial knee joint pain. In addition, he determined that the latent MTrPs in Nora's vastus lateralis may have aggravated her previously inexplicable patellar tracking dysfunction.

Unbeknownst to her previous clinicians, Nora's fall initiated noxious input from her vastus medialis, sensitizing the L3–L4 segments. The convergence of somatic and visceral input at the dorsal horn via WDR neurons then created her new onset of pelvic pain despite the absence of any visceral disease or dysfunction. After initially failing to find any physical abnormalities in her knee joint, these clinicians incorrectly concluded that nothing was physically wrong with her and did not search for and find the myofascial component of her pain and dysfunction.

Bombardment of peripheral noxious input into the dorsal horn from her sports injury likely triggered and perpetuated Nora's back pain condition via several mechanisms including dorsal root reflexes, neurogenic inflammation, ventral horn outflow, and lateral horn outflow. The clinical consequences are increased muscle shortening, pain, and tenderness of her paraspinal and quadriceps muscles (corresponding to the L3–L4 segments).

Her active MTrPs were treated with manual therapy and massage , while the latent ones in her vastus lateralis muscle went unaddressed and therefore persisted. At age 35, Nora developed acute and exquisitely painful cholecystitis for which she underwent a cholecystectomy. Prior to surgery, the sustained noxious input from her cholecystitis was of sufficient intensity and duration to inactivate inhibitory neurons at the segmental level of entry (T6) into the dorsal horn. Fortunately, the gall bladder pain immediately resolved following surgery. However, at the age of 50, nociceptive input from a new, minor but acutely painful injury to Nora's lower back (an area unrelated to her sports injury) activated dorsal horn neurons upon reaching the T6 segmental level. As a result, Nora experienced the same gall bladder pain pattern (i.e., phantom pain) as she did before her gall bladder was removed. While Nora was alarmed by the reoccurrence of her gall bladder pain, her physician explained to her that her gall bladder symptoms likely resulted from death and/or dysfunction of local inhibitory neurons.

In addition, it is noteworthy to mention that, while there were physical stressors that likely triggered Nora's condition, she could have also faced tremendous emotional stressors and hormonal fluctuations that may have exacerbated her condition. When asked about some of the most substantial emotional stressors in her lifetime, Nora mentioned that a month after her soccer injury, her father had passed away and that she was stressed about applying to college. At the onset of her gall bladder pain, she was in the midst of a difficult divorce and had begun menopause. The emotional stress and hormonal fluctuations, as well as the activation of glial cells, could certainly have aggravated Nora's pain conditions and prevented her from recovering. Theoretically, the emotional and hormonal fluctuations could have sensitized latent MTrPs in her pelvic area and lower back, making them active and painful ones.

Considering all of Nora's symptoms and dysfunction, what is the best course of treatment?

The answer required a comprehensive history and physical examination in addition to application of the concepts discussed in this chapter. The examination included a comprehensive musculoskeletal evaluation. First, Nora's physician examined the affected segments corresponding to the area of pain including the L3–L4 (pelvis and knee) and T6 segments (gall bladder) for any signs of sensitization. These included dermatomal allodynia, hyperalgesia, sclerotomal tenderness, and MTrPs within the involved myotomes. To do so, he used the pinch-and-roll test and found allodynia in Nora's L3–L4 and T6 segments. Next, using a Wartenberg pinwheel, the physician found hyperalgesia in Nora's L3–L4 and T6 segments. The physician then applied a pressure algometer to measure the local tenderness (i.e., pain pressure threshold [PPT]) along the affected myotomes. He found active MTrPs in Nora's pelvic area and lower back and latent MTrPs in her vastus lateralis. He explained that the best form of treatment would be dry needling in order to deactivate active and latent MTrPs in the periphery and paraspinous dry needling to desensitize the spinal segments along her areas of pain. He also recommended that Nora supplement dry needling treatments with biofeedback therapy, to gain greater awareness of her physiological functions. As a result of these cognitive–emotional changes, Nora's overall health and performance may improve as well. After three weeks of dry needling (one session per week), Nora and her physician observed significant improvement in her knee and surrounding muscles. She no longer experienced muscle dysfunction and weakness. Upon palpation of her vastus lateralis, the physician noted that the tightness in her muscle improved and the muscle felt softer. Most notably, Nora's range of motion around her knee joint improved. Her physician further confirmed this result by once again measuring her Q angle, which was now in the normal range (<17°), with a result of 15°.

After the paraspinous dry needling sessions in the L3–L4 and T6 segments, Nora's pelvic pain, back pain, and phantom pain decreased dramatically and her clinical findings of allodynia and hyperalgesia also resolved. When an algometer was once again used to measure tenderness along the affected myotomes, there was a significant increase in PPT, suggesting that the area had become desensitized. The active and latent MTrPs in Nora's pelvic area and lower back were also treated in order to prevent resensitization of the spinal segments. She was referred to physical therapy to maintain and improve her range of motion, strength, and flexibility. In the months following her treatment, Nora reports that her mood improved significantly. For the first time in years, she is achieving a full night's rest without waking up in the middle of the night in pain. She is able to re-engage in sports and increase her duration of participation with regained strength. Even years after her treatment, Nora's improvements are sustained, reinforcing the importance of identifying and treating symptoms and signs of peripheral and central sensitization commonly found in chronic pain.

References

1. Sessle, B. J. 2000 Acute and chronic craniofacial pain: brainstem mechanisms of nociceptive transmission and neuroplasticity, and their clinical correlates. *Critical Rev Oral Biol Med*:57–91.

2. Arendt-Nielsen, L., Graven-Nielsen, T. 2002 Deep tissue hyperalgesia. *J Musculoskelet Pain* 10:97–119.

3. Svensson, P., Minoshima, S., Beydoun, A., Morrow, T. J., Casey, K. L. 1997 Cerebral processing of acute skin and muscle pain in humans. *J Neurophysiol* 78(1):450–460.

4. XianMin, Y., Mense, S. 1990 Response properties and descending control of rat dorsal horn neurons with deep receptive fields. *Neuroscience* 39:823–831.

5. Fields, H. L., Basbaum, A. I. 1999 Central nervous system mechanisms of pain modulation, in *Textbook of Pain*, ed. R. Melzack, P. D. Wall. Churchill Livingstone: Edinburgh. pp. 309–329.

6. Wall, P. D., Woolf, C. J. 1984 Muscle but not cutaneous c-afferent input produces prolonged increases in the excitability of the flexion reflex in the rat. *J Physiol* 356:443–458.

7. Stockman, R. 1904 The cause, pathology, and treatment of chronic rheumatism. *Edinburgh Med J* 15:107–116.

8. Froriep R. 1843 Ein Beitrag zur Pathologie und Therapie des Rheumatismus.

9. Gowers W. R. 1904 Lumbago: its lessons and analogues. *Br Med J* 1:117–121.

10. Schade H. 1921 Untersuchungen in der Erkältungstrage: III. Uber den Rheumatismus, insbesondere den Muskelrheumatismus (myogelose). *Müench Med Wochenschr* 68:95–99.

11. Travell J. G., Simons D. G. 1983 Myofascial pain and dysfunction: the trigger point manual. Baltimore: Williams & Wilkins.

12. Travell J. G., Rinzler S. H. 1952 The myofascial genesis of pain. *Postgraduate Medicine* 11:434–452.

13. Robert B. 2007 Myofascial pain syndromes and their evaluation. *Best Pract Res Clin Rheumatol* 21 427–445.

14. Borg-Stein J., Simons D. G. 2002 Focused review: myofascial pain. *Arch Phys Med Rehabil* 83:S40–47, S48–49.

15. Hong C. 1996 Pathophysiology of myofascial trigger point. *J Formos Med Assoc* 95:93–104.

16. Zieglgänsberger, W., Berthele, A., Tölle, T. R. 2005 Understanding neuropathic pain. *CNS Spectrums* 10:298–308.

17. Willard, F. 2008 Basic Mechanisms of Pain: future Trends in CAM Research, in *Integrative Pain Medicine: The Science and Practice of Complementary and Alternative Medicine in Pain Management*, ed. J. F. Audette, A. Bailey, A. Humana Press Inc.: Totowa.

18. Shah, J. P., Gilliams, E. A. 2008 Uncovering the biochemical milieu of myofascial trigger points using in-vivo microdialysis: an application of muscle pain concepts to myofascial pain syndrome. *J Bodyw Mov Ther* 12:371–384.

19. Romero Ventosilla, P. 2007 Consecuencias clínicas de la Estimulación Sensorial persistente: La Sensibilización Espinal Segmentaria Available online at: http://rehab-almenara.org/download/SES%20PRV.pdf [accessed 18 March 2016].

20. Waldman, S. D. ed. 2006 *Physical Diagnosis of Pain: an Atlas of Signs and Symptoms*. 1st edn. Philadelphia: Saunders & Elsevier.

21. Fischer, A. A., Imamura, M. 2000 New concepts in the diagnosis and management of musculoskeletal pain, in *Pain Procedures in Clinical Practice*, ed. T. A. Lennard. Henley & Belfus: Philadelphia. pp. 213–229.

22. Imamura, M., Imamura, S. T., Kaziyama, H. H. S., Targino, R. A., Hsing, W. T., De Souza, L. P. M., Cutait, M. M., Fregni, F., Camanho, G. L. 2008 Impact of nervous system hyperalgesia on pain, disability, and quality of life in patients with knee osteoarthritis: a controlled analysis. *Arthritis Care Res* 59:1424–1431.

23. Shah, J. P., Phillips, T. M., Danoff, J. V., Gerber, L. 2005 An in vivo microanalytical technique for measuring the local biochemical milieu of human skeletal muscle. *J Appl Physiol* 99:1977–1984.

24. Hoheisel, U., Koch, K., Mense, S. 1994 Functional reorganization in the rat dorsal horn during an experimental myositis. *Pain* 59:111–118.

25. Sato, A. 1995 Somatovisceral reflexes. *J Manipulative Physiol Ther* 18:597–602.

26. Sperry, M. A., Goshgarian, H. G. 1993 Ultrastructural changes in the rat phrenic nucleus developing within 2 h after cervical spinal cord hemisection. *Exp Neurol* 120:233–244.

27. Mense, S., Hoheisel, U. 2004 Central nervous sequelae of local muscle pain. *Musculoskelet Pain* 12:101–109.

28. Svensson, P., Minoshima, S., Beydoun, A., Morrow, T. J., Casey, K. L. 1997 Cerebral processing of acute skin and muscle pain in humans. *J Neurophysiol* 78:450–460.

29. Niddam, D. M., Chan, R. C., Lee, S. H., Yeh, T. C., Hsieh, J. C. 2007 Central modulation of pain evoked from myofascial trigger point. *Clin J Pain* 23:440–448.

30. Mense, S. 2010 How Do Muscle Lesions such as Latent and Active Trigger Points Influence Central Nociceptive Neurons? *J Musculoskelet Pain* 18:348–353.

31. Saal, J., Saal, J. 1991 Rehabilitation of the patient, in *Conservative Care of Low Back Pain*, ed. A. White, R. Anderson. Baltimore, Williams and Wilkins. pp. 21–34.

32. Myers H. L. 2006 *Clinical application of counterstrain*. Tucson, AZ: Osteopathic Press.

33. Cantu R. I., Grodin A. J. 2001 Myofascial manipulation: theory and clinical application. 2nd edn. Gaithersburg, Md: Aspen Publishers.

34. Uemoto L., Nascimento de Azevedo R., Almeida Alfaya T., Nunes Jardim Reis R., Depes de Gouvea C. V., Cavalcanti Garcia M. A. 2013 Myofascial trigger point therapy: laser therapy and dry needling. *Curr Pain Headache Rep* 17:357.

35. Simons D. 2002 Understanding effective treatments of myofascial trigger points. *J Bodyw Mov Ther* 6:81–88.

36. Dommerholt J., Huijbregts P. 2011 Myofascial trigger points: pathophysiology and evidence-informed diagnosis and management. Sudbury, Mass.: Jones and Bartlett Publishers.

37. Rayegani S. M., Bayat M., Bahrami M. H., Raeissadat S. A., Kargozar E. 2014 Comparison of dry needling and physiotherapy in treatment of myofascial pain syndrome. *Clin Rheumatol* 33:859–864.

38. Majlesi J., Unalan H. 2010 Effect of treatment on trigger points. *Curr Pain Headache Rep* 14:353–360.

39. Peloso P., Gross A., Haines T., Trinh K., Goldsmith C. H., Burnie S. 2006 Medicinal and injection therapies for mechanical neck disorders *J Rheumatol* 33:957–967

40. Ho K. Y., Tan K. H. 2007 Botulinum toxin A for myofascial trigger point injection: a qualitative systematic review. *Eur J Pain* 11:519–527.

41. Lang A. M. 2002 Botulinum toxin therapy for myofascial pain disorders. *Curr Pain Headache Rep* 6:355–360.

42. Birch S., Jamison RN. 1998 Controlled trial of Japanese acupuncture for chronic myofascial neck pain: assessment of specific and nonspecific effects of treatment. *Clin J Pain* 14:248–255.

43. Chu J. 1995 Dry needling (intramuscular stimulation) in myofascial pain related to lumbar radiculopathy. *Eur J Phys Med Rehabil* 5:106–121.

44. Shah J. P., Danoff J. V., Desai M. J., et al. 2008 Biochemicals associated with pain and inflammation are elevated in sites near to and remote from active myofascial trigger points. *Arch Phys Med Rehabil* 89:16–23.

45. Gerber L. H., Sikdar S., Armstrong K., et al. 2013 A systematic comparison between subjects with no pain and pain associated with active myofascial trigger points. *PM R5*:931–938

46. Fischer, A. A. 2002 New injection techniques for treatment of musculoskeletal pain, in *Myofascial Pain and Fibromyalgia: Trigger Point Management*, ed. E. S. Rachlin, I. S. Rachlin. Mosby. pp. 403–419.

47. Gerwin, R. D. 2005 A review of myofascial pain and fibromyalgia—factors that promote their persistence. *Acupunct Med* 23:121–134.

48. Gerwin, R. D., Dommerholt, J. et al. 2004 An expansion of Simons' integrated hypothesis of trigger point formation. *Curr Pain Headache Rep* 8:468–475.

49. Hägg G. 1991 Static work load and occupational myalgia: a new explanation model. In *Electromyographical Kinesiology*, ed. P. Anderson, D. Hobart, J. Danoff Amsterdam: Elsevier. pp. 141–144.

50. Kaergaard A., Andersen, J. H. 2000 Musculoskeletal disorders of the neck and shoulders in female sewing machine operators: prevalence, incidence, and prognosis. *Occup Environ Med* 57:528–534.

51. Henneman, E., Somjen, G., Carpenter, D. O. 1965 Excitability and inhibitability of motoneurons of different sizes. *J Neurophysiol* 28:599–620.

52. Treaster D., Marras W. S., Burr D., Sheedy J. E., Hart D. 2006 Myofascial trigger point development from visual and postural stressors during computer work. *J Electromyogr Kinesiol* 16:115–124.

53. Stecco, C., Stern, R. et al. 2011 Hyaluronan within fascia in the etiology of myofascial pain. *Surg Radiol Anat* 33:891–896.

NOCICEPTION AND PAIN OF FASCIA

Wilfrid Jänig, Winfried L. Neuhuber

Introduction

Nociception and pain usually focus on well-defined body tissues like skin, skeletal muscle, joints, visceral organs, and the like. Thus pain is subdivided into cutaneous pain, deep somatic pain (skeletal muscle, joints), visceral pain, headache, etc. according to the body tissues. What about nociception and pain in fascial tissues throughout the body? Fascial tissues are fibrous collagenous tissues that are part of a body-wide tensional force transmission system. They are an interconnected tensional network that separates as well as keeps the different component parts of the body tissues together and protects them against overstretching (Langevin & Huijing, 2009; Schleip & Huijing, 2012; Turvey & Fonseca, 2014). Depending on their functions, fascial tissues differ in their structure in terms of the density and directional alignment of the collagen fibers. This implies that fascial tissues also include, in addition to the planar tissue sheaths (such as septa, joint capsules, aponeuroses, organ capsules, or retinacula) other connective tissue structures such as those surrounding blood vessels, perineuria, periosteum, interosseous membranes, epi- and perimysia, fibrous capsules of the intervertebral discs, etc. Whether dura mater, mesenteria, or peritoneal coverings, etc. should be included is debatable (Langevin & Huijing, 2009; Schleip et al., 2012; Schleip & Huijing, 2012). Thus, the definition of facial tissues varies somewhat. We will restrict the discussion of nociception and pain in fascial tissues to deep somatic tissues, including nerves and tissues of the retroperitoneal space.

Although not systematically investigated, practically all fascial tissues are innervated by nociceptive afferent neurons, possibly non-nociceptive afferent neurons and sympathetic (noradrenergic) postganglionic neurons (see Chapter 33). Because there exist only very few (morphological and physiological) investigations of the innervation of fascia, we will base our description mainly on the neurophysiological investigations of the innervation of the knee-joint capsule and skeletal muscle and central integrative processes in spinal cord and supraspinal centers associated with these two groups of tissues (Graven-Nielsen et al., 2008; Mense, 1993, 2013; Schaible & Grubb, 1993; Schaible et al., 2009; Schaible, 2013).

Nociception and pain in all tissues are integral components of the protective behavior of organisms. This behavior consists of the sensory–discriminative, affective, cognitive, and motor (somatomotor, autonomic motor, and neuroendocrine motor) dimensions. These dimensions generated and coordinated by the brain are globally described as pain behavior that serves to protect the tissues against injury and furthers healing. They occur in parallel as well as sequentially. To understand nociception and pain originating in fascial tissues, the following aspects must be kept in mind:

- the biomechanics of the musculoskeletal system including joints, bones, superficial and deep fascia, ligaments, intervertebral discs, etc.

- the afferent innervation of these deep somatic tissues and the encoding of noxious or potentially noxious stimuli by the afferent neurons

- the transmission of nociceptive impulse activity in the spinal cord, caudal trigeminal nucleus, thalamus, and cortex

- the endogenous control of this nociceptive impulse transmission by the brain

- the reactions of skeletomotor, autonomic motor, and neuroendocrine motor systems.

Mechanisms of nociception and pain in fascia are indirectly described in the literature under myofascial pain syndrome (Bennett, 2013; Russell, 2013). We will not discuss mechanisms underlying myofascial trigger points (MTrPs). Most cellular mechanisms discussed on the basis of Simons' 'integrative myofascial trigger point hypothesis' are not based on experimental evidence and measurements (Mense & Simons, 2001; Simons, 2004, 2013). Clinical studies to objectively reproduce the identification of MTrPs, as well as quantitative investigations of the success of therapeutic interventions at the MTrPs, remain incomplete (Lucas et al., 2009; Myburgh et al., 2008; Tough et al., 2009). In fact, the theory of myofascial pain syndrome caused by MTrP is a subject of intense debate (Dommerholt & Gerwin, 2015; Quintner et al., 2014).

The nociceptive system and its cortical control

Figure 28.1 demonstrates schematically and in simplified form the nociceptive system. Primary afferent neurons with Aδ-fibers (conduction velocity 2–30 m/s) or C-fibers (conduction velocity < 2 m/s) encode in their activity noxious mechanical or chemical stimuli. This activity is processed in the spinal and caudal trigeminal dorsal horn and transmitted by ascending tract neurons to centers in the brain stem, hypothalamus, and thalamus. Thalamic neurons involved in processing nociceptive information project to the dorsal posterior insular cortex, the primary interoceptive cortex, and to other cortical areas including the primary and secondary somatosensory cortex. The processing of nociceptive information in the spinal dorsal horn is controlled by centers in the lower and upper brainstem that project to the spinal dorsal horn. These centers are under the control of the limbic system and neocortex. In parallel, the processing of ascending nociceptive information is accompanied at all levels of integration (spinal cord, brainstem, hypothalamus) by activation or inhibition of somatic, autonomic, and neuroendocrine motor systems (only shown for the spinal cord in Figure 28.1), resulting in protective motor behavior. The ascending nociceptive system, endogenous control system, and motor systems are closely welded together at all levels of neural integration.

The peripheral and central nociceptive system is not static, as Figure 28.1 may imply, but underlies

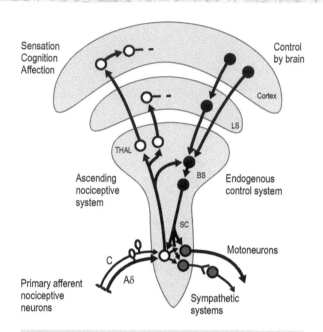

Figure 28.1

The peripheral and central nociceptive system. Aδ and C afferent neurons with thin myelinated or unmyelinated axons. Left: ascending nociceptive system connected to nociceptive primary afferent neurons. Right: endogenous control system of nociception as well as somatic motor system and sympathetic systems. BS = brain stem; LS = limbic system; SC = spinal cord; THAL = thalamus

plastic changes during tissue injury and inflammation leading to acute and chronic pain.

Physiology of primary afferent neurons related to fascial tissues

The primary afferent neuron as an interface between body tissues and brain

Primary afferent nociceptive neurons are equipped with specific molecular mechanisms that are the basis for their activation by noxious physical stimuli (by way of transduction molecules for mechanical or thermal stimuli) or chemical stimuli (e.g., by exogenous or endogenous algogenic substances and inflammatory mediators) (Fig. 28.2). We have some knowledge about transduction channels for thermal (heat and cold) stimuli, but not for noxious mechanical stimuli, about the membrane receptors for inflammatory mediators, about the different types of voltage-dependent ionic channels (sodium, potassium, calcium, chloride) that determine the excitability of the membranes, and about the intracellular pathways connecting the receptors and the cellular effectors (e.g., ionic channels).

The stimuli are encoded by receptor potentials and transmitted in the frequency of the action potentials to the spinal dorsal horn. The central terminals of the nociceptive neurons release at their synapses with the second-order neurons' neurotransmitters (the amino-acid glutamate, the neuropeptide substance P, possibly other neuropeptides, adenosine triphosphate [ATP]), which react with their corresponding subsynaptic receptors in the membranes of the second-order neurons, leading to their activation. The cell bodies of the primary afferent neurons, located in the spinal dorsal root or trigeminal ganglia, synthesize transduction proteins, ionic channels, receptor proteins of the inflammatory mediators, neurotransmitters, and receptors of neurotrophic substances, etc. (Dawes et al., 2013; Gold, 2013; Gold & Caterina, 2009; Woolf & Ma, 2007).

Nociceptive afferent neurons have several functions, depending on the tissues they innervate, and exhibit extraordinary plasticity during peripheral inflammation (see the section later in this chapter on sensitization) or after nerve injury (Hökfelt et al., 2013; Ossipov & Porreca, 2009). They serve as a connecting link between the peripheral body tissues and the central nervous system (CNS). They are possibly

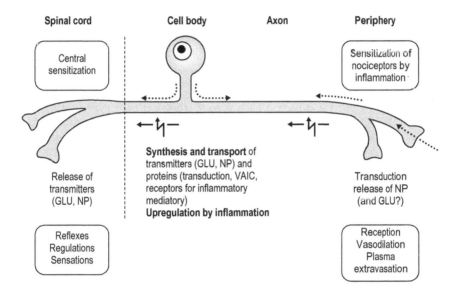

Figure 28.2

The primary afferent nociceptive neuron as a connecting link between body tissues and the spinal dorsal horn or caudal trigeminal nucleus. The cellular functions of the peripheral receptive terminals, axons, cell bodies, and central terminals are shown. The cellular integrative functions are encased. GLU = excitatory amino acid glutamate; NP = neuropeptides like calcitonin-gene-related peptide (CGRP) and substance P (SP); VAIC = voltage-activated ionic channels. Inflammatory mediators are adenosine triphosphate (ATP), bradykinin, histamine, interleukins, prostaglandins, proton ions, and serotonin. Vasodilation occurs at the arteriolar precapillary site and plasma extravasation at the venular postcapillary site of the vascular bed. Solid arrows = excitation; broken arrows = orthodromic or antidromic transport of substances

not only differentiated according to the tissues they innervate and according to the physical stimuli activating them, but also according to their so-called efferent functions:

1. Excitation of peptidergic nociceptive afferent neurons generates, in deep somatic tissues (e.g., joint capsule, fascia, intervertebral discs, perineurium) and visceral tissues, an arteriolar vasodilation and a venular plasma extravasation. Both processes are called neurogenic inflammation and are protective tissue reactions operating independently of the CNS. The vasodilation is generated mainly by release of the neuropeptide calcitonin gene-related peptide (CGRP) and the plasma extravasation by release of substance P from the afferent terminals.

2. Afferent neurons with unmyelinated fibers probably also have trophic functions that are important for the maintenance of the structure of the peripheral tissues.

3. Afferent neurons transport retrogradely from the tissues they innervate to their cell bodies neurotrophic substances such as nerve growth factor (NGF), glial-derived nerve growth factor (GDNF), brain-derived neurotrophic factor (BDNF). These signaling molecules are important for maintaining the structure and function of the afferent neurons, for the upregulation of the synthesis of the different molecules in their cell bodies (see Fig. 28.2), and very likely for the specificity of the synaptic connections between afferent neurons and second-order neurons in the spinal dorsal horn.

The cascade of afferent functions, leading to pain sensations; discomfort; protective reflexes and protective regulations; and efferent functions of nociceptive afferent neurons may serve the same general functional aim: protection and maintenance of the integrity of the body tissues. It is not far-fetched to assume that the nociceptive afferent neurons are subdifferentiated into those having only central functions, those having only peripheral functions, and those having both (Häbler et al., 1990; Jänig, 2006). This general description of the biology of nociceptive primary afferent neurons also applies to those innervating fascial tissues.

Neurophysiology of afferent neurons innervating fascial tissues

Most or all afferent nociceptive neurons innervating fascial tissues are hypothesized to be polymodal, responding to mechanical stimuli, heat stimuli, and chemical stimuli (e.g., bradykinin, capsaicin). This hypothesis is based on several groups of experimental studies:

1. The afferent innervation of the knee joint capsule (cat, rat; Schaible, 2013; Schaible & Grubb, 1993) and of skeletal muscle (mostly gastrocnemius-soleus muscle in cat and rat; Mense, 1993, 2013). In fact, many small-diameter muscle afferents probably innervate fascial tissues of the skeletal muscle.

2. Unmyelinated afferent fibers innervating the paraspinal tissues in rats (Bove & Light, 1995).

3. Afferent C- and Aδ-fibers innervating the retroperitoneal space including blood vessels, nerves, lymph nodes, vertebral column (periosteum, ligaments, intervertebral discs) and fat tissue in cats (Bahns et al., 1986).

4. Afferent C-fibers innervating the pia mater of sacral ventral roots in cats (Jänig & Koltzenburg, 1991). Figure 28.3 demonstrates the discharge of an afferent C-fiber innervating the perineurium of the ventral root to light stretch of the ventral root S2.

Afferent fibers innervating fascial tissues are predominantly excited by mechanical stimuli. Furthermore, many of them are probably also excited by heat stimuli. Finally, all of them are probably excited by chemical stimuli as they occur during inflammation. Whether fascial tissues are innervated by normally mechanoinsensitive (mechanically extremely high-threshold) afferent fibers, we do not know (see Michaelis et al., 1996; Schaible & Grubb, 1993; Schmidt et al., 1995).

Sensitization of nociceptive afferent neurons

Nociceptive afferent neurons innervating fascial tissues are sensitized by mechanical or chemical stimuli

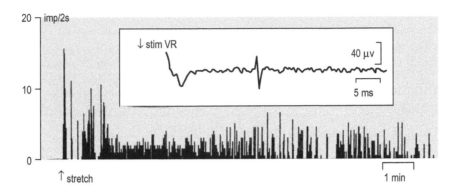

Figure 28.3
Mechanical activation of an unmyelinated afferent fiber innervating the perineurium of a sacral ventral root in a cat. A brief stretch lasting 5 seconds applied to the receptive field activated the fiber. This activation was followed by an after-discharge lasting more than 9 minutes. The activity of the afferent neuron was recorded from the corresponding dorsal root. Its cell body was located in the dorsal root ganglion S2. The inset shows the identification of the afferent unit by electrical stimulation of the ventral root (VR) with single pulses (stim VR). The experiment was conducted on an anesthetized cat. From Jänig & Koltzenburg (1991)

that induce tissue injury or pending injury. Sensitization consists of the following components:

1. Decrease in activation threshold to mechanical stimulation.

2. Increase of responses to mechanical noxious stimuli.

3. Development of spontaneous activity.

4. Recruitment of normally mechanoinsensitive (or extremely high-threshold) afferents for mechanical stimuli.

The cellular and subcellular mechanisms of sensitization of nociceptive afferent neurons are complex and not entirely understood.

A. The endogenous compounds and their receptors involved are:

1. Molecules derived from injured tissues and blood (e.g., proton ions [decrease of pH], potassium ions, prostaglandins, bradykinin, ATP).

2. Neuropeptides released by nociceptive afferent terminals (CGRP, substance P), histamine and other compounds released by mast cells, and serotonin released by platelets.

3. Interleukins (IL) released by cells of the immune system and related cells (macrophages; IL-1, IL-6, IL-8, TNF-α [tumor necrosis factor α]).

4. Neurotrophic substances (e.g., NGF) released by inflammatory cells; they are taken up with their receptors by the nociceptive terminals and transported to the afferent cell bodies.

B. The cellular effectors in the nociceptive terminals that are affected via intracellular signaling pathways during sensitization are:

1. The transduction channels for noxious mechanical or thermal stimuli.

2. The voltage-sensitive ionic channels that determine the excitability of the peripheral afferent terminals, such the sodium channels 1.7 and 1.8, potassium channels, and calcium channels.

3. Receptors for inflammatory mediators.

In essence, sensitization of nociceptive afferent neurons is a plastic adaptation of the nociceptive afferent neurons to the condition of the body tissues, to protect these tissues and enhance healing. It is the main *peripheral* mechanism of acute and chronic inflammatory pain. However, whether the cellular and subcellular peripheral mechanisms operating in acute and chronic conditions are the same is debated (Gold, 2013; Gold & Caterina, 2009; Ringkamp et al., 2013; Woolf & Ma, 2007).

Representation of fascial tissues in the spinal cord

Practically all fascial tissues belong to the deep somatic body domain. Therefore, we assume that nociception and pain, as well as associated protective somatomotor and autonomic reactions, are represented in the CNS in the same way as nociception and pain of joints and skeletal muscle (Schaible, 2009, 2012, 2013; Mense, 1993, 2013). We hypothesize that there exists in the spinal and caudal trigeminal dorsal horn a continuous layer of spinal second-order neurons 1) that receive convergent synaptic input from small-diameter deep somatic afferent neurons, 2) that receives convergent synaptic input from skin and viscera, 3) that is under distinct endogenous control from the brain stem, 4) that is specifically related to somatic and sympathetic protective motor reactions, and 5) that plays a special role in the generation of referred deep somatic pain as well as associated changes in the referred zones generated by somatic and sympathetic efferent systems. This layer of second-order neurons would be an *interoceptive interface* between deep body tissues and brain that is topically organized and reflected in the dermatomes, myotomes, and sclerotomes (see Fig. 28.8).

The spinal dorsal horn

The spinal and caudal trigeminal dorsal horn is organized according to cytological criteria into laminae (Fig. 28.4A) (Todd & Koerber, 2013):

1. Lamina I is located dorsally and is also called lamina marginalis.

2. Lamina II is the substantia gelatinosa of Rolando and is divided into an outer layer and an inner layer.

3. Lamina III and IV form the nucleus proprius.

4. Lamina V and deeper laminae.

Primary afferent neurons project according to their functions into laminae I to V (and deeper):

- Cutaneous afferent neurons: Small-diameter nociceptive myelinated (Aδ-) afferents project in laminae I, II and V. Nociceptive unmyelinated (C) afferents project in laminae I and II. Non-nociceptive afferents project in laminae I and II (Aδ, C, thermoreceptive, mechanoreceptive, other), laminae III and IV (Aβ, mechanoreceptive) and deeper laminae.

- Small diameter deep somatic and spinal visceral afferent neurons (Aδ-, C-) project in lamina I, lamina V and deeper laminae, but only in the outer layer of lamina II.

The neurons of the dorsal horn are about 90% excitatory (60%; transmitter glutamate) or inhibitory (40%; transmitter GABA and/or glycine) interneurons or propriospinal neurons. The remaining 10% or less of the neurons are tract neurons projecting to the brainstem, hypothalamus, and thalamus (Spike et al. 2003). These tract neurons consist functionally of the following groups:

- Nociceptive-specific neurons in lamina I (less so in lamina V) that can only be activated synaptically by noxious mechanical or thermal stimuli mediated by cutaneous afferent neurons with Aδ- or C-fibers.

- Non-nociceptive neurons in lamina I that are specifically activated by innocuous thermal stimuli (cold or warm), itch stimuli, or mechanical stimuli mediated by cutaneous afferent neurons with Aδ- or C-fibers and leading to warm, cool, itch, or sensual touch sensations.

- Nociceptive convergent neurons in lamina I activated by noxious stimuli of the skin, deep somatic tissues, and viscera mediated by afferent neurons with Aδ- or C-fibers (Fig. 28.4B).

- Multireceptive convergent neurons, located mostly in lamina V or deeper lamina, and activated by noxious and innocuous stimuli of skin, deep somatic tissues, and viscera (Fig. 28.4B). These tract neurons are also called wide dynamic range neurons.

This classification of tract neurons is preliminary. It shows that the activity in small-diameter afferent deep somatic and visceral neurons is transmitted to supraspinal centers by convergent neurons

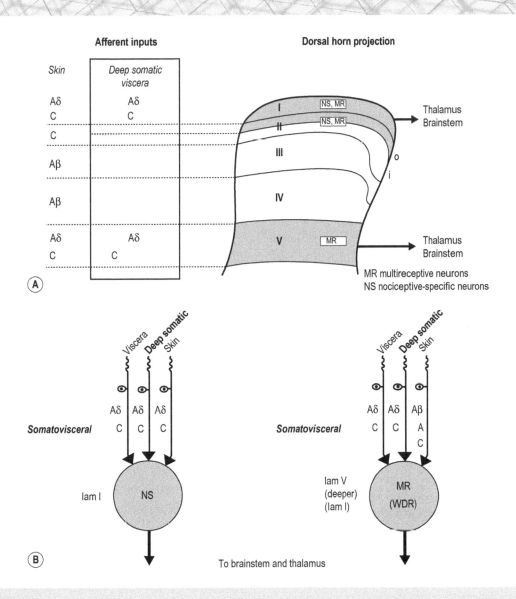

Figure 28.4

Projection of primary afferent neurons from the skin, deep somatic tissues (including fascial tissues), and viscera to the spinal dorsal horn. (A) The dorsal horn is divided according to cytological criteria into laminae: lamina I = lamina marginalis; lamina II = substantia gelatinosa of Rolando (divided into outer layer [o] and inner layer [i]); laminae III and IV = nucleus proprius; lamina V; deeper laminae. Most neurons (≥90%) in laminae I and V are interneurons or propriospinal neurons (Spike at al., 2003). The remaining neurons are tract neurons projecting to the brainstem (tractus spinoreticularis, spino-mesencephalis, spinotectalis), hypothalamus, and thalamus (tractus spinothalamicus). Deep somatic afferent neurons with C- and Aδ-fibers (including afferent neurons innervating fascia) and visceral afferent neurons project to laminae I, IIo and V. (B) Somatovisceral nociceptive specific (NS) and multireceptive (MR) tract neurons are located in laminae I and V. Most synaptic connections from afferent neurons to second-order tract neurons are monosynaptic in lamina I and di- or polysynaptic in lamina V and deeper laminae. lam = lamina; WDR = wide dynamic range

(Fig. 28.5A). Functionally specific tract neurons involved in nociception and pain and activated from deep somatic tissues (or viscera) are rare or do not seem to exist. Most studies of the synaptic afferent input to dorsal horn neurons from deep somatic tissues, skin, and viscera did not test whether the neurons were interneurons or tract neurons. In three studies it was shown that a few rostral lumbar dorsal horn neurons could be activated by stimulation of the thoracolumbar fascia. These neurons were convergent neurons (i.e., they could also be activated from skeletal muscle and/or skin). They were located around lamina V (Hoheisel et al., 2011; Hoheisel & Mense, 2014; Hoheisel et al., 2015).

The activity in afferent neurons with Aδ- or C-fibers is transmitted monosynaptically to tract neurons in lamina I and multisynaptically to tract neurons in lamina V and deeper laminae. Most tract neurons in lamina I project through the contralateral *ventrolateral tract* and tract neurons in lamina V or deeper laminae project through the contralateral *ventromedial tract* to supraspinal centers in the brainstem, hypothalamus, and thalamus (Dostrovsky & Craig, 2013; see Fig. 28.10).

The deep somatic interoceptive interface

The dorsal horn of the spinal cord can be divided functionally into three parts according to Craig (Craig, 2003a; Dostrovsky & Craig, 2013). This division has some explanatory power, but is not generally accepted (see Willis & Coggeshall, 2004a).

1. *Interoception.* The neurons in lamina I serve predominantly interoception and mediate autonomic reflexes. The tract neurons in lamina I mediate information in primary afferent neurons with Aδ- or C-axons that encode in their activity the state of the body tissues (nociceptive neurons of all tissues; thermoreceptive neurons, chemoreceptive neurons of skin [related to itch]; low-threshold mechanoreceptive neurons of skin [related to sensual touch]; metaboreceptive neurons of skeletal muscle; visceral afferent neurons, etc.). Most tract neurons in lamina I receiving nociceptive cutaneous input are nociceptive-specific, many of them with convergent synaptic input from deep somatic tissues and viscera. A few lamina I tract neurons are wide dynamic range (or multireceptive) neurons and can be excited from large-diameter (Aβ) afferent fibers as well as small-diameter afferent fibers.

2. *Exteroception and proprioception.* Neurons in laminae III and IV are involved (together with the dorsal column medial lemniscus system) in somatic exteroception and proprioception.

3. *Somatic and autonomic motor reflexes.* Most ascending tract neurons in lamina V and deeper laminae (VI, VII, VIII, X) can be activated by afferent neurons with Aβ-axons as well as afferent neurons with Aδ- or C-axons innervating deep somatic tissues or viscera. Most of these convergent multireceptive neurons have large receptive fields and ongoing activity. They are probably involved in somatic motor and sympathetic reflexes and regulations, and less so or not at all in the generation of painful and not-painful interoceptive body sensations. This point is a subject of controversy, and is very much debated (Craig & Blomquist, 2002; Willis et al., 2002; Willis & Coggeshall, 2004a, 2004b).

Looking in this way at the spinal dorsal horn one could argue that the dorsal horn neurons form a *myofascial interoceptive interface* between the deep somatic tissues and the brain. Deep somatic afferent neurons with Aδ- and C-axons feed into this interface. It mediates spinal and supraspinal protective reflexes involving somatic motoneurons and sympathetic systems. Tract neurons of this interface project to centers in the brainstem and hypothalamus that are involved in the regulation of somatic, autonomic, and neuroendocrine motor systems, and in the endogenous control of the myofascial interface. Furthermore, the tract neurons project to the thalamus, which is the entrance gate to the cortex. Whether this myofascial interoceptive interface is restricted to the lamina I but includes lamina V and deeper laminae will have to be shown. It is somatotopically organized. We suggest introducing a new concept of *myofasciotomes* that would be a fusion of myotomes and sclerotomes (see Fig. 28.8) and would need to be worked out.

Central sensitization

Synaptic transmission of nociceptive impulse activity in the spinal dorsal horn is changed during acute and chronic pain by the continuous activity in the sensitized nociceptive afferent neurons. These central changes are the expression of the plasticity of the central nociceptive system and are generally called central sensitization. This sensitization involves sensitized nociceptive afferent neurons and the excitatory and inhibitory interneurons in the dorsal horn as well as the excitatory and inhibitory endogenous control systems in the brainstem (Fig. 28.5 and 28.10).

Sensitization of nociceptive afferent neurons (e.g., during tissue inflammation) generates not only an increase of the activation of the central nociceptive specific and convergent neurons but also a change of the central information processing in lamina I, II, V and deeper laminae. This sensitization has the following characteristics:

- Development of or increase in ongoing activity.
- Decrease of threshold to excite the neurons by mechanical or other stimuli.
- Increase of discharge to noxious stimuli.
- Increase of the size of the receptive fields and development of new receptive fields.
- Activation to qualitatively new stimuli.

Figure 28.6 demonstrates as a representative example the sensitization of a dorsal horn neuron during experimental inflammation of the knee joint in the rat. The activation to pressure on the knee joint increased, the neuron was activated from the ankle joint and paw after inflammation and the receptive field of the neuron changed and increased.

The neuronal changes during central sensitization are qualitatively and quantitatively reflected in a changed pain perception as well as reflex activation of motoneurons and sympathetic neurons. Sensitized nociceptive afferent neurons, sensitized dorsal horn neurons, and changed endogenous control neurons as well as efferent somatomotor neurons and sympathetic neurons can now theoretically constitute positive feedback circuits that maintain the activity in the nociceptive afferent neurons and therefore also the pain and the associated motor responses.

The mechanisms underlying central sensitization, that is generated by the changes of the afferent nociceptive neurons (development of ongoing activity, increased release of neuropeptides and neurotrophic factors [e.g., BDNF]), consist of cascades of change that occur in seconds, minutes, hours, and days. They are generated by phosphorylation of glutamate channels and ion channels via intracellular signaling pathways (involving protein kinase A and C, inositol-3-phosphate, intracellular calcium) and by transcription in the cell body (upregulation of the synthesis of receptor molecules for glutamate, neuropeptides, ion channels). Glial cells (particularly the microglia), prostaglandins, and signaling molecules of the immune system (cytokines such as TNFα, IL-2 [IL interleukin], IL-6, IL-8) are involved in the sensitization of spinal nociceptive neurons (Jänig & Levine ,2013).

The mechanisms underlying central sensitization are responsible for the ongoing pain, secondary hyperalgesia, and allodynia as well as the different forms of referred pain (see below). These mechanisms are most likely different for acute and chronic (non-neuropathic) pain. Whether chronic central sensitization is fully reversible when the (chronic) sensitization of afferent nociceptive neurons has been attenuated or terminated, we do not know. Finally, it is hypothesized that central sensitization of the nociceptive system can also be generated without or with rather weak sensitization of afferent nociceptive neurons, such as in chronic widespread pain, including fibromyalgia syndrome, and in other chronic potentially generalizing pain syndromes such as irritable bowel syndrome, interstitial cystitis, chronic low back pain, etc. Finally, sensitization of nociceptive neurons does not only occur in the spinal cord and caudal trigeminal nucleus, but probably also supraspinally in the brainstem, thalamus, and cortex, though this has not been investigated so far.

Referred pain and associated changes in deep somatic tissues

Deep somatic pain is preferentially referred to deep somatic tissues (skeletal muscle, joints, fascia,

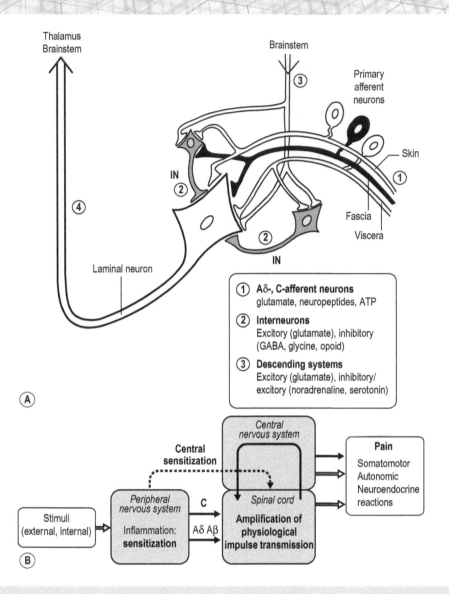

Figure 28.5

(A) Synaptic transmission of the activity from a primary afferent neuron with Aδ- or C-fibers (1) to somatovisceral tract neurons in laminae I or V of the dorsal horn (4) and its modulation. Tract neurons project to the brainstem, hypothalamus, and thalamus. The local (spinal) modulation occurs via excitatory and inhibitory interneurons (IN, 2). The modulation by descending systems (3) occurs via interneurons or directly at the tract neurons. Keep in mind that the interneurons in lamina I (and presumably throughout the dorsal horn) are 10 times more common than the tract neurons. The transmitters are listed in the inset box: ATP = adenosine triphosphate; GABA = γ-amino-butyric acid. (B) Concept of central sensitization following sensitization of nociceptive afferent neurons (e.g., by inflammation). Central sensitization is dependent on sensitization of afferent nociceptive neurons, local excitatory and inhibitory synaptic activity via interneurons, and descending excitatory and inhibitory neurons (1 to 3 in (A)). Aβ = large-diameter myelinated afferents; Aδ = small-diameter myelinated afferents; C = unmyelinated afferents. After Jänig (2014)

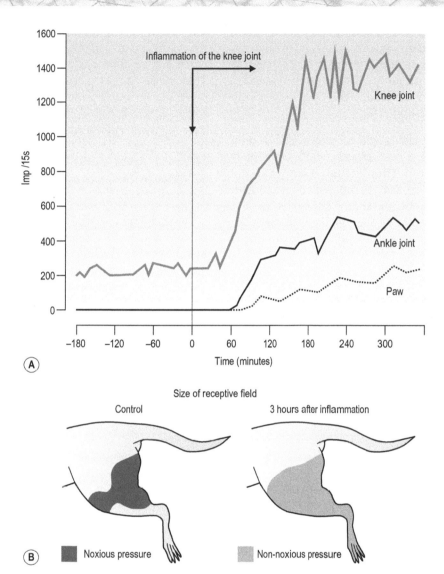

Figure 28.6

Development of the excitability of a dorsal horn neuron during continuous activation of afferent neurons innervating the knee joint in a rat. (A) Activation of the neuron by local noxious pressure lasting 15 seconds applied to the knee joint, to the ankle joint, or to the ipsilateral hind paw before and after inflammation of the knee joint generated by kaolin and carrageenan injected into the knee joint. Ordinate scale, number of action potentials elicited by the noxious pressure stimuli. After inflammation, the responses to noxious pressure applied to the knee joint increased and the neuron could be activated from the ankle joint and the paw. (B) Extension of the receptive field of the neuron after inflammation. Modified after Neugebauer et al. (1993)

AQ3

etc.), and also to visceral organs and (less so or not at all) to the skin. Referred pain consists of ongoing pain and mechanical hyperalgesia or allodynia (somatosomatic hyperalgesia and somatovisceral hyperalgesia, Fig. 28.7) (Mense, 1993; Mense & Simons, 2001; Graven-Nielsen, 2006; Graven-Nielsen

& Arendt-Nielsen, 2008). Visceral pain is referred to other viscera, to deep somatic tissues and to skin (viscerovisceral hyperalgesia, viscerosomatic hyperalgesia) (Giamberardino, 2009; Giamberardino et al., 2010; Foerster, 1933; Head, 1893; Head & Campbell, 1900; Lee et al., 2008).

The spatial extent of the referred zones of deep somatic pain in the deep somatic and visceral body domains are known. They depend on the segmental projections of deep somatic afferent neurons with Aδ- or C-fibers to the spinal cord and the processing of the afferent activity by the convergent dorsal horn neurons receiving synaptic input from the three body domains (Fig. 28.4B).

Figure 28.8 shows the distribution of acute referred deep somatic pain generated experimentally during stimulation of deep somatic nociceptors by injection of a small bolus of hypertonic saline into the ligamenta interspinalia. The local pain is sharp and stinging, appears immediately, and lasts for a few minutes. The referred pain is felt to arise in deep structures, is unpleasant and aching, has a latency of about 30 seconds, is maximal in about 2 minutes and lasts for about 5–10 minutes. Mechanical hyperalge-

sia is delayed for ≥5 minutes and may sometimes persist for ≥1 hour. The interindividual variability is much higher than the intraindividual variability. Thus, repeated injections of hypertonic saline at the same site in the same subject generates consistent responses (Hockaday & Whitty, 1967). Similar results were obtained with the injection of hypertonic saline into skeletal muscles (Graven-Nielsen, 2006; Graven-Nielsen & Arendt-Nielsen, 2008; Kellgren, 1938a, 1938b) as well as fascia, periosteum, tendons or joints (Kellgren, 1939).   AQ1

The innervation of skeletal muscle, including their tendons and fascia, is segmental. The pain generated by stimulation of the interspinal ligaments is referred to several muscles that are innervated via the spinal nerve of the corresponding segment and through spinal nerves of neighboring segments. The group of skeletal muscles innervated by one spinal nerve is called *myotome*. Neighboring myotomes overlap.

The same reasoning can be applied to the afferent innervation of fascia, joints, bone (periosteum), etc. Figure 28.9 shows the segmental afferent innervation of these deep somatic tissues by spinal nerves. Similar to dermatomes and myotomes, there are deep somatic

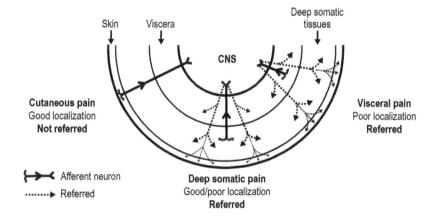

Figure 28.7
Referral of deep somatic and visceral pain. Solid radial lines = afferent neurons. Broken lines and arrows = referrals. Pain of deep somatic tissues is referred to other deep somatic tissues, to viscera, and (less so) to skin. Visceral pain is referred to deep somatic tissues, to other viscera and to skin. The width of the broken arrows indicates the degree of referral. Modified after Ruch (1965)

tissue regions innervated by a spinal nerve called the *sclerotome*. The idea of the sensory innervation of bones goes back to Déjerine (1914). Inman & Saunders (1944) have systematically studied and described the distribution of the sensory innervation of bones, etc. of the upper extremity, the shoulder girdle, the lower extremity, and the pelvic girdle by the spinal nerves in healthy humans (Fig. 28.9). Stimulation of these deep tissues (mechanical, by weak solution of formic acid or by hypertonic saline solution) generates dull and aching pain that may be associated with nausea, vomiting, sweating, and other changes linked to the sympathetic nervous system. This pain is referred to more distally located deep somatic tissues. The distribution of the sclerotomes was never reinvestigated using modern methods (see Ivanusic, 2007).

Chronic deep somatic and visceral pain referred to deep somatic tissues or to skin (and expressed as ongoing pain and mechanical hyperalgesia) is accompanied by changes in the referred zones that are associated with the segmentally organized innervation by sympathetic postganglionic neurons and peptidergic afferent neurons (Box 28.1; Jänig, 1993, 2014):

- Skin blood flow and sweating change – even the pilomotor system may be affected. These changes are hypothesized to be generated by reflex changes of the activity in sympathetic cutaneous vasoconstrictor neurons, sudomotor neurons, and pilomotor neurons (viscerosympathetic, somatosympathetic reflexes). The changes in blood flow may also be dependent on peptides (CGRP, substance P) released locally by peptidergic afferents.

- The skin exhibits edema (swelling) and trophic changes (change in structure and consistency of skin, changes in nails and hairs). Both are hypothesized to be generated by sympathetic neurons (and possibly peptidergic afferent neurons releasing substance P and CGRP). The cellular mechanisms underlying these changes are entirely unexplored.

- Blood flow changes in referred deep somatic tissues mediated by deep somatic vasoconstrictor neurons have never been systematically investigated. However, it is hypothesized that these changes do occur under chronic conditions and have considerable pathophysiological consequences. As in the skin,

blood flow changes may also be locally dependent on peptides (CGRP, substance P) released by peptidergic afferents.

- Referred zones of deep somatic tissues, such as bones (periosteum), joint capsules, planar fascia, and skeletal muscle, may exhibit under chronic conditions edema and trophic (structural) changes. However, these changes and their dependence on the sympathetic innervation, and the peptidergic afferent innervation, as well as their underlying cellular mechanisms have never been systematically investigated – although they may turn out to be very important. After all, the innervation of fascia by peptidergic afferent neurons and sympathetic noradrenergic neurons is not necessarily associated with blood vessels (see Chapter 33, Fig. 33.1).

Supraspinal control of nociception and pain of deep somatic tissues

Pain cannot be reduced to the nociceptive sensations generated by activation of the ascending nociceptive system (Fig. 28.1, left side). Pain or pain behavior is a multidimensional event characterized by the sensory-discriminative, the affective-motivational, the cognitive, and the motor dimensions. The first three dimensions are dependent on the cerebral cortex. The motor dimension consists of the somatic, the autonomic, and the neuroendocrine components, which are potentially also under cortical control. Using modern imaging and other techniques it has been shown that several cortical and subcortical centers are involved in the generation of the pain behavior (Apkarian et al., 2013; Casey & Tran, 2006; Tracey & Mantyh, 2007; Treede & Apkarian, 2009) (see Fig. 28.11, left side). These centers are activated sequentially and in parallel during stimulation of peripheral nociceptive afferent neurons and are sometimes generally described as a 'cerebral signature of pain' (Tracey & Mantyh, 2007). The complexity of cortical and subcortical areas being involved in nociception and pain corresponds to our ability to recognize pain according to its origin in the superficial, deep somatic, or visceral body domains, to recognize spontaneous pain, and to discriminate pain generated by different physiological stimuli, and to discriminate the unpleasantness of pain from the nociceptive aspect (Fig. 28.10).

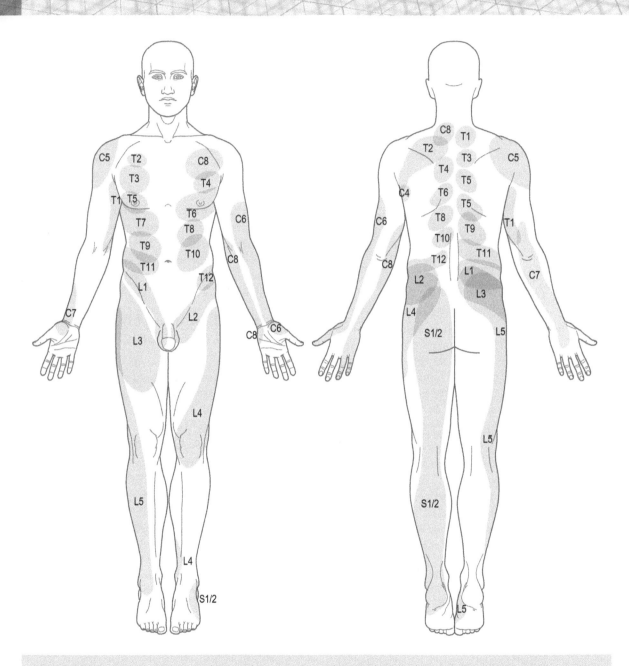

Figure 28.8
Referred pain (ongoing pain, deep mechanical hyperalgesia) in deep tissues produced by activation of nociceptors in the ligamenta interspinalia. The nociceptors were activated by bolus injection of 0.1 to 0.3mL of 6% saline solution into the ligaments. The overlying skin, fascia, and supraspinous ligament were anesthetized by novocaine to avoid stimulating nociceptors other than those in the ligamenta interspinalia. The results were obtained from three trained, healthy subjects. The distribution of ongoing pain and deep mechanical hyperalgesia (deep tenderness) corresponded to each other. After Lewis (1942) and Kellgren (1939)

(Fig. 28.1, right side) has increased considerably with the introduction of the various imaging methods. However, we are far from understanding the cortical mechanisms underlying the biology of pain at the cellular and integrative level. This applies particularly to deep somatic and visceral pain as well as to the categories of chronic inflammatory pain, (chronic) neuropathic pain, and chronic potentially generalizing pain – syndromes that are not triggered by chronically sensitized or injured nociceptive afferent neurons but are most likely the consequence of central dysregulation of the nociceptive system. Figure 28.10 shows the ascending nociceptive system and the endogenous system controlling nociceptive impulse transmission in a schematic and simplified form.

Different cortical areas participate in different aspects (dimensions) of pain (sensation, affection, cognition, somatic and autonomic motor responses). None of these functions can be assigned to only one forebrain structure, that is, each function is represented in more than one brain structure (Casey & Tran, 2006; Treede & Apkarian, 2009) (Fig. 28.11):

- Activation of the ascending nociceptive system in the spinal cord or caudal trigeminal nucleus (in particular neurons in the lamina I [see earlier in this chapter]) and in the thalamus generates nociceptive sensations. These sensations are dependent on the activation of the primary and secondary somatosensory cortices and of the dorsal posterior insular cortex (dpINS) via the posterior ventromedial nucleus of the thalamus (VMpo). The role of the VMpo/dpINS system in the perception of type, localization, duration, and intensity of nociceptive sensations is a subject of controversy (Apkarian et al., 2013; Craig 2003a, 2003b, 2003c, 2004, 2016; Dostrovsky & Craig, 2013) (*1* in Fig. 28.11).

- In parallel with the generation of the nociceptive sensation, protective somatic, autonomic, and neuroendocrine processes are activated via the spinal cord, brainstem, hypothalamus, amygdala, and other brain centers in a stereotyped fashion (*4* in Fig. 28.11).

- The generation of nociceptive sensations is followed and paralleled by a perception of bodily unpleasant

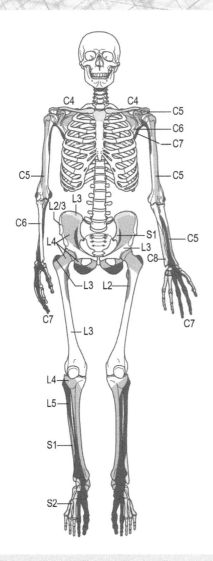

Figure 28.9

Sclerotomes. Segmental innervation of periosteum, inserting ligaments, fascia, interosseous membranes, tendons, and tendinous attachments of ligaments, etc. The results are based on 160 observations made of 26 healthy subjects. The tissues were stimulated mechanically (with needles) and by bolus injections of a weak solution of formic acid or a hypertonic solution of 6% saline. After Inman & Saunders (1944), Déjerine (1914)

Knowledge about the cortical mechanisms of pain and the cortical control of nociception and pain

> **Box 28.1**
>
> ## Characteristics and mechanisms of referred pain (after Jänig, 1993, 2014)
>
> ### A. Characteristics of referred pain and associated changes
>
> 1. *Pain, hyperalgesia, allodynia*: somatosomatic, viscerovisceral, somatovisceral, viscerosomatic.
>
> 2. *Autonomic changes*: blood vessels, sweat glands, erector pili muscles.
>
> 3. *Muscle tension* increase.
>
> 4. *Edema*: skin, subcutaneous, deep somatic. *Trophic changes*: skin, subcutaneous, deep somatic.
>
> ### B. Possible mechanisms underlying referred pain and associated changes
>
> 1. *Sensitization* of spinal somatosomatic and somatovisceral neurons (interneurons, tract neurons).
>
> 2. *Convergence* of visceral, deep somatic, and cutaneous afferent neurons on dorsal horn neurons; subthreshold synapses become *suprathreshold*.
>
> 3. *Balance* between *spinal processing* and *supraspinal control* changed.
>
> 4. *Dichotomizing afferents*: single afferent neurons innervate different tissues (e.g., somatic tissues and viscera).
>
> 5. Somatosympathetic, viscerosympathetic, and viscerosomatic reflexes enhanced.
>
> 6. Changed regulation of *peripheral microcirculation*.
>
> 7. Changed *retrograde axonal transport* of compounds (e.g., trophic factors) in primary afferent neurons.
>
> 8. Generation of edema and induction of trophic changes in tissues by sympathetic neurons.

feelings signaling the injury or impending injury of the body. These unpleasant feelings occur during the activation of the dorsal posterior insular cortex (presumably also the anterior insular cortex), the anterior and posterior cingulate cortex, the inferior parietal cortex, and the premotor cortex. The activation of the medial thalamus (and probably of the hypothalamus) via a parallel pathway including the parabrachial nucleus (not shown in Fig. 28.11) is presumably also involved in the generation of this affective pain component (*2* in Fig. 28.11).

- The secondary (cognitive) appraisal of the nociceptive events and attention to them in the context of experience in the past (memory), expectations, and environmental context leads to the secondary affective pain behavior. This behavior is dependent on the activation of the medial and dorsolateral prefrontal cortices, the orbitofrontal cortex, the hippocampus, and the entorhinal cortex (*3* in Fig. 28.11).

- During the perception of intrusion or threat of the body and secondary (cognitive) appraisal, the (somatic, autonomic, neuroendocrine) motor components are also activated, involving higher brain centers (see broken arrows in Fig. 28.11). These motor components are orchestrated by the anterior cingulate cortex and the amygdala (Neugebauer et al., 2009).

- The transmission of nociceptive impulses in the spinal and trigeminal dorsal horn is controlled by supraspinal centers. Activation of these centers, represented in the periaqueductal gray, in the dorsolateral pontine tegmentum, and in the ventromedial medulla oblongata (including the caudal raphe nuclei) generates antinociception or pronociception depending on the behavioral context. These centers are in turn under the control of the cerebral hemispheres (orbitofrontal cortex, prefrontal cortex, insula, anterior cingulate cortex, amygdala, etc.) (Heinricher & Fields, 2013; Heinricher & Ingram, 2009) (shaded in Figure 28.10).

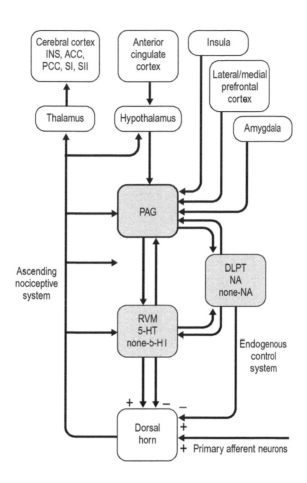

Figure 28.10

The ascending nociceptive system and endogenous system controlling the transmission of impulse activity from afferent nociceptive neurons to second-order neurons in the spinal and trigeminal dorsal horn: a simplified scheme. The ascending nociceptive system is shown on the left; note that the spinothalamic neurons project to the thalamus and to centers in the brainstem and hypothalamus, representing the endogenous control system. Shaded boxes = endogenous control system; note that descending control of nociceptive impulse transmission is inhibitory (antinociception) as well as excitatory (pronociception). ACC = anterior cingulate cortex; DLPT = dorsolateral pontine tegmentum (includes area 5, area 7, nucleus cuneiformis, parabrachial nucleus, and locus coeruleus); INS = insular cortex; PAG = periaqueductal grey; PCC = posterior cingulate cortex; RVM = rostral ventromedial medulla (nucleus raphe magnus, nucleus paragigantocellularis medialis, nucleus parapyramidalis); SI, SII = primary, secondary somatosensory cortex; NA = noradrenaline; 5-HT = 5-hydroxy-tryptamine (serotonin); + = activation; – = inhibition. After Heinricher & Fields (2013)

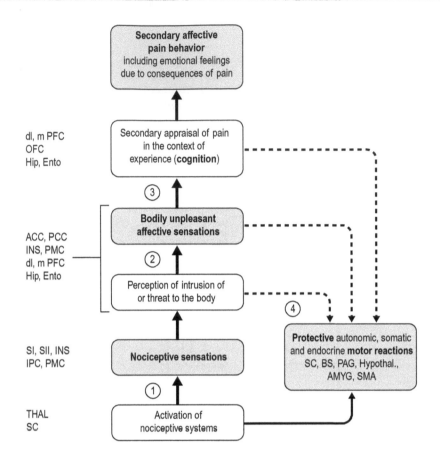

Figure 28.11

The interaction between nociceptive sensations, bodily unpleasant affective sensations, and secondary affective pain behavior and the brain centers possibly involved: a simplified scheme. (1) to (4) refer to the dimensions of pain concerned: (1) sensory-discriminative; (2) affective-motivational; (3) cognitive; (4) motor dimension. Activation of endocrine, somatic, and autonomic motor systems occurs on all integrative levels during activation of the centers representing nociception and pain. The mechanisms of activation of these motor systems by higher centers (see broken arrows) have been little studied. ACC = anterior cingular cortex; AMYG = amygdala; BS = brain stem; dl = dorsolateral; Ento = entorhinal cortex; Hip = hippocampus; Hypothal = hypothalamus; INS = insular cortex; IPC = inferior parietal cortex; m = medial; OFC = orbitofrontal cortex; PAG = periaqueductal gray; PCC = posterior cingulate cortex; PFC = prefrontal cortex; PMC = premotor cortex; SC = spinal cord; SI, SII = primary, secondary somatosensory cortex; SMA = supplementary motor area; THAL = thalamus. Modified from Jänig (2012) and after Casey & Tran (2006) and Price (2000)

This sequential and parallel activation of forebrain centers resulting in pain behavior occurs under biological conditions during transient activation of nociceptors or activation of nociceptors in a recuperative (healing) phase, e.g., in inflammatory pain following tissue injury. The imaging studies on which the data are based show forebrain responses in a correlation manner. They do not tell us in which way individual forebrain centers are causally involved in the generation of the different dimensions of pain.

Conclusion

Fascial tissues are innervated by afferent peptidergic neurons with unmyelinated fibers and sympathetic noradrenergic neurons. Afferent neurons with myelinated axons probably are of marginal importance, in particular in view of their low numbers. The peptidergic afferent neurons are largely polymodal, being involved in nociception and pain of fascia including peripheral neurogenic inflammation. Thus, the peptidergic afferent neurons form, together with the second-order neurons in the spinal dorsal horn, a classical protective interface between fascial tissues and the brain getting into action during noxious stimuli by generating neurogenic inflammation, triggering protective reflexes in sympathetic neurons, and eliciting pain. Most sympathetic neurons innervating fascial tissues are vasoconstrictor in function and are involved in regulation of blood flow. They are probably inhibited during activation of deep somatic nociceptors including those innervating fascia (Kirillova-Woytke et al., 2014) and contribute in this way to the protection of fascial tissues (by increasing blood flow). Whether both populations of neurons are additionally involved in maintaining the trophic functions of fascia is an open question. There is no evidence that sympathetic neurons innervating fascia and nociceptive afferent neurons form feedback circuits.

The afferent and sympathetic innervation of fascia is most likely segmentally organized. This invites speculation that both the innervation of fascia and the innervation of skeletal muscle are organized in some form of fasciomyotomes. This topic is worth investigating in humans.

During painful injury of deep somatic tissues and visceral tissues, referred body tissues exhibit swelling (edema) and trophic changes. These changes are believed to be dependent on the (afferent and sympathetic) innervation of the tissues. The mechanisms underlying these important changes are entirely unknown and need to be explored. Interestingly, similar changes (edema, changes of skin consistency, nails, hair, and osteoporosis) are present in complex regional pain syndrome. Here we have some indirect evidence that these trophic changes are dependent on the sympathetic innervation. After sympathetic blocks or sympathectomy these changes may disappear (Jänig, 2009, 2013; Jänig & Baron, 2002, 2003).

The central representation of nociception and pain associated with fascial tissues seems to be similar or identical to that of skeletal muscle and joints. However, it remains largely unexplored, as illustrated in this chapter, for the spinal dorsal horn and the caudal trigeminal nucleus, the thalamus, the telencephalon, and the central endogenous control system.

AQ2

References

Apkarian, A. V., Bushnell, M. C., & Schweinhardt, P. 2013. Representation of pain in the brain, in *Wall and Melzack's Textbook of Pain, 6th edition*. S. B. McMahon et al., eds, Elsevier, Saunders, Philadelphia, PA, pp. 111–128.

Bahns, E., Ernsberger, U., Jänig, W., & Nelke, A. 1986. Discharge properties of mechanosensitive afferents supplying the retroperitoneal space. *Pflügers Arch* 407:519–525.

Bennett, R. 2013. Myofascial pain, in *Encyclopedia of Pain. 2nd edition*. G. F. Gebhart & R. F. Schmidt, eds, Springer-Verlag, Heidelberg, New York, Dordrecht, London, pp. 2004–2008.

Bove, G. M. & Light, A. R. 1995. Unmyelinated nociceptors of rat paraspinal tissues. *J Neurophysiology* vol. 73:1752–1762.

Casey, K. L. & Tran, T. D. 2006. Cortical mechanisms mediating acute and chronic pain in humans, in *Handbook of Clinical Neurology, Vol 81*. M. J. Aminoff, F. Boller, D. F. Swaab, (series eds), F. Cervero & T. S. Jensen, eds, Elsevier, Edinburgh, pp. 159–177.

Craig, A. D. 2003a. Pain mechanisms: labeled lines versus convergence in central processing. *Annu Rev Neurosci* vol. 26:1–30.

Craig, A. D. 2003b. A new view of pain as a homeostatic emotion. *Trends Neurosci* 26:303–307.

Craig, A. D. 2003c. Interoception: the sense of the physiological condition of the body. *Curr Opin Neurobiol* 13:500–505.

Craig, A. D. 2004. Distribution of trigeminothalamic and spinothalamic lamina I terminations in the macaque monkey. *J Comp Neurol* 477:119–148.

Craig, A. D. 2016. Interoception and emotion: a neuroanatomical perspective, in *Handbook of Emotions, 4th edn*. L. F. Barrett, M. Lewis & J. M. Haviland-Jones, eds, The Guilford Press, New York, NY, pp. 272–288.

Craig, A. D. & Blomqvist, A. 2002 Is there a specific lamina I spinothalamocortical pathway for pain and temperature sensations in primates? *J Pain* 2:95–101.

Dawes, J. M., Andersson, D. A., Bennett, D. L. H., Bevan, S., & McMahon, S. B. 2013. Inflammatory mediators and modulators of pain, in *Wall and Melzack's Textbook of Pain, 6th edn.* S. B. McMahon et al., eds, Elsevier, Saunders, Philadelphia, PA, pp. 48–67.

Déjerine, J. 1914. *Sémiologie du Système Nerveux.* Masson, Paris.

Dommerholt J. & Gerwin R. D. 2015. A critical evaluation of Quinter et al: missing the point. *J Bodyw Mov Ther* 19:193–204.

Dostrovsky, J. O. & Craig, A. D. 2013. Ascending projection systems, in *Wall and Melzack's Textbook of Pain, 6th edn.* S. B. McMahon et al., eds, Elsevier, Saunders, Philadelphia, PA, pp. 182–197.

Foerster, O. 1933. The dermatomes in man. *Brain* 56:1–39.

Giamberardino, M. A. 2009. *Visceral Pain.* Oxford University Press, Oxford.

Giamberardino, M. A., Costantini, R., Affaitati, G., Fabrizio, A., Lapenna, D., Tafuri, E., & Mezzetti, A. 2010. Viscero-visceral hyperalgesia: characterization in different clinical models *Pain* 151:307–322.

Gold, M. S. 2013. Molecular biology of sensory transduction, in *Wall and Melzack's Textbook of Pain, 6th edn.* S. B. McMahon et al., eds, Elsevier, Saunders, Philadelphia, PA, pp. 31–47.

Gold, M. S. & Caterina, M. J. 2009. Molecular biology of the nociceptor/transduction, in *Science of Pain.* A. I. Basbaum & M. C. Bushnell, eds, Academic Press, San Diego, CA, pp. 43–73.

Graven-Nielsen, T. 2006. Fundamentals of muscle pain, referred pain, and deep tissue hyperalgesia. *Scand J Rheumatol Suppl* 122:1–43.

Graven-Nielsen, T. & Arendt-Nielsen, L. 2008. Human models and clinical manifestations of musculoskeletal pain and pain-motor interactions, in *Fundamentals of Musculoskeletal Pain.* T. Graven-Nielsen, L. Arendt-Nielsen, & S. Mense, eds, IASP Press, Seattle, WA, pp. 155–187.

Graven-Nielsen, T., Arendt-Nielsen, L., & Mense, S. eds, 2008. *Fundamentals of Musculoskeletal Pain.* IASP Press, Seattle.

Häbler, H. J., Jänig, W., Koltzenburg, M., & McMahon, S. B. 1990. A quantitative study of the central projection patterns of unmyelinated ventral root afferents in the cat. *J Physiol* 422:265–287.

Head, H. 1893. On disturbances of sensation with especial reference to the pain of visceral disease. *Brain* 16, pp.:1–133.

Head, H. & Campbell, A. W. 1900. The pathology of herpes zoster and its bearing on sensory localization. *Brain* 23, pp. :353–523.

Heinricher, M. M. & Fields, H. L. 2013. Central nervous system mechanisms of pain modulation, in *Wall and Melzack's Textbook of Pain, 6th edn.* S. B. McMahon et al., eds, Elsevier, Saunders, Philadelphia, PA, pp. 129–142.

Heinricher, M. M. & Ingram, S. L. 2009. The brain stem and nociceptive modulation, in *Science of Pain.* A. I. Basbaum & M. C. Bushnell, eds, Academic Press, San Diego, CA, pp. 593–626.

Hockaday, J. M. & Whitty, C. W. 1967. Patterns of referred pain in the normal subject. *Brain* 90:481–496.

Hoheisel, U. & Mense, S. 2014. Inflammation of the thoracolumbar fascia excites and sensitizes rat dorsal horn neurons. *Eur J Pain* 19, no. 3:419–428.

Hoheisel, U., Taguchi, T., Treede, R. D., & Mense, S. 2011. Nociceptive input from the rat thoracolumbar fascia to lumbar dorsal horn neurones. *Eur J Pain* 15:810–815.

Hoheisel, U., Vogt, M.A., Palme, R., Grass, P. & Mense, S. 2015. Immobilization stress sensitizes rat dorsal horn neurons. *Eur J Pain* 19:861–870.

Hökfelt, T. G. M., Zhang, X., Villar, M., Xu, X. J., & Wiesenfeld-Hallin, Z. 2013. Central consequences of peripheral nerve damage, in *Wall and Melzack's Textbook of Pain, 6th edn.* S. B. McMahon et al., eds, Elsevier, Saunders, Philadelphia, PA, pp. 902–914.

Inman, V. T. & Saunders, J. B. M. 1944. Referred pain from skeletal structures. *J Nerv Ment Dis* 99:660–667.

Ivanusic, J. J. 2007. The evidence for the spinal segmental innervation of bone. *Clin Anat* 20:956–960.

Jänig, W. 1993. Spinal visceral afferents, sympathetic nervous system and referred pain, in *New Trends in Referred Pain and Hyperalgesia, Pain Research and Clinical Management, Vol. 7.* L. Vecchiet et al., eds, Elsevier Science Publishers, Amsterdam, pp. 83–92.

Jänig, W. 2006. *The Integrative Action of the Autonomic Nervous System: Neurobiology of Homeostasis.* Cambridge University Press, Cambridge, New York.

Jänig, W. 2009. Autonomic nervous system and pain, in *Science of Pain.* A. I. Basbaum & M. C. Bushnell, eds, Academic Press, San Diego, CA, pp. 193–225.

Jänig, W. 2012. Autonomic reactions in pain. *Pain* 153:733–735.

Jänig, W. 2013. Pain and the sympathetic nervous system: pathophysiological mechanisms, in *Autonomic Failure. 5th edn.* C. J. Mathias & R. Bannister, eds, Oxford University Press, Oxford, pp. 236–246.

Jänig, W. 2014. [Neurobiology of visceral pain], *Schmerz* 28:233–251.

Jänig, W. & Baron, R. 2002. Complex regional pain syndrome is a disease of the central nervous system. *Clin Auton Res* 12:150–164.

Jänig, W. & Baron, R. 2003. Complex regional pain syndrome: mystery explained? *Lancet Neurol* 2:687–697.

Jänig, W., Böhni, U., & von Heymann, W. 2015. Interozeption, Schmerz und vegetatives Nervensystem [Interoception, pain and autonomic nervous system], in *Manuelle Medizin 1: Fehlfunktion und Schmerz am Bewegungsorgan verstehen und behandeln [Manual Medicine 1: Understanding and Treatment of Failure and Pain of the Skeletomotor System].* U. Böhni, M. Lauper, & H. Locher, eds, Georg Thieme Verlag, Stuttgart New York, pp. 69–100.

Jänig, W. & Koltzenburg, M. 1991. Receptive properties of pial afferents. *Pain* 45:77–85.

Jänig, W. & Levine, J. D. 2013. Autonomic, endocrine, and immune interactions in acute and chronic pain, in *Wall & Melzack's Textbook of Pain, 6th edn.* S. B. McMahon et al., eds, Elsevier Saunders, Philadelphia, PA, pp. 198–210.

Kellgren, J. H. 1938a. Observations on referred pain arising from muscle. *Clin Sci* 3:175–190.

Kellgren, J. H. 1938b. A preliminary account of referred pains arising from muscle. *Br Med J* 1:325–327.

Kellgren, J. H. 1939. On the distribution of pain arising from deep somatic structures with charts of segmental pain areas. *Clin Sci* 4:46.

Kirillova-Woytke, I., Baron, R., & Jänig, W. 2014. Reflex inhibition of cutaneous and muscle vasoconstrictor neurons during stimulation of cutaneous and muscle nociceptors. *J Neurophysiol* 111:1833–1845.

Langevin, H. M. & Huijing, P. A. 2009. Communicating about fascia: history, pitfalls, and recommendations, *Int J Ther Massage Bodywork,* no. 4, pp.:3–8.

Lee, M. W., McPhee, R. W., & Stringer, M. D. 2008. An evidence-based approach to human dermatomes. *Clin Anat* 21:363–373.

Lewis, T. 1942. *Pain,* Macmillan, New York, NY.

Lucas, N., Macaskill, P., Irwig, L., Moran, R., & Bogduk, N. 2009. Reliability of physical examination for diagnosis of myofascial trigger points: a systematic review of the literature. *Clin J Pain,* no. 1, pp.:80–89.

Mense, S. 1993. Nociception from skeletal muscle in relation to clinical muscle pain. *Pain* 54:241–289.

Mense, S. 2013. Basic mechanisms of muscle pain, in *Wall and Melzack's Textbook of Pain, 6th edn.* S. B. McMahon et al., eds, Elsevier, Saunders, Philadelphia, PA, pp. 620–628.

Mense, S. & Simons, D. G. 2001. *Muscle Pain. Understanding its Nature, Diagnosis, and Treatment,* Lippincott Williams & Wilkins, Philadelphia, PA.

Michaelis, M., Häbler, H. J., & Jänig, W. 1996. Silent afferents: a separate class of primary afferents? *Clin Exp Pharmacol Physiol* 23:99–105.

Myburgh, C., Larsen, A. H., & Hartvigsen, J. 2008. A systematic, critical review of manual palpation for identifying myofascial trigger points: evidence and clinical significance. *Arch Phys Med Rehabil* 89:1169–1176.

Neugebauer, V., Galhardo, V., Maione, S., & Mackey, S. C. 2009. Forebrain pain mechanisms. *Brain Res Rev* 60:226–242.

Neugebauer, V., Lucke, T., & Schaible, H. G. 1993. N-methyl-D-aspartate (NMDA) and non-NMDA receptor antagonists block the hyperexcitability of dorsal horn neurons during development of acute arthritis in rat's knee joint. *J Neurophysiol* 70:1365–1377.

Ossipov, M. H. & Porreca, F. 2009. Neuropathic pain: basic mechanisms (animal), in *Science of Pain.* A. L. Basbaum & M. C. Bushnell, eds, Academic Press, San Diego, CA, pp. 833–855.

Price, D. D. 2000. Psychological and neural mechanisms of the affective dimension of pain. *Science* 288:1769–1772.

Quintner, J. L., Bove, G. M., & Cohen, M. L. 2014. A critical evaluation of the trigger point phenomenon. *Rheumatology* 54:392–399.

Ringkamp, M., Raja, S. N., Campbell, J. N., & Meyer, R. A. 2013. Peripheral mechanisms of cutaneous nociception, in *Wall and Melzack's Textbook of Pain, 6th edn.* S. B. McMahon et al., eds, Elsevier, Saunders, Philadelphia, PA, pp. 3–34.

Ruch, T. C. 1965. Pathophysiology of pain, in *Physiology and Biophysics.* T. C. Ruch & H. D. Patton, eds, Saunders, Philadelphia, PA, pp. 345–363.

Russell, I. J. 2013. Fibromyalgia syndrome and myofascial pain syndrome, in *Wall and Melzack's Textbook of Pain, 6th edn.* S. B. McMahon et al., eds, Elsevier, Saunders, Philadelphia, PA, pp. 658–682.

Schaible, H. G. 2012. Mechanisms of chronic pain in osteoarthritis. *Curr Rheumatol Rep* 14:549–556.

Schaible, H.-G. 2013. Joint pain: basic mechanisms, in *Wall and Melzack's Textbook of Pain, 6th edn*. S. B. McMahon et al., eds, Elsevier, Saunders, Philadelphia, PA, pp. 609–619.

Schaible, H. G. & Grubb, B. D. 1993. Afferent and spinal mechanisms of joint pain. *Pain* 55:5–54.

Schaible, H. G., Richter, F., Ebersberger, A., Boettger, M. K., Vanegas, H., Natura, G., Vazquez, E., & Segond von, B. G. 2009. Joint pain. *Exp Brain Res* 196:153–162.

Schleip, R. & Huijing, P. A. 2012. Introduction, in *The Tensional Network of the Human Body*. R. Schleip et al., eds, Churchill Livingstone, Elsevier, Edinburgh, pp. xv–xviii.

Schleip, R., Jäger, H., & Klingler, W. 2012. Fascia is alive: how cells modulate the tonicity and architecture of fascial tissues, in *The Tensional Network of the Human Body*. R. Schleip et al., eds, Churchill Livingstone, Elsevier, Edinburgh, pp. 157–164.

Schmidt, R., Schmelz, M., Forster, C., Ringkamp, M., Torebjörk, E., & Handwerker, H. 1995. Novel classes of responsive and unresponsive C nociceptors in human skin. *J Neurosci* 15:333–341.

Simons, D. G. 2004. Review of enigmatic MTrPs as a common cause of enigmatic musculoskeletal pain and dysfunction *J Electromyogr Kinesiol* 14:95–107.

Simons, D. G. 2013. Myofascial trigger points, in *Encyclopedia of Pain, 2nd edn*. G. F. Gebhart & R. F. Schmidt, eds, Springer-Verlag, Heidelberg, New York, Dordrecht, London, pp. 2009–2016.

Spike, R. C., Puskar, Z., Andrew, D., & Todd, A. J. 2003. A quantitative and morphological study of projection neurons in lamina I of the rat lumbar spinal cord. *Eur J Neurosci* 18:2433–2448.

Todd, A. J. & Koerber, H. R. 2013. Neuroanatomical substrates of spinal nociception, in *Wall and Melzack's Textbook of Pain, 6th edn*. S. B. McMahon et al., eds, Elsevier, Saunders, PA, pp. 77–93.

Tough, E. A., White, A. R., Cummings, T. M., Richards, S. H., & Campbell, J. L. 2009. Acupuncture and dry needling in the management of myofascial trigger point pain: a systematic review and meta-analysis of randomised controlled trials. *Eur J Pain* 13:3–10.

Tracey, I. & Mantyh, P. W. 2007. The cerebral signature for pain perception and its modulation. *Neuron* 55:377–391.

Treede, R. D. & Apkarian, A. V. 2009. Nociceptive processing in the cerebral cortex, in *Science of Pain*. A. I. Basbaum & M. C. Bushnell, eds, Academic Press, San Diego, CA, pp. 669–697.

Turvey, M. T. & Fonseca, S. T. 2014. The medium of haptic perception: a tensegrity hypothesis. *J Mot Behav* 46:143–187.

Willis, W. D., Jr., Zhang, X., Honda, C. N., & Giesler, G. J., Jr. 2002. A critical review of the role of the proposed VMpo nucleus in pain. *J Pain* 3:79–94.

Willis, W. D., Jr. & Coggeshall, R. E. 2004a. *Sensory Mechanisms of the Spinal Cord. Primary Afferent Neurons and the Spinal Dorsal Horn, Vol. 1, 3rd edn*. Kluwer Academic/Plenum Publishers, New York, NY.

Willis, W. D., Jr. & Coggeshall, R. E. 2004b. *Sensory Mechanisms of the Spinal Cord. Ascending Sensory Tracts and Their Descending Control, Vol. 2, 3rd edn*. Kluwer Academic/Plenum Publishers, New York, NY.

Woolf, C. J. & Ma, Q. 2007. Nociceptors – noxious stimulus detectors. *Neuron* 55:353–364.

MECHANISMS OF FASCIAL DYSFUNCTION AND TREATMENT

Paolo Tozzi

Overview

This chapter aims to explore the main possible fascia-mediated mechanisms underlying somatic dysfunction and its treatment. The concept of somatic dysfunction, traditionally dominated by the neurological model, is revisited in the light of the several fascial influences that may come into play in its genesis, maintenance, and treatment. A wide range of fascia-related factors is presented, from cell-based mechanisms to cognitive influences, supporting the multidimensional nature of somatic dysfunction and its treatment, intended – at least partially – as a fasciagenic phenomenon.

Introduction

Fascia is a ubiquitous tissue that surrounds and permeates the entire body, from its large to its small constituents. By investing each tissue at all levels, it offers a structural interconnectedness around, within, and between body elements, while allowing sliding and gliding motions at the same time. It appears to play different physiological and functional roles: from joint stability to general movement coordination; from proprioception to nociception (Tozzi, 2012); from transmission of mechanical forces (Huijing, 2009) to wound healing and tissue repair, together with a potential role in many connective tissue pathologies (Gabbiani, 2003).

Instead of consisting of different superimposed layers, gliding on each other, fascia has been proposed as a single architecture at various levels of form and complexity (Guimberteau, 2012). Even at a cellular level, fascia displays an interconnected arrangement with fibroblasts forming an extensively reticular network, via their cytoplasmic expansions, permeating the whole body (Langevin et al., 2004). This soft tissue 'skeleton' has been defined as 'ectoskeleton' (Wood Jones, 1944) in relation to its continuity and function of muscle attachment, enveloping, force transmission, and body-wide proprioception.

Since the foundation of osteopathy, the connective tissue has been traditionally proposed as a fundamental element to be addressed in order to achieve optimal clinical outcomes (Lee, 2006). The role of fascia in particular has always been of key importance: '... this philosophy (of Osteopathy) has chosen the fascia as a foundation of [sic] which to stand ...' (Still, 1899).

Nowadays, the aim of osteopathic medicine remains to promote health and support the inherent self-regulatory capacities, mainly by focusing on the musculoskeletal system as the interface of the homeostatic body potential and of resistance to disease (Hruby, 1992). Therefore, it is paramount to identify and resolve any dysfunction that may compromise health. As such, somatic dysfunction is defined as any 'impaired or altered function of related components of the somatic (body framework) system: skeletal, arthrodial and **myofascial** structures' (ECOP, 2011a), related to neural and/or vascular elements, that might underlie pathophysiologic conditions. The observational and palpatory features of somatic dysfunction include objective findings such as tissue texture change, structural asymmetry, and restriction of motion, together with subjective elements such as tenderness on palpation and/or altered sensitivity (DiGiovanna, 2005).

Since its origins, osteopathic research has focused on the understanding of the mechanisms underlying somatic dysfunction and its features, mainly by exploring the related neurological interactions. Luisa Burns (1907) was the first to conduct scientific studies to investigate the dysfunctional visceral and somatic reflexes associated with osteopathic lesions. Then the experiments of Cole (1951), Denslow (1947), and Korr (1979) advanced the research in the field. The results supported the presence of aberrant somatovisceral reflexes as the scientific basis for the existence of facilitated areas in the spine corresponding to palpable features of osteopathic lesion (the old term for somatic dysfunction). The evidence available has been partly organized into a nociceptive model (Van Buskirk, 1990). This model interprets somatic dysfunction primarily in the light of a neurological perspective, as the result of a neurogenic inflammation, leading to peripheral and central sensitization, including the facilitation of correspondent spinal levels, eventually followed by an adaptive response of the whole organism via the interaction of neuroendocrine pathways (Willard, 1995). Furthermore, the neurological model has represented for decades the dominant explanation for most of the beneficial results obtained by manual intervention. Although it has been only recently integrated into a neurobiological model (Schleip, 2003), it still remains neurologically based in nature.

The rest of this chapter will explore, instead, whether somatic dysfunction and its treatment are partially or even entirely a fasciagenic phenomenon.

Fascia-mediated mechanisms underlying somatic dysfunction

Due to fascial behavior as a tensegritive architecture (Ingber, 2008), any fascial strain may easily cause body-wide repercussions, perceived also at a distance from where it originates, potentially creating stress on any structure enveloped by fascia and thus requiring progressive body adaptation at a local and global level. Various fascia-related mechanisms may underlie somatic dysfunction, aside from the well-known neurogenic influences of the nociceptive model. Such fasciagenic factors might also cause and maintain types of somatic dysfunction that have not yet been classified in the osteopathic field (Tozzi et al., 2012; Bongiorno, 2013).

Fascial architecture

Mechanical forces imposed upon or expressed in the connective tissue seem to regulate collagen organization and deposition along specific lines of tension, at both molecular (Vesentini et al., 2013) and macroscopic (Vleeming et al., 1995) level. The architecture of fascial tissue may show an increased number of stress fibers and coupling to adhesions following nonlinear response of fibroblasts under different magnitude of loading (Faust et al., 2011). This may occur in pathological conditions, too. In chronic musculoskeletal disorders a change in thickness of the related deep fascia has been found and correlated to an increase in the quantity of loose connective tissue lying between dense collagen fiber layers (Stecco et al., 2014). In addition, the micro-architecture of the collagenic network is crucial for determining its mechanical properties. In fact, a D-periodic spacing of collagen structures has been found in various tissues, from higher to lower hierarchical organization, generally ranging from 60 to 70 nm values (Fang et al., 2012). Such structural organization can decrease – as in the case of decreased functional loading – with a consequent reduction in mechanical properties (Thomopoulos et al., 2010), or it can become altered or disrupted in pathological conditions (Fang & Holl, 2013), following a series of fibroblast-mediated mechanisms leading to collagenous remodeling.

This cascade of events affecting fascial micro- and macro-architecture may account for some features of somatic dysfunction such as tissue texture change and positional asymmetry.

Fascial contractility

It has been proposed that fascia may contract in a smooth muscle-like manner (Schleip et al., 2005), independently from skeletal muscle tone. This is possibly related to the presence of smooth muscle cells found in fascial tissue (Staubesand et al., 1997) and the capacity of fascial myofibroblasts to contract via the contractile properties of intracellular alpha-smooth-muscle actin (Hinz & Gabbiani, 2003). Myofibroblast behavior and contraction, in particular in the myocardium, are highly responsive to oxygen levels, vasoactive peptides, autonomic activity, proinflammatory cytokines, and surrounding mechanical tension (Porter & Turner, 2009). Dysfunction of this apparatus may lead to altered myofascial tonus and diminished neuromuscular coordination, potentially leading to several musculoskeletal pathologies and pain syndromes (Klingler et al., 2014). Such changes may take place locally, or might become widespread, causing postural distortions associated with altered force transmissions, especially in the traditionally defined 'postural' fasciae, such as the thoracolumbar fascia, the iliotibial band, and the cervical fascia – among the first to show alterations in the presence of postural defects (Cathie, 1974). The whole series of these events may lead to an abnormal fascial contractility and texture, underlying restriction of motion, and the functional and positional asymmetry found in somatic dysfunction.

Fascial viscoelasticity

Fascia exhibits the potential for both elastic and plastic deformation thanks to the interdependence of the architecture and composition of connective tissue and water content (Woo et al., 1997).

However, an intrinsic and independent viscoelastic property of myofascia has recently been discovered, independently from nervous system activity, as shown by corresponding silent EMG patterns (Masi & Hannon, 2008). Such intrinsic myofascial tone is determined by the molecular interactions of the actomyosin filaments in myofibroblast cells and myosarcomeric units. It may offer a substantial contribution toward maintaining postural stability at a minimal energetic expenditure, differently from neuromotor activation that implies, instead, higher levels of tone to provide stabilization. This is consistent with recent findings in pathological conditions. In fact, persistent static load leads to viscoelastic creep of connective tissue, resulting in a transient neuromuscular disorder, with an intensity directly related to the magnitude of the load (Sbriccoli et al., 2004).

The combination of these events may produce a change in the colloidal consistency of the ground substance to a more solid state, leading to altered myofascial activation. This may account for the tissue texture change, restriction of motion, and asymmetry found in osteopathic dysfunction.

Fascial fluid dynamics

Water content in fascia is dependent on negatively charged glycosaminoglycans as well as on the organization and the stiffness of collagen fibers that resist tissue swelling (Mow & Ratcliffe, 1997). If tensile forces are decreased, fluids are taken in by the constituents of the extracellular matrix (ECM), but if the tension of fibroblasts and fibers is increased, fluids are extruded into the surrounding environment. Therefore, a reciprocal influence exists between mechanical force, fluid dynamics, and cell response. In fact, mechanical forces through the connective tissue may cause changes in interstitial hydrostatic pressure, with the fibroblasts as active modulators of the fluid dynamics by adjusting cell size and matrix tension according to the sensed osmotic pressure changes (Langevin et al. 2013). In the case of inflammation, changes in physical properties of the connective tissue, involving hyaluronic complexes, may influence transcapillary exchange resulting in as much as a hundredfold increase in fluid flow (Reed et al., 2010).

In physiological conditions, a layer of lubricating hyaluronan has been found between the deep fascia and muscle as well as within the loose connective tissue dividing different fibrous sublayers of the deep fascia (Stecco et al., 2011). These hyaluronan layers promote normal fascial function and sliding motion. If compromised, for example following injury or chronic inflammation, they may underlie various types of myofascial dysfunctions and pain.

Fascial pH and influencing factors

Changes in pH, ionic content, and temperature may represent key environmental and metabolic factors influencing fascial viscosity (Thomas & Klingler, 2012). For instance, increased body temperature, such as during physical exercise, may reduce fascial stiffness, while breathing exerts a significant influence on pH. In most breathing pattern disorders, a state of hypocapnia can occur, resulting in elevated pH levels due to respiratory alkalosis (Chaitow et al., 2014). In turn, this may lead to smooth muscle cell contraction and even spasm, with potentially profound effects on fascial, visceral, and vasal tone (Foster et al., 2001). Conversely, a more acidic environment seems to exert a modulating action on connective tissue cells' metabolism and protein synthesis, ranging from predisposing to inflammatory reactions and tissue damage when high levels of acidosis are present (Levick, 1990) up to beneficial effects on composition of both gelatinous and fibrous matrix (Mwale et al., 2011). Therefore, the influence of breathing patterns and temperature – and presumably of nutrition and physical activities, too – should be considered as modulating factors of tissue pH levels, whose oscillations may strongly influence fascial function and be related to fascial dysfunction.

Somatic neurofascial interaction

Benjamin's review (2009) reports several studies showing the presence of primary afferents and nerve fibers within fascia. This may support the property of fascia as a sensory organ. Research also shows that fascia, rather than muscle tissue, is involved in delayed-onset muscle soreness following physical exercise, suggesting its role in pain generation in physiological conditions (Gibson et al., 2009). However, under abnormal mechanical stimulation, a pathological change in fascial innervation may occur, resulting in dysfunctional ingrowth of nociceptive fibers (Sanchis-Alfonso & Roselló-Sastre, 2000) that may generate or maintain inflammation. Irritation of primary afferent fibers in the fascia is capable of initiating the release of neuropeptides, eventually setting up a neurogenic inflammation, peripheral and central sensitization that alters the texture of surrounding connective tissue via the interaction of fibroblast and immune cells (Mense, 2001). Recent studies have also shown that myofascial pain may alter the activity of related superior centers, accounting for a reduction of sensory processing followed by an altered motor output (Schabrun et al., 2013), together with a reorganization of the motor cortex associated with deficits in postural control (Tsao et al., 2008). This suggests fascia as a possible nociceptive source for the establishment of somatic dysfunction and its characteristics, such as tenderness and tissue texture changes.

Autonomic neurofascial interaction

It has been suggested that sympathetic activation may induce myofibroblast contraction in fascial tissue via the release of TGF-β1, hence modulating fascial stiffness (Schleip et al., 2012). This has been proposed in the light of recent evidence in the field of psychoneuroimmunology, reporting TGF-β1 as the missing link between sympathetic activation and altered T3 cell expression (Bhowmick et al., 2009).

The autonomics have also been shown to play a role in pain modulation, by activating sensitized primary afferent fibers either directly or indirectly (Roberts & Kramis, 1990), contributing to the development of chronic myofascial pain syndromes (Malanga & Cruz Colon, 2010).

Therefore, autonomic activity may be involved in the genesis or maintenance of pain and somatic dysfunction in the connective tissue.

Metabolic influences

Different connective tissue cells respond to mechanical loading by inducing collagen expression and remodeling of the matrix under the influence of hormones and growth factors (Kjaer, 2004). Such mechanically induced expression of collagen appears to be mediated in myofascial tissue by specific growth factors, such as insulin growth factors (IGF), mechanogrowth factors, and IGF binding proteins (Olesen et al., 2006). In addition, growth hormone seems to promote matrix collagen tissue (Doessing et al., 2010). Sex hormones, instead, may influence ECM adaptability in mechanical loading, either directly or indirectly, via activation of growth factors and cytokines. Estrogen, in particular, exerts an inhibiting effect on collagen synthesis and fibroblast proliferation (Yu et al., 2001), suggesting that the female cyclical hormonal variations may predispose to injury.

Relaxin, mainly produced during pregnancy, has a strong antifibrotic effect and a key role as inhibitor of collagen turnover in several organs (Samuel, 2005). It has also been shown to reduce alpha-smooth muscle actin expression and cell differentiation, while increasing fibrillar collagenase activity (Bennett et al., 2003), with a plausible effect on myofascial tension and matrix remodeling.

Finally, despite the longstanding belief in its acidosis-induced detrimental effects, lactate is nowadays recognized as an important cell-signaling molecule that can stimulate angiogenesis and collagen deposition in aerobic conditions (Hunt et al., 2007), hence playing a potential role in tissue repair.

In conclusion, various hormonal and metabolic factors may influence myofascial texture and stiffness, playing a possible role in the genesis and maintenance of fascial dysfunction and its features.

Piezoelectricity

Piezoelectricity is a property of a variety of biological structures ranging from bones to proteins and nucleic acids (Fukada, 1982). It is based on an electromechanical coupling by which a mechanical force is converted into an electrical stimulus through a stress-induced polarization, and vice versa. In the connective tissue, thanks to this electromechanical transduction, collagen may exchange physical information from a macroscopic to a cell scale, either directly or via a biochemical process (Stroe et al. 2013). This may work as a modulating mechanism of cell behavior along common pathways with chemical messages and mechanical signals (Grodzinsky, 1983).

With regard to fascia, piezoelectric properties of collagen fibrils have only recently been imaged using piezoresponse force microscopy (Harnagea et al., 2010). The analysis of the signal revealed clear shear piezoelectricity associated with piezoelectric deformation along the fibril axis, with the direction of the displacement being preserved along the whole fiber length, independently of the fiber conformation.

Alterations of collagen architecture, such as may occur following injury, surgery, or chronic inflammation, may lead to changes in piezoelectric responses of the area involved, with consequent repercussions on fascial function and structure.

Water

Interfascial water may activate resonating biomolecules to self-organize through 'coherence domains' (Brizhik et al., 2009), contributing to various tissue functions and structural organization, such as protein folding, cell-to-cell recognition, and behavior (Sommer et al., 2008).

Every collagen fiber in the body is embedded in layers of water molecules that, when associated with proteins, behave in a crystalline manner, that is, in a highly ordered and patterned fashion (Pollack et al., 2006). This water-protein-interaction-based system may offer a dynamic framework for understanding various biological mechanisms, such as DNA transcription and duplication underlying various biophysical processes (Pang, 2013).

It is plausible that fascial dysfunction may be related to structural alteration of the collagen-protein-bound-water network, such as may occur in scar, injury, or inflammation.

Bioenergy

The structural continuum of the collagenous matrix connecting with the intracellular skeleton may work as a semiconductive system, exhibiting coherent vibrations throughout the organism, with a potential regulatory role (Pienta & Coffey, 1991). It also appears to emit other forms of energy.

Biophotons, for instance, have been systematically measured in human bodies, displaying a spectral range from at least 260 to 800 nm (Popp, 2003). They are supposed to be radiations of nonthermal origin, emitted from a delocalized and fully coherent biophoton field within the living system, playing a potential role in cell communication and regulation of cell behavior, including DNA replication and protein synthesis (Chang, 2008). This property may be deregulated or altered in the case of disease and may be associated with many pathogenetic processes underlying various conditions – including those affecting connective tissue – related to a generally high oxidative status of the organism (Van Wijk et al., 2008).

Psychophysiological and cognitive-behavioral influences

Various psychological factors may predispose to the development of chronic musculoskeletal pain and disability (Pincus et al., 2002). In particular fear of pain (or of its potential reoccurrence seems to be more disabling than pain by itself, especially in chronic conditions (Waddell et al., 1993). The result of these events is the strong tendency to avoid activities predisposing to the development of connective tissue fibrosis (inflammation) that in turn reinforces the chronic pain pattern and leads to further decreased mobility (Langevin & Sherman, 2007). The personality type of a given individual (Radnitz et al., 2000) as well as his/her faith and religion (Koenig, 2004) may influence the perception of pain and disability together with the control or treatment of the condition. In fact, as suggested by the cognitive model (Weisenberg, 1984), beliefs, expectations, and generally cognitive and affective components of pain experience are fundamental influences on the development of pain-control and coping strategies. In addition, psychosocial and environmental factors may also generate maladaptive pain behaviors that can be analyzed and changed, as traditionally proposed by the behavioral model (Fordyce, 1976).

In conclusion, all the fasciagenic factors described above may play a role in the genesis and maintenance of somatic dysfunction and of its features, which are certainly related but not exclusively limited to neural influences. Such evidence may explain several local, segmental, and global effects of a given fascial dysfunction, supporting the concept of the osteopathic 'total lesion' (Fryette, 1980) in taking into account the multidimensional aspects of pain.

Fascia-mediated mechanisms underlying the release of somatic dysfunction

In osteopathic practice there exist three main approaches to fascia (see Fig. 29.1), together with a multitude of fascia-related techniques of various levels of aggressiveness (Sergueef & Nelson, 2014). Different manual modalities of intervention on the myofascial complex have shown comparable therapeutic results, possibly due to the common influence and stimulation of fascial tissue (Simmonds et al., 2012). Several mechanisms may underlie fascial release during or following osteopathic maneuvers.

Structural changes

Structural modifications in the connective tissue may occur during or just after treatment, accounting for some palpable changes following manipulation. High-frequency ultrasound measurements applied immediately before and after manual intervention have shown highly significant differences in the structure of the collagen matrix in the dermis, reflecting palpable differences in tension and regularity (Pohl, 2010). These findings are consistent with the proposed property of collagen fibers to self-reorganize and remodel following myofascial work (Martin, 2009).

Since the abnormal palpable findings in connective tissue might be related to abnormal cross-links between collagen fibers, it must be noted that human fibroblasts have been shown to respond to cyclical

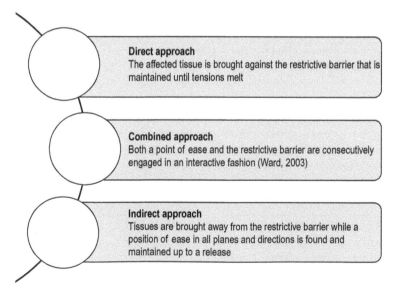

Figure 29.1
Osteopathic approaches to fascia

Direct approach
The affected tissue is brought against the restrictive barrier that is maintained until tensions melt

Combined approach
Both a point of ease and the restrictive barrier are consecutively engaged in an interactive fashion (Ward, 2003)

Indirect approach
Tissues are brought away from the restrictive barrier while a position of ease in all planes and directions is found and maintained up to a release

(3 minutes' stress–3 minutes' relaxation, of about 7% of their length) more than static stretch in the production of collagenase, by increasing it by 200% (Carano & Siciliani, 1996). This enzyme has a potential role in collagen remodeling in dysfunctional tissue, by breaking peptide bonds in collagen.

Cell-based mechanisms

Various forms and degrees of manual loading, ranging from sustained to cyclical, different in direction, speed, magnitude, and frequency, appear to exert a strong impact on cell behavior and gene expression, influencing tissue remodeling through growth factors and enzyme activation.

Several cell-based mechanisms may potentially produce a palpable release during fascial work. Some of these are summarized in Table 29.1. Although most of the proposed mechanisms may take hours or days to produce desirable effects on tissue texture and function, some of them may take effect within minutes of the starting point of a therapeutic maneuver. In fact, in response to sustained changes in tissue length, fibroblasts may rapidly modulate such tension by remodeling their cytoskeleton and changing their contractile apparatus (Langevin et al., 2013). Within minutes they may remodel cell-matrix contacts along the direction of tissue stretch (Ciobanasu et al., 2013), or expand microtubule network and actomyosin activation in order to maintain tensional homeostasis

Cell response	Fibroblasts and myofibroblasts are highly responsive to magnitude (Cao et al., 2013a), direction (Eagan et al., 2007), frequency, and duration (Meltzer & Standley, 2007) of (therapeutic) loading, differentially regulating cell activity, proliferation or apoptosis, ion conductance, gene expression, and also secretion of pro- or anti-inflammatory mediators (Tsuzaki et al., 2003).
Cell nucleus response	Ex vivo and in vivo studies have demonstrated that fibroblasts respond within minutes to mechanical stretching by dynamically remodeling their cytoskeleton with perinuclear redistribution of alpha-actin (Langevin et al., 2005; Langevin et al., 2006).
Cell-to-cell communication	Stimulus in one location leads to a perturbation of distant cells, although these have not received any direct mechanical stimulus (Lu & Thomopoulos, 2013; Wall & Banes, 2005). Therefore therapeutic loading may produce beneficial effects even at a distance from where it is applied.
Effector cell response	Appropriate mechanical loading stimulates protein synthesis at the cellular level, promoting tissue repair and remodeling (Hardmeier et al., 2010; Wang et al., 2012) as well as cell proliferation and migration in wound healing, by sensitizing fibroblasts to nitric oxide (Cao et al., 2013b).
General considerations	Although with differences in degree and form, most of the studies have shown that high-magnitude, heterobiaxial strain may produce inflammatory reactions and increase (or sometimes reduce) fibroblast proliferation, whereas a completely reversed pattern was observed in low-magnitude, equibiaxial strained fibroblasts. This means fascial tissue may respond better to brief, light/moderate magnitude and balanced stretch, than large magnitude and unequal loads.

Table 29.1

Cell-based mechanisms possibly related to manual fascial treatment

through an equal countertension (Eastwood et al., 1998). This might produce a counterforce to the manually induced matrix tension that in turn could be perceived as dropped by the therapist.

Neuromuscular interaction

Fascial work may produce beneficial effects by activating various receptors in the connective tissue able to elicit a series of neuromuscular reflexes. According to Schleip's neurobiological model (2003), this type of event, together with concomitant autonomic and viscoelastic changes, is more likely to explain the immediate effects during fascial release, through activation of Ruffini endings and fascial interstitial mechanoreceptors. Ruffini endings are mainly located in joint capsules and in the dense connective tissue, including fascia (Yahia et al., 1992). They have a slow adaptation to the stimuli being applied, thus they are generally sensitive to slow, sustained or rhythmic, deep pressures, similar to those normally applied in most fascial techniques.

Fascial interstitial mechanoreceptors, on the other hand, have a very low threshold, hence some are responsive to light tissue stretching and others to rapid pressure. It has been suggested that they may exert an influence on autonomic activity and the central nervous system, producing an indirect effect on hemodynamics and tissue viscoelasticity, together with a descending inhibition of muscular tone (Schleip, 2003). Furthermore, low-threshold mechanoreceptors, called 'tactile C-fibers', have recently been discovered in the subcutaneous connective tissue to account for a distinctive system signaling touch in humans (Björnsdotter et al., 2010). Activation of these fibers, as in during gentle touch therapy, relays signals to the insular cortex, the medial prefrontal cortex, and the dorsoanterior cingulate cortex (but not to the somatosensory areas) (McGlone et al., 2014), where sensory and affective information is integrated giving rise to limbic touch. The latter produces a cascade of effects on interpersonal touch, affiliative behavior, psychoendocrine function, the immune system, autonomic regulation, and pain modulation (Olausson et al., 2010).

Finally, the classical nociceptive model proposes that the indirect type of fascial technique may modulate muscle tone and related fascial tension by decreasing physical stress and neural inputs (Van Buskirk, 1990). This may in turn quiet the nociceptors and the correspondent facilitated spinal level, with a consequent modulation of autonomic activity on blood and lymphatic flow.

Autonomic influence

Therapeutic touch may produce stimulation of pressure-sensitive mechanoreceptors in the fascia, followed by a parasympathetic response (Schleip, 2003). This in turn may induce a change in local vasodilatation and tissue viscosity, together with a lowered tonus of intrafascial smooth muscle cells. Such a response has been partially confirmed by evidence. Manual therapy and myofascial osteopathic treatments have been shown to produce an increase in vagal efferent activity, as shown by changes in heart rate (Field et al., 2010), while fascial treatment may produce an upregulation of parasympathetics with an influence on blood shear rate and blood flow turbulence (Queré et al., 2009). At the same time, a modulation of hypersympathetic activity may take place, normalizing various hemodynamic parameters (Henley et al., 2008).

Viscoelastic changes

ECM viscosity changes may take place within minutes while a tensional load is applied, as the result of cell-matrix-induced regulation of fluid flow, independently from neurological activation. In fact, static tissue stretch of areolar connective tissue corresponding to ~20–25% of tissue elongation has been shown to produce fibroblast cytoskeletal remodeling via activation of focal adhesion complexes (Langevin et al., 2011). This in turn leads to remodeling of the cell's focal adhesions and actomyosin activation that develop cell countertension. The latter allows surrounding tissue to relax further and achieve a lower level of resting tension. The study has shown that by changing shape, fibroblasts can dynamically modulate the viscoelastic behavior of areolar connective tissue through specific cytoskeletal mechanisms.

Fluid dynamics

The mechanism explained above may also potentially regulate extracellular fluid flow into the tissue and protect against osmotically-driven swelling when the matrix is stretched (Langevin et al., 2013). In fact, the water flow in the ECM depends on the opposing forces between the osmotic pull of underhydrated glycosaminoglycans and active restraint of the collagenous network exerted by fibroblasts. Therefore, as long as the tension in the matrix is maintained by fibroblasts, water is prevented from entering the tissue (Reed et al., 2010). On the other hand, a (therapeutic) stretch for few minutes would unrestrain the matrix, possibly promoting transcapillary fluid flow and temporary matrix swelling. Interestingly, the fluid pressure might increase more during tangential oscillation and perpendicular vibration than during constant sliding or back-and-forth motion, as predicted by three-dimensional mathematical modeling methods (Roman et al., 2013). Interstitial flow may also be supported by the interplay of calcium ion concentration and unbound water oscillations (Lee, 2008), bringing oxygenation and nutrients in tissues up to a normal concentration. In fact, since fluid flow in the ECM may offer a transport space for nutrients, metabolic wastes, and messenger substances, it may indeed play a role in restoring homeostasis when and where it is compromised.

Endocrine-immunity response

Evidence suggests that manual therapy, including engaging myofascial tissues, might produce sustained and cumulative biologic actions – in part hormonally mediated – that persist for several days or a week, modulating the hypothalamic-pituitary-adrenal axis and immune function (Rapaport et al., 2012; Rapaport et al., 2010; Morhenn et al., 2012). Once-a-week intervention demonstrated patterns of change in circulating lymphocyte markers and cytokine expression, while twice-weekly sessions may increase oxytocin levels and production of proinflammatory cytokines, together with decreased arginine vasopressin and cortisol levels. Hormonal changes were sustained over 3–4 days, while cyotokine changes persisted for 7–8 days. Oxytocin, in particular, could play a role as an endogenous pain-controlling system. In fact, after manual intervention, increased levels of this hormone have been found in plasma and periaqueductal grey matter, exhibiting antinociceptive effects possibly through interaction with the opioid system (Lund et al., 2002). Furthermore, oxytocin appears to be strongly related to the formation of

social bonds as well as interpersonal bonding involving trust (Lieberwirth & Wang, 2014), thus influencing the psychosocial dimension of the individual.

The benefits of osteopathic manipulation, including myofascial work, have also been related to a remarkable increase in haematic nitric oxide (NO) concentration following intervention (Salamon et al., 2004). NO is an important signaling molecule that may be involved, within different actions, in promoting tissue repair and collagen synthesis, in improving clinical symptoms and functions following injury (Bokhari & Murrell, 2012), and in smooth muscle relaxation and angiogenesis (Ziche & Morbidelli, 2000).

Finally, there is a strong possibility that the physiological effects of myofascial work may be in part due to stimulation of the cannabinoid receptors, by producing an anandamide effect on the endocannabinoid system. This system affects fibroblast remodeling, and may play a role in fascial reorganization, diminishing nociception, and reducing inflammation in myofascial tissue (McPartland, 2008).

Bioenergetic interactions

Electromagnetic fields appear to be closely related to the flow and oscillations of ions. In turn, these are highly responsive to mechanical loading, via stretch-activated calcium channels (Follonier Castella et al., 2010). Therefore, mechanical pressure or electricity may be amplified and propagated by proton currents or coherent oscillations and polarization waves throughout the organism, showing properties of nonequilibrium structures under external activation (Mikhailov & Ertl, 1996). In this sense, fascia appears to combine the property of a sol-liquid conductor and of a crystal generator system due to the liquid crystal continuum of the matrix, which can generate and conduct direct currents as well as vibrations (Lee, 2008). An even more interesting possibility is that such a body liquid crystalline continuum may function as a quantum holographic medium, recording patterns of local activities interacting with a globally coherent field. During bodywork an interaction of vibrational, biomagnetic, and bioelectric fields may take place between therapist and client. This may allow an exchange of information about the history and the present status of the living matrix, encoded in cell and tissue structure, accessible holographically by tuning to the appropriate frequencies (Oschman & Oschman, 1994). The result may be the balancing of resonant vibratory circuits.

Cognitive-behavioral factors

Osteopathic intervention should never focus exclusively on the dysfunctional or symptomatic area. Instead, the multidimensional aspect of pain should be considered, especially for chronic patients (Lima et al., 2014), also bearing in mind the osteopathic tenet of the body as a unity with mind and spirit. Therefore, in order to approach the totality of an individual (not just 'a pain'), including his or her social environment, it is necessary to wisely apply biopsychosocial models (Flor & Herman, 2004) – considered as congruous with osteopathic principles (Penney, 2010) – as well as interdisciplinary paradigms (Gatchel, 2005), described as resonating with the osteopathic philosophy (Mackintosh et al., 2011). Instead of just treating a dysfunction, health should be promoted, guiding the patient from the curing of the disease to the protection and potentiation of his/her own health and good quality of life. Maladaptive behaviors, fear, and the emotional experience of pain, catastrophism, helplessness, expectations, trust, cognitive factors, faith, beliefs, and personality – they all need to be addressed in a comprehensive and integrative conceptual model for clinical assessment, treatment, and management of patients with pain, in particular with persistent pain (Keefe et al., 2004).

Conclusion

It is evident that various factors may interplay with myofascial function and its ability to respond to treatment. Furthermore, research in the field of epigenetics may explain some additional aspects of the genesis and release of somatic dysfunction that would also add to the evidence that respiratory-vibratory-oscillatory activating forces, often engaged during osteopathic intervention, affect the connective tissue (Tozzi 2015a, 2015b). What is certain is that the effects of manual fascial interventions are of local, segmental, and global extent, occurring at different times, ranging from minutes to weeks after a given input, via the interaction of several mechanisms influencing tissue properties and behaviors (Tozzi 2015b). Some of these factors are

strongly supported by evidence, whereas others may still need further investigation to be fully understood. Nevertheless, the connective tissue may serve as a *trait d'union* of all these elements, potentially representing a meta-system (Langevin, 2006) that coherently influences structure and function of the whole organism and the interaction between its constituents. In other words, fascia might be the overlooked somatic component interacting with the musculoskeletal system and its function as the 'primary machinery of life' (Korr, 1976) and also because of their shared embryologic origin. Furthermore, it has been proposed to add a connective tissue-fascial model to the existing five models in osteopathic practice (ECOP, 2011b), due to the multifunctional nature and ubiquitous structure of fascial tissue that makes it a unique component in the musculoskeletal apparatus. This sixth osteopathic model is the true interface between all body systems, lying between and acting within the other models; by integrating and coordinating their activity; by pervading their essence, but also transcending their contingent nature; and finally by providing a structural and functional framework for the body's homoeostatic potential and its inherent abilities to heal (Tozzi, 2015b). Therefore, instead of defining bits and pieces of this body-wide fascial structure, as if it is a dead tissue to be surgically dissected, named, and distinguished from surrounding tissues (Stecco, 2014), its form and organization should be considered and understood as a living, pulsating, oscillating, coherent whole, responding and differentiating according to physical, chemical, and psychological forces, as a single structural continuum interacting with a multitude of regulatory functional properties.

References

Benjamin, M. 2009 The fascia of the limbs and back—a review. *J Anat* 214:1–18.

Bennett, R. G., Kharbanda, K. K., Tuma, D. J. 2003 Inhibition of markers of hepatic stellate cell activation by the hormone relaxin. *Biochem Pharmacol* 66:867–874.

Bhowmick, S., Singh, A., Flavell, R. A., et al. 2009 The sympathetic nervous system modulates CD4(+) FoxP3(+) regulatory T cells via a TGF-beta-dependent mechanism. *J Leukoc Biol* 86:1275–1283.

Björnsdotter, M., Morrison, I., Olausson, H. 2010 Feeling good: on the role of C fiber mediated touch in interoception. *Exp Brain Res* 207:149–155.

Bokhari, A. R., Murrell, G. A. 2012 The role of nitric oxide in tendon healing. *J Shoulder Elbow Surg* 21:238–244.

Bongiorno, D., 18 Apr. 2013. Upgrade and improve yourselves: come il dubbio e la curiosità aiutano a migliorarsi. Fascial-motion Ultrasonographic Anatomic Evaluation (FUSAE). Available at: https://davidebongiorno.wordpress.com/2013/04/18/upgrade-and-improve-yourselves-come-il-dubbio-e-la-curiosita-aiutano-a-migliorarsi/ [accessed March 22, 2016].

Brizhik, L. S., Del Giudice, E., Popp, F. A., et al. 2009 On the dynamics of self-organization in living organisms. *Electromagn Biol Med* 28:28–40.

Burns, L. 1907 Viscerosomatic and somatovisceral spinal reflexes. *J Am Osteopath Assoc* 7:51–57.

Cao, T. V., Hicks, M. R., Campbell, D., et al. 2013a Dosed myofascial release in three-dimensional bioengineered tendons: effects on human fibroblast hyperplasia, hypertrophy, and cytokine secretion. *J Manipulative Physiol Ther* 36:513–521.

Cao, T. V., Hicks, M. R., Standley, P. R. 2013b In vitro biomechanical strain regulation of fibroblast wound healing. *J Am Osteopath Assoc* 113:806–818.

Carano, A., Siciliani, G. 1996 Effect of continuous and intermittent forces on human fibroblasts in vitro. *Eur J Orthod* 18:19–26.

Cathie, A. G. 1974 The fascia of the body in relation to function and manipulative therapy. In: The American Academy of Osteopathy Yearbook.. American Academy of Osteopathy, Indianapolis, IN. pp. 81–84.

Chaitow, L., Gilbert, C., Bradley, D. 2014 *Recognizing and Treating Breathing Disorders: A Multidisciplinary Approach. 2nd Edn.* Elsevier Churchill Livingstone.

Chang, J. J. 2008 Physical properties of biophotons and their biological functions. *Indian J Exp Biol* 46:371–377.

Ciobanasu, C., Faivre, B., Le Clainche, C. 2013 Integrating actin dynamics, mechanotransduction and integrin activation: the multiple functions of actin binding proteins in focal adhesions. *Eur J Cell Biol* 92:339–348.

Cole, W. V. 1951 The osteopathic lesion syndrome. In: In: The American Academy of Osteopathy Yearbook. American Academy of Osteopathy, Indianapolis, IN. pp. 149–178.

Denslow, J. S., Korr, I. M., Krems, A. D. 1947 Quantitative studies of chronic facilitation in human motoneuron pools. *Am J Physiol* 150:229–238.

DiGiovanna, E. L. 2005 Somatic dysfunction. In: DiGiovanna, E. L., Schiowitz, S., Dowling, D. J.

(Eds), *An Osteopathic Approach to Diagnosis and Treatment. 3rd Edn.* Lippincott Williams & Wilkins, Philadelphia, PA. p. 16.

Doessing, S., Heinemeier, K. M., Holm, L., et al. 2010 Growth hormone stimulates the collagen synthesis in human tendon and skeletal muscle without affecting myofibrillar protein synthesis. *J Physiol* 588:341–351.

Eagan, T. S., Meltzer, K. R., Standley, P. R. 2007 Importance of strain direction in regulating human fibroblast proliferation and cytokine secretion: a useful in vitro model for soft tissue injury and manual medicine treatments. *J Manipulative Physiol Ther* 30:584–592.

Eastwood, M., McGrouther, D. A., Brown, R. A. 1998 Fibroblast responses to mechanical forces. *Proc Inst Mech Eng H* 212:85–92.

Educational Council on Osteopathic Principles (ECOP) 2011a Glossary of osteopathic terminology usage guide. American Association of Colleges of Osteopathic Medicine (AACOM), Chevy Chase, MD. p. 53.

Educational Council on Osteopathic Principles (ECOP) 2011b Glossary of osteopathic terminology usage guide. American Association of Colleges of Osteopathic Medicine (AACOM), Chevy Chase, MD. pp. 25–26.

Fang, M., Goldstein, E. L., Turner, A. S., et al. 2012 Type I collagen D-Spacing in fibril bundles of dermis, tendon, and bone: bridging between nano- and micro-level tissue hierarchy. *ACS NANO.* 6: 9503–9514.

Fang, M., Holl, M. M. 2013 Variation in type I collagen fibril nanomorphology: the significance and origin. *Bonekey Rep* 2:394.

Faust, U., Hampe, N., Rubner, W., et al. 2011 Cyclic stress at mHz frequencies aligns fibroblasts in direction of zero strain. *PLoS One.* 6:e28963.

Field, T., Diego, M., Hernandez-Reif, M. 2010 Moderate pressure is essential for massage therapy effects. *Int J Neurosci* 120:381–385.

Flor, H., Hermann, C. 2004 Biopsychosocial models of pain. In: Dworkin, R. H., Breitbart, W. S. (Eds.), *Psychosocial Aspects of Pain: A Handbook for Health Care Providers: 27 (Progress in Pain Research and Management).* IASP Press, Seattle. pp. 47–76.

Follonier Castella, L., Gabbiani, G., McCulloch, C. A., et al. 2010 Regulation of myofibroblast activities: calcium pulls some strings behind the scene. *Exp Cell Res* 316:2390–2401.

Fordyce, W. E. 1976 *Behavioral Methods for Chronic Pain and Illness.* C. V. Mosby, St Louis, MO.

Foster, G. T., Vaziri, N. D., Sassoon, C. S. 2001 Respiratory alkalosis. *Respir Care* 46:384–391.

Fryette, H. H. 1980 *Principles of Osteopathic Technique*. Reprint. American Academy Of Osteopathy, Colorado Springs, p. 41.

Fukada, E. 1982 Electrical phenomena in biorheology. *Biorheology* 19:15–27.

Gabbiani, G. 2003 The myofibroblast in wound healing and fibrocontractive diseases. *J Pathol* 200:500–503.

Gatchel, R. J. 2005 *Clinical Essentials of Pain Management*. American Psychological Association, Washington, DC.

Gibson, W., Arendt-Nielsen, L., Taguchi, T., et al. 2009 Increased pain from muscle fascia following eccentric exercise: animal and human findings. *Exp Brain Res* 194:299–308.

Grodzinsky, A. J. 1983 Electromechanical and physicochemical properties of connective tissue. *Crit Rev Biomed Eng* 9:133–199.

Guimberteau, J. C. 2012 [Is the multifibrillar system the structuring architecture of the extracellular matrix?]. [Article in French]. *Ann Chir Plast Esthet* 57:502–506.

Hardmeier, R., Redl, H., Marlovits, S. 2010 Effects of mechanical loading on collagen propeptides processing in cartilage repair. *J Tissue Eng Regen Med* 4:1–11.

Harnagea, C., Vallières, M., Pfeffer, C. P., et al 2010 Two-dimensional nanoscale structural and functional imaging in individual collagen type I fibrils. *Biophys J* 98:3070–3077.

Henley, C. E., Ivins, D., Mills, M., et al. 2008 Osteopathic manipulative treatment and its relationship to autonomic nervous system activity as demonstrated by heart rate variability: a repeated measures study. *Osteopathic Med Prim Care* 2:7.

Hinz, B., Gabbiani, G. 2003 Mechanisms of force generation and transmission by myofibroblasts. *Curr Opin Biotechnol*:538–546.

Hruby, R. J. 1992 Pathophysiologic models and the selection of osteopathic manipulative techniques. *J Osteopath Med* 6:25–30.

Huijing, P. A. 2009 Epimuscular myofascial force transmission: a historical review and implications for new research. International Society of Biomechanics Muybridge Award Lecture, Taipei, 2007. *J Biomech* 42:9–21.

Hunt, T. K., Aslam, R. S., Beckert, S., et al. 2007 Aerobically derived lactate stimulates revascularization and tissue repair via redox mechanisms. *Antioxid Redox Signal* 9:1115–1124.

Ingber, D. E. 2008 Tensegrity and mechanotransduction. *J Bodyw Mov Ther* 12:198–200.

Keefe, F. J., Rumble, M. E., Scipio, C. D. 2004 Psychological aspects of persistent pain: current state of the science. *J Pain* 5:195–211.

Kjaer, M. 2004 Role of extracellular matrix in adaptation of tendon and skeletal muscle to mechanical loading. *Physiol Rev* 84:649–98.

Klingler, W., Velders, M., Hoppe, K. et al. 2014 Clinical relevance of fascial tissue and dysfunctions. *Curr Pain Headache Rep* 18:439.

Koenig, H. G. 2004 Depression in chronic illness: does religion help? *J Christ Nurs* 31:40–46.

Korr, I. M. 1976 The spinal cord as organizer of disease processes: some preliminary perspectives. *J Am Osteopath Assoc* 76:35–45.

Korr, I. M. 1979 The neural basis of osteopathic lesion. In: Peterson, B. (Ed.), The Collected Papers of Irvin M. Korr. American Academy of Osteopathy, Colorado.

Langevin, H. M. 2006 Connective tissue: a body-wide signalling network? *Med Hypotheses* 66: 1074–1077.

Langevin, H. M., Bouffard, N. A., Badger, G. J., et al. 2005 Dynamic fibroblast cytoskeletal response to subcutaneous tissue stretch ex vivo and in vivo. *Am J Physiol Cell Physiol* 288:C747–756.

Langevin, H. M., Bouffard, N. A., Fox, J R., et al. 2011. Fibroblast cytoskeletal remodeling contributes to connective tissue tension. *J Cell Physiol.* 226(5):1166–1175.

Langevin, H. M., Cornbrooks, C. J., Taatjes, D. J. 2004 Fibroblasts form a body-wide cellular network. *Histochem Cell Biol* 122:7–15.

Langevin, H. M., Nedergaard, M., Howe, A. K. 2013 Cellular control of connective tissue matrix tension. *J Cell Biochem.* 114:1714–1719.

Langevin, H. M., Sherman, K. J. 2007 Pathophysiological model for chronic low back pain integrating connective tissue and nervous system mechanisms. *Med Hypotheses* 68:74–80.

Langevin, H. M., Storch, K. N., Cipolla, M. J., et al. 2006 Fibroblast spreading induced by connective tissue stretch involves intracellular redistribution of alpha- and beta-actin. *Histochem Cell Biol* 125:487–495.

Lee, P. R. 2006 Still's concept of connective tissue: lost in 'translation'? *J Am Osteopath Assoc* 106:176–177; author reply 213–214.

Lee, R. P. 2008 The living matrix: a model for the primary respiratory mechanism. *Explore* 4:374–378.

Levick, J R. 1990 Hypoxia and acidosis in chronic inflammatory arthritis; relation to vascular supply and dynamic effusion pressure. *J Rheumatol* 17:579–582.

Lieberwirth, C., Wang, Z. 2014 Social bonding: regulation by neuropeptides. *Front Neurosci* 8:171.

Lima, D. D., Alves, V. L., Turato, E. R. 2014 The phenomenological-existential comprehension of chronic pain: going beyond the standing healthcare models. *Philos Ethics Humanit Med* 9:2.

Lu, H. H., Thomopoulos, S. 2013 Functional attachment of soft tissues to bone: development, healing, and tissue engineering. *Annu Rev Biomed Eng* 15:201–226.

Lund, I., Ge, Y., Yu, L. C., et al 2002 Repeated massage-like stimulation induces long-term effects on nociception: contribution of oxytocinergic mechanisms. *Eur J Neurosci* 16:330–338.

McGlone, F., Wessberg, J., Olausson, H. 2014 Discriminative and affective touch: sensing and feeling. *Neuron* 82:737–755.

Mackintosh, S. E., Adams, C. E., Singer-Chang, G., et al. 2011 An osteopathic approach to implementing and promoting interprofessional education. *J Am Osteopath Assoc* 111:206–212.

Malanga, G. A., Cruz Colon, E. J. 2010 Myofascial low back pain: a review. *Phys Med Rehabil Clin N Am* 21:711–724.

Martin, M. M. 2009 Effects of myofascial release in diffuse systemic sclerosis. *J Bodyw Mov Ther* 13:320–327.

Masi, A. T., Hannon, J C., 2008. Human resting muscle tone (HRMT): narrative introduction and modern concepts. *J Bodyw Mov Ther.* 12(4):320–332.

McPartland, J M. 2008 Expression of the endocannabinoid system in fibroblasts and myofascial tissues. *J Bodyw Mov The* 12:169–182.

Meltzer, K. R., Standley, P. R. 2007 Modeled repetitive motion strain and indirect osteopathic manipulative techniques in regulation of human fibroblast proliferation and interleukin secretion. *J Am Osteopath Assoc* 107:527–536.

Mense, S. 2001 [Pathophysiology of low back pain and the transition to the chronic state - experimental data and new concepts]. *Schmerz*:413–417.

Mikhailov, A. S., Ertl, G. 1996 Nonequilibrium structures in condensed systems. *Science* 272:1596–1597.

Morhenn, V., Beavin, L. E., Zak, P. J. 2012 Massage increases oxytocin and reduces adrenocorticotropin hormone in humans. *Altern Ther Health Med* 18:11–18.

Mow, V. C., Ratcliffe, A. 1997 Structure and function of articular and meniscus. In: Mow, V. C., Hayes, W. C. (Eds.), *Basic Orthopaedic Biomechanics*. Lippincott-Raven, Philadelphia, PA. pp. 113–177.

Mwale, F., Ciobanu, I., Giannitsios, D., et al. 2011 Effect of oxygen levels on proteoglycan synthesis by intervertebral disc cells. *Spine* 36:E131–138.

Olausson, H., Wessberg, J., Morrison, I., et al. 2010 The neurophysiology of unmyelinated tactile afferents. *Neurosci Biobehav Rev* 34:185–191.

Olesen, J L., Heinemeier, K. M., Haddad, F., et al. 2006 Expression of insulin-like growth factor I, insulin-like growth factor binding proteins, and collagen mRNA in mechanically loaded plantaris tendon. *J Appl Physiol* 101:183–188.

Oschman, J. L., Oschman, N. H. 1994 Somatic recall. Part II. Soft tissue holography. *Massage Ther J* 34:66–67, 106–110.

Pang, X. F. 2013 Properties of proton transfer in hydrogen-bonded systems and its experimental evidences and applications in biology. *Prog Biophys Mol Biol* 112:1–32.

Penney, J N. 2010 The biopsychosocial model of pain and contemporary osteopathic practice. *Int J Osteopath Med* 13:42–47.

Pienta, K. J., Coffey, D. S. 1991 Cellular harmonic information transfer through a tissue tensegrity-matrix system. *Med Hypotheses* 34:88–95.

Pincus, T., Burton, A. K., Vogel, S., et al. 2002 A systematic review of psychological factors as predictors of chronicity/disability in prospective cohorts in low back pain. *Spine* 27:E109–120.

Pohl, H. 2010 Changes in the structure of collagen distribution in the skin caused by a manual technique. *J Bodyw Mov Ther* 14:27–34.

Pollack, G. H., Cameron, I. L., Wheatley, D. N. 2006 *Water and the Cell*. Springer, Dordrecht.

Popp, F. A. 2003 Properties of biophotons and their theoretical implications. *Indian J Exp Biol* 41:391–402.

Porter, K. E., Turner, N. A. 2009 Cardiac fibroblasts: at the heart of myocardial remodeling. *Pharmacol Ther* 123:255–278.

Queré, N., Noël, E., Lieutaud, A., et al. 2009 Fasciatherapy combined with pulsology touch induces changes in blood turbulence potentially beneficial for vascular endothelium. *J Bodyw Mov Ther* 13:239–245.

Radnitz, C. L., Bockian, N., Moran, A. 2000 Assessment of psychopathology and personality in people with physical disabilities. In: Frank, R. G., Elliot, T. R. (Eds.), *Handbook of Rehabilitation Psychology*.

American Psychological Association, Washington. pp. 287-309.

Rapaport, M. H., Schettler, P., Breese, C. 2010 A preliminary study of the effects of a single session of Swedish massage on hypothalamic-pituitary-adrenal and immune function in normal individuals. *J Altern Complement Med* 16: 1079-1088

Rapaport, M. H., Schettler, P., Bresee, C. 2012 A preliminary study of the effects of repeated massage on hypothalamic-pituitary-adrenal and immune function in healthy individuals: a study of mechanisms of action and dosage. *J Altern Complement Med* 18:789-797.

Reed, R. K., Lidén, A., Rubin, K. 2010 Edema and fluid dynamics in connective tissue remodelling. *J Mol Cell Cardiol* 48:518-523.

Roberts, W. J., Kramis, R. C. 1990 Sympathetic nervous system influence on acute and chronic pain. In: Fields, H. L. (Ed.), *Pain Syndromes in Neurology*. Butterworth Heineman, Oxford. pp. 85-106.

Roman, M., Chaudhry, H., Bukiet, B., et al. 2013 Mathematical analysis of the flow of hyaluronic acid around fascia during manual therapy motions. *J Am Osteopath Assoc* 113:600-610.

Salamon, E., Zhu, W., Stefano, GB. 2004 Nitric oxide as a possible mechanism for understanding the therapeutic effects of osteopathic manipulative medicine (Review). *Int J Mol Med* 14:443-449.

Samuel, C. S. 2005 Relaxin: antifibrotic properties and effects in models of disease. *Clin Med Res* 3:241-249.

Sanchis-Alfonso, V., Roselló-Sastre, E. 2000 Immunohistochemical analysis for neural markers of the lateral retinaculum in patients with isolated symptomatic patellofemoral malalignment. A neuroanatomic basis for anterior knee pain in the active young patient. *Am J Sports Med* 28:725-731.

Sbriccoli, P., Solomonow, M., Zhou, B. H., et al. 2004 Static load magnitude is a risk factor in the development of cumulative low back disorder. *Muscle Nerve* 29:300-308.

Schabrun, S. M., Jones, E., Kloster, J., et al. 2013 Temporal association between changes in primary sensory cortex and corticomotor output during muscle pain. *Neuroscience* 235:159-164.

Schleip, R. 2003 Fascial plasticity – a new neurobiological explanation. Part 1. *J Bodyw Mov Ther* 7:11-19.

Schleip, R., Klingler, W., Lehmann-Horn, F. 2005 Active fascial contractility: fascia may be able to contract in a smooth muscle-like manner and thereby influence musculoskeletal dynamics. *Med Hypotheses* 65:273-277.

Schleip, R., Jäger, H., Klingler, W. 2012 Fascia is alive – how cells modulate the tonicity and architecture of fascial tissues. In: Schleip, R., Findley, T. W., Chaitow, L., Huijing, P. A. (Eds.), *Fascia: The Tensional Network of the Human Body*. Churchill Livingstone Elsevier, Edinburgh.

Sergueef, N., Nelson, K. 2014 *Osteopathy for the Over 50s. Maintaining Function and Treating Dysfunction*. Handspring Publishing, Pencaitland, UK. pp. 80-82.

Simmonds, N., Miller, P., Gemmell, H. 2012 A theoretical framework for the role of fascia in manual therapy. *J Bodyw Mov Ther* 16:83-93.

Sommer, A. P., Zhu, D., Franke, R. P., Fecht, H. J. 2008 Biomimetics: learning from diamonds. *J Mater Res* 23:3148-3152.

Staubesand, J., Baumbach, K. U., Li, Y. 1997 La structure fine de l'aponévrose jambière. *Phlèbologie* 50:105-113.

Stecco, C. 2014 Why are there so many discussions about the nomenclature of fasciae? *J Bodyw Mov Ther* 18:441-442.

Stecco, C., Stern, R., Porzionato, A., et al. 2011 Hyaluronan within fascia in the etiology of myofascial pain. *Surg Radiol Anat* 33:891-896.

Still, A. T. 1899 *Philosophy of Osteopathy*. A. T. Still, Kirksville, MO. p. 162.

Stroe, M. C., Croit, J. M., Racila, M. 2013 Mechanotransduction in cortical bone and the role of piezoelectricity: a numerical approach. *Comput Methods Biomech Biomed Engin* 16:119-129.

Thomas, J., Klingler, W. 2012 The influence of pH and other metabolic actors on fascial properties. In: Schleip, R., Findley, T. W., Chaitow, L., Huijing, P. A. (Eds.), *Fascia: The Tensional Network of the Human Body*. Churchill Livingstone Elsevier, Edinburgh. pp. 171-176.

Thomopoulos, S., Genin, G. M., Galatz, L. M. 2010 The development and morphogenesis of the tendon-to-bone insertion—what development can teach us about healing. *J Musculoskelet Neuronal Interact* 10:35-45.

Tozzi, P. 2012. Selected fascial aspects of osteopathic practice. *J Bodyw Mov Ther* 16:503-519.

Tozzi, P., 2015a. A unifying neuro-fasciagenic model of somatic dysfunction – Underlying mechanisms and treatment – Part I. *J Bodyw Mov Ther* 19:310-326.

Tozzi, P. 2015b A unifying neuro-fasciagenic model of somatic dysfunction: underlying mechanisms and treatment – Part II. *J Bodyw Mov Ther* 19:526–543.

Tozzi P., Bongiorno, D., Vitturini, C. 2012 Low back pain and kidney mobility: local osteopathic fascial manipulation decreases pain perception and improves renal mobility. *J Bodyw Mov Ther* 16: 381-391.

Tsao, H., Galea, M. P., Hodges, P. W. 2008 Reorganization of the motor cortex is associated with postural control deficits in recurrent low back pain. *Brain* 131:2161-2171.

Tsuzaki, M., Bynum, D., Almekinders, L., et al. 2003 ATP modulates load-inducible IL-1beta, COX 2, and MMP-3 gene expression in human tendon cells. *J Cell Biochem* 89:556-562.

Van Buskirk, R. L. 1990 Nociceptive reflexes and the somatic dysfunction: a model. *J Am Osteopath Assoc.* 90:792-805.

Van Wijk, R., Van Wijk, E. P., Wiegant, F. A., et al. 2008 Free radicals and low-level photon emission in human pathogenesis: state of the art. Indian *J Exp Biol* 46:273-309.

Vesentini, S., Redaelli, A., Gautieri, A., 2013. Nanomechanics of collagen microfibrils. *Muscles Ligaments Tendons J.* 21;3(1):23-34.

Vleeming, A., Pool-Goudzwaard, AL., Stoeckart, R., et al. 1995 The posterior layer of the thoracolumbar fascia. *Spine* 20:753-758.

Waddell, G., Newton, M., Henderson, I., et al. 1993 A Fear-Avoidance Beliefs Questionnaire (FABQ) and the role of fear-avoidance beliefs in chronic low back pain and disability. *Pain* 52:157-168.

Wall, M. E., Banes, A. J. 2005 Early responses to mechanical load in tendon: role for calcium signaling, gap junctions and intercellular communication. *J Musculoskelet Neuronal Interact.* 5:70-84.

Wang, J H., Guo, Q., Li, B. 2012 Tendon biomechanics and mechanobiology—a minireview of basic concepts and recent advancements. *J Hand Ther* 25:133-140; quiz 141.

Weisenberg, J. 1984 Cognitive aspects of pain. In: Wull, P. D., Melzack, R. (Eds.), *Textbook of Pain. 1st Edn.* Churchill Livingston, Edinburgh. pp. 162-172.

Willard, F. H. 1995 Neuro-endocrine-immune network, nociceptive stress, and the general adaptive response. In: Everett, T., Dennis, M., Ricketts, E. (Eds.), *Physiotherapy in Mental Health: A Practical Approach.* Butterworth Heinemann, Oxford. pp. 102-126.

Woo, S., Livesay, G. A. Runco, T. J. et al. 1997 Structure and function of tendons and ligaments. In: Mow, V. C., Hayes, W. C. (Eds.), *Basic Orthopaedic Biomechanics.* Lippincott-Raven, Philadelphia, PA. pp. 209-252.

Wood Jones, F. 1944 *Structure and Function as Seen in the Foot.* Baillière, Tindall and Cox, London.

Yahia, L., Rhalmi, S., Newman, N., et al. 1992 Sensory innervation of human thoracolumbar fascia. An immunohistochemical study. *Acta Orthop Scand* 63:195-197.

Yu, W. D., Panossian, V., Hatch, J D., et al. 2001 Combined effects of estrogen and progesterone on the anterior cruciate ligament. *Clin Orthop Relat Res* 383:268-281.

Ziche, M., Morbidelli, L. 2000 Nitric oxide and angiogenesis. *J Neurooncol* 50:139-148.

ULTRASOUND IMAGING OF FASCIA AND ITS CLINICAL IMPLICATIONS
Davide Bongiorno

Overview

Ever since its foundation, osteopathy has aimed to re-create balance starting from the movement of organs in their classical subdivisions: intrinsic, extrinsic, and their interrelation. The integration of these apparent differences has lead in time to an understanding of fascia and the connective tissue; the former being the sliding surface and the latter providing unity and structure. Ever since echography was introduced in the medical field, it has progressively enabled us to observe not only the organs 'within themselves', but also the relationship between the structures and the organs. This relationship consists of fasciae and their reciprocal movements.

Therefore, it is clear that echography, which enables us to observe tissue movements, is considered to be a very useful 'osteopathic' tool (Syperda et al., 2008).

Originally echography was used to study soft tissues and the musculoskeletal system (skin, fasciae, muscles, tendons, ligaments, joints), but its concept, dynamic specificity, and real-time imaging was progressively implemented in the osteopathic field.

The method fascial motion ultrasound anatomic evaluation (FUSAE) was an attempt to apply echographic dynamic imaging to the field of osteopathy where there was not yet a method able to evaluate and validate the techniques (Bongiorno, 2012).

This chapter will examine the application of echography with the aim of achieving an osteopathic diagnosis, evaluating the results and understanding the causes of pain in the human body.

Introduction

Echography is a diagnostic method that developed rapidly in the musculoskeletal and myofascial field (van Holsbeeck et al., 2001; Lefebvre et al., 1991). It has unique advantages in that it is possible to orientate the ultrasound beam to obtain more specific scans. It also enables 'real-time' imaging, leading to the diffusion of this method, differentiating it from or integrating it with magnetic resonance imaging (MRI) (Sernik & Cerri, 2009). This should not mislead anyone into considering it an easy method to use, as three-dimensional anatomical reconstruction from a plane image is difficult to reproduce (Curry & Tempkin, 1995). It is difficult to recreate topographic relationships (Testut & Jacob, 1904), from anatomical dissections either on cadavers or surgically, as echographic ones (Barozzi et al., 1998). The operator, as well as having clinical experience, should also have an awareness of the limitations of ultrasound (US).

Echography is used in the study of soft tissues to identify palpable formations (Carra et al., 2014). In medical practice, the concept that the ultrasound scanner is becoming the new phonendoscope is well-known. Echography, not only as a diagnostic tool but also as a feedback tool, is finding its role even in the field of classical medicine, among general practitioners. In this chapter, we use it specifically to demonstrate its interest to manual medicine (Whittaker et al., 2007) and its techniques (Luomala et al., 2014). We should also consider that echography results in a method of imaging that is extremely useful in cases that require 'natural' validations, such as tissue changes in the structure/function relationship (Stecco et al., 2014), or to define relationships with other close and deep tissues (Tozzi et al., 2011; Tozzi et al., 2012). I have changed the latter from its surgical aspect, used to estimate what will be the amplitude of the incision on the skin to remove the lesion, to apply it the fascial osteopathic aspect, including myofascial and visceral fascia. In this chapter I will attempt to clarify the role of echography, starting with a physical description of ultrasound, which is fundamental for understanding what anyone 'should' see and what anyone 'can' see with this diagnostic imaging method (Monetti, 2009). I will attempt to highlight the specific qualities of ultrasound and the reason why in the fascial osteopathic field it deserves a place among imaging tools. These qualities are new to osteopathic diagnosis of primary functional alterations, which find in osteopathy a therapeutic relief.

Basic physical mechanisms of ultrasound imaging

The physics of ultrasound is a topic used to recognize its limits and therefore the possibilities of application. Anyone with basic knowledge can 'read' pixels, the elementary units of an image, permitting them to understand the difference between a clinical artefact that is valid and correct and an erroneous one, even if the majority of ultrasound technicians have always declared that 'echography is in reality an artefact!' (Oliva, 1989).

Echographic imaging is realistic but not real, and this should always be considered when anyone is using this tool.

Generally, the first chapters of echographic textbooks have been devoted to the physics of ultrasound (Sasso, 2002; Stramare, 2006). Even if they were all elements converted automatically into 'images' by the scanner, the characteristics of ultrasound, with specific frequencies used to achieve a diagnosis, should be understood because awareness of them allows the user to recognize their limits and to use the characteristics in diagnostic, pathological, or anatomical physiological imaging.

The modality of energy diffusion, in the form of waves, is differentiated as electromagnetic and mechanical. In these, there is the sound. The sound, generating elastic forces, does not diffuse into an empty space but, as a mechanical wave, induces a periodical vibratory movement (period of wave, length of wave, or frequency) of the molecules within matter. Ultrasound has frequencies higher than the upper audible limit (20 kHz) and in medicine it has a frequency value of between 2.5 and 20 MHz. Body

tissues have different molecular structures. This leads to a different and peculiar resistance to the vibration used by ultrasound. The velocity of diffusion of sound depends on the matter that is crossed over. Biological tissues are made up of water, therefore the sound will have a velocity that will oscillate just around the value of 1520 m/s (Stramare et al., 2010). Differences in velocity are related to the quantity of water contained in different tissues: the sound will have a different velocity when it passes over blood, adipose tissue, and bone. When the sound crosses over a tissue it will find a different resistance to its diffusion proportional to a fundamental dimension in echography: the acoustic impedance. Therefore, because of the differences in the acoustic impedance of tissues, the operator can 'see' and distinguish with echography blood from adipose tissue or bone (Table 30.1).

The sound diffuses with different modalities in the space according to the dimension of the source and the values of the length of the waves (frequency). If the acoustic source is bigger than the length of waves, the sound will naturally be collimated and it will become a band that could be orientated by the operator in a

Transmitting substance	Speed of sound (m/sec)	Acoustic impedance
Air	331	0.0004
Fat	1.45	1.38
Water	1.54	1.54
Blood	1.57	1.61
Muscle	1.585	1.70
Cortical bone	4.08	7.8

Table 30.1

The different sound-transmission velocities and the relative 'resistance' to the passage of the sound itself in several different biological structures belonging to our organism and present in our organs (i.e., in a muscle the differentiation of a polymorphic structure depends on the different acoustic impedance of the tissues within it: fat, water, blood, muscle)

specific direction. This is what happens with ultrasound used in diagnostic echography. When an ultrasound band is oriented on a surface, part of the energy is reflexed, partly creating a wave that goes back and is partly transmitted. The first wave that goes back is known as *echo*, while the one that is transmitted will carry on in deep tissues. The greater the acoustic impedance in the tissue, the greater the reflexion will be. This is clear when observing calculi, for example, within the gall bladder or bones.

As with the physics applicable to the principles of optics, there are different modalities of reflexion that are directly related to the angle to which the ultrasound band reproduces on a surface, and secondarily, to the characteristics of the surface itself:

1. *Specular reflexion:* for example, when used with the diaphragmatic surface. This surface is bigger than the length of wave used, so the echo will be entirely reflected toward the source due to its perpendicular position.

2. *Refraction:* when the incidence is not perpendicular to the surface. As in the case of the diaphragm, which is located deeper than the liver (when it is seen from the bottom), where its central part is hyperechoic, whereas the rest of it is less visible. This happens due to the more lateral location of the parts at the central point; they are not perpendicular and therefore only a little part of the reflected wave will go back to the source.

3. *Diffusion:* when the biological structures are smaller than the wavelengths used in echography. The scattering phenomenon will emerge where the energy is sent everywhere and therefore the energy that comes back to the transducer will obviously be very low. The scattering will give life to the parenchymal images, for example, images of the liver, thyroid, or prostate. The degree of scattering of a parenchyma depends on the number and the greatness of the particles crossed over by the ultrasound. The ultrasound will diffuse via these tissues, from outer to inner, progressively reducing its potency.

The reduction depends on these phenomena, and depends even more on the absorption caused by the energy transferred to the single particles. This explains the reason why you can use probes at low frequencies when analyzing deep structures and at high frequencies when evaluating more superficial structures (transverse fascia, muscular fasciae).

We should now consider that when you use an ultrasound probe, you should obtain the 'piezoelectric effect'. This is an effect by which some materials, stimulated by electric energy, can vibrate but also convert the vibration into electrical energy. This effect allows the echographic probe to send and receive the comeback signal at the same time. By converting the entrance signal into an electrical signal it can then be converted into a video signal known as echographic imaging.

Transducers are subdivided into those used for mechanical scans and those used for electrical scans. The sectorial mechanical probes are made up of a single piezoelectric element that oscillates at high velocity, moved by a small electrical source. Mechanical probes are not used any more. Electrical probes, which are modern and more malleable, are now used instead. There are two different shapes:

1. *Linear probes:* in which crystals are attached to each other to form a linear series to a rectangular surface (linear probe to evaluate superficial echography). These probes normally have frequencies between 7.5–15 MHz and are used to study the more superficial structures.

2. *Convex probes:* when the transducer is made up of a curvilinear alignment of crystals. These probes normally have frequencies of between 3.5–6 MHz and are used for studying the deeper structures.

To summarize, there are five concepts of echography that are important in this chapter:

1. The reflexed sound (echo) changes with angle of incidence.

2. When the angle of incidence is 90°, the reflexed wave is identical to the released wave.

3. The echographic image is made up of fundamental elements (pixels). The images in gray (usually 256 levels of gray) are produced by reflexed echo (sound wave) that turns back to the transducer as fundamental elements that vary in brilliance proportionally to the echo intensity.

4. The time between the origin or the departure of sound and its return to the transducer defines the distance of the observed object from its source (echographic probe). This will enhance position and distance on the screen. This highlights the standard echographic image in which from top to bottom there will be respectively objects very close to or very far away from the echographic surface, which will match to the crystals within the probe. The image we see in echography is conditioned by the probe position in relation to the observed object.

5. The echographic image is specular. This means that the left of the reproduced image will correspond to the right-hand side of the patient or of the investigated object, and the right will correspond to the left. This happens when the probe is transversal to the longitudinal axis perpendicular to the organ. For example, in the liver with a transversal scan you can obtain an image that reproduces to the left, the right lobe; and to the right, the left lobe. The same will happen to structures within the organ itself (Fig. 30.1). When the probe is turned,

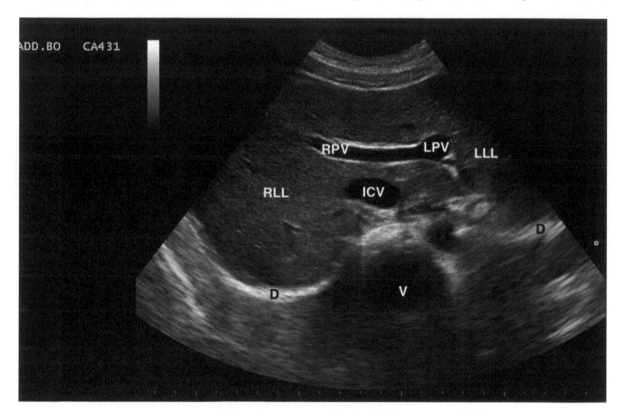

Figure 30.1

A transverse view of the liver. On the left is the (hyperechoic) white arcuate line that shows the right dome of the diaphragm (**D**) with the right lobe of the liver (**RLL**) adjacent to its concave surface. The lower of the two anechoic (black) structures is the retrohepatic inferior vena cava (**IVC**) and the anechoic horizontal structure shows the position of the two portal branches (**LPV**, left portal vein and **RPV**, right portal vein branches). **V** represents a lumbar vertebra and on the right side of the picture you can see a hyperechoic concave image that represents the left diaphragmatic dome (**D**) and anteriorly part of the left lobe of the liver (**LLL**). In the transverse image on the left you can see the structure of the right-hand side and on the right the visceral structures of the left-hand side with a clockwise movement, to achieve a vertical scan, the crystals will lie as if at the top there are cranial regions and at the bottom caudal regions, as if in the image the subject has the head to the left and the feet to the right. In the echographic image we can see that the superior pole of the kidney is lying on the left side of the image while the inferior pole is displayed on the right (Fig. 30.2).

In over 30 years of use, there has never been any scientific evidence of problems relating to the execution of echography on tissues or any contraindications (note: caution is recommended for the use of echo Doppler evaluation during the first 10 weeks of pregnancy). Furthermore, the modern machines are made up of systems

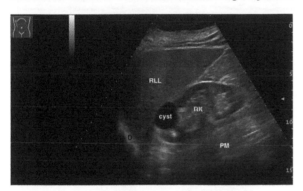

Figure 30.2

A vertical section after the probe was turned clockwise. Therefore, on the left you can see the diaphragm (**D**), the right lobe of the liver (**RLL**) and the right kidney (**RK**) that presents a cortical cystic formation (cyst) at its cranial or superior third anterolateral portion: superior because it belongs to the half of the left organ and anterolateral because it is close to the probe surface and located anterolaterally. Furthermore, it has contact with the hepatorenal border, or Morison's pouch, which is the space between the peritoneal and retroperitoneal cavity. **PM** indicates the typical longitudinal fibril structure of the psoas (on the right) on which the kidney lies and slides during respiration. You can find a cortical cystic formation at the superior third lateral portion

that allow the operator to choose the modality of use that has the least energy emission. The mechanical index (MI) indicates the pressure of ultrasound waves on tissues. The indication to use echography uses the ALARA concept ('as low as reasonably achievable'). This is used to obtain the maximal diagnostic information with the minimal exposure using echography properly. The right use of echography relies on indications established by the consensus conferences and by guidelines (SIUMB, 2005; SIUMB, 2009).

There are some limitations to the method, which cannot be mentioned, that give us a real sense and value of the information obtained with echography:

- *Tissue-related:* The properties of some body structures (e.g., skull, colon) make them inaccessible to US screening.

- *Method-related:* The possibility of scanning all planes prevents any standardization of distance measurements.

- *Examiner-related:* Because of human margins of error, it is almost impossible to reproduce two images, *pre* and *post*, at the same plane and angulation.

- *Patient-related:* Position, breathing, tissue mobility, and viscoelastic changes are all variables that might influence US screening (SIUMB, 2005; SIUMB, 2009).

Description of fascial stratification through US imaging

In soft tissues you can find all the structures related to connective tissue, by which one can understand the connective tissue proper. It is divided into two subclasses: loose connective tissue and dense or compact connective tissue.

1. Loose connective tissue:

    - loose
    - special
        - mucous tissue
        - elastic tissue
        - reticular tissue
        - adipose tissue
        - pigmented tissue.

2. Dense connective tissue:

- irregular compact

- regular compact (tendons, ligaments, and aponeurosis).

One needs to remember that echographic imaging is not histological imaging. You should firstly observe that when you apply the echographic probe on the skin, what you can see is a stratification of tissues on parallel axes.

From outer to inner one can distinguish three axes:

- superficial axis (the skin)

- intermediate axis (fascia superficialis and aponeurosis)

- deep axis (reciprocal tension membranes).

The skin is divided into epidermis, dermis (superficial, medium and deep), and hypodermis in which loose fascia and adipose lobes are found. Below these, on the intermediate axis, one can find the fascia superficialis. The latter is linked to the superficial aponeurosis via the dense pars with some characteristic lobes, but with a greater connective component. Even below this, there is the medium aponeurosis that divides at the neck into the two infrahyoid muscles:

- at the superficial level for the omohyoid and sternocleidomastoid muscles

- deep anteriorly at the level of the thyroid (Fig. 30.3).

Even deeper one can find the deep aponeurosis axis that inferiorly forms the vascular sheath of the neck, continuing at the abdominal level with the fascia proper. And even deeper there are muscular fasciae; connective and muscular stratifications; and bones (if present).

Oblique lines are associated with the parallel stratification of fasciae, especially at the level of the subcutaneous layer that represents a 'better' control of the longitudinal gliding between fascial elements, improving their resistance to physical stresses during body movements. These stratifications form fairly thick laminar elements from outer to inner. On the abdomen one can notice an 'expansion' in

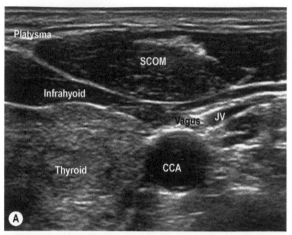

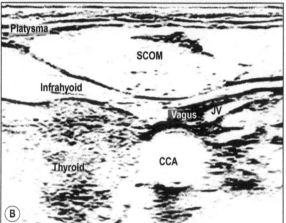

Figure 30.3

These (**A**) positive and (**B**) negative images are from a transverse scan of the anterior portion of the left side of the neck. The probe is linear, as you can see from the superior line of crystals that are 'straight.' Moving from the outer to the inner regions, the image contains the following structures: superficial tissues such as the platysma; the sternocleido-occipital-mastoid muscle (SCOM); the sternothyroid and sternohyoid muscles (Infrahyoid); the anterior common carotid artery (CCA); the jugular vein (JV); the hypogastric vagus nerve (Vagus); and the left lobe of the thyroid (Thyroid). The thin line separating the muscle portion from the vascular–nervous band of the neck is the medial cervical fascia

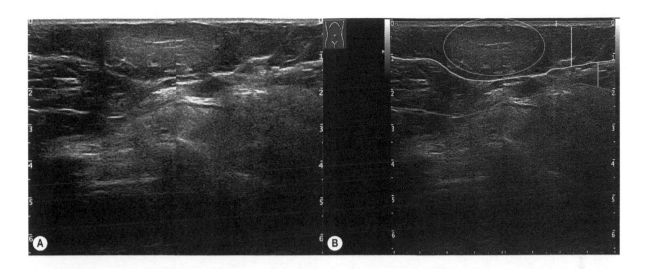

Figure 30.4

These scans of the anterior abdominal wall show the layers, outer to inner, that make up the superficial soft tissues from the epidermis to the hypodermis, to the ventral fascia of the muscles of the abdominal wall. In these images you can see a more echoic formation that is a superficial fibrolypoma, indicated by the oval drawn around it in (**B**). In the oval there are parallel fibrous striae, which contrast with the adjacent adipose area where connective fasciae all lie in the same direction. As you can see, the fasciae lie in the most superficial layer of the hypodermis leading to an invagination of the hyperechoic thin line (between the yellow and purple lines) that is the fascia superficialis. The purple line represents the deep adipose layer that lies on the abdominal muscles

the subcutaneous adipose tissue that shows deformities. The superficial fascia subdivides the hypodermis into two, maintaining its continuity. In the following image, its positive expression (Fig. 30.4) and its negative expression (Fig. 30.5) demonstrate the precise distinction of the main layers.

The secondary layers, the perpendicular and transversal ones, are thin due to their position. If one applies the echographic probe on superficial tissues, such as at the medial third of the anterior compartment of the thigh (rectus femoris muscle), and gradually presses with the probe one can see that the subcutaneous layer, the hypodermis, and the fascia superficialis that divides the hypodermis into two layers maintain their position and relationship. Other structures (such as the rectus femoris muscle) change their thickness, position, angle, and length uninfluenced by forces and glide laterally compared to the force vector that is used (Fig. 30.6).

One should notice that some combinations will emerge maintaining the same direction even when the stimuli are not linear. The fasciae show 3D. The consistency and the acoustic impedance depend on

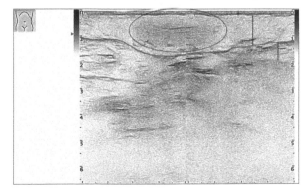

Figure 30.5

Negative image of Figure 30.4 (**B**)

the function that the connective tissue has: elastic, nervous, or adipose. Fascia does not only refer to the structures of the connective tissue, as was once thought, but also to the structures that make up the subcutaneous loose tissue, those of the deep muscular fascia, and those of internal fasciae that separate the different muscular components. There is no apparent continuity between fasciae in our body. This is the reason why we can perform echographic imaging scanning the connective structures, from outer to inner, their connective links between different structures, and their cleavage axis. The word 'cleavage' originates from the French word 'clivage', which in turn originates from the Dutch 'kliven'. It is the natural tendency of structures to separate.

Anatomic cleavage refers to gliding of different organs adjacent to one another or gliding within the same organ, between the structures of which it is made up. It represents the natural tendency to separate of structures made up of the same material that can glide on each other.

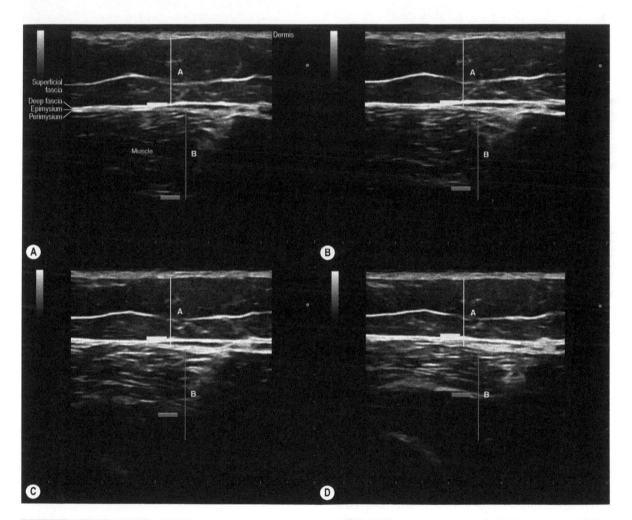

Figure 30.6
The superficial structure of soft tissues. Here the quadriceps are shown. Some fibroconnective formations are in 3D

It is important to understand that one should not consider fascial gliding and anatomical cleavage as synonyms, as one contains the other, even if they are independent. For example, the pulmonary lobes have correspondent anatomical cleavage axes, without a complete fascial gliding to belong to the same anatomical/functional organ. The relations between fasciae, their histological components, and biochemical characteristics (Stecco et al., 2011) are the leading factors in the comprehension of relative movements among connective tissues and their macroscopic characteristics in echographic imaging.

Ultrasound imaging and features of fascial dysfunction

The difficulty in observing fasciae with echography, in particular their mobility, is primarily because their parallel position does not allow us to quantify the distance travelled by horizontal gliding.

It is, however, possible to evaluate any variation in thickness of some fasciae, such as the thoracolumbar fascia (Langevin et al., 2009) and of other fasciae of the neck (Stecco et al., 2014) or fasciae of the upper limb (Stecco et al., 2009).

Any variation in thickness is measured in millimeters. When movement is involved, pixels, as the elementary unit of an image, cannot be used to quantify a movement in the horizontal axis (parallel to the crystals within a probe) unless a 'discrete' element, measurable itself, is measured. The latter is possible when there is an irregularity or thickness of fascia that could be expressed in millimeters from its starting point A to its arrival point B (range of linear movement). This is the case when fascial movement is observable compared to a neutral point, at rest, with oscillations in plus or minus.

Recently some quantifying attempts have been performed (Ichikawa et al., 2013), introducing a concept of tissue distortion in which a fascial distance X is measured at a distance X + t after inducing tension with an attempt to standardize the size of lengthening (in this specific work flexion of the inferior limb from 0 degrees to 45 degrees has been used). The quantitative measurement of distortion in lengthening results is easy to detect as it is visible throughout the external rotation of the adducted humerus (Fig. 30.7). It is more difficult to detect when quantitative data relating to gliding between parallel axes is obtained. In this instance, you should rely on direct *qualitative* observation of reciprocal movement between structures and organs that are related to each other.

As echography is universally recognized as a fundamental method in the study of musculotendinous

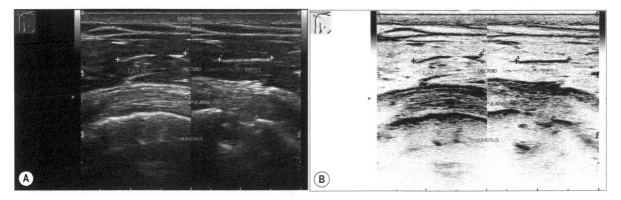

Figure 30.7

In these (A) positive and (B) negative images you can see, from the outer to the inner layers: the epidermis, the hypodermis, the deltoid muscle, the subscapular tendon, and the head of the humerus. In (REST) position you can see a hyperechoic structure within the deltoid muscle that is the endomysium. After an external rotation (EXT ROT) you can see its plastic displacement

structures and of their *quantitative* evaluation, it is well-known especially among echographers that the most common problem is linked to the limited documented *qualitative* results, taking into account the therapeutic pharmacological, physical, or manipulative results. To overcome this dichotomy, it is essential to introduce elastosonographic techniques (Monetti et al., 2012). Some operators who have already started to use these techniques have achieved results, even though the evaluation process applied to superficial fascial structures has only recently been established (Luomala et al., 2014).

In the study of deep fascial movements (focusing on specific viscerofascial relationships obtained by observing kidney movement) gliding is analyzed, following in real time the position between the different pixels that make up the three structures and their reciprocal movements, throughout the physiological movements between the liver and the kidney or between the kidney and the psoas (Tozzi et al., 2012). This valuation has been predominantly qualitative. Its quantification is obtained by measuring the distance between the superior kidney pole and the diaphragm.

Qualitative valuation could be used in observation of gliding among superficial fasciae or between the skin or subcutaneously. The qualitative aspect does not determine any limitation, but it defines an element of valuation in which the numeric value is referred not to a unit of measure of 'space' or of 'time' or a result between the two (velocity), but only 'discrete' values varying from 'present' to 'absent' gradually (i.e., nothing, not good, medium, high). In several works by this author and colleagues (Tozzi et al., 2011; Tozzi et al., 2012) to better identify and standardize the results, it was decided to use two valuations: 'absent' and 'present'. To achieve a better and more detailed subdivision, cardiovascular measures of evaluation can be used to evaluate the strain of vascular structures, even if the algorithms could not be used for our studies.

The dynamic echography of fasciae (i.e., FUSAE) can help us to find and attempt to understand new typologies of somatic dysfunction of which we are not currently aware and for which we do not yet understand the dysfunctional model of correlation. The real-time observation of the kidney–fascia dynamic through fascial release techniques (Tozzi et al., 2011) or the KMI (kidney mobility index) have allowed us to highlight characteristic elements within osteopathic dysfunctions. In 2012 a study was published regarding osteopathic dysfunction in relation to operator reliability, in which echography is used as tool to control and confirm the position and the orientation of the vertebrae, subjected to palpatory tests (Shaw et al., 2012) performed by an osteopath, and then verified using an US device. In this instance the echographic aspect was not dynamic, but just positionally static (Fig. 30.8)

Echographic imaging, improving the positional concept, in relation to palpation, can confirm and clarify which are the palpable structures, either bones (i.e., transverse apophysis and vertebral apophysis), myofascial structures (i.e., sternocleidomastoid muscle [SCM] and arterial–nervous cervical fascia), or visceral structures (i.e., liver border and its movement, kidney movements).

Echographic results in the osteopathic field can be quantified by comparing:

1. The distance (position) of landmarks before treatment and their changes after treatment (for example the distance of a transverse line from the skin and its normalization after the thrust).

2. Echogenic aspects (hypoechoic/hyperechoic) of similar structures in different patients (i.e., the thoracolumbar fascia in patients with chronic lower back pain [LBP] or the shoulder bursae in patients with chronic scapulohumeral arthritis).

As shown in 1), above, the results are hard to visualize as the structures move. Therefore, the dysfunctional definitions are many, considering the restrictions in mobility. Similarly, in the case of 2), you have to consider the ultrasound and the reflexed wave characteristics (see the paragraph on the physics of ultrasound), risking the possibility of having an over- or under-stimulation of different echogenicity of tissues studied in relation to the angle of incidence, known as anisochromia (a different echogenic aspect in relation to the same structure caused by the relation

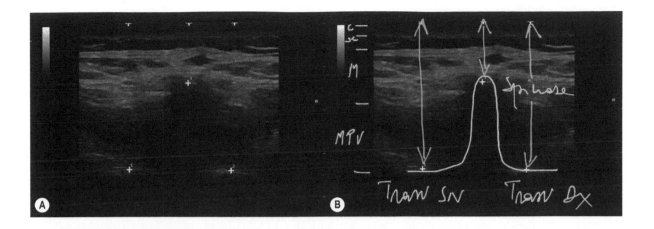

Figure 30.8

(A) Transverse scan with patient lying prone. The probe is orientated on top of the spinous process of a thoracic vertebra. In (B) you can see the structural elements and the distance between the cutaneous border and the transverse line. These images lead to the root of the transverse line at the level of the lamina. C = cutis; M = muscle; MPV = paraspinal muscles; SC = subcutaneous tissue

within the space among constitutive elements and ultrasound). Compared to fascia, scar tissue is not easy to study due to its structural alteration.

Ultrasound imaging and features of fascial tissue following osteopathic manipulative treatment

The echographic observation of fasciae relations has been used to study the correlations between dysfunctions. If we consider one of the most common traumas, for example, whiplash (Schwerla at al., 2013), in which the dysfunctional fascial component (Cisler et al., 1994) represents the element that sustains the presence of symptoms, the study and observation of the cervical viscerofascial structures demonstrates the loss of freedom of movement among different structures within the region (myofascial axis, vascular axis, visceral axis), especially in vertical gliding. When swallowing, assessment of the fascial slips by observing the transition of the pharyngo-esophageal bolus shows that the bolus transition improves after osteopathic treatment. The observation (Fig. 30.9) is focused on the prevertebral fascia (deep cervical fascia) compared to the esophagus (retrovisceral space) and of the latter compared to the perithyroidal fascia or capsule proper.

Real-time observation of the quality of the movements induced by respiration and deglutition confirmed the improvement after osteopathic manipulative treatment in some people suffering with whiplash, both in the quality of movement and in the deglutition. To obtain even better feedback, the time taken by the bolus from pharyngo-esophageal deglutition to the cardio-esophageal junction was recorded. The physiological time taken by the bolus is 7 seconds, so when it is longer than 11 seconds it reveals nonspecific dysphagic aspects.

Why did we use the bolus? Its structural characteristic of mixing liquids and microbubbles of air shows a better 'resonance' when studied with ultrasound and it allows a better visualization even when the bolus is small (Fig. 30.10).

In cases of atypical or nonspecific LBP (not of musculoskeletal origin), many echographic examinations have been carried out to study the 'position' of the kidneys from the 'superficial' to the deep slips. Among the visceral causes of LBP, the kidney position is considered a fundamental element (Tilscher et al., 1977; Schäfer et al., 2013; Lau et al., 2013). The 'osteopathic' observation of fascial slips indicates that kidney position is not the cause of LBP,

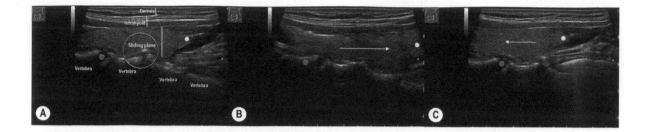

Figure 30.9

This vertical scan was taken using a linear probe at high frequency on the left lobe of the thyroid. The visible structures, from the outer to the inner layers, are: the superficial tissues (epidermis, hypodermis, platysma), the infrahyoid muscular layer, the thyroid gland, and the vertebral column with some cervical vertebrae. On the 'magnifying glass' you can identify the sliding axis between the thyroid and the deep cervical fascia. (A) At rest you can see the structures and the purple dot indicating the anterior border between two cervical vertebrae. The yellow dot represents the inferior lobe of the thyroid. (B) The distance between the purple and yellow dots increases due to the caudal slide of the gland during the first phase of deglutition on the posterior vertical axis. (C) The distance between the purple and yellow dots is reduced to allow cranial sliding during the second phase of deglutition

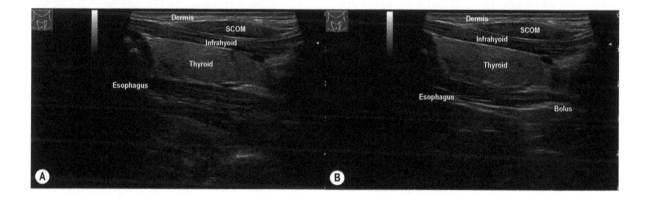

Figure 30.10

This image was obtained with a linear probe at high frequency vertically on the left lobe of the thyroid. The visible structures, from the outer to the inner layers, are: superficial tissues, part of the SCM, part of the infrahyoid muscle, the thyroid gland, the cervical esophagus (the visible part is from the pharyngo-esophageal junction at the left of the picture to the inferior portion of the supraclavicular axis). Posteriorly you can see the vertebral column. If you observe the esophagus at rest (A) and then after the transit of saliva (B) you can identify the presence of the passage of the bolus in the third distal portion of the cervical esophagus throughout the active deglutition. When dysphagia occurs, as shown, the spatial and topographic relationships between the structures are relatively 'fixed' – you can see the invariability of the relationships between the SCM/muscles/thyroid – and this ensures that the passage of the bolus does not interfere with these relationships (see Fig. 30.9) but the loss of sliding is. For example, in the case of a kidney in ptosis, in line with the old medical terminology, but mobile during respiration (induced by the diaphragm), the patient would not have suffered typical LBP; he would have suffered with it if the kidney had been immobile. A published study (Tozzi et al., 2012) revealed that the typology of movement by the kidney (fixed, mobile) had a significant statistical correspondence and a different percentage in the presence of LBP.

Recently, other studies (Stecco et al., 2014) demonstrated a significant correspondence and a validity of echographic imaging in the observation of 'the fascial thickness of the sternal ending of the sternocleidomastoid and medical scalene muscles' and of the 'significant differences between healthy subjects and patients with CNP in the thickness of the upper side of the sternocleidomastoid fascia and the lower and upper sides of the right scalene fascia'.

In a study led by Blanquet in 2010, echographic imaging of the thoracolumbar fascia in patients with LBP, as shown already in Langevin's studies, reveals a thickness and specific aspects of collagen that changes before and after a spinal manipulation. Even Pohl in 2010 confirmed in his study that there could have been changes in the distribution of collagen fibres in the skin after manual treatment.

The usage of elastosonography (Monetti et al., 2012; Langevin et al., 2011) surely confirms the data. In a recent study Glaser et al. (2012) highlighted a new technology that unites elastosonographic algorithms with MRI. This new imaging technology, known as magnetic resonance elastography (MRE), could add new characteristics even in the study of musculoskeletal components and in particular in the study of viscoelastic characteristics in healthy and unhealthy patients.

Comparing MRI with elastosonography (Seo et al., 2014) in the study of fatty muscle degeneration (in this case the supraspinatus) revealed a strict correlation of the two methods and confirmed, in particular, that elastosonography is very important in quantitative evaluation, having either a great diagnostic precision or an excellent correlation with MRI and US.

Clinical implications

Clinical implications are a double diagnostic and therapeutic focalization. Observing fascial dynamics in subjects with rotator cuff syndrome, with negative echographic structural results (tendinitis, calcifications, bursitis, lesions), the dynamic echographic imaging of fasciae allow the introduction of two fundamental functional concepts in obtaining a classification (a 'grading'), prior to the anatomical and pathological assessment, where the tissue damage has already happened. For this reason, by using echographic fascial tests focused on the gliding between the rotator cuff and the space underneath the deltoid muscle throughout active and passive movements in external and internal rotation (rather than the study of the subacromial space in abduction) you can obtain qualitative and quantitative data in the diagnosis and the subsequent therapy. In the case of frozen shoulder or in 'painful shoulders' it is very difficult to obtain diagnostic confirmation (Bongiorno, 2013).

The following are examples of when dynamic observation of fascia could be useful:

• If in dynamic external rotation of the humerus, from a neutral sagittal position, a fast usage of connective and muscular fibers of the deltoid muscle (endomysium) is found. This represents a functional deficit prior to the clinical diagnosis of 'frozen shoulder' in orthopedic tests.

• If when passing from adduction to abduction the movement of the head of the humerus shows a rotation that prevents inferior gliding from happening. The superior position of the humerus leads to a dynamic functional conflict without necessarily the presence of alterations of the inferior acromion preventing any clinical sign of injury, such as the structural damage of the rotator cuff during impingement.

Recently echography has been used to verify osteopathic tests in studies validating osteopathic reliability; even if the investigation was carried out with static imaging because the dynamic 'real-time' evaluation was difficult to execute and not useful to obtain.

Even in the study of anatomy, echographic imaging results can be of great use, especially in the study of deep organs and visceral structures. The most significant example is the pancreas and the vascular structures related to it (the superior mesenteric artery), recognized topographically and with their dynamics during respiration.

Dynamics can illustrate the plastic abilities of vascular structures organized as fascial elements that unite viscera to structure (for example, the relation between the aorta and lumbar arteries and between the latter and the kidneys via renal arteries). The fascial dynamics that can be evaluated via echography correspond to the need in osteopathy to understand and explain the integration of macroarticular, fascial, and visceral environments. It is clear that the central point (fascia) is the most important element of unity between the three environments. Fascia is often evaluated statistically and dynamically, as shown in quantitative aspects, in the analysis of its thickness and in its echogenic characteristics, but less in the qualitative ones where it acts as a topographic element responsible for the gliding between adjacent structures. By focusing on a different area, one can distinguish and assign to each part specific examples:

1. articular and periarticular mobility (soft tissues)
2. scar tissues and fascial density
3. visceral or 'deep' gliding.

In example 1) in a dysfunctional shoulder, fascial and connective tissue stretching visible as endomysium in the deltoid muscle is evident in dysfunctions that can lead to or identify as 'frozen shoulder' (see Fig. 30.7). In example 2), the scar shows tissue changes in their structural alignment and it highlights an evident echogenicity due to an increase in the fibrous component (Fig. 30.11). In example 3) the movements at the kidney on the right-hand side are different due to 'mobility restrictions.' One can differentiate three types: total fixation (V/V/S), structural (V/S), and visceral (V/V).

The aspect that confirms the clinical validity of echographic imaging results is the one in which, even though there is myofascial symptomatology, anomalies, or

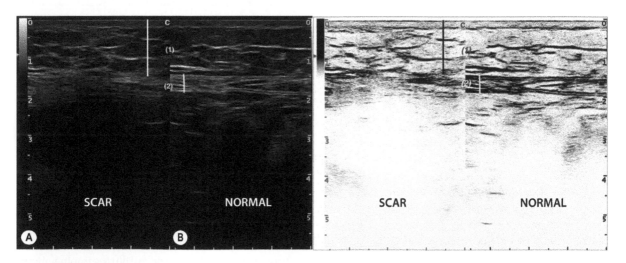

Figure 30.11
This image is obtained by scanning the right hypochondria in a patient who had a right subcostal laparotomy due to cholecystitis. (A) shows 'scarring' and (B) represents the same contralateral area. In (B) you can see a hyperechoic area in the adipose thickening (**1**) with a thin reconstruction of the deep myofascial structures (**2**) without recognizing an adherence of the parietal peritoneum and the adjacent ansa. The image in negative shows a change in the deep fascial structures (muscular aponeurosis, anterior and posterior muscular fascia, and parietal peritoneum) while the thin connective structures in the adipose tissue are similar on both sides

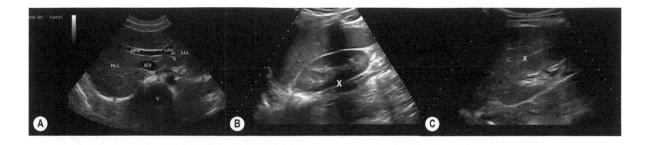

Figure 30.12

This image shows the different level of gliding fixation (**X**). In (A) there is total fixation on both the plane between the liver and the kidney and the plane between the kidney and the psoas muscle. In (B) and (C) only one of the aforementioned planes is free, while the other is fixed

pathologies, themselves contraindications to the manipulation, are identified. One example could be an acute gall bladder osteopathically related to a diminished diaphragmatic dynamic associated with pain (activation of the peritoneum/posterior fascia of the abdominal muscles) either via neurologic connections with the vagus nerve and/or the phrenic nerve. The regional pain, either anterior or posterior at the level of the diaphragm, is linked to the presence of the phrenic nerve at the level of the lung in the supra-retroclavicular fossa. Another example could be pain related to abdominal aortic aneurysms, in which the relation of the periaortic plexus and direct connections with the retroperitoneal fasciae can often lead initially to posterior pain (i.e., LBP).

Conclusion

Echographic imaging with its dynamic implications is of great help not only in the evaluation of structural elements that are fundamental to comprehending the anatomical complexity of living organisms, but also in their qualitative differences among symptomatic and nonsymptomatic patients, the dysfunctional and the nondysfunctional, leading to their becoming predicted elements of pathologies (Harris-Love et al., 2014). There has never been a better time for osteopathy and other manual therapies that focus on fascia to integrate their methods with scientific research. The author understands that these topics may seem 'old' at the time of reading, considering the speed of technological evolution, but, as teachers who contributed to the author's knowledge in echographic clinical medicine thought, only by knowing the past can one improve the future.

References and further reading

Barozzi L., Busilacchi P., Pavlica P. et al. 1998 *Anatomia Ecografica*. Casa Editrice Idelson–Gnocchi s.r.l., Napoli.

Bongiorno D. 2012 Esempi di anatomia dinamica – F.U.S.A.E. (Fascial Motion Ultrasonographic Anatomic Evaluation). Available at: http://www.davidebongiorno.com/esempi-di-anatomia-dinamica-f·u-s-e/ [accessed April 17 2016].

Bongiorno D. 2013 Lo studio della mobilità fasciale nella valutazione dello spazio sub-acromiale (F.U.S.A.E.): nuova prospettiva per la diagnosi nelle algie disfunzionali di spalla. Presented at the XXIV Congresso Nazionale – SIUMB. Rome., November 15–19, 2013.

Cisler T. A. 1994 Whiplash as a total-body injury. *J Am Osteopath Assoc* 94:145–148.

Carra B. J., Bui-Mansfield L. T., O'Brien S. D., Chen D. C. 2014 Sonography of musculoskeletal soft-tissue masses: techniques, pearls, and pitfalls. *Am J Roentgenol* 202:1281–1290.

Curry R. A., Tempkin B. B. 1995 Anatomy layering and sectional anatomy. In: Curry R. A., Tempkin B. B. *Exercises in Ultrasonography: An Introduction to Normal Structure and Functional Anatomy*. Saunders. pp. 27–62.

Glaser K. J., Manduca A., Ehman R. L. 2012 Review of MR elastography applications and recent developments. *J Magn Reson Imaging* 36:757–774.

Harris-Love M. O., Monfaredi R., Ismail C. et al., 2014 Quantitative ultrasound: measurement considerations for the assessment of muscular dystrophy and sarcopenia. *Front Aging Neurosci* 6:1–3.

Ichikawa K., Usa H., Ogawa D. et al. 2013 The reliability of displacement measurement of the deep fascia using ultrasonographic imaging. *J Jpn Health Sci* 16:21–28.

Langevin H. M., Stevens-Tuttle D., Fox J. R. et al. 2009 Ultrasound evidence of altered lumbar connective tissue structure in human subjects with chronic low back pain. *BMC Musculoskelet Disord* 3:151.

Langevin H. M., Fox J. R., Koptiuch C. et al. 2011 Reduced thoracolumbar fascia shear strain in human chronic low back pain. *BMC Musculoskelet Disord* 19:203.

Lau T., Weinstein M., Wakamatsu M. et al. 2013 Low back pain does not improve with surgical treatment of pelvic organ prolapse. *Int Urogynecol J* 24:147–153.

Lefebvre E., Pourcelol L. 1991 *Ecografia Muscolo-Tendinea – Collana di Diagnostica per Immagini.* Editore Masson, Milano.

Luomala T., Pihlman M., Heiskanen J. et al. 2014 Case study: could ultrasound and elastography visualized densified areas inside the deep fascia? *J Bodyw Mov Ther* 18:462–468.

Monetti G. 2009 Semeiotica. In: *Ecografia Muscolo-Scheletrica. Vol. 1. Tecnica, Anatomia e Imaging Integrato.* 1st edition. Timeo Editore, Rastignano, Bologna. pp. 53–147.

Monetti G., Minafra P., Pruna R. et al. 2012 Musculoskeletal system. In: Calliada F., Canepari M., Ferraioli G. et al. *Sono-Elastography: Main Clinical Applications.* EDIMES, Pavia. pp.91–100.

Oliva L. 1989 *Gli Artefatti in Ecotomografia.* Editore Masson, Milano. pp. 1–6.

Pohl H. 2010 Changes in the structure of collagen distribution in the skin caused by a manual technique. *J Bodyw Mov Ther* 14:27–34.

Sasso A. 2002 Cap. 1 Fisica degli Ultrasuoni. In: Bazzocchi M., *Ecografia.* 2nd edition, Vol. 1. Casa Editrice Idelson– Gnocchi s.r.l., Napoli. pp. 3–17.

Schäfer A., Gärtner-Tschacher N., Schöttker-Königer T. 2013 Subgroup-specific therapy of low back pain: description and validity of two classification systems. *Orthopade* 42:90–99.

Schwerla F., Kaiser A. K., Gietz R. et al. 2013 Osteopathic treatment of patients with longterm sequelae of whiplash injury: effect on neck pain disability and quality of life. *J Altern Complement Med* 19:543–549.

Seo J. B., Yoo J. S., Ryu J. W. 2014 The accuracy of sonoelastography in fatty degeneration of the supraspinatus: a comparison of magnetic resonance imaging and conventional ultrasonography. *J Ultrasound* 17:279–285.

Sernik R. A., Cerri G. G. 2009. *Ultrasonografia del Sistema Muscoloscheletrico – Correlazione con la Risonanza Magnetica.* Casa Editrice Piccin, Padova. pp. 1–3.

Shaw K. A., Dougherty J. J., Treffer K. D., Glaros A. G. 2012 Establishing the content validity of palpatory examination for the assessment of the lumbar spine using ultrasonography: a pilot study. *J AM Osteopath Assoc* 112:775–782.

SIUMB 2005 Documento SIUMB per le Linee Guida in Ecografia. *Giornale Italiano di Ecografia.* SIUMB Editore. Vol. 8, n. 4.

SIUMB. 2009 XXI Congresso Nazionale. Standard per una corretta esecuzione dell'esame ecografico. *J Ultrasound* Special Issue 2009.

Stecco A., Macchi V. Stecco, C. et al. 2009 Anatomical study of myofascial continuity in the anterior region of the upper limb. *J Bodyw Mov Ther* 13:53–62.

Stecco C., Stern R., Porzionato A. el al. 2011 Hyaluronan within fascia in the etiology of myofascial pain. *Surg Radiol Anat* 33:891–896.

Stecco A., Meneghini A., Stern R. et al. 2014 Ultrasonography in myofascial neck pain: randomized clinical trial for diagnosis and follow-up. *Surg Radiol Anat* 36:243–253.

Stramare R., SIUMB 2010 Sillabus, Corso Teorico di Formazione in Ultrasonologia. XXII Congresso Nazionale. November. pp. 7–14.

Stramare R., Dorigo A., Velgos F. el al. 2006 Fisica degli ultrasuoni. In: Busilacchi P., Rapaccini G. L. *Ecografia Clinica. Vol. 1.* Casa Editrice Idelson– Gnocchi s.r.l., Napoli, pp. 9-27.

Syperda V. A., Trivedi P. N., Melo L. C. et al. 2008 Ultrasonography in preclinical education: a pilot study. *J Am Osteopath Assoc* 108:601–605.

Testut L., Jacob O. 1904 [1987] *Traité de Topographique Anatomie.* Vols 2 & 3.

II Edition. [Italian translation] UTET, Torino.

Tilscher H., Bogner G., Landsiedl F. 1977 Visceral diseases as cause of lumbar syndromes. *Z Rheumatol* 36:161–167.

Tozzi P., Bongiorno D., Vitturini C., 2011 Fascial release effects on patients with nonspecific cervical or lumbar pain. *J Bodyw Mov Ther* 15:405–416

Tozzi P., Bongiorno D., Villurini C. 2012 Low back pain and kidney mobility: local osteopathic fascial manipulation decreases pain perception and improves renal mobility. *J Bodyw Mov Ther* 16:381–391.

Van Holsbeeck, M. T., Introcaso J. H. 2001 *Musculoskeletal Ultrasound.* 2nd edition. Mosby, Inc. St Louis, Missouri. pp 9–21.

Whittaker J. L., Teyen D. S., Elliot J. M. et al. 2007 Rehabilitative ultrasound imaging: understanding the technology and its applications. *J Orthop Sports Phys Ther* 37:434–449.

MYOFASCIAL MERIDIANS IN PRACTICE

Thomas W. Myers

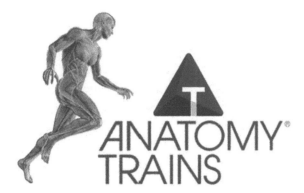

Figure 31.1
Anatomy Trains logo

Preamble: a plea to osteopaths

These are halcyon days for osteopathy! More than a century after the encompassing vision and extraordinary practice of Dr Still, the world is catching up, and osteopaths are set fair to become leaders in the field of 'spatial medicine' (Myers, 1998, 1999a, 1999b). A brief explanation of this term precedes the subject of this chapter: manipulative strategies in the parietal myofasciae. For those in no mood for overarching philosophy or a critique of osteopathic tactics, skip to the end of this preamble.

This writer is not an osteopath, but has been a friend of osteopathy since 1977, when a chain-smoking, greasy-skinned, disheveled but highly skilled osteopath in the American state of Mississippi totally surprised me by sorting my disabling 'flu' with a single elegant cervical manipulation. It was an impressive introduction to the relationship between structure and function. I was introduced to osteopathic vision and principles in 1978 during an intensive training

with Dr Ida Rolf (Rolf, 1977). To this day I regularly cross-refer to and learn from osteopaths on both sides of the Atlantic. The work we profess in our Anatomy Trains school – predominantly shifting adhesed fascial planes – could be considered as a subset of (but no replacement for) osteopathy (Myers, 2014; Earls & Myers, 2010).

Over time, my professional interests have moved away from clinical concerns – pathology or local pain relief, important as they are – to the more educational side of spatial medicine's domain: what programme of activities, exercises, or forms of attention would allow our clients (and more importantly, the next generation) to avoid the widespread pain and pathologies that result from poor body use (Alexander, 1932)?

How do proper movement and sustainable posture develop and mature (Bainbridge-Cohen, 1993)? Where does the 'natural' go wrong (Bateson, 1979)? Or are we simply outliving our joint design (Alexander, 1992)? How much body pain is simply 'mismatch' between the Paleolithic environment in which our species developed versus the self-created urban environment in which most of us live (Lieberman, 2013)? What is the minimal curriculum of movements required to develop and maintain decent biomechanics? These 'spatial medicine' questions have inspired readings in anthropology, biochemistry, developmental movement, embryology, evolutionary biology, biopsychology, and gerontology, and have involved considerable hours of observation of adults and children in a variety of cultures (Konner, 1982).

These 'better use of the self' concerns connect to a more osteopathic question: what is the relationship between intrinsic, cellular, physiological movements (motility) and outer, so-called 'voluntary' movement (mobility)? Somehow a single cell – mostly water – divides and proliferates in an organized, pulsing manner, to become not a tumor but a squalling infant, who against all odds will expand and ossify into a rebellious teenager, who despite your worst fears usually settles into a responsible adult. Considered as a purely mechanical event, the process of embryology and subsequent maturity merits the overused 'Awesome!'.

'Spatial medicine', then, is the study of how our body develops in space, moves through and manipulates the environment, and deals with the perception of inner and outer spatial relationships. We could contrast it to the medicine of Time (psychiatry and psychotherapy, with roots in shamanism), which seeks to orient its patients temporally in the present. It is also contrasts with the predominant medicine of Matter. Material medicine uses the application of matter – principally drugs, but also 'food as medicine' – to change the chemistry of the body. Material medicine so completely occupies the temple of healing at present that both psychiatry and orthopedics have been drawn into its tent to dispense its pharmaceuticals.

Temporal medicine has its Sigmund Freud, and material medicine has its William Harvey, but what of spatial medicine? A. T. Still is the closest we have to a uniting visionary, but his philosophy has yet to spread and unite the entire field. All those who change structure or teach movement lie within spatial medicine's borders – osteopaths, chiropractors, bodyworkers, yoga teachers, personal trainers, physiotherapists, rehabilitation experts, athletic coaches, physical education teachers, even orthopedists – all work in the front lines of changing shape, and the effect of shape change on the structure and function of the person. Currently, these varying fields within spatial medicine are largely isolated, using differing vocabularies, making a unified vision or even inter-profession chatter difficult (Myers & Fredricks, 2012).

This professional isolation of the various branches of spatial medicine is coming to an end with the advent of the electronic era, where the physical demands on the body have so changed from the Paleolithic or even the agricultural era that a coherent theory of human structure and movement function is urgently required – and osteopaths are uniquely positioned to articulate that coherent approach.

It is an imperative of our era that we articulate a new biomechanics that applies consistently from the molecular level to the organismic. Osteopaths are best-positioned to be heralds of coming good by combining the biotensegrity model (explored elsewhere in this volume as well as in Scarr, 2014; Levin, 2003; and Myers, 2014) coupled with the brilliant (if not yet complete) cellular biomechanics of embryology (Blechschmidt, 2004; Willard, 2012).

How does biomechanical development organize the ovum's daughters into the conductors, contractors, supporters, soldiers, and secreters that make up our neurons, muscles, connective tissues, and epithelia? How do we organize some 50 kilograms of water in a thin two-meter column? 'DNA' – the answer since Watson and Crick – has been shown to be a very unsatisfying explanation. Part of the answer lies in the self-regulating properties of gels and fibers of the connective tissue web. Cells themselves cannot organize life on land without the autoregulation in the colloidal extracellular matrix (ECM), compromising dynamically between structural resilience and the necessity for circulatory exchange among all the cells.

Biomechanics has long presumed that muscles pull linearly on tendons between attachment points, running over joints limited by bone shapes, cartilage surfaces, and restricting ligaments. 'If we can understand what each of the 600 muscles are doing in terms of vectors and levers' – or so says the theory – 'we can understand, create, and fix any movement.'

In fact, our whole idea of the body is based on this reductionist, industrial model – the heart is a pump, the lungs are bellows, the kidneys are filters, the brain is a computer, etc. – and no system is more industrially imaged and treated as a machine than the musculoskeletal system. In physical education, we persist in focusing on the industrial concepts of repetition and competition, whereas our electronified era would seem to require sensitivity, lightning reflexes, and originality in movement.

Begun by da Vinci, articulated by Newton, hallowed by Descartes, and set in stone by current textbooks (e.g., Knudsen, 2007), the industrial model of biomechanics has long ago yielded what secrets it possessed. Cracks have appeared in the paradigm – it does not apply well to embryology or high-performance sports, its math is contradicted by research in myofascial force transmission, it makes little allowance for the interaction between emotion and movement, and none for cellular and systemic resonance (Huijing, 2007; Langevin et al., 2006; Sills, 2001). As helpful as the industrial perspective on human movement has been, a more inclusive biomechanics needs its 'Einstein' to articulate a broader vision that will create a 'unified field theory' between mobility and motility.

The 'sensory nerves inform the central nervous system, which then formulates all motor response' is another biomechanical assumption that merits testing – some reactions seem too fast to be coordinated in this telephonic way (Oschman, 2003). Though no mechanism has been proposed to replace it, the unitary fascial net is a likely candidate for certain primitive but speedy forms of signaling (Stecco, 2015; Stecco, 2013). Vibrations in the fascial net are transmitted at the speed of sound (in water), nearly five times as fast as most nerves. Many osteopaths propose inherent rhythms to the fascial membranes contiguous to the organs in the dorsal and ventral cavity and reaching from them around the entire body (Sutherland, 1948; Barrall, 1983). Again, no mechanism for these subtle organizing pulses is yet proven, but clinical experience compels the conviction that the rhythms are present and will eventually be accounted for.

Osteopathy has from its beginning embraced a new biomechanics. Although A. T. Still was not able to express his ideas clothed in today's research or terminology, his intuition previewed much of the paradigm shift we are witnessing today. He wrote a book on 'Fasciae,' that long-ignored 'Cinderella' of body tissues (Still, 1899; Schleip, 2003). These 'fat, greasy membranes,' as the old acupuncture texts accurately call them, are the environment and substrate of every living cell, which cannot function properly without them. What is emerging today from fascial research and movement studies – the medium of structure and stable movement – has been known to osteopathy for some time.

This analysis leads to several pleas from this outsider:

1. Do not forget your roots, and spread its gospel. Osteopathy – the grand tradition of osteopathic manipulative medicine (OMM) – is threatened by medical indoctrination in the USA, and in a number of other countries is closely aligned with physiotherapy (which is in turn closely aligned to the old biomechanics). The strength in osteopathy lies in its original global vision about physical structure and its relation to function.

2. Join the rest of the Spatial Medicine practitioners, especially the front lines of sport medicine and personal training, where exciting new discoveries about human structure and movement are being made (Chek, 2001; Cook, 2010; Earls, 2014). In too many cases, even manipulative osteopaths steer clear of using exercise or even referring patients to movement-based practitioners, largely preferring passive manipulations aimed toward joint alignment or the resonant pulses with the systems. This isolation from other branches of Spatial Medicine is not only hurting the spread of osteopathy, but also denying these other methods the benefit of osteopathic insights.

3. Value muscle tissue's contribution to physiology. In the upper-level bone-setting traditions of both chiropractic and osteopathy, the muscle has been relegated to the low man on the physiological totem pole, the less intelligent end of the sensorimotor track. Still articulated the 'law of the artery,' Palmer 'the law of the nerve' – either way, the skeletal muscles are seen as the end of the command chain, the 'result' of problems up the line, mere servants of higher physiological processes (Still, 1899; Palmer, 2010).

While this last conclusion is understandable, it will not stand. Muscles are 40% of the body weight, testifying to their importance, and could be considered as the beginning of the line for drawing fluid through the body. The right-hand side of the heart pushes the blood through the lungs. The left-hand side of the heart pushes the blood through the arteries (though with their help). It is the skeletal muscles that are the third heart, the venous and lymphatic heart, and lack of use – and our contemporary lifestyle breeds misuse, abuse, and disuse – slows the physiology to where manipulations do not hold, tissues are underhydrated, and other aspects of mens sana in corpore sano are not pulled along.

Osteopaths' ability to create the resonant waves through the various systems is a neat trick of healing requiring developed skills. Without regular activity in the patient's engines of the skeletal muscle drawing circulation, however, these systems will lose energy and tend to track backwards. Balanced muscular activity is a crucial part of spatial medicine, one that osteopathy ignores at its peril.

A complete approach to the body's connective tissue membranes would involve a five-fingered hand:

- cranial osteopathy for the meninges of the dorsal cavity

- visceral manipulation for the coelomic bags that enwrap the organs of the ventral cavity

- joint mobilization and ligamentous release for the periarticular tissues

- myofascial release of muscles and short or adhered tissue in the parietal myofasciae

- taking all those systems into coordinated movement, intrinsic *and* extrinsic.

Combining forces with the exercise, athletic, performance, and physical education professionals would bring osteopathic principles to these educational, essentially preventive endeavors, but can also develop a program to maintain balance, stability, and hydration in the patients – old and young – treated by osteopaths.

Osteopaths are uniquely positioned – with their grasp of physiological motility as well as the new biomechanical concepts of mobility – to contribute to the topology of 'KQ' (kinesthetic intelligence – parallel to IQ and increasingly EQ – emotional intelligence). This exploration could define 'kinesthetic literacy': what curriculum or set of skills does every child need to experience and absorb to develop healthy structure and movement? Osteopaths as a community are well advised to join with others in somatics – trainers, rehab specialists, bodyworkers, yoga and Pilates teachers, and the Phys. Ed. majors teaching our children about their bodies – to formulate a cohesive biomechanics for the twenty-first century.

Anatomy Trains® myofascial meridians defined

To make the myofascial system easier for osteopaths to absorb and utilize, the myofascial system has already been reorganized away from the 'isolated muscle' model to more holistic and osteopathically based ones (Busquet, 1992; Tittel, 1956; Vleeming & Stoeckart, 2007).

Anatomy Trains is one such map among many for linking muscles in kinetic chains – but our myofascial meridians are defined in terms of their fascial linkages and myofascial force transmission as opposed to functional patterns of cocontraction in various common movements (Myers, 2014). To create a myofascial meridian, follow the fibers of the fascial fabric from one muscle to the next; the resulting linear connections have meaning in terms of stability, coordination, and even biopsychology.

To be clear, Anatomy Trains is not a theory of movement, nor a complete theory of structure, it is merely a map of patterns and common global compensations within the parietal myofasciae. It is still of value to the osteopath, however, especially in light of the above considerations and in light of recent research on myofascial force transmission, well-rehearsed in other parts of this book (Franklyn-Miller et al., 2009; Huijing, 2007; van der Wal, 2009; Langevin et al., 2006).

Since the entire system is documented elsewhere (Myers, 2014; or www.AnatomyTrains.com), we present a brief summary of the 12 meridians here. The unitary net enveloping all 600 skeletal muscles can be seen as including the following 12 myofascial continuities, all of which have been dissected intact from both treated and untreated cadavers (Fig. 31.2).

The cardinal lines – running basically longitudinally on the front, back, and sides of the body – provide basic stability, movement, and the joint-saving limitation of movement in the sagittal and coronal planes.

1. *The superficial front line (SFL)* runs from the top of the toes up the anterior surface of the leg, and from the pubic symphysis up the front of the torso to loop over the head with the sternocleidomastoid and its fascial extensions along the lambdoid suture (Fig. 31.2A). The SFL covers our 'soft underbelly' and

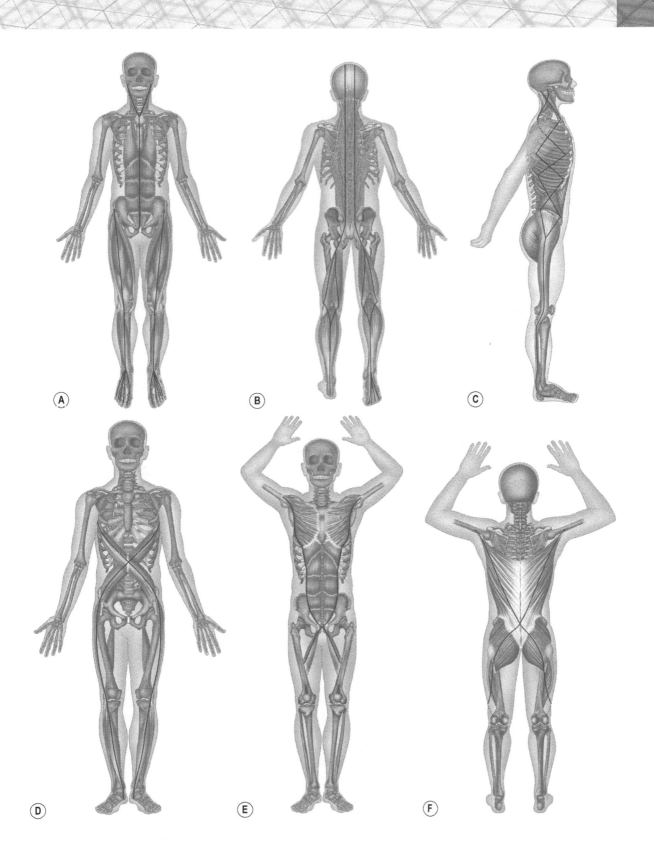

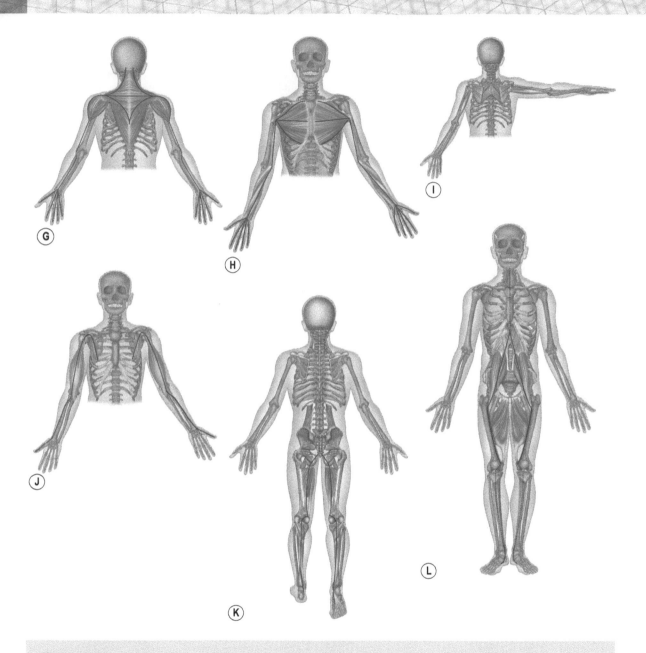

Figure 31.2

Myofascial meridians. (A) The superficial front line. (B) The superficial back line. (C) The lateral line. (D) The spiral line. (E) The front functional line. (F) The back functional line. (G) The superficial back arm line. (H) The superficial front arm line. (I) The deep back arm line. (J) The deep front arm line. (K) The deep back line. (L) The deep front line. Drawings by Amanda Williams. From Earls J. & Myers T. *Fascial Release for Structural Balance*, Chichester: Lotus Publishing and Berkeley, CA: North Atlantic Books, 2010. Reproduced with the permission of Lotus Publishing

tends to over-contract protectively in patterns of fear, insecurity, and trauma (startle response).

2. *The superficial back line (SBL)* runs along the posterior surface from toes to nose, including the plantar fascia, the triceps surae, the hamstrings, and back muscles right down to the powerful suboccipital drivers of spinal movement – all contained within a singular fascial sheet (Fig. 31.2B). The SBL is constantly contracted in upright posture and so tends to have more endurance slow-twitch fibers. Besides lifting the eyes and then the body from the foetal curve, the SBL's principal job is to balance the primary and secondary curves of the spine and legs.

3. *The lateral line (LL)* runs from the lateral arch to the ear up either side of the body (Fig. 31.2C). The LL weaves the front and back lines together like shoelaces and acts to stabilize lateral and rotational movements during walking, running, and other exercise, as well as maintaining imbalances in the coronal plane.

The helical lines – running more obliquely and thus crossing the body's midline, the helical lines create, coordinate, and limit the rotational movements in the horizontal plane, and the more common oblique movements that spiral across the various planes, as well as maintaining postural rotations in the body.

4. *The spiral line (SL)* winds around the torso from skull to hip by way of the contralateral shoulder and rib cage, and winds around the foot and back to the hip like a 'jump rope' under the arches (Fig. 31.2D). The spiral line modulates gait via the contralateral shift of body weight from one foot to the other across the sacroiliac joints.

5. *The front functional line (FFL)* joins the right humerus to the left femur and vice versa by means of the lower edge of the pectoralis major, the semilunar lines between the rectus and oblique muscles, and the short anterior adductors, particularly longus (Fig. 31.2E).

6. *The back functional line (BFL)* similarly joins the contralateral limbs, but across the posterior surface from latissimus through the lumbosacral fascia to the gluteus maximus on the opposite

side (Fig. 31.2F). (These two lines correspond to the *'lignes d'ouverture et fermeture'* in the system of Françoise Mézières, and to the anterior and posterior oblique slings in the work of Andry Vleeming.)

7. *The ipsilateral functional line (IFL)* joins the ipsilateral appendicular complexes, but does so in a spiral manner: from the outer edge of the latissimus dorsi to the posterior edge of the external oblique, on over the attachment at the anterior superior iliac spine with the sartorius connecting to the pes anserinus on the inside of the knee.

The arm lines – all the helical lines augment the force of the arms by extending their lever arm across the trunk to the legs. The arms themselves have four distinct, connected lines designed to facilitate the wide mobility of the upper appendage.

8. *The superficial back arm line (SBAL)* runs from the occiput and thoracic spinous processes out over the shoulder and down over the elbow to the extensor group on the back of the wrist and fingers (Fig. 31.2G). The SBAL could be considered as the top side of a bird's wing.

9. *The superficial front arm line (SFAL)* runs from the trunk – ribs, sternum, hip and spine – out and down the inner and underside of the forearm with the carpal flexors and the longer tendons through the carpal tunnel to the palmar fascia and digits (Fig. 31.2H). The SFAL corresponds to the underside of a bird's wing, and is the principal source of the power we impart to balls, axes, caresses, and manual therapy.

10. *The deep back arm line (DBAL)* runs deep to the SBAL, including the rhomboids, the rotator cuff, the triceps, and the fascia down to the little finger side of the hand (Fig. 31.2I). The scapula is a tethered 'sesamoid bone' within this line. The DBAL corresponds to the trailing edge of the bird's wing, and its misuse in the human arm is very common, leading to many shoulder stability dysfunctions.

11. *The deep front arm line (DFAL)* runs from the ribs via the pectoralis minor and clavipectoral fascia

to the biceps and down the inner arm to the thumb (Fig. 31.2J). The DFAL corresponds to the front of the bird's wing, and similarly controls the arm's angle. Through the thumb it is connected to our grip and stability. Its misuse is also very common, a factor in many 'hunched' upper body postural compensations.

The core line(s) – the remaining line is also the deepest, comprising the body's muscular core and also its myofascial interface with the ventral cavity's viscera. Although it is presented and functions as one line, it is most definitely a 'volume', and one can follow several 'tracks' within this line.

12. *The deep front line (DFL)* begins in the inner arch, including the long toe flexors of the deep posterior compartment, connecting up the tarsal tunnel to the interosseous membrane across the deep back of the knee to the triangular prism of the adductor group (Fig. 31.2L). The adductor group connects posteriorly via the obturatur fascia to the pelvic floor and thus to the anterior longitudinal ligament. Anteriorly it runs from the lesser trochanter at the top of the linea aspera via the psoas complex across the front of the pelvis to the lumbar spine. Both the anterior and posterior tracks join the roots of the diaphragm, spreading upward to include the mediastinal tissues and the deep muscles of the front of the neck and jaw. This line is amazingly rich and complex in its forms and meaning, but still creates a coherent and dissectible fascial continuity from inner ankle to the neuro- and viscerocranium.

Treatment goals in working with the lines

Fascial unity from top to toe and womb to tomb is the fact; these myofascial meridian lines are merely a guiding map within this three-dimensional myofascial 'webwork'. Use the map, but it is no replacement for the actual and personal territory.

1. Within any line, there can be local problems – shortness, adhesion, low muscle tone. The goal of treatment of muscle, neural, or fascial tissues here is to facilitate an even tone (palintonus) across the components of each line. Hypertonicity of the lumbar portion of the SBL, for instance, creates a bow shape from shoulder to ankle, disrupting the entire movement patterning. This lumbar hypertonicity may be linked – again, simply as an example, but common enough – to forward head posture, indicating shortness in the SFL. As both lines approach an even tonal balance, both the forward head posture and the lumbar-generated bow will recede.

2. There can be relational difficulties between the lines – for instance, the fascial plane of the human front (SFL) frequently is pulled down relative to the fascial planes of our back (SBL), which shift up in compensation. The goal in shifting fascial planes is to create the designed, even tensegral balance of the lines for easy, stable, and coherent movement. The remainder of this chapter will focus on this goal.

3. Without making symmetry a god, asymmetrical pulls in any of the lines often create difficulty across the entire system. Progressive and systematic easing, loosening of adhesions, and balancing of fascial planes with their complements can ease global patterns at some distance from the site of pain or restriction. This is especially helpful in chronic cases, where the body has distributed strain in patterns of small adjustments across the fascial net, as opposed to acute pain, where local treatment is generally more appropriate and effective.

Clinical application

This system works well in conjunction with osteopathic philosophy and application. Whether the osteopathic physician takes on this work for him or herself, or assigns it to a competently trained soft-tissue therapist familiar with the meridian system, easing the soft-tissue patterning will allow articular adjustments to maintain, as well as encouraging the psychological and habitual concomitants to resolve at the same time.

Most manual therapists are familiar with techniques to lengthen short tissue, 'comb out' scar tissue, or mobilize static areas. Let us acknowledge the usefulness of those manifold techniques and expand our focus to unique applications of the myofascial meridians for practitioners of osteopathy: adjusting the relationship among fascial and myofascial planes.

This work depends on applying manual pressure in distinct combinations of depth, direction, and duration to 'slide' the myofascial structures, via the hyaluranon-rich gliding layers between adjacent planes, into the relationships required by anatomical design.

Such work may be accompanied by strong sensation as planes shift; either a burning under the skin, or the kind of sensation accompanying a yoga or sport stretch. Unlike the reputation 'rolfing' enjoys, these sensations should not, in this writer's opinion, be permitted to rise to the level of 'pain' (sensation accompanied by the motor intention to withdraw). The only occasions where pain may be necessary is in the restoration of fascial mobility and motility in previously traumatized areas, where the original pain is felt on its way 'out' of the tissues.

Using the set of photos in Figure 31.3 – a frozen moment in time, an inadequate representation of the complexity of a human being, but a necessity in a book – and imagining that we have already adjusted the spine and other joints, how might we work with the soft-tissue planes to support the easy absorption of the desired pattern change?

Looking at the original photos (Fig. 31.3A), we can spot any number of patterns we might like to change, such as the pattern of eversion in the feet and slight varus in the knees. The primary left–right discrepancy comes with a left twist in the mediastinal tissues, requiring a compensatory right rotation in the lower cervicals.

The primary goal of treatment in this case – and our focus for the remainder of this chapter – must be with his highly compensated sagittal balance across the SFL and SBL, with the DFL sandwiched in between. Most of his patterns – and likely later problems – stem from the collapse of the DFL, or his 'core' as it is known these days. 'Collapse' in this case indicating both a loss of tone and a literal falling of the visceral core in relation to the spine.

Prior to lifting and toning the core, however, we need to address myriad imbalances in the SFL and SBL – otherwise none of our 'core' work (or his core exercise) will stick. His compensatory pattern – common enough these days – requires resting the pelvis forward of the feet into the tension of

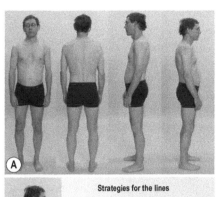

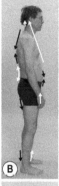

Strategies for the lines

SFL Neck to solar plexus
      Lengthen and lift
      Rectus abdominis
        Shorten
      Rectus femoris
        Lengthen and lift
      Lower leg
        Lengthen and lift

SBL Occiput to C4
      Lengthen and lift
      Erector C4–T12
        Shorten and narrow
      Erectors L1–Sacrum
        Lengthen and widen
      Hamstrings
        Shorten and drop
      Calf and plantar fascia
        Shorten and drop

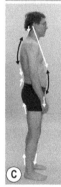

Involvement of the lines

SFL Neck to solar plexus
      Short and down
      Rectus abdominis
        Long and down
      Rectus femoris
        Short and down
      Lower leg
        Short and down

SBL Occiput to C4
      Short and down
      Erector C4–T12
        Long and wide
      Erectors L1–Sacrum
        Lengthen and widen
      Hamstrings
        Short and narrow
      Calf and plantar fascia
        Long and up

Figure 31.3

(A) Subject with common postural patterns. (B) The internal compensatory motion of the soft-tissue planes. White arrows indicate myofascial tissues that are likely to be short. The black arrows show where the front and back myofascial meridians have gone out of relationship with each other. (C) Some aspects of the treatment strategy we might employ to rebalance the lines. White arrows indicate myofascial tissues that are likely to be short and concentrically loaded. Black arrows indicate tissues we are likely to find in a state of eccentric loading

the anterior adductors, pubofemoral ligament, and psoas complex. He drops the rib cage posterior to compensate the anterior pelvic shift, opening the facets in the mid-T-spine, leaning on the posterior longitudinal ligament, and eccentrically loading the erectors in that section. The head comes forward over the pelvis, thus loading the nuchal ligament.

In Figure 31.3B, we diagram this in terms of the internal compensatory motion of the soft-tissue planes. White arrows indicate myofascial tissues that are likely to be short (concentrically loaded in terms of muscle, 'locked short' in terms of fascia). The black arrows show where, regardless of the underlying muscle tone, the front and back myofascial meridians have gone out of relationship with each other.

While everyone is individual, this gentleman demonstrates a very common general pattern in which the frontal plane of myofascia has generally moved caudally relative to the skeleton and the SBL. The posterior plane of fascia has generally moved superiorly relative to the skeleton and the SFL. Many laborers in 'spacial medicine' are trained to look for 'what is short?' (manual therapists) or 'what is weak?' (Pilates and personal trainers). Useful questions both, but here we invite a more rarely asked question: where are the fascial planes in relation to each other? The answer, in this and many other cases (which is why we chose this model), no matter the presenting symptom, is that the front has fallen and the back has hiked up.

In Figure 31.3C, we diagram some aspects of the treatment strategy we might employ to rebalance the lines. White arrows indicate myofascial tissues that are likely to be short (concentrically loaded in terms of muscle, 'locked short' in terms of fascia), while black arrows indicate tissues we are likely to find in a state of eccentric loading ('locked long' in terms of fascia). Our own methods employ direct technique, moving the fascial plane in the direction we would like to see it move, being sure to apply slow, gentle, and firm contact at the correct level of fascial plane, allowing time for the release along the areolar hyaluronic planes. This may be accompanied by exercise in the session or as homework to provide increased muscle tone and awareness where necessary.

Generally, as you can see, this will involve upward movement in the front and downward movement in the back. Lifting the plane of the SFL in the front of the leg and thigh while dropping the plane of the SBL in back will allow the client to center the pelvis once more over the ankle instead of in front of it. Lifting the upper SFL will both free the breath from the costal arch in front and allow the head to float back up over the rib cage, rather than so far in front of it.

Greater strength and tone in the thoracic erectors (while fascially bringing them medially, as they are often spread laterally in a kyphotic T-spine) will help open the front of the rib cage and bring it forward over the pelvis and under the head. Progressive release of the suboccipital muscles will be necessary with this and likely every session, given the neurological importance of these muscles to his eyes and eyeglasses, as well as the whole sagittal imbalance we are detailing here.

Interestingly, although he shows no strong imbalance in the spiral lines (the twist in the rib cage and lower cervicals is much deeper in the DFL), he will benefit from increased tone in the spiral line complex, such as that martial artists or CrossFit® adherents get from boxing. Because the spiral lines cross the body's midline between the shoulder blades and over the navel, increased tone in these lines will tend to pull the belly in and push the T-spine forward.

In the lumbars, the SBL, expressed as erectors within the laminae of the thoracolumbar fascia, needs to be dropped as well, but also lengthened and widened. Adding some exercise for the lower abdomen will help maintain these changes. Lifting the inseam of the leg (anterior adductors and medial intermuscular septum) and dropping the posteromedial portion of the thigh (medial hamstrings, the intermuscular septum between hamstrings and adductors, and the adductor magnus complex) will restore a neutral pelvis over the femur and under the spine.

Many other items could be detailed for this gentleman, but this will suffice to give the practicing osteopath some idea of how global postural assessment, analysis in terms of these myofascial connections, and treatment in terms of these larger patterns of planar relationship can be helpful in supporting the osteopathic manipulations you are already using.

Treatment is always modified to fit the individual pattern, and is modified in terms of continual observation of how the pattern is changing in response. Our school professes an entire treatment protocol of 12 sessions, progressively working through loosening and harmonizing the lines, though many practitioners use our assessments, strategies, protocols, and techniques in much shorter applications in conjunction with their primary manual therapy or movement education approach. You can find a variety of approaches to these sets of skills in the Anatomy Trains book, website, DVDs, seminars, and online learning courses.

Osteopathy sits in the middle of spatial medicine, connecting the inner world of motility to the outer world of mobility, and connecting physiology to functional movement. It is very important that osteopathy turn outward to embrace and inform all the adjunct methods of spatial medicine – such as the one we have outlined here – into a unifying whole.

References

Alexander F. M. *The Use of the Self*. London: Methuen, 1932. Reissued: London: Orion Books, 2001.

Alexander R. M. *The Human Machine*. New York: Columbia University Press, 1992.

Bainbridge-Cohen B. *Sensing, Feeling, and Action*. Northampton MA: Contact Editions, 1993.

Barrall J.-P., Mercier P. *Visceral Manipulation*. Seattle: Eastland Press, 1983.

Bateson G. *Mind and Nature*. New York: Dutton, 1979.

Blechschmidt E. *The Ontogenetic Basis of Human Anatomy*. Berkeley, CA: North Atlantic, 2004.

Busquet L. *Les Chaines Musculaires, Vols 1–4*. Paris: Frères Mairlot, 1992.

Chek P., *Movement That Matters*. Lansing MI: CHEK Institute, 2001.

Cook G., Burton L., et al. *Movement: Functional Movement Systems: Screening, Assessment, Corrective Strategies*. Norfolk, VA: On Target Publications, 2010.

Earls J. *Born to Walk: Myofascial Efficiency and the Body in Movement*. Chichester: Lotus Publishing and Berkeley, CA: North Atlantic Books, 2014.

Earls J. & Myers T. *Fascial Release for Structural Balance*. Chichester: Lotus Publishing and Berkeley, CA: North Atlantic Books. 2010.

Franklyn-Miller A., et al. The strain patterns of the deep fascia of the lower limb. In: *Fascial Research II: Basic Science and Implications for Conventional and Complementary Health Care*. Munich: Elsevier GmbH, 2009.

Huijing P. A. Epimuscular myofascial force transmission between antagonistic and synergistic muscles can explain movement limitation in spastic paresis. *Journal Biomech*. 2007;17:708–724.

Knudsen D. *Fundamentals of Biomechanics*, 2nd edition. New York: Springer, 2007.

Konner M. *The Tangled Wing*. New York: Henry Holt, 1982.

Langevin H. M., Bouffard N.A., Badger G. J. Subcutaneous tissue fibroblast cytoskeletal remodeling induced by acupuncture: evidence for a mechanotransduction. *J Cell Physiol*. 2006;207:767–774.

Levin S. The tensegrity-truss as a model for spine mechanics. *Mech Med Biol*. 2003;2:374–388.

Lieberman D. *The Story of the Human Body*. New York: Pantheon Books, 2013.

Myers T. Kinesthetic dystonia, Part 1. *J Bodyw Mov Ther*. 1998;2:101–114.

Myers T. Kinesthetic dystonia, Part 2. *J Bodyw Mov Ther*. 1999a;2:231–247.

Myers T. Kinesthetic dystonia Parts 3a & b. *J Bodyw Mov Ther*. 1999b;3:36–43.

Myers T. W. *Anatomy Trains: Myofascial Meridians for Manual and Movement Therapists*. Edinburgh: Churchill Livingstone, 2014.

Myers T., Fredricks C. Stretching and fascia. In: Schleip R. Findley T. W., Chaitow L., et al. (eds) *Fascia: The Tensional Network of the Human Body*. Edinburgh: Churchill Livingstone, 2012, p. 433–439.

Oschman J. *Energy Medicine in Therapeutics and Human Performance*. Edinburgh: Butterworth Heinemann, 2003.

Palmer D. D. *Chiropractic: A Science, an Art and the Philosophy Thereof*. Whitefish, MT: Kessinger Publishing, LLC, 2010.

Rolf I. *Rolfing*. Rochester: Healing Arts Press, 1977.

Scarr G. Biotensegrity. Pencaitland: Handspring Publishing, 2014.

Schleip, R. Fascial plasticity—a new neurobiological explanation. *J Bodyw Mov Ther*. Part 1: 2003;7:11–19; Part 2: 2003:104–116.

Sills F. *Craniosacral Biodynamics*. Berkeley, CA: North Atlantic, 2001.

Stecco C. *Functional Atlas of the Human Fascial System*. Edinburgh: Churchill Livingstone, 2015.

Stecco L., Stecco C. *Fascial Manipulation for Internal Dysfunction*. Padua: Piccini, 2013.

Still A. T. *Osteopathic Research and Practice*. Kirksville, MO: Kirksville Press, 1910.

Still A. T. *Early Osteopathy in the Words of A. T. Still*. Kirksville, MO: Truman State University Press, 1991.

Sutherland W. G. The cranial bowl: A treatise relating to cranial articular mobility, cranial articular lesions and cranial technic, 2nd edition. London: Free Press Company, 1948.

Tittel K. *Beschreibende und Funktionelle Anatomie des Menschen*. Munich: Urban & Fischer, 1956.

van der Wal J. The architecture of connective tissue in the musculoskeletal system. In: Huijing P. A., et al. (eds) *Fascia Research II: Basic Science and Implications*. Munich: Elsevier GmbH, 2009.

Vleeming A., Stoeckart R. The role of the pelvic girdle in coupling the spine and legs: a clinical anatomical perspective on pelvic stability. In: Vleeming A., Mooney V., Stoeckart R. (eds) *Movement, Stability and Lumbopelvic Pain*. Edinburgh: Churchill Livingstone, 2007.

Willard F. Visceral fascia. In: Schleip R., Findley T. W., Chaitow L., et al. (eds) *Fascia: The Tensional Network of the Human Body*. Edinburgh: Churchill Livingstone, 2012, pp. 53–56.

THE CONTRACTILE FIELD AND FASCIA

Phillip Beach

Clinical implications and integration of fascia as an organ

The contractile field (CF) model is a whole-organism approach to understanding human movement. The 'fields' are derived from primary vertebrate movement patterns. The model offers new insights into the interaction of large fields of contractility.

Fascia, from this whole-organism perspective, can be assessed via a series of deeply embedded postures that the human body uses for repose. Losing ease in these archetypal postures will stress the fascial web.

Manual therapy directed toward fascia should target the regions where fascia converges and emerges, for example, the bones and cartilage around the sensory capsules, the modiolus of the mouth, the palmar fascia, the plantar fascia, and the perineal body are such convergent regions. Contractile fields interact via emergent borders. They can be palpated and will include the spinous processes and the sacrum; rib angles and the lumbar lateral raphe; the costochondral junctions; the linea semilunaris; and the linea alba.

Introduction

A colleague enters the room. You stand and turn to greet your friend. This simple act of greeting involves hundreds of named muscles informed by neurological cascades of remarkable complexity. Joints and fascia help shape the movement toward the handshake, whilst at deeper levels of physiological function blood pressure and visceral mobility go largely unnoticed unless painful.

These whole-organism movement patterns are the concern of the CF model. It is a quest to discern the primary movement patterns that the human body employs, seamlessly blended, to produce the movements of life. It is a quest that has drawn little attention from the human movement fraternity. Most of our analysis to date is a joint-by-joint approach, as exemplified brilliantly by Kapandji (1974), or a focus on named tissues such as IVDs; facet or skull joints; the multifidus, etc.; or more recently fascia. There is some work toward a regional approach proposing the various slings, cores, and anatomy trains. These approaches are predicated on a cadaveric model where anatomical exposure is thought to provide a form of proof.

To best understand whole-organism contractility we need to think about modeling. What would a model of movement function look like that binds together many tissues and regions into something more coherent? To do this we need to turn to that crucial thought structure used by science when dealing with complexity – the modeling process. This chapter will outline a new model of movement, and then, from that context, consider the role of fascia.

Modeling

Human movement is obviously multidimensional and complex. Many anatomical entities and concurrent physiologies contribute to our every movement. Thus our goal, faced with the complexity of the world, is to create and test models that, at their best, are simple and elegant. Good models have both explanatory and predictive power (Holland, 1998). In short, if we cannot model the system under study, we really do not understand it.

From the outset the thoughtful use of analogy and metaphor is vital to the development of a model. When looking at a complex system the process of understanding and modeling must involve the identification of what are called in modeling theory the 'crucial building blocks'. These are not always apparent. Teasing out building blocks that are not of central significance to the system being studied will yield models that are of little theoretical value or practical use.

Once those primary building blocks are discerned, their interaction becomes the subject of interest. Meaningful relationships between the building blocks are looked for and mapped. The product of this is a model that then proves its worth in the roles of insight and understanding, prediction of future scenarios, and thus planning for those possible consequences. Models help discern nodal points where the system complexly converges, or regions where the system may bifurcate, invert, or display critical phenomena.

Importantly, we will not develop whole-organism movement models from the study of cadavers. Fritjof Capra (1996) describes it thus:

'The study of **pattern** is crucial to the understanding of living systems because systemic properties, as we have seen, arise from a configuration of ordered relationships. Systemic properties are properties of a pattern.

What is destroyed when a living organism is dissected is its pattern. The components are there, but the configuration of the relationships between them–the pattern–is destroyed, and thus the organism dies.'

The human form, derived from 500+ million years of vertebrate evolution, will not yield its patterns casually. But there is pattern – those patterns can be searched for via evolutionary biomechanics, allied with that most personal of studies, embryology.

So to model human movement patterns we come back to 'building blocks'. The CF model suggests these are important for a whole-organism model of movement. They are:

• *Mesoderm:* This forms the skeletal muscle, the skeleton, the dermis of skin, the connective tissue (fascia), the gonads and kidneys, the heart, the blood, the lymph cells, and the spleen. Notice how gonads, kidneys, and blood are part of the mesodermal system. These organs need to be incorporated into the model.

• *Mammalian movement patterns:* It is useful in the modeling process to widen our scope beyond the human example. A good model is portable to other, related species. Fish, characterized by a backbone, employ a lateral flexion pattern. Dolphins, a tetrapod that returned to the water circa 60 million years ago, move via a flexion/extension pattern. Human gait patterns are characterized by a contratwisting of the shoulders and pelvis – we torque.

• *Sense organs:* We are not mapped by our central nervous system with all body parts weighted equally. The nose, eyes, ears, lips, tongue, hands, nipples, feet, genitals, and anus are massively over-represented. We move in life to place those crucial organs where we need them in space. Movement without sense organs is nonsensical.

• *The suboccipital region and the 'spinal gearbox':* During vertebrate evolution the spine gradually became more regionalized. The suboccipital, cervical, thoracic, lumbar, sacral, and coccygeal regions emerged (Kardong, 1998). The suboccipital region is unique in its complexity. That, along with a lumbar spine that torques differently in flexion and extension (Gracovetsky, 1998), must be embedded in the biomechanics of the CF model.

• *Limb rotation:* Human limbs are derived from the fins of fish (Carroll, 2005). Fish, the archetypal vertebrate, employ the body wall for propulsion and the fins to then steer that power. A terrestrial existence modified that pattern as the limbs assumed the dual responsibilities of lifting the ventral body away from the terrain and assuming a propulsive role. In our species the upper limbs are said to externally rotate whilst the lower limbs rotate and twist internally. Our bipedal gait is only possible because of this long-axis twist of the lower limbs.

• *The coelom and kidneys:* The earliest life on this planet was either tethered into place or drifted in water currents. The evolution of mesoderm (Erwin et al., 1997) facilitated movement in the aquatic environment. With volitional movement came choice – movement toward warmth, friend, or prey. Sense organs emerged to respond to this challenge. In our vertebrate body plan (*Bauplan*) the mesoderm split to allow the external body wall movement to be semi-independent of gut mobility and motility. This created a fluid-filled cavity, the coelom. When one reads about the evolution of movement on this planet, the advent of the coelom was a crucial innovation. In the adult human the embryonic coelom morphs to become the pericardium, the pleural, and the peritoneal cavities. If these cavities stick (e.g., peritonitis) you will not feel like moving.

- *Pulsatile and peristaltic movements*: Mesoderm wraps the heart/blood vessels and the gastrointestinal tract with contractile tissue. A blood pressure lowering drug or a strong laxative can undermine months of strength and conditioning training. A model that acknowledges only the myofascial aspect of movement is incomplete.

The contractile field model

Each CF courses from the rostral pole to the caudal pole of the body, somewhat like a magnet. Each CF has a warp and weft like a textile. Therefore there is no 'core' in the model, as deep tissue will surely rise to a more superficial fascial layer. Likewise, each field can be seen as 'riverlike' in that it can widen and 'slow' in some body regions, then narrow and 'speed up' in another. For example, the rectus abdominus is wide at the costal cartilage but narrow as it inserts onto the pubis. So the abdominal region, possibly with a recent meal on board, will move with less speed than the pubic region that is employed for gait. Borders between fields are important to consider. At every level of the biological hierarchy borders define relationships.

A novel aspect of the CF model is the embedding of a sense organ in a field of contractility. The neuroarchitecture of the vertebrate body plan has been remarkably stable over 500 million years. The cranial nerves were first described from human dissection and the same pattern has been described across the vertebrate phyla (fish do not have CN XI and XII as they do not have a moveable tongue or a neck). We all adhere

to a sensory platform where the nose leads, eyes are intermediate, and ears further back and lateral. So as the vertebrate body biomechanically responded to the transition from an aquatic to a terrestrial environment, the coupling between sense organs and movement patterns could not be reinvented. The ancient vertebrate body plan imposed limits that evolution has had to work within. So the model suggests the sense organs and vertebrate fields of contractility are evolutionarily and developmentally coupled. Within a CF the embedded sense organ acts as a nodal region or, to use a metaphor, as a lighthouse that helps guide early embryological development of the field.

Importantly, the fields are totally interpenetrative and interactive. The movements of life use all the fields. Teasing these fields out is for our intellectual pleasure.

The model has a:

- lateral contractile field (L-CF)
- dorso/ventral contractile field (D/V-CF).

Interaction of these fields produces:

- helical contractile fields (H-CF) with a left twist and a right twist
- limb contractile fields (limb-CFs) that emerge from, and empower, the H-CF
- a radial contractile field (R-CF)
- a fluid field (F-F)
- chiralic contractile fields (C-CFs) with *pulsatile* and *peristaltic* functions.

Below is a brief introduction to each field. For the purposes of the model it is best to consider the body and limbs as initially separate. Snakes and dolphins lost limbs and they are still vertebrates. For a fuller description, refer to my text (Beach, 2010).

Lateral contractile field (L-CF)

This CF is derived from the lateral undulation of fish. It courses from the lateral rectus of the eye to the otic region, decusses (to cross) to the contralateral side, and then down the lateral aspect of the body wall to the perineal body.

Remarkably, the early vertebrate brain devoted a cranial nerve to the lateral rectus of the eye. This muscle is then closely coupled with the medial rectus. The eyes would have needed this left/right mobility prioritized, as fish would need to counter the lateral undulation of the propulsive lateral body wall. As fish do not have a cervical region the decoupling of the eyes from the body wall would have been essential for visual tracking.

The human ear has an evolutionary history that is associated with the lateral jaw and the lateral line found in fish. Thus the lateral body wall has always been associated with the otic region. It is part of the vertebrate body plan. So the model places the ear in the L-CF as a nodal region, along with the lateral skull and the lateral jaw. As vertebrates faced the biomechanical challenges of a terrestrial environment regional specializations of the vertebrae emerge in the fossil record. The L-CF is modeled as crossing from the left to the right, and vice versa, in the suboccipital region. This decoupling of the head from the neck is essential to the righting reactions that babies must master for normal development.

So if we are considering the (left) lateral eye, ear, and jaw, the L-CF in the movements of life will usually decuss to the contralateral (right) side. Our bipedal gait will use this pattern. We can now follow the field caudally with the scalenes. Note that the three scalenes are embryologically the same muscles as the trilaminar body wall muscles of the thorax and abdomen. The L-CF is modeled as employing the posterior and middle scalene, the external and internal intercostals, and the external and internal obliques. These muscles drape over the lateral body wall with oblique fibers at right angles to each other. When both act together we get a pure lateral flexion, but most of the time one or the other will dominate so that a torque forwards or backwards is coupled to the lateral flexion.

The posterior border of the L-CF is the angle of the ribs and the lateral raphe of the thoracolumbar fascia. The anterior border is the costochondral junction of the ribs and the linea semilunaris of the abdominal wall. The L-CF exhibits the biodynamic slowing and speeding effect discussed above by being wide in the ribs 6/7/8/9 region, to then narrow to the lateral neck via the scalenes or to the iliac crest below.

From the iliac crest the L-CF will follow the ilia internally to then emerge as the iliococcygeal muscle, the tail-wagging muscle of a dog. From the sacrum the bilaminar L-CF will course to the perineal body to then twist and cross to the contralateral side. From an embryological perspective the internal oblique *is* the external oblique on the contralateral side. The musculature does not form via separate muscles. Rather the image is more that of an embryological wind that carries the pioneer myoblasts until they are too heavy and drop out. The CFs have their developmental roots in these wind like morphogenic fields.

In summary this is a lateral, bilaminar, twisted ring of contractility that has nodal points in the otic region, decusses at the suboccipital region, to then course over the lateral body wall to twist in the perineal body to the contralateral side.

Dorso/ventral contractile field (D/V-CF)

Just as we cannot have a left L-CF without a right L-CF, we cannot have a dorsal CF without a ventral CF. The dorsal aspect of the D/V-CF originates just below the nose, the embedded sense organ in this CF. The field continues around the nose to the supraorbital notch to then pass up to the vertex of the skull. From there the field passes down the posterior skull to the insertion of the suboccipital spinal muscles. The D-CF courses down the spinal column as the cascade of the erector spinae, with a strict left/right division, to insert on the posterior medial aspect of the iliac crest and the sacrum. Contractility then losses that strict left/right division as it passes from the sacrum to contribute to the musculature of the external anal muscle, and coursing then onto the perineal body where left and right blend.

During embryonic folding this contractile tissue is drawn toward the future lower abdominal wall. In effect the lower abdominal wall is of dorsal derivation. Note that if this caudal migratory process is disrupted the lower abdominal wall may be deficient and the bladder then exposed.

Below the navel the D-CF fuses with the V-CF to then carry on as the rectus abdominus, again with a left/right separation. The field is then modeled as carrying on as the parasternal interchondral intercostal muscles that are a regional specialization of the intercostals.

As the CFs approach the head the complexity increases. At the top ribs the V-CF bifurcates. The V-CF may continue bilaterally as the sternocleidomastoids or it may pursue the midline infra- and suprahyoid muscles to converge on the root of the tongue. The bifurcation of the CF allows for contractility to decuss from the front body to the back body and vice versa, again via the suboccipital complex. This allows for the righting reflex.

Thus the D/V-CF is a bilateral, para-axial twisted ring of contractility that has the nose as the embedded sense organ, the suboccipital region to decuss dorsal and ventral when needed, the fusion of dorsal and ventral below the navel, and the perineal body blending left and right.

Helical contractile fields (H-CFs)

The H-CF is the interaction of a left- and a right-handed helical contractility that is characterized by crossing of the midline via fascial depth change. The eyes are the embedded sensory organs in this CF. It is a CF that does not use different muscles to those found in the L-CF and the D/V-CF but rather biomechanically couples those fields together.

The words 'oblique' and 'intermediate' are associated with the H-CF. 'Oblique' as this orientation in the contractile tissue facilitates helical biomechanics. The word 'intermediate' because intermediate lines on the body wall are the control points for this CF. If you need to manually twist someone, the best hand holds are not on the dorsal or ventral body wall, nor on the lateral body wall, but the intermediate holds between (i.e., the rib angles of the dorsal body and the costochondral junction/linea semilunaris of the ventral body).

The H-CF places the intermediate sense organ, the eyes, as the embedded sense organ of the fields. The neurology of the optic nerve, allied with the complexity of oculomotor, trochlear, and abducens nerves, blends the left and right helixes into a functional whole. The eye, a ball in a socket, is the ideal sensory organ to integrate the complex biomechanics and weight shifts that helical motion demands of a terrestrial vertebrate.

From the occiput and the spinous processes of the vertebrae the H-CF can be visualized as a whole-organism, oblique left and right wrap. It is not a line or a ribbon that can be wrapped about the torso; rather it is an oblique sheet of tissue that extends the entire length of the spine. Contractility that originates in the upper spine has more opportunity to cross the midline, whereas a caudal spine origin offers less space to helix around the torso. As the contractility crosses the anterior or posterior midline it changes fascial depth. The external oblique is continuous with the contralateral internal oblique via both fascial depth change and neurological decussation.

Helical contractility is so important to our movement that the model suggests that not only are the eyes embedded, but also the nipples, with the caudal root of this pattern being the tip of the genital. Moore et al. (2012) has a photo of a newborn male with dual penile tips, thus hinting that the single genital tip is a nodal fusion of left and right biodynamics.

Limb contractile fields (limb-CFs)

It is time to add limbs to the CF model. The limbs are modeled as extruding from and then empowering the H-CF. To understand this aspect of the model we need to look to the embryonic origins of the limbs.

The limbs emerge from an extraordinary embryonic structure called the ectodermal ring, also known as the Wolffian ridge as J. Wolff first noted the ring in 1759. The ectodermal ring is a transient structure in early embryonic development. The ring, a thickening of the ectoderm, covers the earliest manifestations of the mouth, nose, eyes, ears, vagus nerve, hands, nipples, feet, genital tip, and anus. In short, everything that your brain takes a keen interest in. The ectodermal ring is described as being intermediate because it is placed between the somites of the dorsal embryonic body and the visceral swellings of the ventral body. As the limb buds emerge the ring regresses. The limb buds are initially paddle-shaped with the early muscular system divided into a dorsal and ventral moiety (half). The limb buds then contrarotate. The arms are described as externally rotating whereas the legs internally rotate with an additional long-axis twist.

Because of this long-axis twist the dorsal torso contributes to the quadriceps, the anterior compartment of the leg, and the ankle/toe extensors. The ventral torso contributes to the adductors, hamstrings, the posterior compartment of the lower leg, the plantar flexors, and the flexors, of the foot. This twist of the leg musculature adds considerable complexity to the interaction between the H-CF and the lower limb.

Within the dual left and right H-CFs are zones that have been reinforced as preferred biomechanical pathways. The oblique upper and lower limb muscles such as the pectoralis and the gluteus maximus offer this reinforcement. Humans have profoundly exploited helical motion patterns. We use contratwisting of the upper and the lower torso for the quintessential human movement patterns of walking, running, and throwing.

In summary the limbs empower the H-CF via their large, obliquely inclined muscles such as the pectorals, the latissimus dorsi, the gluteals, and the psoas. The hands and feet are the embedded sense organs of the limb-CFs.

Radial contractile field (R-CF)

The word 'radial' is used here to describe a cross-section of the torso that can compress and dilate. We can squeeze our torso when needed, for example during a heavy lift, but we must also be able to dilate our torso with breath and food. To stress one function over the other is not correct.

The vertebrate spine does not like to be shortened and buckled. All the CFs outlined above will impose those buckling loads on the spinal column. To offset this the R-CF will squeeze the body wall to thus maintain the longitudinal integrity of the spine. This involves a system-wide response that is far larger than the transverse abdominus (TA). Note that the TA itself is a deep muscle only in the upper abdomen. Below the navel it rises in the fascial layers to become superficial above the pubis. The R-CF will employ the pelvic floor, the TA, the diaphragm, the intercostal intimi, the anterior scales, the platysma, the buccinators, and the orbicularis oris and occuli – all involved in a ceaseless contracting and expanding of the whole organism.

The R-CF is not 'deep' or 'core'. The concept of a distinct core is alien to the CF model, where musculature warps and wefts within a seamless fascial web (see also Lederman, 2007). The embedded sense organs in this field are modeled as the mouth and anus.

Fluid field (F-F)

Kidneys, a mesodermal organ, have had a long and complex evolutionary history that is reflected in their complex embryological development. Those histories are associated with the coelom. The advent of a coelom, a fluid-filled cleft within the mesodermal layer, facilitated the movement of early life on this planet (Clark, 1964). Kidneys that evolved within a seawater environment will function quite differently to those needed for movement within a freshwater environment. A terrestrial environment was another challenge for an organ that must ensure every cell is bathed in physiologically appropriate fluids.

The F-F creates space in the model to factor in the central role fluid physiology has on our movement. For example, a fine athlete with years of training presents for a race. A small diuretic tablet slipped into his water will undermine all that preparation. Our modern lifestyle has profoundly challenged our F-F via our salt and sugar consumption.

Chiralic contractile fields (C-CFs)

The trilaminar body wall and the limbs are derived from the somatic mesoderm. The deeper layer of mesoderm (splanchnic) forms the majority of the visceral musculature.

The external musculature is bilaterally symmetrical. Every muscle we have on the left side we have on the right side. At the external level bilateral symmetry is seen as a good thing. At the visceral level this is not the case. Visceral organs are 'handed'; each organ has a place on the left or the right. This handedness in chemistry is called chirality. Gloves are an example of this, as a left glove will not fit on a right hand. At international mathematics and physics conferences there is huge debate about the relationship between symmetry and asymmetry. One must presume the first picoseconds of the Big Bang were symmetrical but the universe came into being because of the breaking of this initial symmetry. We have embodied this debate as our bilaterally symmetrical body wall/limbs interact with a bilateral visceral system.

The CF model has a pulsatile and a peristaltic component within the C-CF. Our ability to move with grace and facility requires a hemodynamic that can respond to imposed loads but return to resting norms, and a gut/respiratory tube that extracts and transits nutrients in the normal manner. Our patients present to us with musculoskeletal distress but the case history often reveals concomitant blood pressure or pulmonary/gastrointestinal distress.

The interaction of the CFs creates the movement patterns we use in life. If, for example, one was supine and wanted to roll up to a sitting position, the CF model helps us understand why the obliques are the first to activate. If the abdominal flexors alone contracted, the body shape would try to escape laterally. To counter this the L-CF will act bilaterally to first create the lateral bracing that then allows the contracting rectus abdominus to act coherently.

Without the lateral bracing the roll-up would buckle to the left or right. So the L-CF and the D/V-CF are coupled together to manage shape change. That coupling is then further enabled via the facet joints of the lumbar spine to create a form of gearbox. Lateral flexion is the initiator; this movement is then coupled with flexion or extension of the lumbar spine to yield a twist of the torso to either the left or the right. Serge Gracovetsky clarified the biomechanics of this in 1998. Our bipedal gait is built around this coupling.

Modality of assessment

A whole-organism model of movement gradually encourages a different approach to assessment and treatment. The assessment approach taken here includes the examination of 'archetypal postures of repose' (APs).

The flip side of movement is repose. For millions of years, after exercise we would have returned to the ground to rest and recuperate. These postures of rest are as deeply embedded in our biomechanical health as temperature (about 37°C) and blood pressure (about 120/80 mmHg) are in our physiological health. If you lose access to biomechanical ease on the floor, and the strength to arise from the floor with ease and facility, musculoskeletal distress will surely follow.

APs are central to a concept of biomechanical 'tune'. If the human body was a guitar, instead of the standard six strings, we have 600, and they are arranged in three dimensions rather than two. In addition, our instrument is designed to fold into resting patterns that have emerged from six million years of human evolution. Out of that extraordinary complexity emerges postures that are characteristic of our species. They act to retune the physique after movement. Two postures I will routinely examine are the full squat and cross-legged postures. Learning to read the pattern and nuance of these postures takes time.

The full squat

The ability to fully squat is a posture rooted in our biomechanical design. Jonathan Kingdon (2003), a world expert on the mammals of East Africa, suggests our evolution toward the modern condition started with an ape that could fully squat. It is a posture that we all master as youngsters (Fig. 32.1) but then tend to lose as we come to rely on heeled shoes, chairs, and sitting toilets.

Cross-legged sitting

The many variants of cross-legged sitting are the alternatives to the more linear postures as exemplified by the squat. Cross-legged sitting opens the vascular tree so that blood can course within the leg following deeply coevolved fascial pathways.

The contractile field model and fascia

Fascia, because of its investment across tissues, plays a crucial role in both delineating and integrating the CFs described above. For a treatment to target fascia, the CF model indicates the following:

- The sensory capsules. The regions around the nose, eyes, and ears need to be palpated. The nose is a control point for extension, the eyes for helical motion, and the ears for lateral flexion.

- The modiolus of the mouth is located just lateral to the mouth. These are fibromuscular masses that nine facial muscles spiralize into in a complex manner (Williams, 1995). They are best palpated with the opposed thumb and forefinger compressing the skin and mucosa. Once a light compression is applied, the patient is instructed to make facial and neck movements.

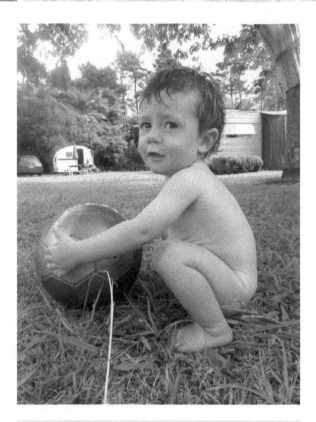

Figure 32.1
The full squat

- The palmar and plantar fascia. The plantar fascia in particular is a tissue that we render weak and dysfunctional via our shoe-based lifestyle, and when the shoes are removed the foot is only exposed to flat surfaces or carpet. Place a value on being barefoot more often.

- The dorsal and ventral midline. In embryology the midline is considered to be a special developmental field.

- The intermediate lines that mark the borders between fields. The dorsal intermediate lines course over the eyes, the intermediate head and neck, the rib angles, and the lateral raphe of the lumbar region.

- The anterior intermediate line is represented by the sternocleidomastoid, the root of the axilla, the costochondral junctions, the linea semilunaris, and the root of the groin.

- The sacrum. Here the spinous processes, the facet joints, and the transverse processes arise from the deep to become superficial. To palpate bone, use the knuckle as an applicator for a bone-to-bone touch.

- The perineal body.

Summary

The fascial web acts as an integrative matrix within which the contractile fields are enmeshed. Each CF will course over many named tissues that cooperate to form the patterns of movement we have inherited from over 500 million years of movement drama. Bipedal gait is a relative newcomer to this long party. It required a contratwisting of the shoulders and pelvis. From this pattern we then learnt to throw, so that both the upper and lower limbs became enmeshed in our species' exploitation of helical patterns. The CF model provides an insight into those biomechanics that have endowed us with great power.

The concept of APs has been introduced. All people, all cultures, and all age groups have historically used these postures to enable rest and recuperation. Only recently has the use of chairs became ubiquitous. Our culture places value on many things, but resting on the floor is not one of them. The simple act of floor sitting, and then getting up from the floor is of real value to our biomechanical well-being. The simple act of taking one's shoes off and exposing the plantar fascia to the terrain is likewise of real value to our well-being. In the author's clinical experience, these simple changes to lifestyle have a profoundly normalizing, 'tuning' effect on our fascial web.

References

Beach, P. (2010) *Muscles and Meridians: The Manipulation of Shape.* Churchill Livingstone, Edinburgh.

Capra, F. (1996). *The Web of Life: A New Synthesis of Mind and Matter.* Harper Collins, London.

Carroll, S. B. (2005) *Endless Forms Most Beautiful.* Weidenfeld & Nicolson, London.

Clark, R. B. (1964) *Dynamics in Metazoan Evolution: The Origins of the Coelom and Segments.* Clarendon Press, Oxford.

Erwin, D., Valentine, J. and Jablonski D. (1997) The origin of Animal body plans. *American Scientist.* 85(2):126–137.

Gracovetsky, S. (1988) The Spinal Engine. Springer-Verlag Wein, New York.

Holland, J. H. (1998) *Emergence-From Chaos to Order*. Oxford University Press, Oxford.

Kapandji, I. A. (1974) *The Physiology of the Joints: The Trunk and the Vertebral Column, Volume 3. 2nd edition*. Churchill Livingstone.

Kardong, K. V. (1998) *Vertebrates. 2nd edition*. McGraw-Hill.

Kingdon, J. (2003) *Lowly Origin: Where, When, and Why Our Ancestors First Stood Up*. Princeton University Press, Princeton and Oxford.

Moore, K. L., Persaud, T. V. N., Torchia, M. G. (2012) *The Developing Human: Clinically Oriented Embryology. 9th edition*. Saunders.

Lederman, E. (2007) The myth of core stability. *CPDO Online Journal*. June, 1–17.

Williams, P. L. (ed.) (1995) *Gray's Anatomy. 38th edition*. Churchill Livingstone.

THE INNERVATION OF FASCIAL TISSUES: FOCUS ON THIN-CALIBER AFFERENTS AND SYMPATHETIC EFFERENTS

Winfried L. Neuhuber, Wilfrid Jänig

Introduction

Recent years have seen a significant surge in what is called by some authors 'fascia research' in order to make the distinction from 'connective tissue research' in its broader sense (Schleip et al., 2012). In this context, 'fascia' is used as an umbrella term not only for a variety of classically rather well-defined connective tissue structures such as cervical; upper and lower limb fasciae; thoracolumbar fascia; intermuscular septa, etc. but also to include joint and organ capsules; ligaments; epi-, peri- and endomysium; epi- and perineurium; vascular sheaths; periosteum and tentatively even tendons, mesenteries, and dura into a 'fascial net' (Langevin & Huijing, 2009; Schleip et al., 2012). The advantage of this appealing concept certainly lies in the emphasis on the connectivity of a 'tensional network of the human body' as heralded in a recent book (Schleip et al., 2012). However, the need for such a far-reaching terminological turn is to be questioned as it is not able to resolve problems of distinction between heterogeneous structures in a better way, or may even be worse than classical anatomic terminology and result in more confusion (Benjamin, 2009; FCAT, 1998; Standring et al., 2008; Stecco et al., 2013b). In this chapter we will describe the innervation of fasciae. We will use the term 'fascia' for those structures that were classically referred to as such (e.g., thoracolumbar fascia) and for all other structures their established terms (tendon, joint capsule, periosteum, perineurium, mesentery, dura, etc.).

Innervation of fascial tissues by afferent and efferent neurons

Axons in the peripheral nervous system are conventionally classified according to diameter, degree of myelination, and conduction velocity, the latter being closely linked to the former. Erlanger and Gasser introduced a mixed Latin/Greek classification (Aα, Aβ, Aγ, Aδ, B, and C), for both motor and sensory fibers, whereas Lloyd and Hunt considered only muscle afferents, defining groups I to IV. In the present context, axons connected to corpuscular sensors are belonging largely to the thick myelinated Aβ class (diameter 6–12 μm, conduction velocity 36–72 m/s), while thin-caliber axons terminating as free nerve endings (FNEs) are thin myelinated Aδ (diameter 1–6 μm, conduction velocity 4–36 m/s) or unmyelinated C (diameter 0.2–1.5 μm, conduction velocity 0.4–2.0 m/s) fibers. Afferent Aδ and afferent C axons are equivalent to group III and IV afferents, respectively (Gardner & Johnson, 2013). Postganglionic sympathetic axons are unmyelinated and belong to the C fiber class.

Myelinated afferent nerve fibers from corpuscular mechanosensors

Myelinated afferent axons from fascial structures are derived from rapidly adapting simple lamellated corpuscles; large Pacini corpuscles, sometimes of the Golgi-Mazzoni type (with several inner cores); and slowly adapting Ruffini corpuscles, all displaying a low threshold to mechanical stimulation. Axons from Ruffini and Pacini corpuscles belong to the Aβ class, those from simple lamellated corpuscles are in the Aδ range (Halata & Strasmann, 1990). They are connected to large and medium-sized dorsal root and cranial ganglion cells and project, as can be surmised from studies on their cutaneous counterparts, to dorsal horn laminae III, IV, and VI (Brown et al., 1981). The long central axons continue through the ipsilateral dorsal columns, contributing to the medial lemniscal system, ultimately terminating in contralateral somatosensory cortices SI and SII. Thus, these afferents most likely serve a proprioceptive function. As muscles frequently originate from fasciae, intermuscular septa, joint capsules, and associated ligaments (van der Wal, 2009), where Golgi tendon organs are also found, they should also be included in this set of fascia-related sensors. Their Ib axons measure up to 15 microns and are fast conducting (Halata & Strasmann, 1990).

There are both classical and more recent studies on the occurrence and distribution to different tissues of these specialized sensors in various mammalian species, including human (see Halata & Strasmann, 1990 for a review of the older literature). Lamellated and Pacini corpuscles were described, for example, in interosseous membranes of the cat (Silfvenius, 1970), in the knee joint capsule of both cat and human, and in the human anterior cruciate ligament (Halata, 1977; Halata & Strasmann, 1990), in ligaments of the human wrist (Hagert et al., 2005), in the retinacula of the human leg (Stecco et al., 2010), in the human plantar aponeurosis (plantar fascia, Stecco et al., 2013a), within the capsule of Golgi tendon organs (Halata & Strasmann, 1990), and, last not least, in the mesenteries (Kubik & Szabo, 1955). They detect rapidly changing local compression (Proske & Gandevia, 2012). Ruffini corpuscles belong to the typical repertoire of joint capsular and ligament innervation (Halata, 1977; Halata & Strasmann, 1990; Lee et al., 2012) but were also found in retinacula (Stecco et al., 2010) and plantar aponeurosis (Stecco et al., 2013a). Ruffini corpuscles signal tissue stress in joint capsules, ligaments, and fasciae. Both rapidly and slowly adapting joint and fascia sensors appear to merely detect the limits of movement range, while muscle spindles subserve the moment-to-moment monitoring of joint position (Proske & Gandevia, 2012).

While many of these studies were *anecdotal* or *semiquantitative*, there exist a few that attempted to quantify corpuscular and also free (see below) nerve endings as well as to map their distribution to particular areas of fasciae and joints in order to promote a deeper understanding of their role in both physiology and pathophysiology. One of these notable exceptions studied the lateral elbow region, the aponeurotic origin area of the supinator muscle of the rat and the opossum (Strasmann et al., 1990a, 1990b). It was in this location where striking differences were noted between species. In the rat, there were about ten lamellated corpuscles embedded in the aponeurotic muscle origin. No Ruffini corpuscles were detected. In the opossum, only three lamellated corpuscles were found in a superficial connective tissue layer covering the aponeurosis; in the capsule of the humeroradial joint; and between the radius periosteum and the supinator muscle. A cluster of Ruffini corpuscles was found in the joint; capsule of this animal. The authors attempted to relate these differences in sensory equipment to differences in the motor behavior of these species (precise tension monitoring of small groups of muscle fibers during quadrupedal locomotion in the rat versus monitoring of joint capsule overstretching during climbing in the opossum, Strasmann et al., 1990b). Another study from the same group mapped corpuscular sensors in the mouse shoulder joint (Backenköhler et al., 1997). Here, lamellar corpuscles and Golgi tendon organs dominated over Ruffini corpuscles. In a detailed investigation of human wrist ligament innervation, dorsal ligaments and the scapholunate interosseous ligament were found to be densely supplied with corpuscular endings, whereas palmar ligaments received much less or almost no nerve fibers (Hagert et al., 2005). This corresponds to the pivotal role of the scapholunate and dorsal ligaments in wrist alignment and stability. Strikingly, both Ruffini and lamellar corpuscles were absent from the mouse temporomandibular joint (Dreessen et al., 1990) and the rat thoracolumbar fascia (Tesarz et al., 2011). Although not dealing with terminal sensory structures but rather with nerve-fiber bundles, three-dimensional reconstructions of the thoracolumbar fasciae (TLF) and crural fasciae (CF) showed nerves confined to the superficial layer of the TLF but concentrated in the middle and deep layers of the CF (Benetazzo et al., 2011). These studies exemplify the importance of a close look at both structure and architecture (van der Wal, 2009) but also caution against premature generalization of anecdotal observations.

Thin myelinated and unmyelinated afferent nerve fibers

By far the most numerous afferent axons from fascial and other deep somatic structures belong to the thin myelinated Aδ/group III and unmyelinated C/group IV classes (Halata & Strasmann, 1990). As there is almost no structure in the body that is not innervated, it was to be expected that fascial structures are also supplied by thin caliber axons that give rise to 'free nerve endings' (FNEs) (Halata & Strasmann, 1990). Many thin-caliber afferents are proven or at least suspected nociceptors, either specific for particular nociceptive stimuli (mechanical, heat, cold, acid) or polymodal (see Chapter 28). They derive from small- to medium-sized dorsal root and sensory cranial ganglion cells and split into several subpopulations that contain a mixture of various peptides, prominently calcitonin gene-related peptide (CGRP) and substance P (SP), or are non-peptidergic (Snider & McMahon, 1998). In both deep somatic structures and viscera, peptidergic neurons dominate over the nonpeptidergic population (Ivanusic, 2009; Robinson et al., 2004). A significant feature of the peptidergic subpopulation is the ability to release the peptides upon stimulation from their peripheral terminals, executing a so-called local effector function on blood vessels and other tissue components, such as mast cells (Holzer, 1988; Lennerz et al., 2008). Further subdivisions of primary afferent neurons were based on expression profiles of functionally relevant receptor and other molecules (Usoskin et al., 2015). The central axons of these neurons terminate in the superficial (laminae I and II) and deep (lamina V) spinal and medullary dorsal horns. From there, secondary tract neurons (about 10% of the neurons) send their axons contralaterally via the anterolateral system to specific targets in the brainstem and thalamus, the latter relaying these messages to the insular cortex, the primary interoceptive cortex, and the cingulate cortex, part of the 'pain matrix' (see Chapter 28).

Painstaking analysis of ultrathin serial sections, partly fed into three-dimensional reconstructions, of small nerves in joint capsules, muscles, tendons, dura, and mesenteries (Dreessen et al., 1990; von Düring & Andres, 1990; Heppelmann et al., 1990; Kerjaschki & Stockinger, 1970; Meßlinger et al., 1993; Strasmann et al., 1990a) revealed consistent general morphological features of FNEs. Many of them were closely related to small blood and lymphatic vessels, though others coursed through the extracellular matrix without noticeable vascular relationships. The perineurium of the small nerve fiber bundles ended as an open sleeve several hundred microns before the terminal bulge, and the myelin sheath of group III axons was lost shortly

before the end of the perineurium. Thus, the terminal receptive portion of group III and IV axons communicated freely with the surrounding tissue, not shielded by a blood–nerve barrier. Although the axons were still accompanied by Schwann cells, they displayed more and more bare surface areas where the axolemma, covered only by the basal lamina, was facing the surrounding extracellular matrix.

Thoracolumbar fascia

In a recent detailed study on the innervation of the superficial lamina of the thoracolumbar fascia of the rat, immunohistochemistry for the general neuronal marker PGP 9.5 showed a very inhomogeneous distribution of nerve fibers. The overwhelming majority of single varicose terminal axons were detected in the subcutaneous tissue and the thin outer layer of this fascia bordering the subcutis, whereas only a few were found in the thick middle and thin inner layers (Tesarz et al., 2011). Immunostaining for CGRP and SP was used to specifically label presumed nociceptive axons. Again, a distribution bias to the subcutis and outer fascial layer was seen. This was particularly evident for SP axons, which were completely absent from both the thick middle and thin inner layers. Peptide-containing varicosities were frequently seen without any vascular relation (Fig. 33.1 and 33.2). Preliminary data were also presented for the human thoracolumbar fascia documenting peptidergic presumably nociceptive varicose axons close to collagen fiber bundles.

Peri- and intramuscular connective tissue, tendons, and joint capsules

Nerve fibers of group III and IV and FNEs derived from them were studied using electron microscopy in the knee joint capsule, gastrocnemius-soleus muscle, and Achilles tendon of sympathectomized cats (von Düring & Andres, 1990; Heppelmann et al., 1990). In the branches of the cat tibial nerve to the gastrocnemius muscle, group IV afferents account for about 40% of all unmyelinated axons (von Düring & Andres, 1990). They were frequently related to small blood and lymphatic vessels in the perimysium externum and internum but not to the endomysium, which contains the capillaries and motor axons traveling to motor endplates (Fig. 33.3A). FNEs were also found

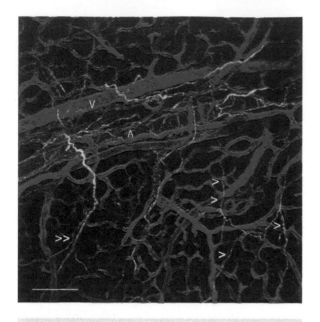

Figure 33.1

Overview of the peptidergic afferent and sympathetic innervation of the superficial layer of the rat thoracolumbar fascia bordering the subcutis. An artery (**A**) accompanied by a vein (**V**) gives rise to a dense network of arterioles and metarterioles, which are stained blue due to immunohistochemical detection of smooth muscle actin. Sympathetic postganglionic axons (red, TH immunoreactive) form a perivascular plexus around the artery and follow the arterioles for some distance. Afferent axons (green, CGRP immunoreactive) accompany both the artery and arterioles and also the vein. The double arrowhead points to bundles of afferent and sympathetic axons that appear to detach from arterioles; single arrowheads point to varicose CGRP-positive afferent axons that course without apparent relation to blood vessels through the tissue. Whole-mount preparation, three-channel immunofluorescence, extended focus projection of a stack of 52 confocal single optical sections taken at a z-step of 0.35 μm. Bar is 100 μm

was supplied with endings of group IV axons. Intramuscular thin-caliber afferent axons predominantly accompanying small blood vessels were also identified using immunohistochemistry for CGRP and SP (Reinert et al., 1998). In particular, the SP fibers underwent significant sprouting in experimental myositis.

Group III and IV axons were found in all portions of the rat supinator muscle (Strasmann et al., 1990a). They were particularly prominent in its proximal third and the aponeurotic origin close to the lateral epicondyle. Some were also found in the capsules of lamellar corpuscules. In the temporomandibular joint of the mouse, FNEs derived from group III and IV axons were the only type of afferent axons (Dreessen et al., 1990). They occurred mainly dorsolaterally in the stratum fibrosum and subsynoviale of the joint capsule.

Thin-caliber primary afferent axons were labeled by anterograde tracing from cervical dorsal root ganglia to the sternomastoid muscle of the rat. They were frequently in close vicinity to mast cells and predominantly distributed to the red portion of this muscle (Zenker et al., 1988). This is remarkable as muscle spindles and Golgi tendon organs were also confined to the red portion. Since thin-caliber muscle afferents monitor, among other parameters, the chemical milieu within the muscle, this distribution bias of thin caliber afferents may indicate that metaboreceptive signals from a muscle originate mainly in its red portion, thus having possibly more impact on homeostatic regulation than those from its white portion.

Neurovascular tracts

Blood and large lymphatic vessels are typically bound together by connective tissue sheaths that subserve important functions (e.g., supporting the return of venous blood from the lower extremities to the heart). In some regions (e.g., the neck, arm, and leg), nerve trunks are included in these vascular-nerve bundles or neurovascular tracts. The collagenous nature of these sheaths provides them with a significant ability to transmit traction to surrounding structures (Huijing, 2009). Vascular

without any contact to blood vessels but frequently in close relationship to mast cells (Fig. 33.3B). Remarkably, the endoneurium of small intramuscular nerves

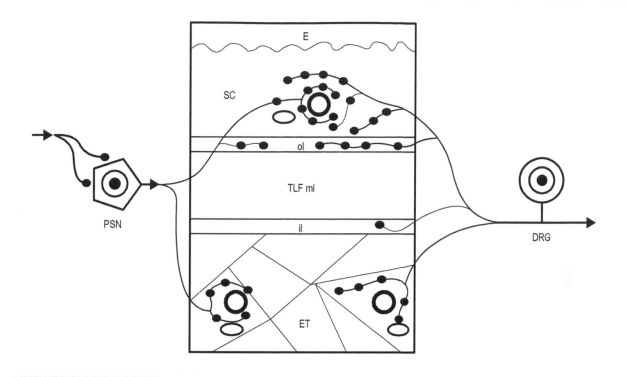

Figure 33.2

Diagram of the distribution of thin-caliber afferents and sympathetic postganglionics to the rat thoracolumbar fascia (TLF) in a schematized transverse section through this fascia with overlying skin (**E** denotes epidermis) and erector trunci muscle (**ET**) beneath. Varicose terminal axons of both neuron types are primarily distributed to blood vessels in the subcutis (**SC**) and the perimysium internum of the muscle, but also to the connective tissue of the subcutis and the outer layer (**ol**) of the fascia. Note that the middle (**ml**) and inner (**il**) layers of the fascia are almost devoid of innervation. This scheme does not intend to suggest that all these collaterals originate from the same neuronal cell bodies. DRG = dorsal root ganglion neuron; PSN = postganglionic sympathetic neuron; circular profiles = small arteries; ellipsoid profiles = small veins. Based on data from Tesarz et al. 2011

sheaths and the adventitia of both arteries and veins are well supplied with thin-caliber afferent fibers (Michaelis et al., 1994).

Compared to the fascial sheaths of blood vessels, the sheaths of peripheral nerves display a more sophisticated architecture (Peltonen et al., 2013). In particular, the perineurium, by virtue of tight junctions between its multiple layers of flat epithelial cells, provides an efficient diffusion barrier. The nervi nervorum represent fine bundles mostly of group IV axons and distribute in the epineurium (Fig. 33.4), from where they penetrate the perineurium to enter the endoneurium (von Düring & Andres, 1990). Many peptidergic afferent axons in the epineurium innervate blood vessels, but this vascular innervation stops at the perineurium (Appenzeller et al., 1984). Within the endoneurium, free peptidergic group IV fibers are able to release CGRP and appear to function as nociceptors (Sauer et al., 1999).

Periosteum and bone

The periosteum covers the skeleton, providing blood and nerve supply to the bones. At the origin and insertion of muscles, there is connective tissue continuity from the periosteum to the peritenoneum and the fascia of muscles. The innervation of the periosteum by mechanosensory nociceptive afferents is high,

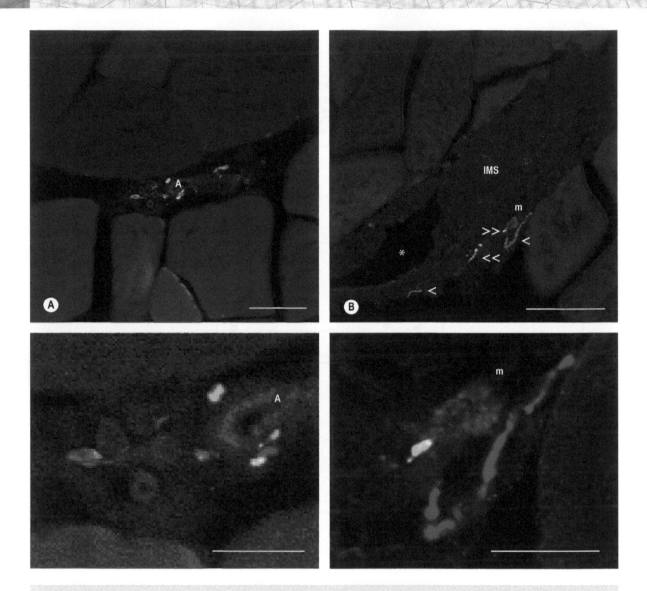

Figure 33.3

Distribution of thin-caliber afferents and sympathetic postganglionics to muscular connective tissue. (A) An arteriole (**A**) in the perimysium internum of the rat erector trunci is accompanied by both sympathetic (green – TH-immunoreactive) and afferent (red – CGRP-immunoreactive) varicosities. The endomysium between single muscle fibers is devoid of nerve fibers. The striated muscle fibers and the wall of the arteriole stain blue due to autofluorescence. (B) 'Free' sympathetic (double arrowheads, green – TH positive) and afferent (single arrowheads, red – CGRP positive) varicosities between erector trunci muscle fibers and an intramuscular septum (**IMS**) obviously unrelated to blood vessels but in close vicinity to a mast cell (**m** – the red granular staining most likely results from unspecific binding of the CGRP antibody). Asterisk indicates artificial cleft in the septum due to sectioning. Zoom-ins of the central areas are mounted below the respective overviews. Cryostat sections, three-channel immunofluorescence, extended focus projection of a stack of 7 (A) and 9 (B) single confocal optical sections taken at a z-step of 0.50μm. Bars are 50μm in (A), 100μm in (B), and 20μm in both zoom-ins

as known from experience. Thin-caliber afferents immunoreactive for CGRP and tropomyosin receptor kinase A (TrkA) form a rather dense network in the periosteum of the mouse femur, from where some axons enter the trabecular bone and bone marrow (Castaneda-Corral et al., 2011; Martin et al., 2007). Most of these periosteal sensory axons are unrelated to blood vessels, in contrast to tyrosine hydroxylase (TH) immunoreactive sympathetic fibers, which typically follow small arteries and arterioles. Retrograde tracing experiments from the rat tibia demonstrated dorsal root ganglion cells from segmental levels L1 to L6 with a peak at L3 and L4 (Ivanusic 2009). The majority of these sensory neurons were small to medium-sized and immunoreactive for either CGRP/neurofilament 200 or IB4. This is compatible with group III/IV peptidergic and group IV nonpeptidergic presumably nociceptive axons. Studies on the development of bone innervation suggested a role for CGRP containing sensory neurons in bone development and remodeling also (Gajda et al., 2005).

Visceral fascia, mesenteries, and serosa

Connective tissue enveloping the viscera of the neck, thorax (mediastinum), abdomen (mesenteries, retroperitoneal organs), and pelvis (endopelvic fascia), and their related vascular tracts, also including the endothoracic and endoabdominal fasciae, were suggested to represent a tensional continuum from the base of the skull to the pelvic floor (Willard, 2012). The pleura and peritoneum are intimately linked to these 'visceral fasciae' and the adhesive forces created by the humidity of adjacent serosal surfaces may significantly contribute to this visceral 'tensional network'. Therefore, the innervation of serosa will also be considered here. The rat parietal pleura is innervated by small- to medium-sized dorsal root ganglion neurons immunopositive for the acid-sensitive channels TRPV1 and ASIC3 compatible with nociceptive function (Groth et al., 2006). They are distributed over a wide segmental range from C3 to T12, peaking around C4/C5 and from T1 to T6, indicating pleural innervation by phrenic and intercostal nerves. In a study combining anterograde tracing and electrophysiological recording from the mesenterium of the guinea pig ileum, nociceptive spots were confined to the mesenterial attachment, where labeled nerve fiber bundles entered the wall of the gut along with

arteries (Song et al., 2009). This confirmed an earlier electrophysiological demonstration of receptive fields of lumbar colonic afferents at the mesenterial attachment (Blumberg et al., 1983). The rat parietal peritoneum is innervated by group III and group IV axons from lower thoracic and some mid-cervical spinal ganglion neurons (Tanaka et al., 2002). The terminal portions of group III axons penetrated the peritoneal mesothelium after having lost their myelin sheath reaching into the peritoneal cavity, while group IV axons remained within the peritoneal cell layer (Tanaka et al., 2011).

Meninges

The dura and leptomeninges (arachnoid and pia) provide a protective envelope for the brain and spinal cord. They continue along the roots of spinal and cranial nerves, blending with the capsule of sensory ganglia and the sheaths of peripheral nerves. In contrast to most other 'fascial' structures, the dura represents a highly vascularized tissue that plays a pivotal role in reabsorption of cerebrospinal fluid and brain cooling (Zenker & Kubik, 1996). The cranial dura displayed a rich innervation by thin-caliber afferent axons derived from cell bodies in the trigeminal ganglion, and, in the posterior cranial fossa, from neurons in the jugular ganglion of the vagus (Andres et al., 1987; Neuhuber, 2004). Many of these afferent axons were immunoreactive for CGRP and SP (Keller & Marfurt, 1991; Meßlinger et al., 1993) and were heavily distributed to branches of meningeal arteries, dural sinus, and connective tissue without any vascular relation. The distribution of the CGRP receptor complex to meningeal arteries (but not veins) and mast cells is well compatible with the role of CGRP released from afferent terminals in the control of meningeal blood flow and inflammation (Lennerz et al., 2008). These peptide-containing axons frequently displayed complex terminal formations with laminar expansions (Meßlinger et al., 1993) reminiscent of low-threshold mechanosensory terminals in viscera (Phillips & Powley, 2000). An interesting and probably clinically significant subpopulation of trigeminal axons innervating the cranial dura penetrated the sutures between calvarial bones and projected to extracranial periosteum and even muscle (Schueler et al., 2013, 2014). The spinal dura was comparably less densely innervated; the nerve fibers concentrated on its ventral aspect and were almost completely lacking posteriorly (Groen et al. 1988). The pia mater of spinal nerve roots was supplied by unmyelinated afferent axons that possibly represent a significant portion of so-called 'ventral root afferents' (Hildebrand et al., 1997; Jänig & Koltzenburg, 1991).

Postganglionic sympathetic nerve fibers

Postganglionic sympathetic neurons innervate virtually all tissues including bone and bone marrow. Deep somatic structures appear to be particularly densely innervated. In the cat gastrocnemius-soleus muscle nerve, between 60–75% of unmyelinated axons were sympathetic postganglionics (von Düring & Andres,

1990; McLachlan & Jänig, 1983), while in rat muscle nerves the values were slightly lower (gastrocnemius-soleus nerve: 42%, Baron et al., 1988; sternomastoid nerve: 40%, Sandoz & Zenker, 1986). In the rat thoracolumbar fascia, a majority of nerve fibers staining for the general marker PGP 9.5 were sympathetic (Tesarz et al., 2011). This is in stark contrast to cutaneous nerves where only between 16–29% of all unmyelinated nerve fibers were sympathetic (Baron et al., 1988; McLachlan & Jänig, 1983). In all tissues studied so far, most sympathetic postganglionics as identified by immunohistochemistry for TH or dopamine beta hydroxylase (DBH) or, in older investigations, by the formaldehyde or glyoxylic-acid-induced histofluorescence, accompanied blood vessels forming

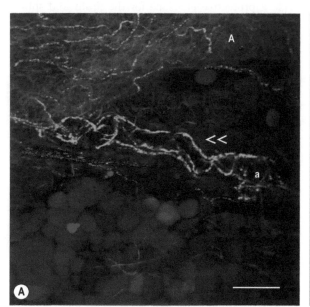
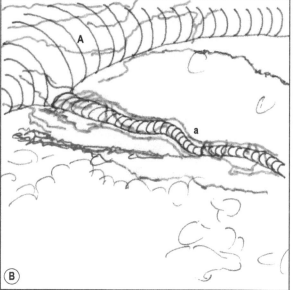

Figure 33.4

(A) Innervation of the epineurium of the human cervical vagus nerve by peptidergic primary afferents (red – CGRP-immunoreactive) and sympathetic postganglionics (green – TH-immunoreactive). Varicose sympathetic axons form a plexus (double arrowhead) around a small artery (**a**) and are abundant in the adventitia of a larger artery (**A**). A bundle of CGRP-positive axons travels parallel to the sympathetic plexus at a greater distance from the small blood vessel. Adipocytes stain blue, and smooth-contoured connective tissue fibers between the adipocytes in the lower half stain green due to autofluorescence. (B) Corresponding drawing emphasizing the wall of both arteries. Whole-mount preparation from a body donated to the Institute of Anatomy of the University Erlangen-Nürnberg; three-channel immunofluorescence, extended focus projection of a stack of 17 single confocal optical sections taken at a z-step of 0.50 μm. Bar is 100 μm

a perivascular plexus (Fig. 33.1–33.4). Of note, one of the 'fascial' tissues (i.e., the periosteum) induces, similar to sweat glands, during ontogeny a change from an adrenergic to a cholinergic phenotype in sympathetic postganglionic neurons (Asmus et al., 2000). However, there are several reports on sympathetic axons that appeared to terminate in the extracellular matrix unrelated to any vessels (Fig. 33.1, 33.2, 33.3B) (rat cranial dura, Keller et al., 1989; rat and human thoracolumbar fascia, Tesarz et al., 2011). This raises the question of what function these 'free' sympathetic axons may subserve. Clues might be provided by studies indicating that sympathetic neurons are involved in bone development and bone remodeling (Gajda et al., 2010, Karsenty & Ferron, 2012). Similar mechanisms may be at work in the extracellular matrix of soft 'fascial' tissues.

Is there a mystery in fascial innervation?

As shown in this section, fascial tissues are supplied by the full range of myelinated and, probably even more important, unmyelinated afferents as well as adrenergic and also (in the case of the periosteum) cholinergic sympathetic postganglionics. Depending on their topographical relationships to other structures, both thin-caliber afferent and sympathetic fibers are involved in a variety of functions, from mechanoreception, chemoreception, and nociception through vasoregulation to immunomodulation and possibly also remodeling of the extracellular matrix. Some of these functions may appear at present to be as mysterious as the effects of manual therapy or osteopathic treatments sometimes might be. However, elucidating the morphofunctional basis of fascial innervation in its context with other tissues of the body, ranging from the macroscopic to the molecular level, will demystify these functions.

Conclusion

Both the physiological and pathophysiological roles of fasciae depend probably to a large extent on their innervation. However, there are many differences with respect to density and distribution of the various sensory structures, even within confined areas (e.g., the wrist ligaments or the thoracolumbar fascia), as well as between the same anatomical structure (e.g., the lateral elbow region), in different species. The full extent of these differences and how they relate to the representation of fasciae in the brain is unknown, even for small mammalian 'model' species, and premature generalizations should be avoided. Likewise, the extent and significance of nonvascular sympathetic innervation of connective tissue are unknown. Nevertheless, these differences most likely have an impact on both the physiology and pathophysiology of fasciae and on manual therapy or osteopathic strategies. An understanding of these phenomena will certainly be furthered by careful combined anatomical and physiological research.

Acknowledgements

The skilful help of Dr Thomas Buder in preparing the tissue for Figure 33.4 and of Karin Löschner and Hedwig Symowski in performing the immunohistochemistry for Figures 33.1, 33.3, and 33.4 is gratefully acknowledged.

References

Andres K. H., von Düring M., Muszynski K., Schmidt R. F. 1987. Nerve fibres and their terminals of the dura mater encephali of the rat. *Anat Embryol* 175:289–301.

Appenzeller O., Dhital K. K., Cowen T., Burnstock G. 1984. The nerves to blood vessels supplying blood to nerves: the innervation of vasa nervorum. *Brain Res* 304:383–386.

Asmus S. E, Parsons S., Landis S. C. 2000. Developmental changes in the transmitter properties of sympathetic neurons that innervate the periosteum. *J Neurosci* 20:1495–1504.

Backenköhler U., Strasmann T. J., Halata Z. 1997. Topography of mechanoreceptors in the shoulder joint region – a computer-aided 3D reconstruction in the laboratory mouse. *Anat Rec* 248:433–441.

Baron R., Jänig W., Kollmann W. 1988. Sympathetic and afferent somata projecting in hindlimb nerves and the anatomical organization of the lumbar sympathetic nervous system of the rat. *J Comp Neurol* 275:460–468.

Benetazzo L., Bizzego A., De Caro R., Frigo G., Guidolin D., Stecco C. 2011. 3D reconstruction of the crural and thoracolumbar fasciae. *Surg Radiol Anat* 33:855–862.

Benjamin M. 2009. The fascia of the limbs and back – a review. *J Anat* 214:1–18.

Blumberg H., Haupt P., Jänig W., Kohler W. 1983. Encoding of visceral noxious stimuli in the discharge patterns of visceral afferent fibres from the colon. *Pflügers Arch* 398:33–40.

Brown A. G., Fyffe R. E. W., Rose P. K., Snow P. J. 1981. Spinal cord collaterals from axons of type II slowly adapting units in the cat. *J Physiol* 316:469–480.

Castaneda-Corral G., Jimenez-Andrade J. M., Bloom A. P., Taylor R. N., Mantyh W. G., Kaczmarska M. J., Ghilardi J. R., Mantyh P. W. 2011. The majority of myelinated and unmyelinated sensory nerve fibers that innervate bone express the tropomyosin receptor kinase A. *Neuroscience* 178:196–207.

Dreessen D., Halata Z., Strasmann T. 1990. Sensory innervation of the temporomandibular joint in the mouse. *Acta Anat* 139:154–160.

Federative Committee on Anatomical Terminology (FCAT). 1998. *Terminologia anatomica*. Stuttgart New York: Thieme.

Gajda M., Litwin J. A., Cichocki T., Timmermans J. P., Adriaensen D. 2005. Development of sensory innervation in rat tibia: co-localization of CGRP and substance P with growth-associated protein 43 (GAP-43). *J Anat* 207:135–144.

Gajda M., Litwin J. A., Tabarowski Z., Zagólski O., Cichocki T., Timmermans J. P., Adriaensen D. 2010. Development of rat tibia innervation: colocalization of autonomic nerve fiber markers with growth-associated protein 43. *Cells Tiss Org* 191:489–499.

Gardner E. P., Johnson K. O. 2013. The somatosensory system: receptors and central pathways, in *Principles of Neural Science*, 5th edn. E. R. Kandel, J. H. Schwartz, T. M. Jessell, S. A. Siegelbaum, A. J. Hudspeth eds, McGraw Hill, New York, NY, pp. 475–497.

Groen G. J., Baljet B., Drukker J. 1988. The innervation of the spinal dura mater: anatomy and clinical implications. *Acta Neurochir* 92:39–46.

Groth M., Helbig T., Grau V., Kummer W., Haberberger R. V. 2006. Spinal afferent neurons projecting to the rat lung and pleura express acid sensitive channels. *Respir Res* 7:96–111.

Hagert E., Forsgren S., Ljung B. O. 2005. Differences in the presence of mechanoreceptors and nerve structures between wrist ligaments may imply differential roles in wrist stabilization. *J Orthop Res* 23:757–763.

Halata Z. 1977. The ultrastructure of the sensory nerve endings in the articular capsule of the knee joint of the domestic cat (Ruffini corpuscles and Pacinian corpuscles). *J Anat* 124:717–729.

Halata Z., Strasmann T. 1990. The ultrastructure of mechanoreceptors in the musculoskeletal system of mammals, in *The Primary Afferent Neuron*. W. Zenker,

W. L. Neuhuber, eds, Plenum Press, New York, NY, pp. 51–65.

Heppelmann B., Meßlinger K., Neiss W. F., Schmidt R. F. 1990. The sensory terminal tree of 'free nerve endings' in the articular capsule of the knee, in *The Primary Afferent Neuron*. W. Zenker, W. L. Neuhuber, eds, Plenum Press, New York, NY, pp. 73–85.

Hildebrand C., Karlsson M., Risling M. 1997. Ganglionic axons in motor roots and pia mater. *Prog Neurobiol* 51:89–128.

Holzer P. 1988. Local effector functions of capsaicin-sensitive sensory nerve endings: involvement of tachykinins, calcitonin gene-related peptide and other neuropeptides. *Neuroscience* 24:739–768.

Huijing P. A. 2009. Epimuscular myofascial force transmission. Historical review and implications for new research. *J Biomech* 42:9–21.

Ivanusic J. J. 2009. Size, neurochemistry, and segmental distribution of sensory neurons innervating the rat tibia. *J Comp Neurol* 517:276–283.

Jänig W., Koltzenburg M. 1991. Receptive properties of pial afferents. *Pain* 45:77–85.

Karsenty G., Ferron M. 2012. The contribution of bone to whole-organism physiology. *Nature* 481:314–320.

Keller J. T., Marfurt C. F. 1991. Peptidergic and serotoninergic innervation of the rat dura mater. *J Comp Neurol* 309:515–534.

Keller J. T., Marfurt C. F., Dimlich R. V., Tierney B. E. 1989. Sympathetic innervation of the supratentorial dura mater of the rat. *J Comp Neurol* 290:310–321.

Kerjaschki D., Stockinger L. 1970. Zur Struktur und Funktion des Perineuriums. Die Endigungsweise des Perineuriums vegetativer Nerven. *Z Zellforsch* 110:386–400.

Kubik I., Szabo J. 1955. Die Innervation der Lymphgefäße im Mesenterium. *Acta Morphol Acad Sci Hung* 6:25–31.

Langevin, H. M., Huijing, P. A. 2009. Communicating about fascia: history, pitfalls, and recommendations. *Int J Ther Massage Bodywork* 2:3–8.

Lee J., Ladd A., Hagert E. 2012. Immunofluorescent triple-staining technique to identify sensory nerve endings in human thumb ligaments. *Cells Tiss Org* 195:456–464.

Lennerz JK, Rühle V, Ceppa EP, Neuhuber WL, Bunnett NW, Grady EF, Messlinger K. 2008. Calcitonin receptor-like receptor (CLR), receptor activity-modifying protein 1 (RAMP1), and calcitonin gene-related peptide (CGRP) immunoreactivity in the rat trigeminovascular system: differences between peripheral and central CGRP receptor distribution. *J Comp Neurol* 507:1277–1299.

Martin C. D., Jimenez-Andrade J. M., Ghilardi J. R., Mantyh P. W. 2007. Organization of a unique net-like meshwork of CGRP+ sensory fibers in the mouse periosteum: implications for the generation and maintenance of bone fracture pain. *Neurosci Lett* 427:148–152.

McLachlan E. M., Jänig W. 1983. The cell bodies of origin of sympathetic and sensory axons in some skin and muscle nerves of the cat hindlimb. *J Comp Neurol* 214:115–130.

Meßlinger K., Hanesch U., Baumgärtel M., Trost B., Schmidt R. F. 1993. Innervation of the dura mater encephali of cat and rat: ultrastructure and calcitonin gene-related peptide-like and substance P-like immunoreactivity. *Anat Embryol* 188:219–237.

Michaelis M., Göder R., Häbler H., Jänig W. 1994. Properties of afferent nerve fibres supplying the saphenous vein in the cat. *J Physiol* 474:233–243.

Neuhuber W. 2004. Hirnnerven, in *Benninghoff/ Drenckhahn Anatomie, Vol. 2, 16th edn.* D. Drenckhahn, ed, Urban & Fischer, München, pp. 547–565.

Peltonen S., Alanne M., Peltonen J. 2013. Barriers of the peripheral nerve. *Tissue Barriers* 1:e24956.

Phillips R. J., Powley I. L. 2000. Tension and stretch receptors in gastrointestinal smooth muscle: re-evaluating vagal mechanoreceptor electrophysiology. *Brain Res Rev* 34:1–26

Proske U., Gandevia S. C. 2012. The proprioceptive senses: their roles in signaling body shape, body position and movement, and muscle force. *Physiol Rev* 92:1651–1697.

Reinert A., Kaske A., Mense S. 1998. Inflammation-induced increase in the density of neuropeptide-immunoreactive nerve endings in rat skeletal muscle. *Exp Brain Res* 121:174–180.

Robinson D. R., McNaughton P. A., Evans M. L., Hicks G. A. 2004. Characterization of the primary spinal afferent innervation of the mouse colon using retrograde labeling. *Neurogastroenterol Motil* 16:113–124.

Sandoz P. A., Zenker W. 1986. Unmyelinated axons in a muscle nerve. Electron microscopic morphometry of the sternomastoid nerve in normal and sympathectomized rats. *Anat Embryol* 174:207–213.

Sauer S. K., Bove G. M., Averbeck B., Reeh P. W. 1999. Rat peripheral nerve components release calcitonin gene-related peptide and prostaglandin E2 in response to noxious stimuli: evidence that nervi nervorum are nociceptors. *Neuroscience* 92:319–325.

Schleip R., Findley T. W., Chaitow L., Huijing P. A., eds. 2012. *Fascia. The Tensional Network of the Human Body.* Churchill Livingstone, Elsevier, Edinburgh.

Schueler M., Messlinger K., Dux M., Neuhuber W. L., De Col R. 2013. Extracranial projections of meningeal afferents and their impact on meningeal nociception and headache. *Pain* 154:1622–1631.

Schueler M., Neuhuber W. L., De Col R., Messlinger K. 2014. Innervation of rat and human dura mater and pericranial tissues in the parieto-temporal region by meningeal afferents. *Headache* 54:996–1009.

Silfvenius H. 1970. Characteristics of receptors and afferent fibres of the forelimb interosseous nerve of the cat. *Acta Physiol Scand* 79:6–23.

Snider W. D., McMahon S. B. 1998. Tackling pain at the source: new ideas about nociceptors. *Neuron* 20:629–632.

Song X., Chen B. N., Zagorodnyuk V. P., Lynn P. A., Blackshaw L. A., Grundy D., Brunsden A. M., Costa M., Brookes S. J. H. 2009. Identification of medium/high-threshold extrinsic mechanosensitive afferent nerves to the gastrointestinal tract. *Gastroenterology* 137:274–284.

Standring S., Ellis H., Healy J., Johnson D., Williams A., eds. 2008. *Gray's Anatomy, 40th edn* Churchill Livingstone, London.

Stecco C., Corradin M., Macchi V., Morra A., Porzionato A., Biz C., De Caro R. 2013a. Plantar fascia anatomy and its relationship with Achilles tendon and paratenon. *J Anat* 223:665–676.

Stecco C., Macchi V., Porzionato A., Morra A., Parenti A., Stecco A., Delmas V., De Caro R. 2010. The ankle retinacula: morphological evidence of the proprioceptive role of the fascial system. *Cells Tiss Org* 192:200–210.

Stecco C., Tiengo C., Stecco A., Porzionato A., Macchi V., Stern R., De Caro R. 2013b. Fascia redefined: anatomical features and technical relevance in fascial flap surgery. *Surg Radiol Anat* 35:369–376.

Strasmann T., van der Wal J. C., Halata Z., Drukker J. 1990a. Functional topography and ultrastructure of periarticular mechanoreceptors in the lateral elbow region of the rat. *Acta Anat* 138:1–14.

Strasmann T., van der Wal J. C., Halata Z., Drukker J. 1990b. Sensory innervation patterns of the origins of the supinator muscles in the rat and the gray short-tailed opossum in relation to function, in *The Primary Afferent Neuron*. W. Zenker, W. L. Neuhuber, eds, Plenum Press, New York, NY, pp. 67–72.

Tanaka K., Hayakawa T., Maeda S., Kuwahara-Otani S., Seki M. 2011. Distribution and ultrastructure of afferent fibers in the parietal peritoneum of the rat. *Anat Rec* 294:1736–1742.

Tanaka K., Matsugami T., Chiba T. 2002. The origin of sensory innervation of the peritoneum in the rat. *Anat Embryol* 205:307–313.

Tesarz J., Hoheisel U., Wiedenhöfer B., Mense S. 2011. Sensory innervation of the thoracolumbar fascia in rats and humans. *Neuroscience* 194:302–308.

Usoskin D., Furlan A., Islam S., Abdo H., Lönnerberg P., Lou D., Hjerling-Leffler J., Haeggström J., Kharchenko O., Kharchenko P. V., Linnarsson S., Ernfors P. 2015. Unbiased classification of sensory neuron types by large-scale single-cell RNA sequencing. *Nat Neurosci* 18:145–153.

van der Wal J. 2009. The architecture of the connective tissue in the musculoskeletal system – an often overlooked functional parameter as to proprioception in the locomotor apparatus. *Int J Ther Massage Bodywork* 2:9–23.

von Düring M., Andres K. H. 1990. Topography and ultrastructure of group III and IV nerve terminals of the cat's gastrocnemius-soleus muscle, in *The Primary Afferent Neuron*. W. Zenker, W. L. Neuhuber, eds, Plenum Press, New York, NY, pp. 35–41.

Willard F. H. 2012. Visceral fascia, in *Fascia. The Tensional Network of the Human Body*. R. Schleip, T. W. Findley, L. Chaitow, P. A. Huijing, eds, Churchill Livingstone, Elsevier, Edinburgh, pp. 53–56.

Zenker W., Kubik S. 1996. Brain cooling in humans – anatomical considerations. *Anat Embryol* 193:1–13.

Zenker W., Sandoz P. A., Neuhuber W. 1988. The distribution of anterogradely labeled I-IV primary afferents in histochemically defined compartments of the rat's sternomastoid muscle. *Anat Embryol* 177:235-243.

MYOFASCIAL RELEASE

Carol J. Manheim

Introduction

Myofascial release is a specific set of muscle and soft tissue stretching techniques that are guided entirely by feedback from the targeted tissues (Manheim, 2008). The term 'myofascial' recognizes that muscles and muscle fibers are surrounded by fascia and neither can be stretched independently of the other. Any limitation of the muscle, the individual muscle fibers, or the surrounding fascia can prevent efficient movement and may cause pain. Feedback allows the expert practitioner of myofascial release to distinguish the sensation of a restriction in the fascia or in the muscle fibers.

Technically, all muscle stretching is myofascial stretching. The term myofascial release has been used to describe a variety of stretching techniques. However, these other techniques are not guided by feedback.

Origins and history of myofascial release

The origins of myofascial release date back to the beginning of the profession of osteopathy. Although many different osteopathic physicians used and taught soft tissue stretching techniques, none wrote them down or developed a textbook from which to teach. Dr Robert Ward and colleagues gathered the stretching techniques that were guided by feedback, coined the term 'myofascial release' to describe them, and gave the first formal course in 1981 (Manheim, 2008). The first commercially published textbook was released in 1989 (Manheim & Lavett, 1989).

Principles and method of application

The technique of myofascial release on the surface is quite simple. Stretch is applied to the targeted tissue until resistance is felt. The stretch is maintained until the tissue elongates (releases). Without breaking contact, additional stretch is applied until resistance is felt again. The sequence is repeated until no further stretch can be applied and an end-feel is reached. The end-feel indicates a new or different resting length of the muscle spindles in the myofascial unit. Myofascial release is learned initially by applying stretch in line with the muscle fibers (Fig. 34.1). Feedback may change the direction of stretch to diagonal when the targeted tissues still need to elongate but are prevented by anatomic limitations (Fig. 34.2). When feedback can be consistently recognized, stretch may be applied using a vertical lift, moving the targeted muscle perpendicular to the body (Fig. 34.3), or a vertical stretch down into the muscle (Fig. 34.4). The vertical stretch down is also used during 'myofascial trigger point releases', and 'scar releases'. Stretch is applied in a variety of ways using the fingertips, the

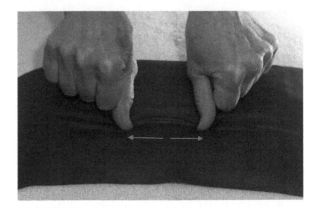

Figure 34.1
The initial stretch of a muscle is applied in line with the muscle fibers

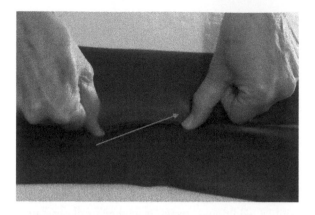

Figure 34.2
When an anatomical limitation prevents further stretch in line with the muscle fibers and a final end-feel has not been achieved, (in response to feedback and without breaking contact) the stretch is moved diagonally

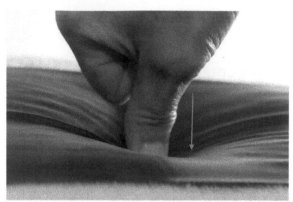

Figure 34.4
When the practitioner can accurately monitor a release, stretch can be applied to a thick muscle (e.g., gastrocnemius, quadriceps femoris) using a vertical stretch down into the muscle belly. The vertical stretch down is also used to release tender and trigger points

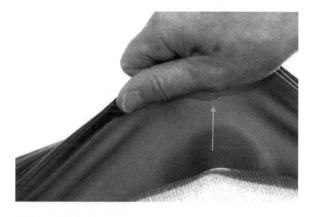

Figure 34.3
When the practitioner can accurately monitor a release, stretch can be applied to some muscles (e.g., sternocleidomastoid, brachioradialis) using a vertical lift

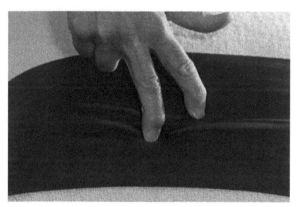

Figure 34.5
A small muscle or a small section of a muscle may be stretched using two fingers of one hand or one finger and the thumb of one hand

palm, or the ulnar border of the hands (Fig. 34.5–34.9). The comfort of the practitioner and the patient determines the specific way stretch is applied.

Depending upon the specific myofascial release being used, the patient may exhibit spontaneous movement as the practitioner is applying stretch. This movement is the body's way of positioning the targeted tissue at the correct angle to allow the release to occur. Arm, leg, and head spontaneous movements

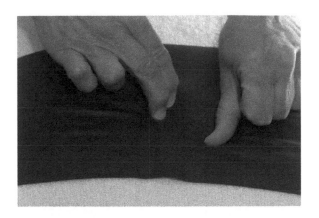

Figure 34.6
Stretch may be applied using one, two, or three fingers of one hand and the thumb of the other hand, or between multiple fingers on each hand

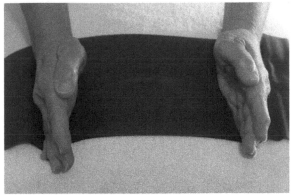

Figure 34.8
Stretch may be applied using the ulnar border of both hands

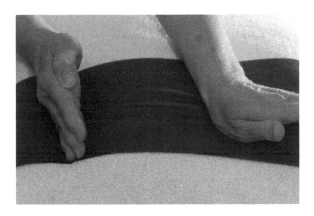

Figure 34.7
Stretch may be applied using the ulnar border of one hand and the heel of the other hand, or using multiple fingers of one hand and the heel of the other hand

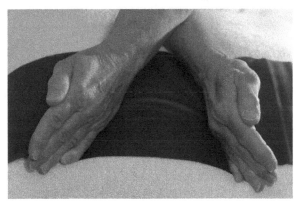

Figure 34.9
When more force is needed to apply stretch, crossing the arms allows the practitioner to use a more powerful pushing motion. The practitioner may find that crossing arms is a more comfortable and energy-efficient way to apply stretch

may take the patient into a painful range of motion before a release can be achieved.

The mechanics of myofascial release can be taught and learned in a short period of time. However, the critical component of being able to accurately monitor feedback can only be learned with practice while treating patients. Each patient will benefit from treatment with myofascial release while the practitioner develops greater skill utilizing the technique. Myofascial release is not appropriate for all practitioners. The effective practitioner 1) must be able to stay mentally present and focused on the feedback felt in the hands, 2) can recognize the sensation of a release in different tissues and positions, 3) is comfortable allowing the patient to direct the treatment by feedback, and 4) does not need to be in total control.

Physiological response to treatment

Both touch and the length of the muscle spindles are mediated by the autonomic nervous system. Therefore, the physiological body responses to treatment are autonomic in nature. The common response to myofascial release is vasodilatation, giving the sensation of heat being released from the patient's body. This vasodilatation can be localized to the area being treated or can appear in other areas of the body. The distal vasodilatation may indicate another area that requires treatment or areas that have also released at the same time. A patient who responds with excessive vasodilatation can actually lower core temperature and must be monitored closely. Infrequently, vasoconstriction will occur, giving the sensation of cold.

The emotional response to treatment can vary widely. The most common response is a feeling of calm and contentment. The patient may feel a special bond or closeness with the practitioner. Professional boundaries must be made clear to avoid a misunderstanding of the nature of this (nonsexual) bond. When the area being treated has been injured during a traumatic event, the treatment may reawaken the body's memory of the event and the emotions engendered. The patient must be allowed to express these emotions to avoid retraumatization.

Trigger points

The practitioner of myofascial release should have a competent knowledge of trigger points and their radiation patterns (Simons et al., 1999; Travell & Simons, 1993; Dommerholt & Huijbregts, 2011). The pattern of vasodilatation or vasoconstriction in response to myofascial release often mimics the patterns of trigger points. The pain pattern from scar and skin adhesions may also be similar to the radiation patterns of trigger points. When a patient has a pain complaint that cannot be reproduced with direct palpation, knowledge of trigger point radiation patterns may direct the practitioner to the source of the patient's pain. As the practitioner's hands become more sensitive to feedback from the patient's body, feedback will lead the practitioner from the locus of the pain complaint to its source, particularly if the pain does not follow a known radiation pattern. The reader is referred to Chapter 27 by J. Shah and N. Thakker for an in-depth discussion of trigger points.

Concept of the 'good hurt'

The paradox of the 'good hurt' is easily understood after the patient has experienced it for the first time. While it seems contradictory for a pain to feel good at the same time, this happens often during treatment with myofascial release. If the patient is only experiencing pain without an underlying sensation of 'rightness', then the technique should be stopped.

Process of change

When first seen, the patient's soft tissue holding pattern and posture is the 'normal' state monitored in his/her central nervous system. For an elongated resting length achieved during treatment to become permanent, the central nervous system must accept the new length and change the internal image of 'normal'. Therefore, the changes achieved during the initial treatments may not last until the central nervous system recognizes the new resting length and posture as more comfortable and energy efficient.

Goals of myofascial release

The long-term goal of myofascial release is for the patient to achieve the most energy-efficient posture possible with the least amount of pain that can be maintained during daily activities. There are many intermediate goals that must be achieved before the long-term goal. The first, most important, goal is for the patient to recognize the sensation of a release. The second, equally important, goal is for the patient to recognize the sensation of a relaxed muscle versus a tense muscle.

Indications, contraindications, precautions

Indications

1. Myofascial release should always be used prior to joint manipulation.

2. The patient has a chronic soft tissue pain complaint that has not responded to other treatments (e.g., fibromyalgia, post-polio syndrome, chronic low back and/or neck pain).

3. The patient has asymmetrical posture due to soft tissue restrictions.

4. The patient has chronic pain from active myofascial trigger points.

5. The patient has referred pain without an easily identified origin.

6. The patient has pain from scar adhesions.

Contraindications

1. The patient cannot tolerate the close contact needed for myofascial release.

2. A trust relationship between the practitioner and the patient does not exist.

3. The patient has a contagious skin condition.

4. The patient does not understand the concept of the 'good hurt'.

5. The patient has chronic fatigue syndrome. Treatment with myofascial release can increase the fatigue and severely limit the patient's ability to perform any activities of daily living.

Precautions

1. Myofascial release may drop blood glucose levels in patients with diabetes. The patient should check blood glucose levels before and after treatment with myofascial release. Most patients with diabetes will respond to treatment in much the same way they respond to exercise. When the patient's blood glucose levels drop too low during treatment, the expert practitioner will be able to recognize the change in muscle tension and take appropriate action.

2. Myofascial release consistently drops blood pressure, so all patients must rest in place immediately following treatment when treatment is initiated. When the patient's pattern of blood pressure variation is determined, the rest period may be able to be eliminated.

3. A patient who responds with vasodilation throughout the body may need shorter treatment times to avoid dropping core temperature.

4. A patient who is on anticoagulant therapy may bruise easily.

5. The patient may enter a hypnotic state and re-experience a traumatic situation and emotional state.

Clinical cases

These case vignettes are presented to illustrate some of the problems for which patients sought treatment by the author. As can be seen, sometimes treatment clarified the source of the patient's pain and required referral to another medical practitioner. Sometimes the best outcome was to reduce the patient's chronic pain level to a tolerable range. The most satisfying outcome was to permanently eliminate the problem that brought the patient to treatment.

Clinical case 1

Mrs R. was in her middle 50s and suffering from severe pain in her 'teeth' even after all her teeth had been extracted. She was unable to tolerate wearing dentures because it increased her pain. Pain medications provided no relief, so she had stopped taking them. Since she was unable to chew, she had been on a liquid diet for the past year.

Mrs R. was very distressed and depressed. She admitted she had considered suicide due to her unremitting pain. She had lost a significant amount of weight and had not purchased any clothes that fit. While she was talking, her jaw movement was observed to be asymmetrical and traced a zigzag pattern with opening. She had not been diagnosed with temporomandibular joint (TMJ) dysfunction before her tooth pain began.

Palpation found multiple active trigger points in the temporalis, masseters, and other facial muscles that immediately reproduced her 'tooth' pain. Myofascial trigger point releases significantly decreased her pain, but did not alleviate it. She was referred to an oral surgeon who traced her remaining pain to bone exostoses. Injection of novocaine into the exostoses temporarily relieved her pain. Surgical excision of the exostoses finally eliminated her pain and allowed her to be successfully fitted with dentures.

Clinical case 2

Mr M. was a retired military officer who had chronic atypical back pain that made it difficult for him to ride in a car. Abdominal surgery as a young man had left him with a scar that was retracted four centimeters into his abdomen when he was supine. When he was upright, the folded skin over the retracted scar looked like a closed eye. Mr M. said his back pain always felt like it was related to this scar. He had tried many different treatments while he was still on active military duty and after he retired, without any lasting relief.

Palpation of his back and abdominal muscles did not locate any active trigger points or any other reason for his back pain. Partial reproduction of his pain complaint was achieved when mobility of his deeply retracted scar was tested. Treatment began with indirect scar releases to decrease the retraction of the scar and gain mobility of the surrounding tissues. When no further progress was possible with indirect treatment, direct vertical scar release was begun. Many treatment sessions were needed to slowly release the deep adhesions until the retraction had been reduced to 1 cm. By then, Mr M. was able to ride in a car without discomfort and he no longer needed to limit his activities due to back pain.

Clinical case 3

Mrs Z. had been diagnosed with Type 1 diabetes as a child and had experienced many complications associated with diabetes. She had undergone a kidney transplant approximately 15 years earlier and was on low-dose immune suppression. While working at a local hospital, she was injured when the elevator malfunctioned and dropped several floors before the emergency brakes stopped it. Mrs Z. had received inadequate treatment for her injuries and developed chronic pain that limited her daily activities. In spite of her pain, she continued to work full-time. Three years after her initial injury, Mrs Z. was referred to the author.

Palpation revealed multiple active myofascial trigger points throughout the muscles in her arms and legs in addition to her neck, entire back, and anterior chest wall. Testing the mobility of scar adhesions from her multiple surgeries also caused an increase in her pain complaints. Prior to each treatment, Mrs Z. would record her blood glucose level and rate her pain in specific body areas. She would repeat the process at the end of each treatment session.

Treatment with myofascial release began three times a week. Mrs Z.'s initial goal was to regain enough neck rotation so she would not have to turn her entire body to look behind her while backing up her car. When that goal was achieved, treatment was decreased to twice a week. She was unable to take pain medications due to side effects and interactions with her other medications. Mrs Z. was able to continue working full-time as long as she received treatment twice a week.

Clinical case 4

Ms C. was a woman in her middle 50s who had been diagnosed with fibromyalgia by a physician at a hospital's pain clinic. She was unable to tolerate the physical therapy program associated with the pain clinic. Like many people with fibromyalgia, she had tried many different medications without success. Some medications did nothing. Others caused intolerable side effects or she would have an adverse response to them. What she did not tell this author until four months later was she could only get out of bed long enough to come to her therapy appointments. Ms C. could not take care of her home and her husband had to do all the cooking and cleaning. Prior to her illness, Ms C. ran her own business in addition to caring for her home and husband.

Ms C.'s passive range of motion at all joints was within normal limits, but her active range was not. Her strength was barely within functional range and her endurance was poor. She had tender points and trigger points throughout her soft tissue and had difficulty tolerating the contact needed for treatment. Treatment was begun twice a week but had to be decreased to once a week due to 'transportation' problems.

Gradually, Ms C. began to walk with more confidence and her smile no longer looked forced. After four months of treatment, Ms C. said she was doing so much better because she was 'in bed for only three days' after treatment the previous week. She was able to unload, but not load, the dishwasher and she was able to set the table for dinner each night. Ms C. explained she had been afraid to set goals because that would have revealed how little she could do and she was afraid the author would not continue to treat her. Ms C. continued to improve and to achieve the short-term goals she set for herself over the next four months. She was able to take short trips with her husband and began looking for part-time work. Twelve months after beginning treatment with myofascial release, Ms C. was able to resume working full-time.

Conclusion

Myofascial release is a safe, effective treatment for soft tissue dysfunction that cannot be successfully treated with more conventional physical treatment. This technique can be learned easily during a weekend course. The practitioner will continue to learn with each patient treatment, gaining expertise one patient at a time. Confidence in and mastery of the technique is communicated to the patient through touch. In time, the practitioner will find patients responding more rapidly to treatment compared to when the practitioner first began using myofascial release.

Acknowledgements

Rhonda Ferris RN read and edited each draft of this chapter, providing valuable feedback and suggestions. Michael Phillip Manheim gave his time and expertise to provide the photographs for this chapter.

References

Dommerholt, J. & Huijbregts, P., 2011, *Myofascial Trigger Points: Pathophysiology and Evidence-Informed Diagnosis and Management,* Jones and Bartlett Publishers, Sudbury, MA.

Manheim, C. J., 2008, *The Myofascial Release Manual,* 4th edition, Slack Incorporated, Thorofare, NJ.*

Manheim, C. J. & Lavett, D. K., 1989, *The Myofascial Release Manual,* Slack Incorporated, Thorofare, NJ.

Simons, D. G., Travell, J. G. & Simons, L. S., 1999, *Myofascial Pain and Dysfunction: The Trigger Point Manual, Volume 1. Upper Half of Body, Second Edition,* Lippincott Williams & Wilkins, Baltimore, Md.

Travell, J. G. & Simons, D. G., 1993, *Myofascial Pain and Dysfunction: The Trigger Point Manual, Volume 2. The Lower Extremities,* Lippincott Williams & Wilkins, Baltimore, Md.

*The *Myofascial Release Manual,* 4th *edition* has been translated into German, Korean, and Polish. The 3rd edition has been translated into Italian.

THE FASCIAL DISTORTION MODEL ORIGINATED BY STEPHEN P. TYPALDOS[1]

Georg Harrer

Introduction

Whoever gets hurt or feels pain somewhere in the body has a clear perspective of this pain. Roughly half of the peripheral nervous system is dedicated to conducting the information gained in the tissue to the central nervous system. In the spinal cord more than 50% of the fibers are afferent. Some of them conduct superficial sensations, such as touch or temperature, but the vast majority are preserved for the deep sensitivity of tension, position, acceleration, and pain.[2] The tissue responsible for this sensitivity, including pain, is fascia. The fascia hosts all the sensors for the perception of the body. Proprioception and nociception, together known as the so-called sixth sense, remained undiscovered until the beginning of the twentieth century.[3] Neuroscience later divided nociception from proprioception, a common approach in Western medicine. But in fact they never seem to work separately. Whenever we feel pain, we feel tension and position at the same time. So this adds specific impressions to the pain, like color to a painting.

When it comes to mechanical forces at the level of tissue, fascia is the only tissue that is susceptible to injury. All other tissues are hosted by the fascia and more or less amorphous without it. A muscle, for instance, is organized with endomysium, epimysium, and perimysium. The muscle fibers themselves are unable to maintain shape without the fascia and can therefore only be injured on a cellular or chemical level. All physical forces are applied to the fascia.

Fascia is deformed by harmful forces. The nociceptors are mechanoreceptors detecting fascial deformation. There is also chemical sensitivity of nociceptors, but many of the chemical messengers activating the nociceptors are results of mechanical cellular damage. The nociceptors detect these mechanical and chemical changes within the fascia and transform them into electrical potentials. The brain interprets these signals as pain. The pain is always interpreted together with proprioceptive information and hence every pain feels different.

So the individual complaining of pain, in general known as the patient, equipped with the most advanced and accurate sensory system, has a clear perspective concerning the specific pain. In the history of medicine this information has mostly been ignored by physicians. Lacking a language in common, patients and physicians were doomed to misinterpretation.

Philosophical considerations

Disease, injury, or malfunction cannot be understood by the physician, only interpreted. Mankind developed numerous approaches to this interpretation. The condition itself is too complex to be comprehended by the human mind. We are forced to reduce its complexity in order to contemplate and understand the condition of the patient. Natural science calls this reduction in complexity a model. Worldwide over the centuries there have been innumerable models of vast variety in terms of etiology, pathogenesis, diagnostics, and treatment.[4] In general the proponents of these medical models are unaware of the fact that they are utilizing a model. Physicians always intend to consider the local contemporary model to be the truth (a term unsuitable for the description of nature) and therefore all other models have to be false. In contrast to medicine, models are widely used in natural science and allow contemplation and constant progress through adjusting the model. The term 'truth' in its scientific sense is focused on accurate measurement and valid experiment, and is not a judgment on the entire underlying model.[5]

The fascial distortion model

One of these medical models is the fascial distortion model (FDM), originated by the American physician Stephen P. Typaldos (1957–2006).

Within the FDM all injuries and other conditions causing pain, disability, and other malfunctions are envisioned as one or more of six specific distortions of the connective tissue. A distortion means an alteration in shape from perfect to inadequate.

Number six is the present state, since there have been six distortions described so far. Maybe in the future research will lead to more than six.

Envisioning all injuries and other conditions as distortions allows new treatment approaches since differences to damaged, distorted fascia can be reshaped to restore function and ease.

Diagnostics according to the FDM

Basic considerations on FDM diagnostics

Each of the six fascial distortion types feels different, since each one stresses different structures of the sensory system and leads to specific vectors of force within the three-dimensional, seamless, and continuous fascial network. The person hurting has no difficulty whatsoever in distinguishing the type of pain. The barrier is communication.

Visual diagnostic system

In all spoken languages there is a deficit in communicating proprioceptive impressions and pain. The vocabulary is too limited by far to express the perception.

In the early 1990s Typaldos found through thorough observation that his patients described their pain and discomfort with distinct, reproducible, and recognizable gestures. Those with similar gestures responded well to similar treatment. It took him two years of specific research and categorization to determine a set of six specific pathologies with specific gestures, verbal descriptions of the conditions, and treatment responses. He was unable to match these pathologies to any disorders he was introduced to in his medical and osteopathic education. Typaldos

spent many hours discussing his findings with pathologists and anatomists. In dissection he found fascial tissue to be the only tissue that was present in all locations of complaints.

The pain-related gestures described by Typaldos as 'body language' are interpreted as subconscious movements, not directly controlled by the mind. This makes this source of information very reliable, considering that it is the expression of proprioceptive and nociceptive impressions. In behavioral science, behavior that is considered to be undeliberate is rated higher in terms of authenticity. The polygraph, a device to detect lying in law enforcement is a good example of this high rating of subconscious actions, since the device is especially designed for detection of undeliberate phenomena.

Evolutionary considerations on pain gestures

Since the early 1990s, when Typaldos published the body language of fascial distortions, this diagnostic approach has been applied in various continents among various races. All displayed the same gestures when asked about their pain. This behavior suggests that the pain gestures are inborn. This question is always difficult to prove scientifically but most other gestures used for nonverbal communication vary from country to country. Repetitive horizontal movements of the head mean 'no' in some cultures; in others this gesture means 'yes'. The pain gestures seem to be different since they do not require socialization. Children have a clear body language in terms of pain gestures in conditions, which none of their family members had in the lifetime of the child. So from whom did the little boy or girl learn how to gesture? The same applies to blind patients. As for all innate human behavior, we do not know why our patients do as they do. We can only categorize and interpret the behavior.

Verbal communication of fascial distortions

Verbal expressions, such as 'burning' or 'numb', are also helpful to identify the specific distortion. These expressions vary from language to language and are therefore more difficult to evaluate than gestures.

Verbal communication is different to gestures in that it is widely under the control of the mind. That makes it a far less reliable source of information. Only a small part of the content is representing the proprioceptive sensation. The vast majority is information gained from other medical professionals, media, and medical illustrations. As an example a patient might say 'I suffer from a herniated disc!' but in reality he suffers from pulling pain in his leg and numbness in two of his toes. The bulged disc is the interpretation of the patient's neurologist and so the patient adopts this theoretical interpretation in his verbal expression. The bulged disc itself is based on imaging strategies, can be found in MRI scans in up to 75% of the population, and is rarely in correlation with symptoms.[6] Another patient might say 'I suffer from low blood pressure!' and in fact suffers from dizziness. It is likely that dizziness has been a common complaint since the birth of mankind, but systolic blood pressure was first measured in 1896[7] and diastolic blood pressure in 1905.[8] So people have only suffered from 'low blood pressure' since then.

Palpation as a diagnostic tool

In the FDM palpation is considered as a helpful tool to locate the distortion once diagnosed. Not all of the six distortion types are palpable. The inter-rater reliability of palpation is very poor, so it is rated as a very unreliable tool for primary qualitative diagnosis.[9–13]

Imaging of fascial distortions

Imaging strategies do not play any role in FDM diagnostics in its present state. They do not seem to improve the diagnostic process.

General considerations on diagnosis

All diagnostic techniques can be tested, rated, and compared. The concerns are 'inter-rater reliability' and 'relevance'.

Inter-rater reliability means: How many examiners with a certain standardized amount of training and experience come to the same diagnosis in the same patient? Studies have shown that the inter-rater reliability of 'pain gesture reading' is with a $\varkappa$ (kappa) value in good range comparable with many radiologic techniques.[14,15] Pain gesture reading has a

short tradition so far and probably the inter-rater reliability of pain gesture reading can be improved with more research on pain gestures.

Relevance means: How relevant is my finding? How likely is it that this finding leads to different treatment or a different outcome. This has not been specifically studied for gesture reading so far, so there is only indirect evidence for the relevance of pain gesture reading from clinical studies.[16,17] With imaging this is different. Several studies have been done on imaging in back pain and have shown evidence of very low or zero relevance.[18,19] This suggests that there is evidence that imaging does not lead to higher relevance in back pain. The same applies to many other musculoskeletal complaints.

It has to be emphasized that there is no correlation between the level of inter-rater reliability and the level of relevance. One does not lead to the other.

Fascial distortions

The trigger band (TB)

One type of connective tissue is banded fascia (Fig. 35.1). This means almost all fibers are aligned in the same direction in order to resist forces along this direction. Due to their architecture these fascial bands are prone to injury caused by shearing forces. When a shearing force is applied to banded fascia the long fibers lose their coherence and separate longitudinally. The bands then become shorter and the edges along the separation become twisted.[20] The cross-links are fibers with different alignment than the vast majority of the banded fascia. They attach the longitudinal fibers to each other and are doomed to break under shearing forces. The natural limitations for this pathology are bones and cross-bands (Fig. 35.1). Both prevent the fibers from separating further even under shearing forces. Because of its form-stability, bone keeps the fibers in place with its mineral matrix. If the forces are beyond the stability of the bony matrix the TB may enter the bone, resulting in fracture. Cross-bands resist shearing forces and are therefore natural limitations for this pathology.

The best analogy of the TB concept is probably the Ziploc® bag.

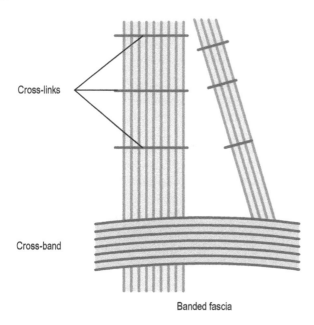

Cross-links

Cross-band

Banded fascia

Figure 35.1
Banded fascia

Without treatment nature has the ability to heal trigger bands by wound healing. This involves a wide variety of cellular actions stimulated by chemical messengers. The main work seems to be done by the fibroblasts. This is the only cell that maintains the ability to produce collagen fibers after the period of growth. These cells are chemotactically attracted to wounds and climb along fibrin polymers to reattach the separated fibers. In general, the correct alignment to restitutio ad integrum is guided by motion. Only tissue in motion can heal properly since the formation of nonfunctional fibers, commonly called adhesions, is mechanically prevented by movement. Fibroblast activity connecting two elements that are not supposed to move together is counteracted by movement since this will rupture the adhesions as long they are not strong enough to prohibit the movement. Fibers that reattach elements supposed to move together are not stressed by movement, so the fibroblast activity is supported by a selective process repeatedly rupturing nonfunctional collagen fibers. All immobilized tissue under fibroblast activity is doomed to develop adhesions and end up with persistent defect after healing. Unfortunately, many patients are immobilized in this

crucial phase, driven by other medical models. In nature immobilization is rare and always counteracted by mobilizing forces such as thirst and starvation. Deprived of these activating forces our patients are inclined to rest or follow immobilizing strategies to avoid pain. This by no means implies that we should introduce starvation and thirst into modern treatment or cease fulfilling the basic needs of the injured. However, it is important to understand that the evolutionary history of wound healing shows that we are not genetically designed or prepared for healing while immobilized.

Chronicity

Once adhesions are formed between two sets of banded fascia, which are not supposed to move together biomechanically, shearing forces are introduced to the fascia as soon as movement is commenced. This will repeatedly produce new trigger bands in new locations adjacent to the initial trigger band. These new trigger bands heal again and lead to rest, forming adhesions and so maintaining a vicious circle of healing with persistent defect. Within the terminology of the fascial distortion model this is a chronic trigger band (Fig. 35.2). Conversely, a trigger band that has not formed adhesions is therefore acute. We see that time (Χρόνος [khrónos] in Greek, commonly considered to be the determining factor for chronicity) is a minor player. Rest and immobilization are the main causes of the formation of adhesions. Hence these treatment strategies are considered to be inadequate and are therefore not applied in FDM treatment.

All these thoughts apply exclusively to trigger bands. The five distortions below are not considered to be wounds, so healing is not involved and there is no potential for adhesions leading to chronicity.

The herniated trigger point (HTP)

All compartments of the human body are separated by fascia. The architecture of this kind of fascia allows the cavities to be sealed and prevents the enclosed organ from protruding out of the cavity. In general, (apart from the thorax) the pressure gradient makes tissue and fluids prone to protrude toward the surface as soon as a gap in the sealing fascia allows the

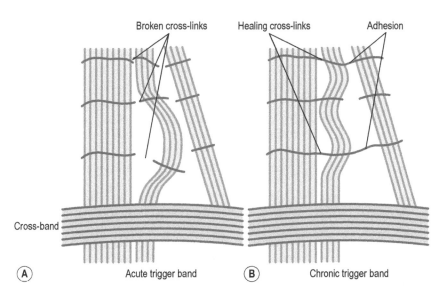

Figure 35.2
(A) Broken cross-links
(B) Healing cross-links

Broken cross-links   Healing cross-links   Adhesion

Cross-band

(A)   Acute trigger band   (B)   Chronic trigger band

content to pass. Some of these hernias (e.g., inguinal hernia) are well explored and there are successful (mainly surgical) treatments available. Others are less well known and the complaints are not understood as a herniation in the medical community. Only the concerted occurrence of an opening of the canal, a pressure peak, and the protrusion of tissue through the fascial plane can be identified as pathology. Each component occurring on its own is physiological. It has to be emphasized that all fascial plains can form herniation when tissue protrudes through them. Not all are understood as compartments so far.[21] For example, fat tissue in the upper arm might protrude through a set of fascial fibers and so becomes protruded within the same tissue. Once a herniated trigger point is formed, it is maintained by the pressure gradient. Spontaneous healing is not expected but reduction leads to repair. In the FDM herniated trigger points within the musculoskeletal system play a major role in explaining patients' complaints, and allow entirely new treatment options utilizing the concept of reduction.[22–24]

The natural progression of an HTP is uneventful. Once it has occurred the HTP is permanent. There seems to be no natural repair strategy. HTPs remain protruded until reduced. The success rate of the treatment does not correlate with the duration of the condition. Since the hernial opening is considered to be a natural orifice there is no wound. The ramifications of this are that there is no wound healing, and

there are no fibroblasts, and no adhesions. Therefore, the HTP cannot be considered as chronic in the terminology of the FDM.

The continuum distortion (CD)

To understand CD, it is necessary to look into the nature of bone and ligament in a fundamental way.[25] In the traditional model the point where bone and ligament come together is understood as an 'insertion.' A junction of two obviously different structures is postulated. This is contradictory to the enormous stability of this junction. In the continuum theory, as part of the FDM, bone and ligament are envisioned as one structure. Ligament is accordingly considered to be nonmineralized bone and bone-calcified ligament. Single bones are not considered to be components of 'in vivo anatomy' and only come into existence after collagen biodegradation, or in medical dissection studies. The same principle applies for ligaments.

The fact that, according to the continuum theory, the vast majority of fibrous pathways are within bone suggests an important role for collagen fibers in bone stability. Fascial fibers can be considered as the highly tensile component of this compound, analogous to the steel in ferroconcrete. A purely mineral-based material can never be resistant to bending forces. Different to bone, it is only resistant to compression forces. The FDM postulates that the tissue in the transition zone has the ability to shift between two states (i.e., between bone and ligament). Depending on the demands it can become ligamentous or osseous by shifting calcium matrix out of or into the bone. Since the calcium concentration is high in the bone and low in the ligament, the soluble mineral is prone to spread into the ligamentous zone, driven by the force of entropy. Physical activity forces the calcium back into the bone by osteoblast activity in the bone and mechanical stress on calcium that has shifted into the ligament. Conversely, it is common for this not to happen when immobilized patients experience a lack of physical activity in intensive care units and in space flight. Osteoporosis in the bones and calcifications in the ligament are the manifestations of this.[26–29]

According to the FDM this phenomenon occurs several times a day on a small scale when physical activity leads to a small shift of the transition zone toward its ligamentous configuration and inactivity leads to a small shift toward osseous configuration. This shift can only be synchronized in the entire 'insertion'. As soon as one part of the transition zone shifts in the osseous configuration while the rest shifts into the ligamentous configuration continuum, distortion occurs. CD is envisioned as a pathological step in the transition zone between bone and ligament.

Envisioning bones and ligaments as one structure (the continuum) with calcified and noncalcified zones allows an entirely new perspective on injury and complaints located in or adjacent to 'insertions'.

The natural progression leads to a slow repair by the osseous metabolism. Lacking a wound, inflammation or wound healing is not involved. So chronicity is not possible in CD.

The folding distortion (FD)

In the body there are numerous flexible junctions. These flexible junctions, generally termed joints, are surprisingly durable, even with repetitive movement. A knee joint, for instance, can be bent and straightened over many years without damage or resistance against the movement. The motion appears to be well guided by multiple structures. In FDM we consider the sum of all these protective structures to work like bellows. The folds facilitate the guided movement,

stabilize it three-dimensionally, and bring all components to the correct spot on reduction. The folds of this structure are very stable in the mid-range of their motion. The closer it comes to the limits in terms of unfolding or refolding, the more two-dimensional the system becomes, losing the folded arrangement. This leads to vulnerability and the folding fascia becomes distorted in a wrinkled way. This concept applies to all moving zones within the body, including joints, intermuscular septum, and interosseous membranes.

Once wrinkled, the body has little chance to restore the folds. In capsuled joints effusion can be understood as a repair mechanism. Nature inflates the bellow to come to a new starting point without wrinkles or folds and then gradually the natural folding restores itself once the wrinkles are eliminated. Without the effusion FD is doomed to wait for a restoring force vector introduced randomly by activity or targeted by therapy.

The cylinder distortion (CyD)

All structures in the body are held in place by connective tissue. In blunt dissection we observe a cobweblike tissue in all gaps between the anatomical structures. It is in general widely removed in dissection studies. Following these cobweb fibers of the loose connective tissue we find cylindrical pathways around organs, extremities, and the trunk, forming tubular patterns.[30] These tubes and cylinders are in general ignored by anatomists, since they focus on the content and not the surrounding cylinders. This fascial tissue is tensile in all directions. In contrast with other manifestations of connective tissue, the specific arrangement of the collagen fibers allows far more elasticity. The cylindrical coils go in virtually all directions. Although interwoven, all the fibers of the cylindrical fascia have to move separately to allow equal distribution of tension to all coils in any movement. If these coils become entangled in each other, the ability to move separately decreases, leading to disturbed proprioception and nociception in the entire region. In the FDM this condition is called cylinder distortion (CyD).

The geometry of the entanglement is very complex, therefore prognosis and duration of the condition vary significantly. In CyD the continuity of the fibers is intact. Hence inflammation and wound healing does not come into action, so without adhesions we do not expect chronicity.

Tectonic fixation (TF)

All joints in the body are considered to be slide bearings. All these slide bearings consist of fascia. Some of these slide bearings possess anatomical features such as cartilage or synovial fluid and are therefore termed 'joints'. Other slide bearings lack these anatomical features but have similar functional ability. All slide bearings of the body show a similar construction. They consist of two corresponding sliding faces and a layer of lubricant in between. This may be a non-Newtonian fluid such as synovial fluid or a more Newtonian fluid like extracellular fluid that freely corresponds with the surrounding tissue.[31–33] In so-called joints these sliding faces are cartilage and the lubricant is synovial fluid. In other slide bearings, such as the scapulothoracic articulation, the lubricant is interstitial fluid. All work the same way and perform a tectonic movement, a horizontal gliding.

TF is the loss of this ability to glide. The production of synovial fluid is triggered by motion. It needs only a short immobilization to omit the production of synovial fluid. This causes stiffness of the joint. As soon as the joint is moved again the production of synovial fluid recommences. This restores the ability to glide.

Apart from joints there are numerous slide bearings surrounding tendons or between the lungs and the thorax. In these slide bearings the interstitial fluid is the lubricant and the same rules apply.

A lack of fluid leads to stiffness. Movement leads to more fluid. TF is always secondary either to other fascial distortions or immobilization due to external reasons. Once the reason for the immobilization is eliminated, children need only a few days to get back to their normal mobility, but in elderly people this may take longer. The permanent correction of the TF is only possible once the causative fascial distortion (one or more of the other five) is eliminated.

General considerations on treatment

It is obvious that all treatment techniques, be they manual, surgical, pharmaceutical, or based on other strategies, are to some extent applied to fascia. There is no way to perform a manual treatment without applying forces to fascia. The same applies virtually to all treatment approaches since fascia surrounds and divides all other tissues. So the term 'fascial technique' can be seen as a pleonasm and is therefore redundant. If used, the term expresses more the focus of the therapist and so displays the medical model underlying the treatment.

In the fascial distortion model all treatment techniques are highly specific in terms of the forces applied and specific in the way these forces are introduced to the body. All techniques, no matter the origin (manual, surgical, exercises ...), that apply forces to the body can be classified and so linked to one or more of the fascial distortions. In general, the technique should be applied to a single, specific distortion, but since the forces are also applied to types of fascia other than the target fascia, effects on other distortions can be observed.

Trigger band (TB) treatment

The treatment of trigger bands is aimed to untwist the twisted fascial band, break the adhesion, and reapproximate the separated fibers. The technique introduced by Typaldos utilizes firm pressure applied with the thumb, gliding along the fascial pathway.

Stretching, weight-training, and other types of exercises can be used to improve the outcome and prevent adhesions.

Herniated trigger point (HTP) treatment

The treatment of HTPs consists of reducing the tissue that is protruding through the fascial plane and moving it into the original position. The same principle is applied to herniation in surgery. Please note that not all herniations are HTPs in the narrower sense, and vice versa, but the pathophysiological concept is similar. Unfortunately, many well-documented herniations are rarely treated surgically in modern surgery (femoral, gluteal, and lumbar hernias), even though there have been attempts in the past.[23,24] Typaldos suggested manual techniques with the goal of reduction. The thumb is utilized to reduce the tissue through the fascial plane using brawn and finesse. Once reduced, ease and function is restored immediately.

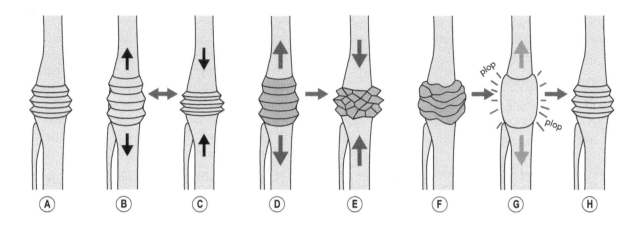

Figure 35.3

(A) Normal folding fascia. (B) Folding fascia adapting to traction. (C) Folding fascia adapting to compression. (D) Folding fascia losing folds due to too much traction. (E) Folding distortion: folding fascia becoming crumpled by unguided compression, due to a lack of folds. (F) Folding distortion. (G) Folding distortion resolving due to therapeutic traction. (H) Restored folding

Continuum distortion (CD) treatment

In CD the pathology is envisioned as an inadequate distribution of calcium in the transition zone between bone and ligament, in both zones of the skeletal continuum. The goal of the treatment is to shift the calcium matrix to adequate distribution. This can be achieved by firm pressure applied on the transition zone with the thumb, or in some cases by manipulation technique. In the latter the short traction force on the ligament is utilized to shift the bony matrix.

Folding distortion (FD) treatment

In FD it is essential to apply the treatment force in the same direction as the force that caused the folding distortion (Fig. 35.3). Hence traction injury, known as unfolding distortion (uFD), is treated by traction therapy. Compression injury, known as refolding distortion (rFD), is treated by applying compression forces. These therapeutic forces can be applied manually or by gravity (e.g., inversion therapy for uFD or horseback riding for rFD. If the direction of force is unknown, as in the majority of cases, the most comfortable position is the best. The patient is the guide. In contrast to TB, HTP, and CD, the treatment of FD is always expected to be pain free.

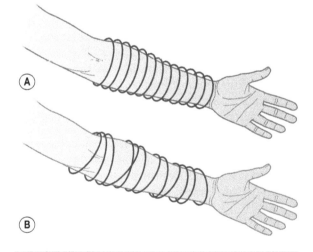

Figure 35.4

(A) Normal cylinder fascia. (B) Cylinder distortion

Cylinder distortion (CyD) treatment

In cylinder distortion (Fig. 35.4) the goal is to untangle the entangled fibers of the cylinder fascia. In general, shearing forces applied to the skin either manually or with tools are efficient. The tools allow angles of force that are difficult to achieve with the hands. Suction cups, clamps, and other tools are used.

Tectonic fixation (TF) treatment

In tectonic fixation the goal is to restore the ability of the gliding fascia to glide. Mobilization and manipulation concentrate on movement. Other techniques concentrate more on the joint fluid. Joint replacement with endoprothesis is classified as an ultima ratio tectonic treatment. This does not suggest joint replacement as first-line treatment, but it illustrates that all techniques can be classified and linked to fascial distortions. This improves interdisciplinary cooperation.

General considerations on side effects and communication

In TB treatment bruising is a common side effect. The more chronic the TB, the more likely it is that bruising occurs as a visual ramification of adhesiolysis. In TB, CD, and HTP pain is also experienced by the patient during the treatment and in TB there is also some soreness over the following days.

Other side effects are rare and can be studied in detail in FDM textbooks. The same applies to relative contraindications against the different specific techniques used to counteract fascial distortions.

Evaluation of treatment

In general, the evaluation for the treatment of fascial distortions is functional. Mobility tests and stress tests using weights are common and are performed immediately after every technique. Since the criteria for evaluation of the outcome are range of motion, force, stability, and balance, they are equally available both to patient and therapist.

Final considerations

At present, the musculoskeletal system is the focus of the fascial distortion model. This is probably for historic reasons, since Typaldos first described musculoskeletal complaints and their treatment. Later in his textbook he states that he expects the main impact to be in cardiology, since fascial distortions in the human heart are far more dangerous than in the ankle or knee.

So it is to be expected that the fascial distortion model will be applied to a growing number of complaints in the future.

References

1. Typaldos S. *FDM: Clinical and Theoretical Application of the Fascial Distortion Model within the Practice of Medicine and Surgery.* Orthopathic Global Health Publications, 2002.

2. Duus P. Propriozeption. In: *Neurologisch-topische Diagnostik, 7 Auflage.* Thieme Verlag. 2001, pp.10–30.

3. Sherrington, C. S. *The Integrative Action of the Nervous System.* New York: Charles Scribner's Sons, 1906.

4. Rotschuh K. *Konzepte der Medizin in Vergangenheit und Gegenwart.* Stuttgart: Hippokrates Verlag, 1978.

5. Huber H. 'Was ist Wahrheit?' Überblick zu aktuellen Wahrheitstheorien. *Aufklärung und Kritik.* 2002;1:96–103.

6. Jensen M. C., Brant-Zawadzki M. N., Obuchowski N. et al. Magnetic resonance imaging of the lumbar spine in people without back pain. *N Engl J Med.* 1994, 14;331(2):69–73.

7. Riva-Rocci S. Un nuovo sfigmomanometro. *Gazz Med Torino.* 1896;47:981, 1001.

8. Korotkow N. S. On methods of studying blood pressure. *Bull Imperial Acad Med (St Petersburg).* 1905;4:365.

9. Stochkendahl M. J., Christensen H. W., Hartvigsen J. et al. Manual examination of the spine, a systematic critical literature review of reproducibility. *J Manipulative Physiol Ther.* 2006;29(6):475–485.

10. Seffinger M. A., Najm W. I., Mishra S. I. et al. Reliability of spinal palpation for diagnosis of back and neck pain: a systematic review of the literature. *Spine.* 2004;29(19):E413–425.

11. Haneline M. T., Young M. A review of intraexaminer and interexaminer reliability of static spinal palpation: a literature synthesis. *J Manipulative Physiol Ther.* 2009;32(5):379–386.

12. Rogers J. S., Witt P. L., Gross M. T. et al. Simultaneous palpation of the craniosacral rate at the head and feet: intrarater and interrater reliability and rate comparisons. *Phys Ther.* 1998;78(11):1175–1185.

13. Meredith G. A study of the inter-rater reliability of passive spinal motion palpation of the cervical spine in an asymptomatic student population

when assessed by experienced osteopaths. Thesis. British School of Osteopathy, 2011.

14. Anker S. Interrater-Reliabilität bei der Beurteilung der Körpersprache nach dem Fasziendistorsionsmodell (FDM). Master Thesis zur Erlangung des Grades Master of Science in Osteopathie an der Donau Universität/Wiener Schule für Osteopathie, Wien, Juni 2011.

15. Stechmann K. Intertester-Reliabilität der Distorsionsklassifizierung anhand der Körpersprache nach den Prinzipien des Fasziendistorsionsmodells. These zur Erlangung des Grades Bachelor. HAWK Hochschule für Angewandte Wissenschaft und Kunst. Hildesheim, 2011.

16. Stein C., Fink M. et al. Untersuchung der Wirksamkeit einer manuellen Behandlungstechnik nach dem Faszien-Distorsions-Modell bei schmerzhaft eingeschränkter Schulterbeweglichkeit. Dissertation zur Erlangung des Doktorgrades der Medizin in der Medizinischen Hochschule, Hannover, 2008.

17. Rossmy C. Der Effekt desFasziendistorsionsmodells (FDM) auf die schmerzhaft eingeschränkte Abduktion der Schulter. Wissenschaftliche Arbeit zur Erlangung des 'DO-DROM' des Deutschen Registers Osteopathischer Medizin. College für angewandte Osteopathie. 2002.

18. Balagué F., Mannion A. F., Pellisé F., Cedraschi C. Non-specific low back pain. *Lancet.* 2012;379(9814):482–491.

19. Chou R., Fu R., Carrino J. A., Deyo R. A. Imaging strategies for low-back pain: systematic review and meta-analysis. *Lancet.* 2009;373(9662):463–472.

20. Typaldos S. P. Introduction to the Fascial Distortion Model. *AAO Journal.* Spring 1994; 17–34.

21. Bond D. Low back pain and episacral lipomas. *Dynamic Chiropractic.* 2000;18(19).

22. Copeman W. S. C., Ackerman W. L. 'Fibrositis' of the back. *Quart J Med.* 1944 April–July;13:37–51.

23. Dittrich R. J. The role of soft tissue lesions in low back pain. *The British Journal of Physical Medicine.* 1957 Oct; 233–238.

24. Dittrich R. J. Soft tissue lesion as cause of low back pain. *American Journal of Surgery.* 1956 Jan;80–85.

25. Typaldos S. P. Continuum technique. *AAO Journal.* Summer 1995;15–19.

26. Orford N. R., Saunders K., Merriman E. et al. Skeletal morbidity among survivors of critical illness. *Crit Care Med.* 2011 Jun;39(6):1295–1300.

27. Fukuoka H., Nishimura Y., Haruna M. et al. Effect of bed rest immobilization on metabolic turnover of bone and bone mineral density. *J Gravit Physiol.* 1997 Jan;4(1):75–81.

28. Scratcherd T., Grundy D. Calcium metabolism and the osteopenia of space flight. *J Br Interplanet Soc.* 1989 Aug;42(7):371–373.

29. Smith S. M., Zwart S. R., Heer M. et al. Men and women in space: bone loss and kidney stone risk after long-duration spaceflight. *J Bone Miner Res.* 2014 Jul;29(7):1639–1645.

30. Guimberteau J. C. 'Strolling under the skin.' Movie showing in vivo microscopic studies by J. C. Guimberteau MD.

31. Wright V., Dowson D. Lubrication and cartilage. *J Anat.* 1976 Feb;121(Pt 1):107–118.

32. Roques C. F., Bellet D., Boyer P. Biorheologic study of pathological synovial fluids, [Article in French] *Rev Rhum Mal Osteoartic.* 1978 Jun;45(6):383–387.

33. Goudoulas T. B., Kastrinakis E. G., Nychas S. G. Rheological study of synovial fluid obtained from dogs: healthy, pathological, and post-surgery, after spontaneous rupture of cranial cruciate ligament. *Ann Biomed Eng.* 2010 Jan;38(1):57–65.

PRACTICAL APPLICATION OF THE STILL TECHNIQUE

Christian Fossum

It was by the virtue of technique that the public came in contact with osteopathy, a statement that probably held true a hundred years ago as it does today. The practical value of osteopathy, its ability to make good, and a great deal of its professional identity has been through hands-on care. A. T. Still actualized his theories through treatment. Furthermore, each technique was distinct to the actual problem at hand, with a profound respect for the welfare of the tissues under his hands. There was no sameness of execution, nor did his technique have anything in common with routinism. He did not apply techniques to treat somatic dysfunction, but to treat the person. His method of working consisted of a careful search for abnormal tissue tensions and reactions, which was not confined to single tissues with immediately related nerves and vessels, but also included distant parts and tissues. When treating patients, he was acutely aware of nature's attempt to compensate the initial problem or suffering, and he spent time discovering and unraveling problems within problems based on the concatenation of mechanisms that make up the totality of the living organism. It was a constant search, which started with the train of pathophysiological processes, manifestations, and registrations, elevating technique far above drudgery or any semblance of routinism. Something new, something essentially different, was discovered in every case, and indeed, in every succeeding treatment. This complex way of thinking is often abstracted into Still's much-quoted axiom of 'find it, fix it and leave it alone'. Using this and extending it slightly, the purpose of treating a patient from Still's perspective seemed to be that of 1) 'finding' whatever tissue (or part) may be disturbing or interfering with the health-ful and comfortable functioning of the complete man, and 2) 'fixing' that tissue (or part) so that it can answer properly and adequately when the roll is called for duty in the overall economy of the patient. Furthermore, in the 'fixing', the techniques or manipulations in each case were devised on the spot while developing through the senses or their extension an awareness of the functioning patient as he changed from moment to moment. Thus, in the early days of teaching, students were introduced early to the clinic with the patient as the primary object of study, and manipulative technique was not included as a subject of study because of the need to devise individualized and dynamic techniques of manipulation minutely suited to the idiosyncrasies of the individual patient. In Still's perspective, technique developed from palpation and an awareness of the patient as a whole rather than 'manipulations' to correct 'lesions'.

Assessment

To a large extent, current osteopathic literature uses various theoretical and prescriptive biomechanical models to describe assessment and treatment of loss of function or motion as a part of the somatic dysfunction. Notable examples include the principles of coupled spinal motions based on the observations of Fryette, as well as the motions hypothesized to take place in the pelvic girdle during walking and the activities of daily living, as initially described by Mitchell Sr. However, in the early part of the osteopathic profession it seems that a more pragmatic approach to assessment and treatment, of a more experimental and immediate nature, was used. Using motion and tissue responses as criteria, the palpatory feed-back to the introduction of motion in all planes was more important in determining treatment direction and positioning than prescriptive, biome-chanical models. Such models may be 'operational boot-straps', preventing the appreciation of non-linear tissue behavior and responses in assessment and treatment.

When using any variants of the Still technique, several types of palpatory clues are used to detect areas of tissue distortions, including tissue texture

variation, subjective sensitivity to pressure, and increased resistance to both local pressure and shearing, as well as the introduction of passive motion. This is usually done with the palpating hand as the receiver and the other hand introducing motion in the tissues and joint complexes. Palpatory impressions and discrimination of areas with myo-fascial and fascial strain and stress is essential in the application of the technique. And, at the same time, while palpating and assessing local structures it is essential to appreciate functional relationships and

---

Box 36.1

Summary of assessment principles

Illustration of assessment principles

Using the principles of 'listen', 'look', 'feel', and 'move', the clinician should have focused on the area of significance. Then, after determining the area to treat (somatic dysfunction with fascial tissue distortion), specific assessment is used prior to the application of any of the variants of the Still technique. Most methods, including evaluation of motion, tissue and motor responses, fascial ease and bind to tissue tension and traction, inherent motions, or fascial listening posts can be used. The key is that evalua-tion needs to be dynamic and not static, evaluating tissue behavior and motion rather than position or holding pattern. Though the latter may be of importance, motion and tissue response informs the technique.

Although this picture illustrates the Cartesian coordination system, it is important to keep in mind the nonlinear behavior of tissues and tissue responses during assessment and treatment.

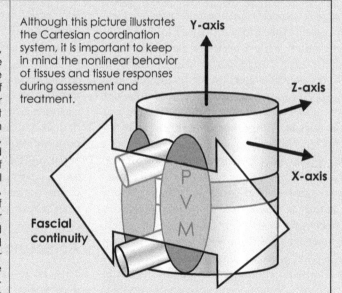

Receiving hand	Motion hand
Sensing tissue texture variations, sensitivity to local pressure, increased resistance to pressure and shearing of tissues, and abnormal tissue responses to the introduction of passive motion.	Introduces motion through either bony or fascial leverages: • Y-axis: rotation, traction, and compression • Z-axis: side-bending, anterior and posterior translation • X-axis: flexion and extension, lateral translation.

tissue continuity, as they may be important in the abnormal fascial tension. It is also clinically useful to palpate and assess both the superficial and deep areas of suspected dysfunction in both upright and lying-down positions to see how the tension and patterns of tension alter with changes in position and respiration.

A summary of assessment principles can be found in Box 36.1.

Examples of treatment techniques

See Tables 36.1 and 36.2 for examples of treatment techniques.

Table 36.1

Treatment of Sibson's fascia and first rib in seated position (see Fig. 36.1)

Applied anatomy	This fascial covering of the pleural dome develops embryologically from the deep prevertebral fascia. Sibson's fascia can be considered in two parts: 1) the fascial tent covering the dome (the suprapleural membrane), and 2) the several fibrous-ligamentous attachments to the lower cervical region and the inside of the first rib (the suprapleural bands). Through the latter passes the lower part of the brachial plexus (the C8–T1: the ulnar nerve). There is also a close topographical relationship between Sibson's fascia and the stellate ganglion. The thoracic duct pierces the Sibson's fascia twice before it joins the union of the internal jugular and subclavian vein where the lymph enters into the systemic circulation (Fig. 36.2 and 36.3).
Patient position	The patient is sitting with the clinician standing behind him. Example: treatment of the right side.
Technique positioning	• The thumb of the left hand palpates the posterior head of the first rib, and the fingers monitor the tissues in the region of the shaft of the same rib. • With the right hand contacting the patient's right elbow, the patient's arm is moved in a posterior direction while at the same time the first rib is gently pushed in an anterior–inferior direction with the left hand. This disengages the rib from the vertebrae. • From its posterior position, the patient's elbow is brought behind the back of the patient while simultaneously gently externally rotating the glenohumeral joint. • Compression is added between the elbow of the patient and the posterior contact on the head of the first rib.
Activating force	Articulatory: • While maintaining the compression, the elbow of the patient is moved upwards while keeping it behind the back of the patient to maintain tension. • When the glenohumeral joint naturally forces the elbow outward, the compression is eased, and, in a sweeping motion, the arm is brought across the chest of the patient. • The whole movement from start to finish looks similar to that of a 'crawl swim'. Bouncing of the barrier: • After positioning and adding compression, introduce rhythmic and gentle compression combined with a minimal or slight increase in external rotation at the glenohumeral joint. This gentle and rhythmic activating force is continued until a release is palpable in the area of the posterior first rib head.

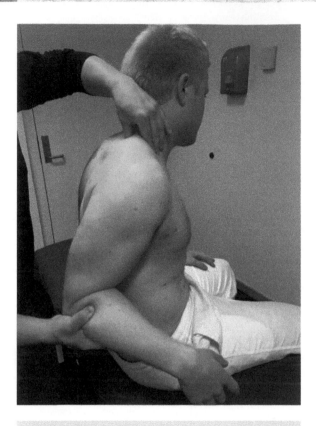

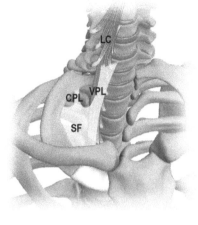

Figure 36.2

The suprapleural membrane and the suprapleural ligaments. CPL = costopleural ligament; LC = longus colli muscle; SF = Sibson's fascia; VPL = vertebropleural ligament

Figure 36.1

Illustration of treatment of the first rib with Sibson's fascia. Articulatory activating force. The clinician contacts the head of the first rib on the right side with the thumb of the left hand. The right hand grabs the patient's right elbow. The rib is gently disengaged from the vertebrae by pushing it anteriorly and inferiorly while at the same time moving the patient's elbow in a posterior direction. Then the elbow is brought behind the back of the patient while simultaneously doing a gentle external rotation of the glenohumeral joint. Compression is added between the first rib and the elbow, and this is maintained while the elbow is moved upward, and released when when it is moved outward through the natural rotation of the shoulder, and then the arm in its totality is moved in front and across the chest of the patient

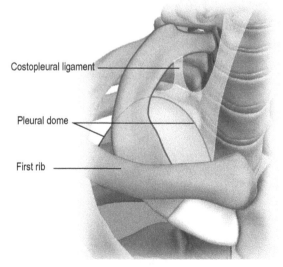

Costopleural ligament

Pleural dome

First rib

Figure 36.3

The first rib with the costopleural ligament (CPL) and the pleural dome. The CPL is a part of Sibson's fascia (suprapleural membrane) and attaches it to the first rib or to one of the suprapleural bands

Applied anatomy	The diaphragm separates the thoracic cavity from the abdominal cavity and consists of three major parts, attaching to the lower ribs and the thoracolumbar junction and upper lumbar spine. Both sides are covered by fascia, the endothoracic fascia and the transversalis fascia, and it is an important muscle in both respiratory and circulatory dynamics, as well as through its fascial and fascial–ligamentous continuity.
Patient position	The patient is sitting.
Technique positioning	• The clinician contacts the lower ribs with both hands using anterior and posterior contact and a gentle anterior–posterior compression is introduced. • The motion preference is tested in flexion and extension, side-bending through lateral translation and rotation. • The three directions with less resistance to motion are exaggerated and stacked and additional anterior–posterior compression is added to stabilize.
Activating force	Exaggeration of the lesion: • Maintaining the compression in the three directions that are stacked, and then reversing in an articulatory fashion 2–3 times. Example: • The right hemidiaphragm is treated. The position is exaggerated in flexion, lateral translation to the left and rotation to the right. Anterior–posterior compression is added. In the reversal phase, the initial motion is moving the patient into extension, followed by lateral translation to the right coupled with rotation to the left. This is repeated 2–3 times in a continuous motion.

Table 36.2
Treatment of the respiratory diaphragm (see Fig. 36.4)

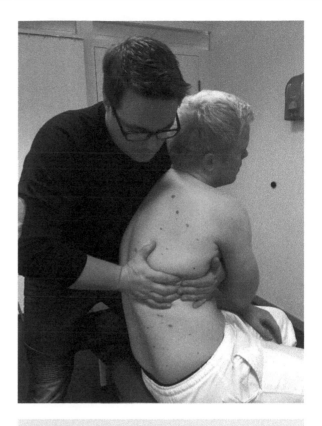

Figure 36.4
Demonstration of treatment of the right hemidiaphragm. Exaggeration of the lesion. The clinician contacts the lower ribs anteriorly and posteriorly with an anterior–posterior (AP) hold. Gentle compression is added. Then the directions of ease are tested in all three available places, and they are exaggerated onto the physiological barrier, stacking all three planes. In this example flexion, translation to the left, and rotation to the left are used. Then more AP compression is added, followed by an articulatory motion through the lower ribs and the diaphragm with its fascial connections. The movements used in this example are extension and right translation with right rotation. This is smoothly and fluently repeated 2–3 times before retesting

Further reading

Van Buskirk R. L. (2006) *The Still Technique Manual: Applications of a Rediscovered Technique of Andrew Taylor Still, M.D. 2nd edition.* Indianapolis: American Academy of Osteopathy.

Soft tissue work

Laurie S. Hartmann

Introduction

Soft tissue work is an essential manual approach in osteopathic practice, although occasionally overlooked in osteopathic education or underestimated in its therapeutic potential. Instead, soft tissue work should be emphasized throughout training and as a foundation of osteopathic practice. Since the effectiveness of this approach often leads to the effectiveness of other techniques, its rationale should be appropriately revisited. Many aspects of soft tissue work have the effect of producing a good relaxation in the patient and in the tissues and consequently prepare the way for the next approach to be used without causing trauma, discomfort, or an adverse reaction.

There are countless methods of soft tissue techniques, although only a few are commonly taught in osteopathic education. Yet they are all efficient and effective and therefore successful in producing the required relaxation.

Comprehension

Indications

- Firstly, it needs to be discovered why we are using soft tissue techniques on the patient. It can be to relax the patient and give the patient confidence in the practitioner.

- Secondly, it gives the practitioner a good feel for what is going on in the tissues. This will allow better control of the joints and soft tissues in other techniques.

- Thirdly, it prepares the tissues for the next approach, which is to be more specific and will then make a change and improvement in the function of the joints and tissues.

- Finally, it is a good choice at the end of a treatment to give the patient and the tissues that 'feel-good' factor.

The main objective of using good, specific soft tissue techniques is to achieve more muscle relaxation and patient cooperation in the problem area being dealt with.

Using soft tissue work to relax the patient will also give a good 'feel' and feedback from the tissues. This 'feel' and feedback will be immensely useful in any further application of techniques. The tissue's response is paramount in choosing which approach to use in treatment (Fig. 37.1, 37.2).

Contraindications

If the tissues are inflamed other than from the initial strain, then soft tissue work is not indicated until the reason for the inflammatory response is found. If the patient is in such pain that merely touching them causes more pain, then we should wait until they are more relaxed and able to get the full benefit from the approach. If one puts one's hands on the patient and they are clearly uncomfortable, then we must stop and get their full appreciation of what we are trying to do with the tissues. If there is swelling in the area that we are working on, then we need to find out what is causing the swelling.

Methods of applying soft tissue work

Schools teach different methods of applying the force to the patient. Some emphasize:

- *Inhibitory pressure:* This is a pressure applied until the muscles relax. It is usually applied for up to 30 seconds and is an effective treatment if the patient is in a lot of pain or scared of moving.

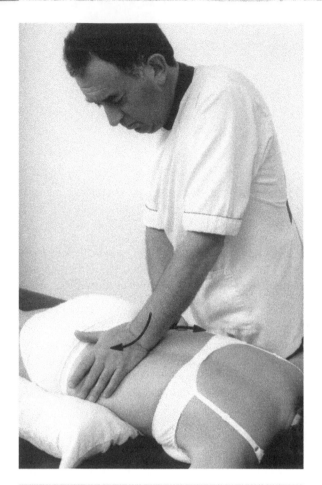

Figure 37.1
Deep soft tissue work on the lumbar spine.
Note the use of a pillow under the abdomen
and the use of the other hand to restrict
movement of the spine

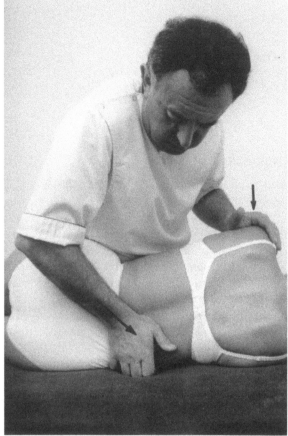

Figure 37.2
Soft tissue work on the lower side of the
lumbars with the patient side-lying. This can
be applied on the side nearer the table.
Please note the use of the other hand to
stabilize the patient and that the practitioner
remains upright

- *Stretching and kneading:* This is the method that
  will be explored in this chapter. It is the main
  method used by osteopaths throughout the
  world. It can be applied slowly or quickly. The
  best result occurs with a much slower method
  than we usually apply.

- *Petrissage:* This is a method used by physiotherapists, but it has a use for tissues that are
  very tight as it stretches the underlying tissues quite a bit and is useful for getting them
  to relax.

- *Skin rolling:* This is a method that most osteopaths
  do not use, but it has a use when the patient is in
  a lot of pain and as a prelude to deeper pressure on
  the tissues as time goes by.

- *Deep friction:* This is useful over tendons and muscle
  ends to produce a reaction to the pressure of
  increased circulation.

- *Effleurage:* This is a method that uses deep pressure
  over muscles. It is sometimes used with a lubricant

to make it more comfortable. It does not go very deep so will not produce the relaxation that we can achieve with other methods.

These methods all have a place in osteopathy. Some osteopaths will prefer one or another, but what we are discussing here is the usual method of application of a pressure that relaxes muscles with deep pressure and then a release of the pressure.

Possible mechanisms during soft tissue application

Most patients seem to like soft tissue work done on painful areas. This is a natural approach and seems to help them quite a bit. Some do not like this method and prefer a more vigorous method of work on the tissues. One has to find the method that the patient likes and then concentrate on that method. If one slows down the method of approach, the patient will usually relax very quickly and the tissues will cooperate with the practitioner. Much of this is a psychological method, but there may be other reasons why this works so well. The mere fact of touching the patient is a very powerful method of first getting them to relax and allowing us to finish the job in process.

General principles

Treatment table height

There are four aspects of good, specific soft tissue work. The first aspect to look at is the balance of the operator. Most practitioners nowadays have adjustable-height treatment tables. This is most beneficial for preventing fatigue and dysfunction in the practitioner, however, the table height must be adjusted for individual techniques as well. Many practitioners work without thinking of what the table height is for each technique and they may well be working at an inefficient height for the particular technique being used. So the first thing that improves soft tissue work is making sure the table height is correct for the morphology of the patient, the height of the practitioner, and the technique being applied.

Operator posture

The operator's feet should be about shoulder width apart. If the table is too high the operator brings their feet closer together, and if the table is too low the operator's feet are too wide-apart. These two postures make for a less stable base, reducing the effectiveness of the technique and tiring the operator unnecessarily. Also, the operator's lumbar curve will be more normal if the feet are shoulder width apart. This sets the body in the right position for the technique and, therefore, raises the level of success. The operator's leg muscles are much better at keeping the operator's body centrally positioned over their feet and these muscles do not tire as easily as the muscles of the operator's trunk.

Handling

The third aspect to investigate is the handling of the patient. This, again, is very important in giving confidence to the patient. The operator's arms should be in the middle of their range, without using full extension of the elbows. There is a useful experiment one can do to prove this is an important aspect. Ask the patient to close their eyes, apply soft tissue work to the patient with full extension at the elbow, and then apply the same technique with slightly flexed elbows and ask the patient which felt more comfortable, more in control, and more effective. They will always choose the flexed-elbow approach! If there is a choice, patients will always choose the practitioner with the best handling (Fig. 37.3).

Tension sense

Tension sense has also to be acquired when treating patients. If practitioners do not have tension sense then more force than is necessary may be used to perform techniques. This is very important for patient comfort and patient safety when it comes to areas such as high-velocity thrust techniques. When one achieves good handling and good posture it is easier to feel tissue tension. If one's balance is good, the tension can be felt using proprioceptors coming right up from the feet through knees, hips, and thorax through the arms to the hands.

As an aside, a nonslip floor covering helps greatly in producing good soft tissue work and other techniques.

Sense of barrier

A sense of rhythm produces relaxation in the patient. If soft tissue work is the choice for producing relaxation,

Creating this barrier at a focal point maximizes the effect of the technique. If one is using thrust techniques it takes time to feel the sense of barrier. Some practitioners will acquire this barrier sense very quickly; for others it may take more time and practice to get a good sense of barrier. Take time to develop this skill and you will be rewarded with a higher rate of success in improvement in the patient's signs and symptoms. In soft tissue technique a sense of barrier allows the practitioner to feel when the muscles will 'give' and then the maximum effect will result. If one is asked to break a piece of wood, one will first attempt to bend the wood a little to see how much force is required to break the wood. To get the tension at the optimum to break the wood one then takes the flexibility out of the wood by twisting it or bending it, and then a final thrust or impulse is applied at the barrier point. The wood will then break at the point of the applied tension. This same method is needed to create a soft tissue tension/barrier as at this tension point the practitioner will achieve the optimum result with the least force and, therefore, the least chance of damage or trauma to the tissues. Somehow soft tissue work has not been regarded highly enough as needing to be as specific as any other technique.

Try applying the heels of the hands first and then rolling the rest of the hand onto the patient. Patients find this very reassuring, especially if they are unable to see the practitioner approach (as in treatments to the back, for instance).

Summary

As one progresses in the profession and more and more patients are booked in for consultations and treatments, the operator must learn to conserve energy. The best way to conserve energy is good balance, correct table height, and *slowing down* the time of each stroke of soft tissue technique. It has been proven that the optimum length of *each* stroke should be between 5 and 7 seconds! This allows for fluid interchange to occur (Fig. 37.4).

This seems a long time, but in the end it actually works on the patient and tissues much faster. However, to maintain this slower time for each stroke, it is essential to have the correct balance, posture, and stance.

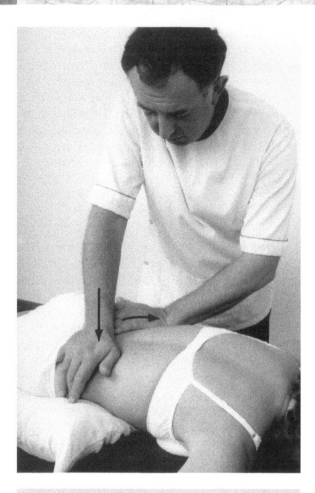

Figure 37.3
The elbows are bent and the other hand is restricting movement. Note the use of a pillow under the abdomen to reduce the pressure into extension

then the method of applying the hands to the patient will have a big influence on the ability to achieve this. One aspect that takes time to learn is the sense of 'barrier' that one is achieving in the patient's tissues. To achieve this 'barrier' the practitioner must focus on the area of dysfunction by restricting movement at that point. This is achieved by applying levers (i.e., side-bending, side-shifting, rotation, compression, or using patient breathing). The aim is to use a maximum number of levers but a minimum amount of each lever. This concept and principle applies to soft tissue work and thrust techniques.

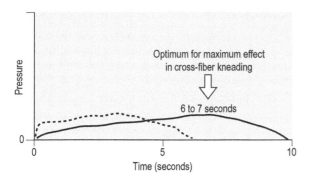

Figure 37.4
Soft tissue work on the spine. The practitioner only achieves the optimal result if he or she waits for a total of 7 seconds instead of the 5 that most will use

Procedure

The actual technique

The soft tissue technique itself starts with the application of the hand as mentioned above. Say we are working on erector spinae – push this muscle gently for a few seconds, and then by changing the angle of the hand and the point of the hand that is applying the pressure we can home down on a smaller area. The muscle will relax very much in line with the area to which we are applying pressure. This same force applied too quickly will be uncomfortable and may well meet an uncomfortable resistance felt by the patient. This slower, refined-down method is very effective in producing a good relaxation in the patient and the soft tissues. So, to reiterate, apply pressure on the muscles you are working on, then push against this muscle until one meets resistance. Then hold for a few seconds until the muscle is felt to relax, often around 3 or 4 seconds, change the direction of the push slightly for a further 1 or 2 seconds, gently release the pressure until you can slide the hand along, and repeat this process on an adjacent area. Do not remove the hands as this can be very irritating to the patient and the tissues. As an experiment, the first few times you try this method you can palpate the muscle you have been working on to check the amount of relaxation you have produced. You will be pleasantly surprised at the effect you will

have had. This method appears slow and pedantic but produces amazingly quick results. With practice it becomes the automatic, subconscious method to use and the one that produces long-lasting, quick results. One other aspect to be covered is the practitioner's head position. Keep the head up in line with the spine. This is another experiment you can try by using the patient's cooperation to prove the point. Apply your soft tissue stroke with your head down looking at the patient's back, and then try the same procedure with your head in line with your spine and ask the patient which way felt better: the first or the second stroke. Without fail, the patient will prefer the method with the practitioner's head up!

Operator posture and stance

The position of the operator's legs is also important. Face the table with the front of your thighs parallel and gently touching against the table edge, come up on your toes, and swivel so that you are facing the head of the table. You now have a front leg and a back leg. If your back leg is your right leg then your right hand will be stronger than your left hand. So if you want to be powerful use your right hand, but if the patient is in a lot of pain you need to be more gentle so you can use your left hand. Obviously the opposite applies if you are standing on the other side of the table! Once again, when you start thinking this way and using this method, try asking the patient if they notice any difference between your two hands and which they prefer. Most practitioners seem to prefer having the rear heel off the floor. What this gives is the ability to increase the feel for the tissues in the patient. Feedback is very important in our profession (Fig. 37.5).

Using the table to gently support the practitioner makes the technique more effective and avoids using the patient as a means of balance – not a good idea! This support from the table also takes some of the strain from the practitioner and reduces practitioner fatigue.

Variants to consider in practicing soft tissue work

If the patient is still finding it difficult to relax, a gentle holding of the practitioner's breath for one or

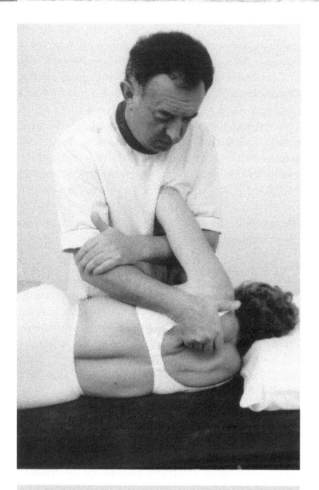

Figure 37.5

Soft tissue work on the shoulder muscles with the patient side-lying. This is a useful hold for the patient. It means the practitioner is upright and thus fatigues less than with the usual method

two seconds before the end of the stroke, timing the letting go of the breath with the end of the stroke, can often help.

If you feel you must use the point of your elbow for added pressure to reach very tight muscles, you can make this more comfortable for the patient by using the other hand to spread a load over a wider area at the same time.

Another tip if the practitioner is finding it difficult to achieve patient relaxation is for the practitioner to close their eyes for a while during the application of soft tissue techniques. Try different methods to see what works for you. If something is not working, don't abandon it as it may be useful on a different patient. After a time, you will soon learn what is best for which type of patient. The author has found that 70% of practitioners find that closing their eyes during treatment will relax the patient very well. Another little experiment to prove that whatever the practitioner does will influence the result in the patient is for the practitioner to focus their mind on their own back. The patient will notice that something is 'different' – maybe better, maybe not – but definitely 'different'. This is a very useful method if one is having difficulty in getting the muscles to relax. Put the feeling of tension in one's own back and the patient will then relax very quickly. If one is working on the thorax, concentrate on the thoracic area of one's own spine. If one is working on the lumbar area, concentrate on the lumbar area of one's own lower back. With practice this will work very quickly to produce a better operator pressure on the patient. After a few weeks practicing this, it will turn on automatically and the patient will let the muscles relax very quickly.

Practical exercise

Most students will use the hands as a tool and do not feel much happening to the patient. This can be overcome by getting the student to use the hands to apply pressure to a pillow for a while, then to do the technique without a patient. This will make sure that their posture is effective and that they will be in the right position for the procedure. If they then feel unstable, their posture needs work to get it better. Often this can be achieved by raising the table by a few inches when working on patients. For the following exercise we need to raise the table by a few inches to make this possible.

Firstly, have the patient in a pain-free (if possible) position on the table. Soft tissue techniques can be applied with the patient side-lying, supine, or prone. Prone can often be a problem for patients and can cause even more problems. If you are going to work prone, make sure there is a small pillow under the abdomen to prevent lumbar lordosis. Side-lying is often the preferred position for muscle relaxation. Have the patient nearer the edge of the table as the center of the table is too far away to allow the practitioner to work with a good posture. The aim is not to slide the hands across the skin but to contact the muscle through the skin and work directly on it. Sliding the hands in soft tissue work is only skin rubbing and will not create fluid interchange in soft tissues. Soft tissue techniques should feel natural after a while using these methods and this will produce speedy, effective, and comfortable results.

Do not try to change all these aspects at the same time. Introduce one or two a day until you feel 'at home' with them before adding another one. This way you can assess which aspect is best for you to use or is not suitable for you, in which case you can try it at a later stage.

Conclusion

So we can see that there are a great number of ways we can change what the practitioner does during soft tissue techniques that will considerably influence the outcome and how the patient feels toward the treatment and the practitioner. So to reiterate the point: these techniques will enable you build on what you learnt as a student and will help you improve and move on.

Further reading

Hartman, L., 1997. *Handbook of Osteopathic Technique*. 3rd edn. Cengage Learning.

Lederman, E., 1997. *Fundamentals of Manual Therapy*. 1st edn. Edinburgh: Churchill Livingstone.

VIBRATORY TECHNIQUE ON FASCIAL TISSUE

Fabio Schröter

'... when an Osteopath attempts to write, I suggest that he confines himself to what he knows to be the facts, the results of his own experience, not a transcript of what old authors have said and quotations from papers.'

A. T. Still (1899)

The author personally applies the modality of treatment by using oscillations and vibrations used in osteopathy since 1998, after Dr Fulford who studied the application of these methods, and due to the experience gathered in the field, considers this modality very beneficial for the patient and extremely safe for the operator.

Working on fascia is classically considered to be of vital importance even by the founder of osteopathy, A. T. Still. The same applies in modern research by modern osteopaths, for example Comeaux (Comeaux, 2002, 2008), Koss, (Fulford & Koss [n. d.]), O'Connell, (O'Connell, 2000), who think that giving freedom to fascia is very beneficial, not only for overall patient health but also for the various systems that make up the human body.

One of the elements lost in osteopathic medicine is rhythm. This author, either in his role as an operator, an examiner, or a teacher over the years, appreciates the diagnostic and therapeutic ability of many other operators and colleagues. We have all experienced both success and setbacks in the application of our philosophy and in the therapeutic essence of osteopathy. So, based on techniques that have proved successful, this author would like to recommend this rhythmical and dynamic element, which was the one of the original aspects of osteopathic treatment used by the *first* generation of osteopaths.

This rhythmical and dynamic element, also defined as vibratory, can be performed either with the hands or by using tools. It is perfectly suited to use in osteopathic practice and I am grateful to my precursor Dr Fulford for his unsurpassed value and geniality.

Vibration has a great effect on the fluid dynamic within the human body, on its metabolic function, on some specific properties of connective and fascial tissues, and on the bioelectrical components of the human body. I would like to mention in relation to this some studies published by Judith A. O'Connell DO FAAO in Chapters 2 and 3 of her book *Bioelectric Fascial Activation and Release* (O'Connell, 2000). These very interesting papers emphasize the mechanic and bioelectrical ability of fascial tissue.

Fascia is a band or sheet of fibrous tissue that envelops the whole body, including muscles and their many layers. This tissue has continuity. This means that any movement or stress in an area of the body is never an isolated phenomenon, but has a global impact.

Any stress, or after any stress, whether this is chemical, traumatic, or iatrogenic in nature, will be responsible for changes in the fascial tissue, in its viscosity, and in some of its own characteristics, giving it a reduced mechanical ability and lowering its chances of producing endocrine and enzymatic secretions. Therefore, this process will manifest as the body's inability to maintain autoregulation.

When this dynamic property is lacking, no movement occurs. So it reduces the normal body functions, creating pathology. Pathology in the osteopathic sense can be defined as an extreme way to allow dynamism to flow again.

The application of vibration is not a means of finding a definitive answer to the human dilemma of disease, but it could represent a way to make the right changes with the aim of recuperating the spontaneous and autonomous abilities of the human body, taking into account the osteopathic philosophy originated by A. T. Still.

The vibratory technique, as explained above, must be considered in all respects as a manual therapy, and then included in the therapeutic procedures used in the national health system. Therefore, the operator with an osteopathic background will get closer to it and introduce it in his treatment approach, keeping in mind that, even if it is a secure form of treatment approach, there are still risks and contraindications related to it.

Even though vibration is used on all parts of the body currently there is no research confirming the benefits or risks. It is common sense, for example, that an osteopathic treatment using vibration applied to some internal organs, or even to the fasciae that surround or contain them, requires a thorough knowledge of anatomy and the ability of the operator to keep in mind not only the general health status of the patient and the time of day the treatment is given, but also the patient's diet and many other factors.

The factors mentioned above need to be taken into special consideration, especially in relation to the hemodynamic effect the technique has on the lymphatic system. The practitioner has to make up his mind whether to entirely embrace osteopathic philosophy and use vibration in order to stimulate the patient, or apply vibration in a very analytical and defined way on a specific structure. This author thinks that the real solution is somewhere in between these two extremes. On the one hand, an analysis that is confined to a specific area will reduce the possibility of applying vibration as a modality of treatment in osteopathy for many extremely valid therapeutic options. On the other hand, a too-global approach does not take into account the momentaneous specific needs that could lead to therapeutic flows.

Therefore, considering the several thousands of cases I have treated over the years, my aim nowadays is to focus on the freedom the technique creates within the human body, enabling continual evaluation of the patient globally and in an analytical way.

The main focus of the therapeutic approach to fascia using vibration is the present movement or minimal movement, which is the spontaneous movement we can observe in a patient without using any external forces. This movement, according to Dr Fulford, represents the vital energy within every human being. His ideas were based on the research of Dr Harold Burr– a neuroanatomist at the University of Yale, known for his studies of the L-Field. Nowadays, the osteopathic scientific community has to aim to make as objective as possible the sensorial feelings gained by osteopaths using tissue palpation. This author thinks that therapeutic efficacy and the ability to make osteopathic approaches objective, especially when referring to fascial tissue, has to be the indiscriminate result of a balanced relationship between science and knowledge. Rational ability, made perfect over many years: ideas, clinical thoughts, and laboratory tests have to be combined with the experience we have gained in this field, such as total presence in the moment and in the place where the treatment is taking place, in which intention and visual representation are inseparable. This has to be taken into account especially when we would like to 'give' kinetic vibratory energy to a tissue.

In accordance with the ideas developed by Still, Sutherland, and Fulford, working on fascia should mean working globally: analyzing every detail does not mean allowing the operator to lose focus on the global complexity of the individual. The fundamental idea of these men is that the vital force can dominate the whole individual only if fascia tissue is free and healthy and able to express its own physiology globally. Fascia as bone is able to conduct electricity. We are now considering the piezoelectric property of these tissues. Therefore, their effects rely on movement, as do many other metabolic processes occurring in the body. This piezoelectric property depends on the connective component of fascia and bone, which can have a negative or positive charge depending respectively on whether they are compressed or distended/tensed.

The aim is to improve the ability of the respiratory system and the musculoskeletal system, allowing freedom of movement of body fluids and keeping in mind the biodynamic complexity of the individual. We need to remember that this complexity is functionally integral only if the fascial continuity allows its own ability to conduct electricity (O'Connell, 2000).

Dr Fulford said that the aforementioned electrical field can be activated by applying vibration to the fascia and that vibration technique, if well applied, can free the energy locked within fascia and activate the normal physiological processes within the tissue. This vibration can be therefore used to start a healing process from trauma, independently from the different types of trauma (chemical, emotional, and physical).

At this point we should remind ourselves that in the concept of osteopathy there is no division of the physical, emotional, and physiological components of the individual and that a person is a unit of body, mind, and spirit. This concept was well known to the first generation of osteopaths, who treated with equal success pathologies that nowadays would be considered to be of a psychiatric nature, taking into account the data collected years ago (Hildreth, 1942).

The protocol

As explained above, this author does not like to talk about protocols in the osteopathic field, but if you would like minimal guidance on the procedure of evaluating a patient, we can follow the classical approach as follows.

Starting from the lower extremities to the patient's head, we try to find the areas of the body that do not move correctly according to the parameters published by the AOA (TART – tenderness, asymmetry, range of motion, and tissue texture changes). Furthermore, you should try to evaluate every system by its intrinsic involuntarily motility: every evaluated segment needs to be able to show temperature and expansion or contraction, if it has a normal metabolism. As mentioned above, we would like a new scientific language to grow, to allow this new sensorial language to have its own objective dignity, in order to for it to become verifiable from practitioner to practitioner.

The 11 points that follow are this author's ideas (developed from 25 years' experience) based on Dr Fulford's modality, and on considerations and improvements published and discussed by Drs Zachary Comeaux, Paula Eschruth, and Richard Koss. After having discussed the technique with these doctors, it is impossible to quantify in this short chapter the thoughts, philosophy, and concepts studied by Dr Fulford on the vibratory aspect of the human body. Therefore, what follows is exclusively an idea or stimulus for more modern and developed research, following the most modern physical and metaphysical philosophical knowledge available today.

1. Observe the respiratory function while the patient lies supine. The presence of an area of dysfunction such as ribs 5, 6, and 7 on the left-hand side (the anterior portion) are the result of traumatic shock. Dr Fulford would diagnose this as diaphragmatic asymmetry (Fig. 38.1) caused by the larger extension of the left lung. The author recommends a gentle and nonlengthy touch, due to the fact that the area is quite sensitive and often emotional shocks can be created, as the tissues are a 'deposit' of the individual's life story. Therefore, an aggressive and lengthy palpation of some areas of the body can have major effects on the person.

2. Bilateral palpation of the rib cage (Fig. 38.2), focusing the attention either on thoracic respiration or on primary respiration in healthy subjects. Primary respiration and thoracic respiration will not find any resistance in the fasciae within the thorax and will try to become similar in rhythm and amplitude, and respiration will be homogenous on both sides.

3. The lower extremity: evaluate the knees, then the malleoli, and the interosseous membrane. Globally, if any of these elements is in dysfunction it can have an effect either on the pelvic mechanism or, through the fascia, on the diaphragm, and this is termed an ascending lesion.

4. Check the stability of the navicular bone, the cuboids, the metatarsal joints, and the anteroposterior relationship with the cuneiform bones. Mobility of the plantar fascia should be the primary aim to allow free circulation of the

Figure 38.1
Assessing respiratory function

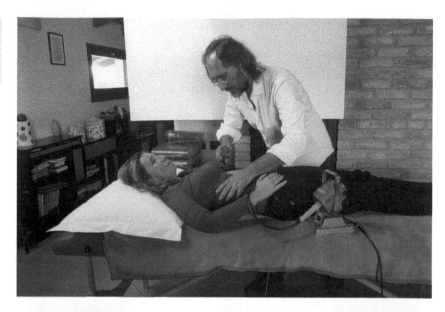

Figure 38.2
Bilateral palpation of the rib cage

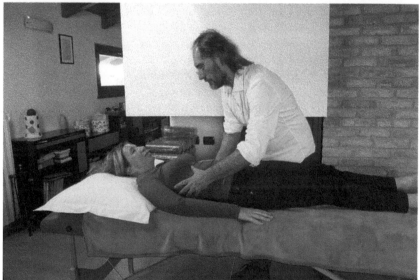

lymphatic and vascular fluids and for its own property of providing a spring while walking.

5. Evaluate the ability of the femurs to internally and externally rotate and to move anteriorly and posteriorly (Fig. 38.3). It is recommended that you perform the mobility tests either using wide movements, such as circumduction, or using a more localized movement to the joint itself. An operator without much experience could perform these tests in order to obtain clinical evidence that is more objective and safe. After a while, pal-

pation will become more ergonomic and easy to use if based on pressure test.

6. With the patient in supine position, evaluate the mobility of the sacroiliac joints with anterior–posterior movements. Keep in mind the visceral connections with the kidneys, the bladder, and so on.

7. Working on the sacroiliac joint, lay the patient on their side, and apply a more analytic palpation on the coccyx. Evaluate the transition area T12/L1 (diaphragm), considering the sev-

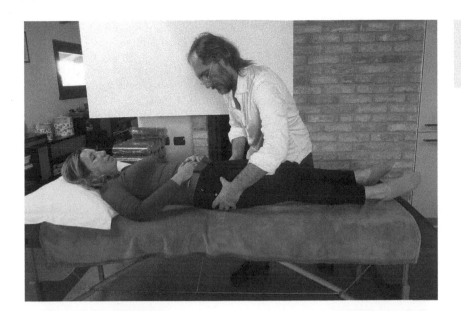

Figure 38.3
Performing mobility tests on the femur

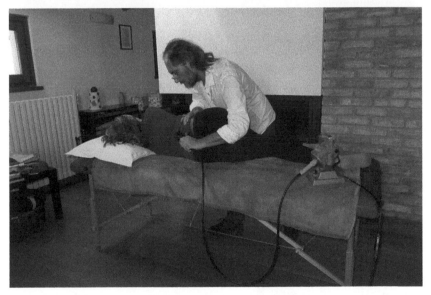

Figure 38.4
Working on the sacroiliac joint

eral joints between the thoracic spine and the ribs (C7-D1 – superior thoracic diaphragm). Dr Fulford highlighted also the importance of L3 (Fig. 38.4) and C3 due to the presence of strong folds of fascia. Working on the sacroiliac joint or the sacrococcygeal joint will help to free the pelvic diaphragm completely.

8. Evaluate the upper limb with the patient in a supine position. The upper limb needs to be elevated to its full range of movement. Evaluate the clavicles and the ribs palpable just beneath the subclavius and the pectoral muscle. Keep an eye on the respiration, as it needs to be free and quantitatively symmetrical between the two sides (as mentioned above).

9. Evaluate the upper limb: move the elbow outward and inward and vice versa, test pronation and supination, feel the interosseous membrane and the anteroposterior movement of the carpal and metacarpal bones. Here the aim is to evaluate the palmar fascia, as the repetitive movements of the hand can lead to restrictions

in this area, which is very important in creating a pumping effect for the fluids in the upper extremity.

10. Evaluate with a gentle pressure the cranial and facial bones (Fig. 38.5). Keeping the patient in a supine position, try to find a rigid area within the bones and/or sutures. The author recommends that even in the adult subject the pressure should be extremely gentle, even though after years those structures become more rigid. Keep in mind that the greater the pressure used when palpating, the less the clinician will gain in terms of perception. Try to focus on the tentorium and the falx.

11. Evaluate the area C0/C1/C2. The exchange between the dura mater and the rectus capitis posterior makes this area extremely interesting due to their fascial connection. Keep the patient in a supine position. Evaluate also the temporomandibular joints, either by asking the patient to open her mouth or by gently applying translatory movement from one side to the other.

Note: When there are dysfunctional areas, it is important to find balance above and below the foramen magnum, especially when using vibratory techniques, either with the hands or with tools (Fulford's percussor). It is always ideal that the fluctuations above and below the foramen magnum are similar in amplitude and quality, so that we can contain the collateral effects of the treatment.

Osteopathy is not the only discipline which believes that every trauma is stored in the body. Several other traditional medicines both in the East and West recognize that a traumatic event, be it physical, chemical or emotional, is stored in the human body fascia, changing its bioelectrical, enzymatic, mechanical and physiological characteristics (Reich, 1963; Nicholls, 2012; Johari, 1996).

Whatever the nature of the trauma, through the piezoelectric effect mentioned previously, kinetic energy is converted into electricity. This concept can be used when treating someone. Therefore, we can give the tissue mechanical stimulations, which can positively alter the energy potential of the treated area.

Materials

The author uses Fulford's percussor (Fig. 38.6) combined with manual vibrations. Manual vibration requires more effort from the operator. The vibration generated by the tool is not necessary to create a therapeutic effect on its own. This is the reason why the combination of Fulford's percussor with manual vibrations has become the preferred way.

The choice of the tool frequency is toward the medium gamma of the tool, especially during the

Figure 38.5
Evaluating the cranial and facial bones

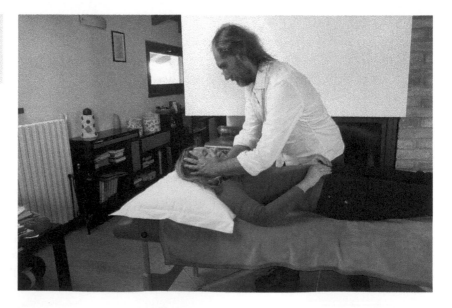

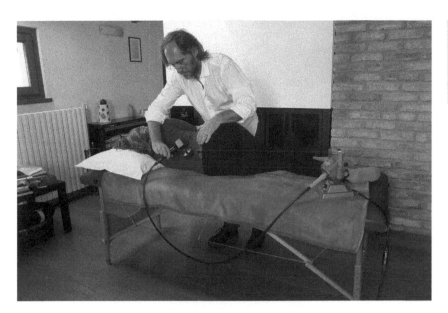

Figure 38.6
Fulford's percussor combined with manual vibrations

first treatments. It rarely goes over 75% of the tool velocity. Over the years many practitioners have developed confidence in using the tool and a better understanding of its pros and cons. As already mentioned, the ability to use it depends on the individual who decides to train in order to use it, as Dr Fulford required of anyone who wanted to use this osteopathic approach.

Patients treated had different health conditions, with good results and very minimal contraindications. Many patients in the paediatric and geriatric age groups revealed high tolerance and good results, especially on the fascia that appeared to be in chronic dysfunction. With the development of diagnostic tools and with the focus more on the area needing treatment, improvements increased and the duration of the application was decreased. A well-trained operator can treat completely and make the right corrections in 30 minutes.

The technique has been applied not only to the high-density areas of fascia within the musculoskeletal system, but also to the viscera. In some cases, there will be contraindications when treating sick patients. Even if the contraindication is not high risk, special care and minimal treatment time are required. Treatment is contraindicated especially for those patients suffering from an oncological disorder because the vibration can facilitate cell proliferation.

The same applies for patients who have recently had fractures or surgery.

It is important to avoid fascia areas associated with high sensitivity, such as the eyes. If necessary, you can treat pregnant women with very low frequencies far away from the abdomen.

What is outlined above applies to the application of vibration using a tool and also to manual application. As mentioned at the beginning of this chapter, it is very important to introduce into the fascial system the rhythmical and dynamic element that we tend not to use in a traumatic event. Too much force or elevated frequencies when using vibration are useless and sometimes dangerous. The operator needs to aim for a rhythmical and balanced exchange. Today's research reveals that the accumulation of histamine, prostaglandins, and other proinflammatory protein secretions tends to weaken the tissue. Therefore, it is worthwhile working on adjacent areas in order to improve drainage.

References and further reading

AAA Convocation. Bioelectric Fascial Activation and Release: A Bioenergetic Holographic Approach. 2013.

Anthroposophical leading thoughts: from nature to sub-nature. Online since July, 30, 2002. Available at: http://wn.rsarchive.org/Books/GA026/English/RSP1973/GA026_c29.html [accessed April 6, 2016].

Attlee T. *Cranio-Sacral Integration: Foundation*. Springing Dragon, 2012.

Comeaux Z. *Robert Fulford, D.O. and the Philosopher Physician*. Seattle, WA: Eastland Press, 2002.

Comeaux Z. *Harmonic Healing*. North Atlantic Books, 2008.

Fulford R. C. *Are We on the Path? The Collected Works of Robert C. Fulford D.O.* Cranial Press, 2003.

Fulford R. C. Koss R. W. Dr. Fulford's Basic Percussor Course with Drs. Fulford and Koss. DVD. (Distribution and duplication authorized by Drs. Fulford and Koss.) [n. d.]

Hildreth A. G. *The Lengthening Shadow of Dr. Andrew Taylor Still*. Mrs. A. G. Hildreth and Mrs. A. E. Van Vleck, 1942.

Johari H. *Ayurvedic Massage: Traditional Indian Techniques for Balancing Body and Mind*. Healing Arts Press, 1996.

Jealous J. The Emergence of Originality: A Biodynamic View of Osteopathy in theCranial Field. Self-published. Franconia, 2008.

Nicholls C. *The Posture Workbook: Free Yourself from Back, Neck and Shoulder Pain with the Alexander Technique*. D & B Publishing, 2012.

O'Connell J. *Bioelectric Fascial Activation and Release, The Physician's Guide to Hunting with Dr. Still*. Indianapolis, IN: American Academy of Osteopathy, 2000.

Reich W. *Selected Writings: An Introduction to Orgonomy*. Farrar, Straus and Giroux, 1963.Still A. T. Dr. Andrew T. Still's papers. A. T. Still University. Museum of Osteopathic Medicine. Available at: http://www.atsu.edu/museum/stillpapers/index.htm [accessed April 6, 2016].

Still A. T. Personal note to Henry Bunting Journal of Osteopathy editor, 1899. Extract from Lewis J. *From the Dry Bone to the Living Man*. Dry Bone Press, 2012.

Van Buskirk R. L. (2006) *The Still Technique Manual: Applications of a Rediscovered Technique of Andrew Taylor Still, M.D.* 2nd edition. Indianapolis: American Academy of Osteopathy.

THE BIOENERGETIC MODEL OF FASCIA AS RELATED TO TRAUMA

Judith A. O'Connell

Bioelectric fascial activation and release: an evolution in myofascial release

Historical perspective

Fascia has been an integral part of osteopathic medicine since its inception by A. T. Still in the 1800s. Since that time it has inspired osteopathic thought and caused an evolution in osteopathic technique. In his text *Philosophy of Osteopathy*, Still speaks frequently on the importance of fascia, admonishing his followers to look closely there for the causes of death that do the destruction of life (Still, 1899).

In the 1980s a group of osteopathic physicians gathered to discuss new thoughts and approaches to the treatment of disease that was not joint based. Chila, Ward, and Peckham began to investigate and evolve their understanding of how fascia interfaces with the human condition, and applied new techniques influenced by the muscle energy and cranial osteopathy models that became known as myofascial release. Ward contributed his biomechanical model (Ward, 2003) and Chila contributed his big bandage fascial continuum model (Chila, 2006).

In the 1990s as a significant renaissance of osteopathic technique emerged there was a resurgence of Sutherland's cranial methods and extracranial applications of balanced membranous and ligamentous tension, of visceral manipulation, of Fulford's percussion vibratory techniques and the 'breath of life' (Fulford, 1997), and of a renewed interest in lymphatic techniques.

Influenced by this evolution in osteopathic thought, O'Connell in the late 1980s and early 1990s began to integrate nonosteopathic bioenergetic concepts, both physical and metaphysical, into a new understanding of the bioenergetic nature of fascia. Tensegrity concepts as taught by Stiles and Buckminster Fuller, the new physics, metaphysics, and new understandings of the integrated nature of structure and function led to an osteopathic refocusing on homeostasis that emerged as a holographic model for understanding diagnosing and treating in the fascia (O'Connell, 2010). This brought together three myofascial models: the biomechanical model of Ward, the fascial continuum model of Chila, and the bioenergetic model of O'Connell (O'Connell, 2010).

Holographic model of diagnosis and treatment in the fascia

From its humble beginnings osteopathy has been firmly rooted in direct relationships between structure and function within the human condition. The physical container with compartments, diaphragms, and longitudinal structural components responds to tensegrity, fluidity, visceral, and mechanical constructs. Changes in the structure are reflected in changes in function and changes in function cause alterations in structural components. Balance is the key and homeostasis the goal.

Fascia is an active, intelligent tissue involved in homeostasis by acting as an interface between internal and external environs (O'Connell, 2000). Fascia is bioelectric, acting as a transducer between mechanical and biological events as a piezoelectric interface. Through osteopathic palpation applied thoughtfully and compassionately, coupled with a firm understanding of the structure and function of the human being, homeostasis can be affected through the application of osteopathic manipulative techniques. As such, the whole of an individual is contained within the components and the components define the whole within the holographic being.

Holographic palpation

Fascia is a holographic tissue acting as a coordinator and communicator of events and responses in support of homeostasis. Homeostasis is a holographic, dynamic set of processes seeking health. As such, any distortion in structure or function will be reflected in homeostasis and the fascia. Through intelligent palpation by a skilled clinician this holographic fascial system allows for the identification and assessment of function and dysfunction through: the integrity, relationships, and function of all structures; the status and function of viscera and systems; and the capacity of homeostasis to be activated and supported (O'Connell, 2010).

Holographic perception

To begin to perceive holographically, an understanding of three-dimensional anatomy coupled with heightened physical palpation skill is required. A. T. Still carried bones in his pockets and would palpate them often to create a clear mental image of the structure in his mind. Coupling the study of anatomy, imaging, and palpation are the foundations for holographic perception. The following are the steps in bioelectric fascial activation and release:

1. Use the fascia as a portal of entry to the whole person.

2. Hold an image of the anatomy to be examined in your mind.

3. Use a deep breath to set the fascia in motion.

4. Follow the patterns of motion created by the alterations in structure and function (somatic dysfunction), allowing the system to lead you.

5. Once identified, record the patterns of dysfunction.

6. Activate the fascia with three deep respiratory cycles.

7. Release is innate and occurs through direct or indirect fascial compression or distraction within three deep respiratory cycles.

Trauma in the fascia: undoing the damage and supporting the healing

Trauma: a tale told in the fascia

Fascia is a bioenergetic, bioresponsive interface that responds directionally and proportionally to biologic and biomechanical distortions. Any trauma that occurs is written in the fascia, waiting for discovery. Trauma is multidimensional and affects every aspect of the person – physical, emotional, mental, and spiritual. Fascia acts as a recorder and a reactor, absorbing and disbursing trauma leaving identifiable patterns of dysfunction to be discovered through intelligent palpation (O'Connell, 2003). Through the fascial interface with homeostasis balancing internal and external events, metabolic and cellular traumatic events are converted into discoverable patterns of dysfunction.

Fascia is truly where 'the causes of death do the destruction of life' (Still, 1899).

Trauma: more than just physical

Trauma affects us on many levels. We see examples of this daily with military trauma creating post-traumatic stress disorders, sports injuries with post-concussion syndrome, and socioeconomic traumas causing debilitating mental and emotional stress disorders. Trauma impacts physical, emotional, mental, and spiritual health and causes impairments at all levels, increasing physical disease and contributing to a sense of spiritual despair. No matter what the cause, trauma leaves a discernible trail in the fascia. Through intelligent palpation and by choosing an appropriate fascial portal of entry the clinician has the opportunity to positively affect homeostasis by helping to reduce dysfunctional loads affecting all bodies.

Trauma in one body affects all bodies, physical through metaphysical (Fig. 39.1).

Recognizing the whole: Still (A. T.) the gift of osteopathy

An understanding now emerges of the true gift of osteopathy: the body is a unified whole; the body has

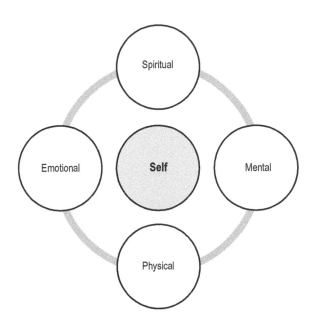

Figure 39.1
Interacting bodies

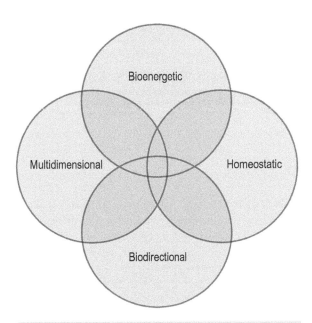

Figure 39.2
Trauma characteristics

the innate ability to heal; structure and function are interdependent and interrelated; through the examination and treatment of the musculoskeletal system the whole of the person is assessable; and humans are triune in nature, composed of a body, mind, and spirit. In addition, we have discovered all trauma interfaces in the fascia affecting homeostasis in and between all bodies of a human being.

Trauma from all sources is written through the bioenergetic responsiveness of fascia. Physical compressive and distractive forces cause a biodirectional absorption and distribution of force within compensation patterns that are discoverable through intelligent palpation. Emotional, mental, and spiritual traumas affect homeostatic processes to create physical patterns of dysfunction discoverable through intelligent palpation. It is in the fascia that homeostasis monitors, acts, and reacts to internal and external events from the physical through the metaphysical (Fig. 39.2).

Identifying the trauma pattern

It is essential to successful treatment that the trauma pattern be identified correctly so that the appropriate techniques necessary to support homeostasis can be applied. This begins with a good trauma history. In Table 39.1 components of the trauma history are given. Collecting a good trauma history paints a picture of the patient at the time of trauma and how things have evolved since that point in time. This is important as the longer trauma exists, the greater the compensation load is throughout all levels of the person. These deep-seated trauma patterns may be difficult to eradicate (O'Connell, 2000).

Physical examination takes into consideration the trauma history and helps in identifying the primary trauma site, components of the reaction to the event, and relationships in the fascia and the whole person as a result. Trauma should be suspected when physical findings are not consistent with the history, somatic dysfunctions do not resolve with appropriate treatment, symptoms continue to evolve into chronic conditions, repetitive activities occur in the work setting, and overt signs of trauma such as bruises, abrasions, and dislocations occur.

Trauma history	Examples
Chronology of trauma	Chronic, acute, age, length of symptoms
Events surrounding the start of signs and symptoms	State of health, illness, stressors, overt trauma, life changes, depression
Mechanism	Fall, MVA, blunt force, surgery, birth, concussion
Direction of force	Hit in right side of head, rear-ended and thrown into steering wheel, fall on ice onto left hip
Signs and symptoms of original trauma	Swelling, pain, loss of function, fractures, dislocations, loss of consciousness, visceral symptoms
Evolution of symptoms	Radiation, migration, transformation of symptoms, functional changes, constitutional changes, overflow to other systems
Imaging and testing related to the trauma	Medical record review from previous providers, ER records, MRI, CT, X-rays, labs
Types and responses to treatment	Improved, worsened, unchanged, ER visit, OTC and prescribed medications, surgery, PT, CMT, injections, supplements, acupuncture
Pretrauma disease and any changes since trauma	Diabetes, hypertension, IBS, mental function, organ function
Post-trauma disease emergence	Chronic pain, IBS, RSD, fatigue, fibromyalgia
Other traumas prior to or since the presenting trauma	Multiple falls, other MVA, surgeries, fractures, etc. with or without known continuation of symptoms
Disability associated with this trauma	Worker's compensation, short- or long-term disability, poor cognitive function, personal injury
Disability not associated with this trauma	Worker's compensation, short- or long-term disability, social security disability, poor cognitive function, personal injury

CMT = chiropractic manipulative treatment; CT = computed tomography; ER = emergency room; IBS = irritable bowel syndrome; MRI = magnetic resonance imaging; MVA = motor vehicle accident; OTC = over the counter; PT = physiotherapy; RSD = reflex sympathetic dystrophy

Table 39.1

Trauma history components

The fascia may reveal to you on examination evidence of traumatic events that will need further evaluation. The body memory of trauma patterns recorded in the fascia will remain there until released. Cognitive memory may be faulty of distant traumatic events or of severe trauma that is often repressed, such as abuse of any type. Remember that physical symptoms may have roots in emotional, mental, or spiritual trauma, much like an iceberg where the physical trail is only the tip and the true root is left to be discovered below the surface (O'Connell, 2000).

The process of diagnosing in the fascia involves an intelligent dialogue based on understanding the anatomy. The fascial anatomy is a system of diaphragms and cables that act as a dynamic adaptive structure based on the design of tubes within tubes within tubes. It recalls the embryologic development from a grapelike collection of cells to an ovoid disk centered on a tubular notochord. The development continues three-dimensionally, evolving into a tubular structure containing developing organs and systems. Diaphragms create compartments and cross-structures allowing the developing embryo to resist the forces of entropy and enthalpy. This structural design provides a continuous system of interrelated and interdependent parts where nothing is isolated.

When palpating and diagnosing in the fascia, this tubular design with strategically placed horizontal diaphragms (centrally respiratory, tentorium, thoracic inlet, and pelvic) gives the clinician the ability to access the whole system from any portal of entry on the body. In essence, the structure of the fascia creates a communication network and a clinician using intelligent palpation can access the system for diagnosis and treatment purposes (O'Connell, 2010).

Diagnosing and treating in the fascia is much like floating in a pool. Imagine being on a raft in the pool and being totally passive not trying to direct any motion. The natural motion of the water and its response to the environment causes you to move. If you are passive in this endeavor, floating will follow a path created by the water. This is much like diagnosing and sensing motion within the fascia, where the clinician is a passive observer and traveler, allowing the intelligent fascia to lead you to dysfunctions based on the system's present needs. It is important to remember that diagnosing in this fashion the clinician must:

1. First be an observer

2. partner with the patient

3. not question the path traveled

4. remember and record the pattern and dysfunctions identified.

Treatment dance

Putting all these pieces together, the clinician is now ready to enter a therapeutic encounter. Based on the diagnosis and recognition of the trauma pattern identified through history and physical examination, a portal of entry is identified and contacted. The clinician holds an intention to focus on the patient's innate healing capacity and surrenders their ego. The clinician places their attention to sensing the pattern without question, and following it to its primary dysfunction. Activation using respiratory assistance of three respiratory cycles allows for the release.

- Choose a portal of entry into the fascia with the intention of activating self-healing properties and homeostasis.

- Pay attention to the pattern presented, resisting the desire to direct.

- Activation and release with respiratory assist is patient mediated.

The holographic nature of fascia allows for traumatic events to be recorded and assessable, from any portal of entry. The human condition is holographic, with all levels of being (physical, emotional, mental, and spiritual) being nested and available through intelligent palpation in the fascia. Releases in the physical are attached to emotional, mental, and spiritual relationships and releases within the whole (O'Connell, 2000).

Compensation patterns

In a traumatized system compensation patterns evolve, allowing the continuation of functions necessary to engage life. *Functional compensation* occurs when the compensatory, distributive, and absorptive mechanisms of the fascia are intact. Treatment concerns in this type of pattern are for decompensation and inability to maintain normal function. As the trauma pattern is resolved, flare-ups of symptoms and dysfunction are very common. *Dysfunctional compensation* occurs when the compensatory, distributive, and absorptive mechanisms of the fascia are compromised. Treatment concern is for addressing the most significant dysfunction first, which chronologically may not be the most recent pattern of dysfunction. Caution should be taken to limit the intervention in order to respect the system's need to recoup and rebalance.

Complex trauma

Often, patients present with a very complex traumatic event or multiple traumas noted in their history. It is important to understand the effects these traumas have on the whole person. Multiple trauma vectors may occur in one event, such as a motor vehicle accident where the vehicle slid on the ice, spun, and then rolled in a ditch, causing multiple events within one traumatic incident. There may be a history of multiple traumatic events with multiple trauma vector patterns within the same person. This is very common where a patient may report a recent fall on the ice, a remote motor vehicle accident, a traumatic birth, and present-day significant emotional stressors. In either of these cases there are multiple trauma vectors affecting function. These may cause an accumulation trauma vector based on the interactions of each of these primary and compensatory dysfunction patterns. This interaction will produce one emergent accumulation vector (O'Connell, 2000). This is very common in a situation where multiple traumas occur or their patterns intersect in the same region. The accumulated trauma vector does not follow anatomic or physiologic patterns of motion.

Methodical treatment approach

Once the trauma patterns are identified, a methodical approach to treatment yields the best results. This approach can be best thought of as like peeling an onion. The intelligent fascia prioritizes the trauma patterns and presents them to the skilled clinician in the proper order of need for release based on the maintenance of homeostasis. As the presenting trauma pattern is released, the fascia presents the next layer for treatment. This process continues until all layers are resolved, just like peeling an onion!

The most dysfunctional trauma pattern has the most significant changes in motion, tissue texture, tenderness, structural integrity, and physiologic asymmetry. Chronology of traumatic events should not restrict the consideration of which pattern to treat. The clinician should rely upon the system's direction and selection to treat the most dysfunctional trauma pattern first (O'Connell, 2000).

It is important to note that, while it is tempting to treat multiple trauma patterns in a session, multiple treatment sessions that allow homeostatic adjustment are preferable. Imagine the game of pick-up sticks where a stack of sticks that contain one uniquely colored stick are released and form a pile. This pile attains a balance of multidirectional sticks, much like the multiple trauma vectors within the fascia. This weblike design is stable.

The object of the game is to remove the uniquely colored stick without destabilizing the web, much like the clinician treating the trauma vectors seeking the core dysfunction. These sticks form patterns that are interwoven, interdependent, and interrelated so that removal of a stick may destabilize the web, causing it to collapse. Within the web there is a stick that can be removed without destabilizing the whole web based on the physics of the structure. This stick may not be the uniquely colored one. To be successful and win the game each stick that the structure frees up must be removed, allowing the structure to rebalance between moves until the uniquely colored stick is freed. The same occurs with multiple trauma vectors.

The analogy of pick-up sticks illustrates important considerations in the treatment of multiple-trauma vectors. The clinician must always be concerned for metabolic integrity. The treatment of multiple trauma vectors begins with treatment of the most emergent pattern chosen by the intelligent fascia. Allowing time between treatments for system balance to occur respects homeostasis. Treatment intervals of one week or more should be tailored to the patient's condition and response to treatment. Remember that treatment in the physical affects the emotional, mental, and spiritual self, which are layered just like the pick-up sticks and will need time to adapt. Never forget that overtreatment risks decompensation in all systems and may have dire consequences for the patient.

Evaluating treatment effectiveness

Another analogy useful in understanding treatment effectiveness is a swing. Imagine your patient is on a swing. Somatic dysfunction causes alterations in motion that are readily identified through the processes already discussed. Push the swing by creating an impulse in the fascia through respiratory assistance or the application of compressive or distractive forces and analyze the response in the fascia. Choose the most dysfunctional pattern, apply the appropriate osteopathic manipulative technique, activate homeostatic mechanisms, release the dysfunction, and support motion (O'Connell, 2003). Resolution of the somatic dysfunction allows the swing to move freely.

Trauma load adds drag to the system, resulting in loss of motion over time and causing the swing to stop moving. This is perceived as a change in the innate motion of the fascia. Using the swing to assess the vitality and resilience of the system pre- and post-treatment is an indicator of homeostatic stability and the effectiveness of treatment. Repeat the process of pushing the swing on each visit while peeling the onion. Homeostasis is reached when the system is able to maintain momentum between visits.

Chronic management of traumatized patients

Chronic effects of trauma may be permanent, with alterations in structures, functions, and relationships created by the trauma directly or the interventions needed to address the trauma in the acute state. These alterations create continuous drag, preventing the system from achieving and maintaining momentum and motion. This causes a (natural) decompensation cycle even in the face of appropriate treatment. Signs of decompensation include (but are not limited to) fatigue, increasing pain, increase in stiffness, return of symptoms, decrease in system and/or organ function, ineffectiveness of previously helpful activities (yoga, stretching, lifestyle changes), and a lack of a sense of well-being. Teach patients to recognize their signs and symptoms of decompensation and intervene before the system crashes. Treatment schedule is customized to each individual based on their decompensation cycle and the use of the swing analogy can help to identify this pattern. Extend time between treatments incrementally, allowing patients to come in sooner if they begin to decompensate.

> **WARNING!** Iatrogenic trauma is the hardest to rectify. Common causes of iatrogenic trauma are:
>
> - well-intentioned manual treatment with misapplied forces
> - shotgun techniques with poor localization
> - inappropriate technique for the dysfunction
> - over-treating
> - not respecting the individual's homeostatic mechanism.

OMT releases the trauma and supports healing

The fascia provides the clinician with unparalleled access to the whole person. Osteopathic manipulative treatment (OMT) offers a menu of multiple techniques and myriads of combinations to meet the needs of the system using joint-based, muscle activation, subtle techniques, bioenergetics, and inherent motion approaches (O'Connell, 2003). Diagnosis in the fascia provides access to all bodies (physical, emotional, mental, and spiritual), identifies trauma and compensation patterns, and stratifies the patterns based on homeostatic need (O'Connell, 2010). Treatment is tailored to the individual's need with the activation of homeostatic mechanisms and release of dysfunction through the application of OMT affecting the continuum of self.

This continuum is a reflective relationship often recognized as the dynamic of 'as above so below' and exists between all bodies (physical, emotional, mental, and spiritual) and the metaphysical. Expressed in osteopathic terms:

1. The unity of all systems.
2. Dysfunction in one body is manifest throughout the whole.
3. Access to all bodies is found in the fascia.

Within the fascial continuum intracellular function is connected with extracorporeal events, and the metaphysical is related to the physical. This continuum extends to all creation, where the most seemingly insignificant event affects all that is.

The challenge of the multilayered release

Understanding the continuum, the holographic nature of the individual, and the potency of releases in the fascia is essential for treatment success. The clinician understands the concepts of body memory and the consequences of physical releases triggering emotional, mental, and spiritual releases. Anticipating the need for appropriate resources to address these issues as they arise during treatment is prudent. Respect for the patient's culture and belief is essential to creating a healing environment and trusting relationship. Remember that you are a partner, not a director, in this dance (O'Connell, 2000).

The clinician is also a part of the continuum and is affected by the healing intervention. Treating at this level is transformative for patient and clinician. Be ready for personal enlightenment as you continue on the path of an osteopathic healer.

The object of the doctor is to find health – any fool can find disease!

References and further reading

Chila A. G. *Connective Tissue Continuity: Membranous and Ligamentous Articular Dysfunction.* Athens OH: Ohio University College of Osteopathic Medicine. 2006, p. 48.

Chila A. (ed.) *Foundations of Osteopathic Medicine.* 3rd Edition. Philadelphia, PA: Lippincott Williams and Wilkins. 2010.

Fulford R. C. *Touch of Life.* Pocket. 1997.

O'Connell J. *Bioelectric Fascial Activation and Release: The Physician's Guide to Hunting with Dr. Still,* Indianapolis, IN: American Academy of Osteopathy. 2000.

O'Connell J. Bioelectric responsiveness of fascia: a model for understanding the effects of manipulation. *Techniques in Orthopaedics.* 2003;18(1):67–73

O'Connell J. Myofascial release. In: *Foundations of Osteopathic Medicine.* 3rd Edition. Chila A. (ed.). Philadelphia, PA: Lippincott Williams and Wilkins. 2010.

Still, A. T. *Philosophy of Osteopathy.* Indianapolis, IN: American Academy of Osteopathy. 1899.

Ward R. C., Hruby R. J. et al. *Foundations for Osteopathic Medicine.* 2nd Edition. Philadelphia, PA: Lippincott Williams and Wilkins. 2003.

FASCIAL UNWINDING TECHNIQUE

Paolo Tozzi

Overview

Fascial unwinding (FU) is a relatively common osteopathic technique, specifically addressing fascial dysfunctions, with the aim of releasing tension, reducing symptoms, and restoring function. Despite the fact that some kinds of precursors of this approach have been around since the early years of osteopathy, the origins of FU are still uncertain, with its protocol of application being only recently defined. It has been indicated for a variety of conditions mainly affecting myofascial tissue, ranging from inflammatory processes to chronic disorders. In fact, its gentle application as well as its safe and indirect nature has made it suitable for acute presentations, while it can also be successfully applied for long-term symptoms. Technically speaking, FU is a dynamic, indirect fascial technique: indirect, since it disengages the tissue barrier and follows patterns of ease; dynamic, because it involves a constant monitoring while motion is applied in response to fascial tension that needs to be acknowledged, amplified, and unwound until a release is felt. These principles can be clinically applied from the smallest joint in the body, such as an interphalangeal joint, to an entire limb or throughout the spine, up to and including the whole body simultaneously. In any case, a discrete amount of palpatory skill and experience are necessary to appropriately perform the technique and to gain the desired clinical outcomes. The versatility of this approach extends its potential effectiveness to most fascial dysfunctions in patients of any age. However, not everyone seems to be responsive to the unwinding method, considering that patient relaxation is a crucial requirement for its application. Few theories have been advanced to explain its therapeutic results, although many other fascial mechanisms could come into play. Furthermore, research has offered some evidence on the efficacy of this technique, although further investigation is still required to better understand its clinical implications and physiological effects.

Introduction

The osteopathic origins of unwinding methods are still unclear, although they have been described for decades by several osteopathic practitioners (Ward, 2003a). Since the early 1920s, William Neidner, a student of Sutherland, who defined his approach as *fascial twist*, applied specific direct manipulative techniques to the myofascial tissue in the osteopathic field. Neidner was engaged at that time in researching effective treatment for muscular dystrophy in children. By observing and palpating the entire fascial organization of the body, he noticed that people in good health tend to show a clockwise fascial torsional pattern from head to feet (Centers et al., 2003). He then proposed that myofascial tissue dysfunctions could be globally released by various types of techniques relying on the use of the limbs as long levers for the untwisting maneuver (DeStefano, 2011). This approach employed mainly torsional forces to the extremities, aimed at restoring a balanced fascial tension by finding and maintaining a myofascial barrier until it yields. This would also promote symmetry of the transitional areas of the spine as well as reinstate compensatory postural patterns. Mitchell himself, in his first published work (1958), suggested applying such direct methods of treatment to the myofascial tissue before addressing any articular dysfunctions. Lately, this procedure has been indicated at the conclusion of a treatment program, after more local strain patterns have been released (Centers et al., 2003), since it induces a profound relaxation in the patient.

The idea of 'twisted' fascial patterns existing in healthy conditions as a result of postural adaptation was then re-evoked and readapted in the 1970s by Gordon Zink. He hypothesized alternating myofascial patterns occurring in healthy individuals at the level of the body diaphragms, showing preferential rotations and inclinations at around the corresponding transitional areas of the spine (Zink & Lawson, 1979). This included the tentorium motion at around the C0–C2 articular complex, the superior thoracic diaphragm at the C7–T1 level, the thoracoabdominal diaphragm at T12–L1, and the pelvic diaphragm rotating at the level of the L5–S1 junction. Zink defined as common patterns that showed, from the top down, a preferential left–right–left–right rotation. He then named as uncommon those oriented in the opposite direction. Ideally, diaphragms should be aligned and move in a rhythmic, coordinated fashion during breathing. However, they commonly rotate and side-bend around their structural pivots to compensate for various physiological forces (uneven foetal positions during pregnancy, motor cerebral dominance, etc.) or unphysiological stressors (leg length discrepancy, etc.) (Pope, 2003). According to the Zink model (1973), the health status of an individual is equal to his/her ability to compensate to any given stressor, in such a way that the total homeostatic potential would remain basically the same. In other words, the greater the individual's capacity for adaptation, the better his or her state of health will be. This is why central myofascial patterns, alternating in a functional manner, are so important and useful in maintaining the autoregulation of the organism. When this function is overwhelmed or disrupted, the myofascial structures lose their alternating pattern, showing signs of rotation and side-bending consecutively in the same direction. This results in loss of adaptive abilities in the area involved, increasing energy expenditure, altering function, and affecting posture by overloading the correspondent spinal transitional areas (Defeo & Hicks, 1993). These patterns can be manually assessed and treated (Zink & Lawson, 1979), either positionally or by means of patient cooperation through voluntary muscle contraction (Chaitow, 2005).

Elaine Wallace developed the so-called *torque unwinding* (Dowling, 2011): a theoretical construct of the body imagined as a collection of adjacent and overlapping cubes, whose alignment may get disrupted after injury, bringing the cubes into a dysfunctional state of torsion. The treatment consists of applying oscillating torsional pressures directed centrally from two opposed theoretical cube faces, mirroring the position of the original trauma and allowing the release to occur.

Nevertheless, although the Neidner and Zink models were both addressing myofascial patterns, they proposed mainly static manual approaches to resolve dysfunctions present at that level. Instead, a more dynamic concept based on the unwinding of the intrinsic fascial tensions was probably recently introduced by Viola Frymann:

'The principle of this profound technique is to place the patient in the position that they were in at the moment of injury, and permit fascia to go through whatever motions are necessary to eliminate all the forces imposed by the impact.'

(Frymann, 1998a)

Nowadays, FU is formally described as: 'a manual technique involving constant feedback to the osteopathic practitioner who is passively moving a portion of the patient's body in response to the sensation of movement' (ECOP, 2011). In this sense, FU has been considered as a form of indirect myofascial release: 'the dysfunctional tissues are guided along the path of least resistance until free movement is achieved' (Minasny, 2009).

In spite of the different definitions that have been proposed, FU remains a dynamic, indirect technique usually applied to the myofascial–articular complex, aimed at releasing fascial restrictions and restoring tissue mobility and function. The operator engages the restricted tissues/joint by unfolding the whole pattern of dysfunctional vectors associated with the inherent fascial motion: a shearing, torsional, or rotational component may find the opportunity to express in a complex three-dimensional pattern that needs to be supported, amplified, and unwound, until release is perceived. If you consider the tissues being targeted, FU might be viewed as within the concept of the osteopathic biomechanical model, in the light of its impact on the musculoskeletal system, and of its consequent beneficial influence on posture, articular mobility, myofascial tension, structural alignment, and balance. However, it can also be seen as falling under the respiratory–circulatory model. In fact, by releasing myofascial tensions, the major obstacles to venous–lymphatic drainage are removed, and the action of the thoracoabdomino-pelvic pump becomes unimpeded (Zink, 1977). The restoration of free circulation of fluids, from arterial to venous, from lymphatic to cerebrospinal and interstitial, guarantees adequate tissue oxygenation, healthy cellular function, and high homeostatic potential. By balancing myofascial tension, the pressure gradients within and between tissue layers are re-established; hence a functional fluid motion is restored. This would promote the removal of inflammatory mediators and metabolic wastes, as well as the resolution of edemas and congestions, in both acute or chronic conditions (Kuchera, 2011), while tissue repair and regenerative processes will be supported, too.

Aims, indications, and evidence

Thanks to its safe and gentle application, as well as its broad versatility, FU has been used for decades by osteopaths, craniosacral therapists, and myofascial workers. However, its origin and main application remains within the osteopathic field. It has been usually described in relation to the release of physical features associated with fascial restrictions, and it has also been indicated for unwinding the so-called craniosacral mechanism (Frymann, 1998b). In this sense, the main aims are to correct somatic dysfunction, to release pain, musculoskeletal tension, and fascial restriction (Ward, 2003b), especially following injury (Frymann, 1998b) or surgery. More recently, a somatoemotional component has been included, suggesting that FU might release trauma-induced energy stored in the myofascial system (Upledger, 1987).

FU is generally indicated for any myofascial condition, including those related to surgery or sports injury, such as tennis elbow, plantar fasciitis, shin splints, muscular and tendinous injury rehabilitation (Weintraub, 2003), or any repetitively strained or overused joint and related myofascial structures. Furthermore, it has been advanced as an integrative approach for a variety of visceral techniques, aimed at releasing tension in and around serous membranes, visceral ligaments, and capsules (Stone, 2007a). In a very subtle and gentle form, it has been proposed for pregnant patients too, in the prepartum or intrapartum period, to promote an optimal fetal position in a more accommodating and tensionally balanced environment (Stone, 2007b).

Finally, FU may be also suitable for approaching scar tissues. A scar is considered to be active if at least one of its layers does not move freely and resistance to passive movement in at least one direction can be palpated (Lewit & Olsanska, 2004). FU may be used within hours or days from surgery, as it requires no significant range of motion through the scar or incision sites (Stone, 2007c). It aims to restore mobility by releasing tissue adherences and fibrotic material, so as to improve sliding motion between the involved tissue layers and enhance fluid circulation, cell nutrition, and tissue regeneration.

FU can be performed on any single articulation or group of articulations, or even the whole body. For the latter, the simultaneous cooperation of two operators may be required if the patient is an adult, but in the case of infants or children a single practitioner is usually sufficient. Most of the time FU is addressed to the neck, arms, or legs, as these are mobile regions where strain and trauma easily manifest. However, not everyone is responsive to FU. Patients who are unable to relax may not be responsive. Therefore, alternative strategies should be used. In some cases, unwinding may happen spontaneously while the therapist is applying other techniques. For instance, neck unwinding may occur spontaneously during the performance of myofascial release technique (Weintraub 2003) or suboccipital decompression. Finally, some patients may be so particularly predisposed to respond to this method, that they can even be instructed on how to gently self-unwind. In fact, following a guided meditation session, patients may learn how to connect with their own myofascial system, feeling for any tension within, and for the ways such tension wants to release. This experience, under the operator's guidance, may allow a spontaneous and effective body unwinding, bringing tissues back to their natural tensional state, often resulting in emotional – as well as physical – release.

FU has been demonstrated to be a beneficial integrative technique:

- to reduce pain and improve sliding fascial mobility in patients with non-specific neck pain (Tozzi et al., 2011)

- to reduce pain and improve visceral mobility in people with low back pain (Tozzi et al., 2012)

- in the treatment of adult scoliosis (Blum, 2002), spondylolisthesis (Kuchera, 2003), and tension-type headaches (Anderson & Seniscal, 2006).

No injuries have been reported in the literature as being attributed to indirect or fascial techniques (Vick et al., 1996) apart from an isolated, documented case (Kerr, 1997) following the Rolfing method. However, it has been speculated that adverse reactions are not fully or adequately reported in the osteopathic scientific literature (Vick et al., 1996). In addition, it must be noted that a myalgic flare may occur within the first 12 hours after treatment, usually lasting not more than 24–48 hours (DiGiovanna, 2005), similar to muscle pain after a vigorous workout.

As regards applying most of the indirect techniques to a local site, the absolute contraindications are: recent closed head injury; acute vascular accident; bleeding or aneurysm; and acute visceral infections (WHO, 2010). Relative contraindications are malignancy, open wound, severe osteoporosis, infection, bone fracture, joint dislocation, and gross instability (Nicholas & Nicholas, 2008).

Protocol

The unwinding process can be applied to the whole body or to any part of the body, especially the limbs and neck. The neck or extremities can be treated regionally or used as levers to manipulate the trunk. 'Unwinding methods refer to operator-induced spontaneous bending and twisting maneuvers affecting both upper and lower limbs' (Ward, 2003a).

FU application can be described by the following phases:

1. *Evaluation:* that implies a thorough assessment of the myofascial system to identify any sign of fascial restriction. In this process it is fundamental to consider the entireness of fascial tissue, extending mostly in a spiral pattern from the extremities to the axial part of the body. Due to its ubiquitous nature and structure, any disruption of fascial function at any level may potentially produce an effect elsewhere in the organism. Abnormal areas of tension within this system, following a recent or longstanding injury, surgery, or any sort of repetitive strain, creates adaptive compensatory patterns, following the path of least resistance. This can lead to altered structural alignment, impaired movement patterns, joint restrictions, pain, poor energy levels, and decreased vitality (Hruby, 1992). Therefore, a body-wide postural evaluation should be accurately performed, together with hands-on assessment of the tone and texture of the myofascial tissue, joint range of motion, muscle testing, and subjective complaints of pain and/or loss of function. The ultimate goal for the operator is to identify the dysfunctional body region to be worked on, including the dysfunctional vectors in the fascia. These are preferential patterns of tissue motion, perceived by the practitioner as movements toward 'ease', usually mirroring directions of past injury or trauma.

2. *Induction:* at this stage, in particular, a state of relaxation from the patient is required. The operator approaches the involved area with a gentle touch, reinforcing the procedure by visualizing the anatomy of the region being worked. He or she initially induces motion, usually by lifting and holding the area in a relaxed position, so as to reduce the influence of gravity and overcome reactive proprioceptive postural tone (Minasny, 2009). Alternatively, a distraction or compression force on related joints can be added to prompt the process. For example, in leg unwinding, with the patient supine, the operator lifts and supports the leg under the ankle, while a mild compression toward the hip joint can be added to promote the unwinding motion. The scope is to hold tissues in a balanced and relaxed state, remaining sensitive to fascial clues that suggest any direction of spontaneous expression of inherent tensional patterns.

3. *Unwinding:* the operator supports the patient while focusing on the area of major fascial tension, allowing any spontaneous movement to manifest. This is probably the most difficult phase of the procedure, because of its dynamic

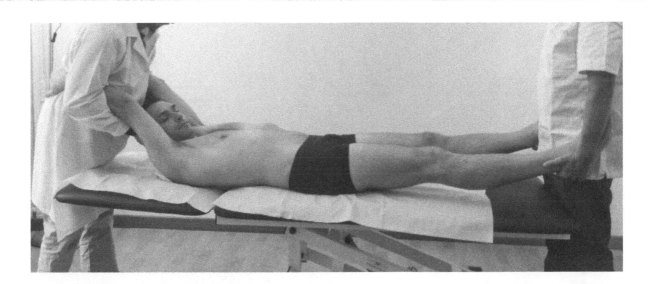

Figure 40.1

FU technique with two operators. The picture shows a common hold for applying a total body FU on an adult patient with the cooperation of two osteopaths. The patient lies supine on the couch. One operator stands at the feet, lifting and holding the legs at the ankles. The second operator stands on the opposite side, lifting and holding the head. Alternatively, he/she may leave the head of the patient on the couch and use the arms as levers instead. In this case, the arms of the patient should be raised up and supported from the elbows, with the hands resting on the osteopath's flanks. If a strong leverage is needed, both head and arms may be employed as levers, as shown in the picture

nature that requires high sensitivity, kinesthetic appreciation, and fine palpation skills from the practitioner. The latter should sense movements arising from the inherent motion of dysfunctional tissues that should not be directed or forced but just acknowledged and followed. Such patterns of motion are mostly unpredictable: shearing, torsional or rotational components may arise, usually following a spiral path, sometimes very subtle, sometimes extremely vigorous, either rhythmic or random, but always at their own individual pace. The unwinding process should never be allowed to occur as a 'fulcrumless' circular motion, since that would be unlikely to produce any therapeutic effect. Instead, a precise fulcrum should be identified, around which tissues may express their dysfunctional pattern. Such a fulcrum should be the point of major fascial restriction being addressed. During the entire procedure, the patient gives constant feedback to the operator, while the latter supports and amplifies the range and intensity of movement, guided by inherent fascial tensions, until a spontaneous release is perceived. During this process, it may happen that the therapist feels uncomfortable with keeping the same hold of a given structure in unwinding mode or, even worse, that the maneuver becomes unsafe by making the patient unstable on the couch. In both cases, the operator should stop the technique to choose a more effective hold, and by instructing the patient to assume a safer position.

4. *Still point:* this is only occasionally present. It involves a cessation of the unwinding process, resulting in a still point where no motion occurs and tissues are 'silent'. The patient's cooperation may be requested at this stage, such as forced respiration, to promote tissue changes and release.

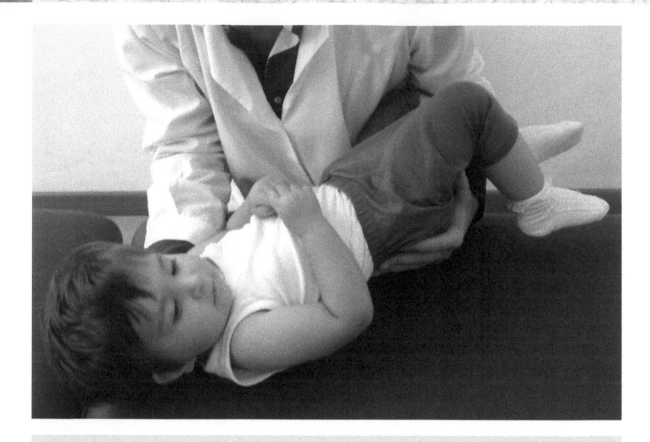

Figure 40.2
Common FU hold on infants. The patient lies supine, while the operator takes an occiput–sacral hold. The induction process may trigger a complex unwinding throughout the body, focused at the base of the skull and sacrum in particular, while forces might be conveyed towards the thoracoabdominal diaphragm at some point. The unwinding process needs always to be addressed and focused on the fulcrum of major fascial density and restriction. A still point may occur during the maneuver. The hand-hold may need to be changed to allow a more effective performance and/or to better control movement, keeping the infant in a safe position

5. *Release:* a collapse of myofascial tension may be felt together with warmth and a 'melting' sense in the tissues that are being worked on. A release may take seconds to be obtained when working on recent and mild restrictions, whereas long-standing or severe injuries may require more than one session. In some cases, an emotional release may occur, or be induced, during the unwinding method.

6. *Reassessment:* tissue should be re-examined after release has been achieved, and a sense of bal-

anced tension within and around the myofascial tissue should be verified. Any combined therapeutic exercise and traditional manual modalities may then be found to be more effective in achieving enhanced function.

If total body unwinding needs to be performed on an adult patient, normally the cooperation of two operators is required. In this case, with the patient lying supine, one practitioner lifts and holds both legs at the ankles; while a colleague lifts and holds the head, with the patient's arms raised up in between the osteopath's elbows and trunk, and the patient's hands resting on the osteopath's flanks (Fig. 40.1). Both operators focus on the areas of major fascial restriction in the respective halves of the body. A simultaneous unwinding may then take place, usually requiring a change of hand-hold and constant monitoring of patient position. If the adult patient is constitutionally smaller than the operator, or if the patient is a child, a single practitioner can easily perform total body unwinding. In the case of an infant patient, full body unwinding can be started through an occipitosacral hold with the baby in a supine position (Fig. 40.2). Again, the effective movement will be felt as a spontaneous expression of tension from dysfunctional tissues, until the release is felt.

Finally, if scar tissue needs to be worked, the procedure remains basically the same, although FU is applied in a combined manner in this case (i.e., by simultaneously performing a direct and an indirect maneuver). One operator's hand takes a contact on the dysfunctional scar, with a focus on the points of major restriction, fibrosis, and tension. He or she then chooses the most appropriate lever to unwind the scar tissue – that is usually a limb or the head and neck, depending where the scar is located. Whatever structure has been selected as leverage, it is held and maintained in a relaxed position with the other hand. The combined fascial unwinding can now be performed: with one hand the practitioner applies a direct fascial technique on the scar, by engaging and holding the tissue barrier; then the locally gathered tension is unwound in indirect fashion by means of the lever being supported by the other hand. Once the barrier yields, the operator looks for any further tissue restriction. Once this is found, the lever will be used again to unwind the given tension. The procedure goes on until a complete release of the scar is achieved. A still point may occur, requiring some form of patient cooperation to allow change to occur.

Mechanisms

Although fascia has been demonstrated to contract in a smooth-muscle-like manner (Schleip et al. 2005), its ability to unwind has not yet been investigated. In the literature, FU is usually explained as an expression of the body's ability to self-correct from functional disturbances, with the muscles, ligaments, and fascia being ascribed as the agencies for such motion (Frymann 1998b). However, a variety of interacting electromechanical events affecting central, peripheral, autonomic, and even physiologic functions have been proposed to come into play in generating the unwinding process (Ward, 2003c). Yet the mechanism behind it is still unknown.

Minasny (2009) has advanced an interesting theory to explain the unwinding process:

- When applying FU, the operator initiates the unwinding through a gentle touch and an induction along directions of ease. This may produce a stimulation of pressure-sensitive mechanoreceptors in the fascial tissue followed by a parasympathetic response (Schleip, 2003).

- The latter may induce a state of relaxation in the patient, possibly associated with rapid eye movement or deep breathing (Bertolucci, 2008). A change in local vasodilatation and tissue viscosity, together with a lowered tonus of intrafascial smooth muscle cells, may also take place under parasympathetic influence (Schleip, 2003).

- In response to the proprioceptive input from the induction process, the central nervous system (CNS) changes muscle tone and allows muscle action and movements along paths of least resistance.

- At this point of relaxed central activity, ideomotor reflexes occur (Dorko, 2003). These are unconscious reflexes that imply involuntary muscle movement, mostly ascribed to an external force and possibly caused by prior expectations or suggestions. The ideomotor action is generated through voluntary motor control, but is altered and experienced as an involuntary reaction. This is why the patient usually assumes that the therapist is guiding the movement during FU, although when made aware of it can consciously stop it. This indicates dissociation between voluntary action and conscious experience.

- This unconscious movement or stretching sensation stimulates a response in the tissue, providing feedback to the CNS, which, in turn, will generate the movements again, as outlined in the theory of ideomotor action (Elsner & Hommel, 2001).

- The process is repeated until a release is achieved.

Since tissue release seems to be unrelated to viscoelastic deformation of fascia (Chaudhry et al., 2008), which would, in fact, require much stronger or longer duration forces, neurological reflexive changes in tissue tonus have been proposed to explain the effects of fascial work (Schleip, 2003). Minasny concludes that FU occurs when a physical induction by a therapist prompts ideomotor action experienced as involuntary by the patient. However, other mechanisms may come into play.

Masi & Hannon (2008) have proposed an interesting model to understand myofascial tone. It is described as the passive tension of skeletal muscles producing a resistance to a given stretch. Such tension is supposed to derive from intrinsic molecular viscoelastic properties. This has been demonstrated to be independent from nervous system activity, as shown by corresponding silent EMG patterns. In other terms, this tone, defined as *human resting myofascial tone* (HRMT), is an intrinsic and independent viscoelastic property of the myofascia, resulting from molecular interactions of the actomyosin filaments in myofibroblast cells and myosarcomeric units. It may offer a substantial contribution to maintaining postural stability with minimal energetic expenditure, in contrast with neuromotor activation that implies instead higher levels of tone to provide stabilization. From a functional point of view, HRMT is integrated with the fascial and ligamentous tensional complex, thereby constituting a biotensegrity network (Levin & Martin, 2012). Therefore, the tension is transmitted to the complexity of the myofascial unit via various matrix fibrils and molecular elements in the connective tissue. Different musculoskeletal conditions and dysfunctions seem to be related to a change in normal levels of HRMT that would in turn affect the tension on surrounding fascial and ligamentous structures with an influence on joint mobility, movement control, and posture stability (Masi at al., 2010). This might also be self-maintained by intramuscular connective tissue capable of active contraction and consequently able to influence passive muscle stiffness, especially in tonic muscles (Schleip et al., 2006). Consequently, the altered distribution of tension might lead to a consistent tissue microinjury and maladaptive repair reactions (Masi at al., 2010), although these mechanisms are currently unexplained. FU might produce beneficial effect on releasing any alteration of the HRMT, by allowing the inherent tension to express under the facilitating guidance of the operator. This concept may well integrate with Minasny's theory: while CNS activity is reduced and parasympathetic tone is upraised, inducing patient relaxation, the HRMT may find the ideal neurophysiological context to unwind its tensions along paths of least resistance. The ideomotor action may occur in the meantime, allowing for involuntary muscle movement to occur, although the HRMT will be the force that dictates the direction of such motion.

Furthermore, some studies have demonstrated the effect of myofascial work on upregulation of parasympathetic tone with an influence on blood shear rate and blood flow turbulence (Queré et al., 2009). Others have shown a modulation of hypersympathicotonia with an improvement in a variety of visceral and psychosomatic features as demonstrated by hemodynamic functions (Rivers et al., 2008), heart rate variability (Henley et al., 2008), and anxiety levels (Fernández-Perez et al., 2008) following osteopathic fascial work.

Some therapeutic changes following FU may also be related to the anandamide effect on the endocannabinoid system: an endorphin system constituted of cell membrane receptors, endogenous ligands, and ligand-metabolizing enzymes. This system affects fibroblast remodeling, and may play a role in fascial reorganization, diminishing nociception and reducing inflammation in myofascial tissues (McPartland et al., 2005). Cannabinoids are also linked to cardiovascular changes, smooth muscle relaxation, and perhaps to mood changes through their role on the CNS (Ralevic et al., 2002).

Traditionally, it has been suggested that most of the changes following fascial work may be the result of a transformation of the ground substance from its densified state (gel) to a more fluid (sol) state (Rolf, 1962). Such thixotropic changes seem to increase the production of hyaluronic acid, together with the flow within the fascial tissue, thanks to the interplay of calcium ion concentration and unbound water oscillations (Lee, 2008). Such interfascial flow may play a role in improving drainage of inflammatory mediators and metabolic wastes; and in decreasing chemical irritation of the autonomic nervous system endings, and nociceptive stimuli to somatic endings, also via oxytocinergic mechanisms (Lund et al., 2002). Finally, these fluidic motions applied to vascular and nerve tissue following manipulations can cause a remarkable increase in hematic nitric oxide concentration (Salamon et al., 2004), whose known beneficial effects (Tota & Trimmer, 2011) may explain some of the therapeutic results following fascial work.

Other authors, instead, have considered piezoelectric properties as an alternative explanation of the change in fascial plasticity. The fascia presents crystalline collagen strands that display a polarity within their molecular structure and can then generate piezoelectricity: applying an electric stimulus causes mechanical motion (vibration) and applying physical force (tension, compression, or shear) generates electricity (Lee, 2008). Therefore, fascia seems to combine the properties of a sol-liquid conductor and a crystal generator system, which can generate and conduct direct currents, including the ability to store memories and traumas (Oschman, 2009) by using energy transmissions as information (Pischinger, 1991).

Clinical case

A 30 year-old secretary presented with a constant dull ache in the coccygeal region, with occasionally acute episodes when sitting for more than 2–3 hours. No other symptoms were associated with this pain. The onset was a year before, two months after she gave birth to her first child, following a caesarean section. Since then, she also suffered with recurrent haemorrhoids and cystitis. The examination revealed: a pelvic positional unbalance (tilted right and rotated left); a remarkable dysfunction of the pelvic diaphragm (R>L); a dysfunction of the right broad ligament of the uterus, causing a torsion of the organ toward the right side; an active suprapubic scar (R>L); a somatic dysfunction of L1–L2; a reduction in most planes of the sacrum and coccyx mobility and motility; an SBS right torsion; and a left TMJ dysfunction. The pelvic region was primarily addressed during the first treatment. The scar was released with FU combined application using the hold shown in Fig. 40.3. Once the scar tension yielded, the same technique was continued to release the right broad ligament of the

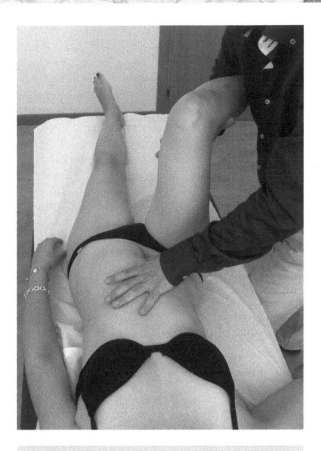

Figure 40.3

FU applied to scar tissue. When applied to actively dysfunctional scar tissues, FU can be performed in a combined manner. One hand takes a contact on the scar tissue, right where the points of major restriction are perceived. In this case, the contact will be suprapubic, on the scar that resulted from the caesarean section. The other hand supports the better leverage that can be used to unwind the scar. In this case, it will be the lower limb closer to the side where major scar restriction has been found. While the cranial hand performs a direct fascial technique on the scar tissue, moving against the barrier, the caudal hand will be using the limb as leverage to unwind any tension that has been locally gathered. The maneuver is continued until a full release of the tension is achieved

uterus. Then the pelvic diaphragm was approached by the use of inhibitory pressure and direct myofascial release. Articulatory techniques were applied to the lower limbs, pelvis, and lumbar spine. The patient was instructed to perform every day specific exercises for reinforcing lower abdominal muscles and pelvic muscle tone. The second visit was planned after one week. The symptoms improved consistently, appearing only in a mild form after 5-6 hours of sitting. No signs of dysfunction were found in the areas worked during the first treatment. The lumbar dysfunction and the craniosacral alterations, although still present, were showing a mild improvement of palpatory features. The former was corrected by the application of a direct manipulation through a sitting lift technique, while the latter was normalized though a TMJ decompression manoeuvre, followed by an SBS decompression technique and an occipitosacral balancing. The patient was then asked to return for a third check in two weeks' time, while water gym and general stretching were recommended twice a week for at least three months.

References

Anderson, R. E., Seniscal, C. 2006 A comparison of selected osteopathic treatment and relaxation for tension-type headaches. *Headache*. 46:1273–1280.

Bertolucci, L. F. 2008 Muscle repositioning: a new verifiable approach to neuro-myofascial release? *J Bodyw Mov Ther*. 12(3):213–224.

Blum, C. L. 2002 Chiropractic and pilates therapy for the treatment of adult scoliosis. *J Manipulative Physiol Ther* 25:E3.

Centers, S., Morelli, M. A., Vallad-Hiz, C., et al. 2003 General pediatrics. In: Ward, R. C. (Ed.), *Foundations for Osteopathic Medicine*. 2nd Edn. Lippincott Williams & Wilkins, Philadelphia, PA. p. 324.

Chaitow, L. 2005 *Cranial Manipulation: Theory and Practice: Osseous and Soft Tissue Approaches*. Elsevier Health Sciences. pp. 370–372.

Chaudhry, H., Schleip, R., Ji, Z., et al. 2008 Three-dimensional mathematical model for deformation of human fasciae in manual therapy. *J Am Osteopath Assoc* 108:379–390.

Defeo, G., Hicks, L. 1993 A description of the common compensatory pattern in relationship to the osteopathic postural examination. *Dynamic Chiropractic*. 11:24.

DeStefano, L. A. 2011 Greenman's principles of manual medicine. 4th Edn., Williams and Wilkins, Baltimore, MD. p. 155.

DiGiovanna, E. L. 2005 The manipulative prescription. In: DiGiovanna, E. L., Schiowitz, S., Dowling, D. J. (Eds), An Osteopathic Approach to Diagnosis and Treatment. 3rd Edn., Lippincott Williams & Wilkins, Philadelphia, PA. Ch. 118.

Dorko, B. L. 2003 The analgesia of movement: ideomotor activity and manual care. *J Osteopath Med* 6:93–95.

Dowling, D. J. 2011 Progressive inhibition of neuromuscular structures. In: Chila, A. (Ed.), *Foundations of Osteopathic Medicine*. 3rd Edn., Lippincott Williams & Wilkins, Philadelphia, PA. p. 822.

Educational Council on Osteopathic Principles (ECOP) 2011 Glossary of osteopathic terminology usage guide. American Association of Colleges of Osteopathic Medicine (AACOM), Chevy Chase, MD. p. 29.

Elsner, B., Hommel, B. 2001 Effect anticipation and action control. *J Exp Psychol Hum Percept Perform* 27:229–240.

Fernández-Perez, A. M., Peralta-Ramírez, M. I., Pilat, A., et al. 2008 Effects of myofascial induction techniques on physiologic and psychologic parameters: a randomized controlled trial. *J Altern Complement Med* 14:807–811.

Frymann, V. M. 1998a The collected papers of Viola M. Frymann, DO. Legacy of osteopathy to children. *Am Acad Osteopath.*, Indianapolis, IN. p. 82.

Frymann, V. M. 1998b Fascial release techniques. In: *The Collected Papers of Viola M. Frymann, DO. Legacy of Osteopathy to Children*. American Academy of Osteopathy, Indianapolis, IN. pp. 72-82.

Henley, C. E., Ivins, D., Mills, M., et al. 2008 Osteopathic manipulative treatment and its relationship to autonomic nervous system activity as demonstrated by heart rate variability: a repeated measures study. *Osteopath Med Prim Care* 2:7.

Hruby, R. J. 1992 Pathophysiologic models and the selection of osteopathic manipulative techniques. *J Osteopath Med* 6:25–30.

Kerr, H. D. 1997 Ureteral stent displacement associated with deep massage. *WMJ* 96:57-58.

Kuchera, M. L. 2003 Postural considerations in coronal, horizontal and sagittal planes. In: Ward, R. C. (ed.), *Foundations for Osteopathic Medicine*. 2nd Edn. Lippincott Williams & Wilkins, Philadelphia, P. A. pp. 629–630.

Kuchera, M. L. 2011 Lymphatics approach. In: Chila, A. (Ed.), *Foundations of Osteopathic Medicine*. 3rd Edn. Lippincott Williams & Wilkins, Philadelphia, PA. Ch. 51.

Lee, R. P. 2008 The living matrix: a model for the primary respiratory mechanism. *Explore* 4:374–378.

Levin, S., Martin, D. 2012 Biotensegrity: the mechanics of fascia. In: Schleip, R., Findley, T. W., Chaitow, L., Huijing, P. A. (Eds.) *Fascia: The Tensional Network of The Human Body*. Churchill Livingstone Elsevier, Edinburgh. pp. 137–142.

Lewit, K., Olsanska, S. 2004 Clinical importance of active scars: abnormal scars as a cause of myofascial pain. *J Manip Physiol Ther* 27:399–402.

Lund, I., Ge, Y., Yu, L. C., et al. 2002 Repeated massage-like stimulation induces long-term effects on nociception: contribution of oxytocinergic mechanisms. *Eur J Neurosci* 16:330–338.

Masi, A. T., Hannon, J. C. 2008 Human resting muscle tone (HRMT): narrative introduction and modern concepts. *J Bodyw Mov Ther* 12:320–332.

Masi, A. T., Nair, K., Evans, T., et al. 2010 Clinical, biomechanical, and physiological translational interpretations of human resting myofascial tone or tension. *Int J Ther Massage Bodywork* 3:16–28.

McPartland, J. M., Giuffrida, A., King, J., et al. 2005 Cannabimimetic effects of osteopathic manipulative treatment. *J Am Osteopath Assoc* 105:283–291.

Minasny, B. 2009 Understanding the process of fascial unwinding. *Int J Ther Massage Bodywork* 2:10 17.

Mitchell, F. L., Sr. 1958 Structural pelvic function. In: Barnes, M. W. (Ed.), *Yearbook of the Academy of Applied Osteopathy*. American Academy of Osteopathy, Indianapolis. p. 79.

Nicholas, A., Nicholas, E. 2008 *Atlas of Osteopathic Techniques*, 2nd Edn. Lippincott Williams & Wilkins, Philadelphia. p. 116.

Oschman, J. L. 2009 Charge transfer in the living matrix. *J Bodyw Mov Ther* 13:215–228.

Pischinger, A. 1991 *Matrix and Matrix Regulation: Basis for a Holistic Theory of Medicine*. Haug International, Brussels. p. 53.

Pope, R. E. 2003 The common compensatory pattern: its origin and relationship to the postural model. *J Am Acad Osteopath* 13:19–40.

Queré, N., Noël, E., Lieutaud, A., et al. 2009 Fasciatherapy combined with pulsology touch induces changes in blood turbulence potentially beneficial for vascular endothelium. *J Bodyw Mov Ther* 13:239–245.

Ralevic, V., Kendall, D. A., Randall, M. D., et al. 2002 Cannabinoid modulation of sensory neurotransmission via cannabinoid and vanilloid receptors: roles in regulation of cardiovascular function. *Life Sci* 71:2577–2594.

Rivers, W. E., Treffer, K. D., Glaros, A. G. et al. 2008 Short-term hematologic and hemodynamic effects of osteopathic lymphatic techniques: a pilot crossover trial. *J Am Osteopath Assoc* 108:646–651.

Rolf, I. 1962 *Structural Dynamics*. British Academy of Applied Osteopathy Yearbook.

Salamon, E., Zhu, W., Stefano, G. 2004 Nitric oxide as a possible mechanism for understanding the therapeutic effects of osteopathic manipulative medicine. *Int J Mol Med* 14:443–449.

Schleip, R. 2003 Fascial plasticity: a new neurobiological explanation. Part 2. *J Bodyw Mov Ther* 7:104–116.

Schleip. R., Klingler, W., Lehmann-Horn, F. 2005 Active fascial contractility: fascia may be able to contract in a smooth muscle-like manner and thereby influence musculoskeletal dynamics. *Med Hypotheses* 65:273–277.

Schleip, R., Naylor, I. L., Ursu, D., et al. 2006 Passive muscle stiffness may be influenced by active contractility of intramuscular connective tissue. *Med Hypotheses* 66:66-71.

Stone, C. A. 2007a *Visceral and Obstetric Osteopathy*. Elsevier Churchill Livingstone, Edinburgh.

Stone, C. A. 2007b *Visceral and Obstetric Osteopathy*. Elsevier Churchill Livingstone, Edinburgh. p. 297.

Stone, C. A. 2007c *Visceral and Obstetric Osteopathy*. Elsevier Churchill Livingstone, Edinburgh. p. 278.

Tota, B., Trimmer, B. (eds) 2011 *Nitric Oxide*. Elsevier Health Sciences.

Tozzi, P., Bongiorno, D., Vitturini, C. 2011 Fascial release effects on patients with non-specific cervical or lumbar pain. *J Bodyw Mov Ther* 15:405 416.

Tozzi P., Bongiorno, D., Vitturini, C. 2012 Low back pain and kidney mobility: local osteopathic fascial manipulation decreases pain perception and improves renal mobility. *J Bodyw Mov Ther* 16:381-391.

Upledger, J. E. 1987 *Craniosacral Therapy II: Beyond the Dura*. Eastland Press, Seattle.

Vick, D. A., McKay, C., Zengerle, C. R. 1996 The safety of manipulative treatment: review of the literature from 1925 to 1993. *J Am Osteopath Assoc* 96:113-115.

Ward, R. C. 2003a Integrated neuromusculoskeletal release and myofascial release. In: Ward, R. C. (Ed.), *Foundations for Osteopathic Medicine*. 2nd Edn. Lippincott Williams & Wilkins, Philadelphia, PA. p. 960.

Ward, R. C. 2003b Integrated neuromusculoskeletal release and myofascial release. In: Ward, R. C. (Ed.), *Foundations for Osteopathic Medicine*. 2nd Edn. Lippincott Williams & Wilkins, Philadelphia, PA.

Ward, R. C. 2003c Integrated neuromusculoskeletal release and myofascial release. In: Ward, RC. (Ed.), *Foundations for Osteopathic Medicine*. 2nd Edn. Lippincott Williams & Wilkins, Philadelphia, PA. p. 961.

Weintraub, W. 2003 Tendon and ligament healing: a new approach to sports and overuse injury. Paradigm Publications, Herndon, VA. p. 66-67.

World Health Organization (WHO) 2010 Safety issues. In: Benchmarks for training in osteopathy. WHO, Geneva, Switzerland. p. 17.

Zink, J. G. 1973 Applications of the osteopathic holistic approach to homeostasis. *Am Acad Osteopath Yearb* 37–47.

Zink, J. G. 1977 Respiratory and circulatory care: the conceptual model. *Osteopath Ann* 5:108-112.

Zink, J. G., Lawson, W. B. 1979 An osteopathic structural examination and functional interpretation of the soma. *Osteopath Ann* 7:12-19.

MYOFASCIAL INDUCTION THERAPY (MIT)

Andrzej Pilat

Introduction

There are contrasting opinions as to which structures can be defined as fascia (Langevin, 2014; Langevin & Huijing, 2009; Schleip et al., 2012; Swanson, 2013; Stecco, 2014). This chapter analyzes fascial classification in manual therapy from a functional approach. Thus, we recommend using the expression 'fascial system'. This *system* gathers various types of cells with different activities (similarly to the digestive system or the nervous system) and relates to other body systems through an uninterrupted and innervated structure of functional stability (Pilat, 2014), shaped by the 'three-dimensional collagenous matrix' (Kumka & Bonar, 2012).

The fascial system represents a complex communicational architecture, which provides mechanoreceptive information. This process occurs not exclusively because of its topographic distribution, but mainly through the pattern of *how* it interrelates with other body structures, especially muscles. In its fibrous construction, it has the ability to align with and accommodate the intrinsic and extrinsic tensional body requirements. The tensional paths, created outside the appropriate biomechanical movement patterns, can thus redirect the body's dynamics. The density, distribution, and organoleptic characteristics of the system differ throughout the body but its continuity is essential, allowing the fascia to act as a synergistic whole, absorbing and distributing local stimuli to the entire system. The inherent synergy of the structured fascial system enables the human body to adapt, according to requirements from outside and inside the body, or in relation to the availability of energy and nutrients in the immediate environment. Besides its structural role, fascia also distributes stimuli to the body. Its sensory network registers thermal and chemical changes, pressure, vibration, and movement impulses, and analyzes, categorizes, and transmits them to the central nervous system. The central nervous system receives, absorbs, transforms, evaluates, and consolidates these impulses and sends the instructions to other body systems (Pilat, 2014).

Considering the basic functional analysis, we recognize the existence of the superficial and deep fascia (Fig. 41.1). The deep fascia can be subdivided into myofascia, viscerofascia, and meninges. This classification may differ in some aspects (e.g., the

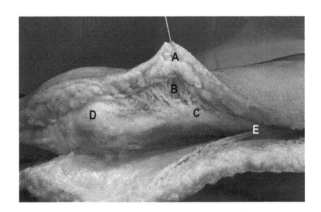

Figure 41.1

Anterior aspect of the knee and thigh in a dissection of an unembalmed cadaver with a high percentage of body fat. Note the two levels of superficial fascia: superficial and deep. **A** Superficial layer of superficial fascia (honeycomb fascia) with a large amount of cuboidal fatty nodes; **B** Deep layer of superficial fascia with flat fatty nodes; **C** Deep fascia (myofascial layer); **D** Patella; **E** Iliotibial band

relation between the fascial planes and layers) from the viewpoint of experts in gross anatomy and histology (Lancerotto et al., 2011).

Myofascial therapy is not exclusive to any profession. There are a variety of approaches and techniques, generally based on similar conceptual principles. Although its exact mechanism is not yet fully understood, myofascial therapy applications are emerging with a solid and growing base of evidence and broad therapeutic potential. A unification and validation of clinical procedures, via research, is required (Ajimsha et al., 2012; Remvig et al., 2008).

Myofascial force transmission

The universal model of muscular contraction based on the gliding of filaments of actin and myosin, described over 40 years ago by Huxley & Simmons (1971), supports the Newtonian analysis of body movement, characterized by the action of levers. In this model, the myofibrils, arranged in series, act as independent motors that approximate myotendinous/myoaponeurotic junctions, therefore triggering movement. However, the discovery of the ultrastructure and the mechanobiology of the sarcomeral unit, have given shape to a new model of myofibrils, embedded inside the extracellular matrix, which, at the same time, participates (from its own dynamic) in the contractile phenomenon (Yucesoy, 2010). The shortening of the myofibril exerts a force from within the myofascial structure (endomysium, perimysium, and epimysium) and resembles more the principles of the tensegrity model (Gillies & Lieber, 2011) rather than a simple linear analysis (movements arranged in series). Most of the contractile forces are destined for myotendinous units, however; approximately 30% of them use the 'epimysial' transmission paths, that is, parallel to tendinous ones (Huijing, 2007). In this model the muscle does not act as an isolated and independent entity. Instead, collagenous linkages between epimysia of adjacent muscles, such as the neurovascular tracts, provide indirect intermuscular connections. Usually, these lateral connections and the consequences of their presence are not taken into consideration in most models related to body movement. Nevertheless, in recent years, several studies have indicated mechanical interactions between adjacent muscles, including myofascial force transmission in research models and clinical analyses.

Innervation

Fascia is a mechanosensitive structure (Vaticón, 2009; Langevin, 2011). Usually, neuroanatomical studies focus mainly on discs, facet joints, muscle fibers, tendons, or ligaments, and there is limited information relating to the innervation of fascia. Our interest focuses on the functional connection, which involves mainly communication through the loose connective tissue structures through the unique network of mechanoreceptors known as interstitial mechanoreceptors (type III and IV free nerve endings). Each receptor has two subgroups with low or high levels of mechanosensitivity related to cell architecture. The presence of these types of receptors has been confirmed in recent studies:

- Group III muscle afferents are found in perimuscular fascia and the adventitia of muscle blood vessels and respond to a variety of stimuli, including pressure and stretch (which results in matrix deformation after mechanical impulse application) (Lin et al., 2009).

- Thoracolumbar fascia (TLF) is a highly innervated tissue (Taguchi et al., 2009).

- Substantial innervation of nonspecialized connective tissue through the A δ and/or C fibers (Corey, 2011; Tesarz et al., 2011).

- Strong link between fascia and the autonomic nervous system (Haouzi et al., 1999).

- Many fibers – especially in the superficial fascia – expressed tyrosine hydroxylase, an enzyme characteristic of postganglionic sympathetic fibers (dopamine secretion control). This finding may explain why patients with low back pain report increased intensity of pain when they are under psychological stress (Chou & Shekelle, 2010).

- Neural action potentially firing through nerve terminals is linked to specific mechanical deformation and extracellular matrix interactions (Lin et al., 2009).

- Stimulation of group III and IV muscle afferents has been shown to have important reflex effects on both the somatic and autonomic nervous systems. These include an inhibitory effect on alpha motor neurons, an excitatory effect on gamma motoneurones, and an excitatory effect on the sympathetic nervous system (Kaufman et al., 2002).

- Encapsulated nerve terminations may be involved in the proprioceptive role of fascia (van der Wal, 2009).

Definition of myofascial induction therapy

MIT is a hands-on, full-body approach, focusing on restoration of body function. In this process of assessment and treatment the practitioner applies gentle manual mechanical stress transfer (traction and/or compression) to targeted dysfunctional tissue. The outcome is a reciprocal reaction from the body that involves biochemical, signaling, metabolic, and finally physiological responses. This process aims to remodel the tissue matrix responsiveness and to facilitate and optimize information transfer to, and within, the fascial system. The term 'induction' relates to the recovery of movement facilitation, rather than a passive stretching of the fascial system. This is primarily a learning process in the search for a restored homeostasis to recover range of motion, appropriate tension, strength, and, mainly, movement coordination. The general goal of MIT application is to restore the internal balance of the fascial system and improve the body's movement ability in musculoskeletal, neural, vascular, cranial, and visceral body components. It is a focused process, controlled by the central nervous system, in which the clinician acts as a catalyst (facilitator). The therapeutic action focuses on the provision of resources for homeostatic balance adjustment. The final aim of the therapeutic process is not settlement of stable hierarchies, rather facilitation of optimal adaptation to environmental demands (Pilat, 2014). Figure 41.2 summarizes the MIT conceptual reasoning process. We should emphasize the importance of integration (active engagement) of the patient in the process. The outcome (body image changes, improvements in functional skills) should be assessed not only by the therapist but also the patient).

MIT application: indications and contraindications

The indications and contraindications for the application of MIT generally coincide with those applied in manual therapies in general. Table 41.1 summarizes the most relevant indications and contraindications.

Myofascial dysfunction

Definition

Fascial system dysfunction is defined as alteration of the highly organized assortment of specialized movements, and as an incorrect transfer of

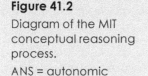

Figure 41.2

Diagram of the MIT conceptual reasoning process.

ANS = autonomic nervous system; CNS = central nervous system; MIT = myofascial induction therapy

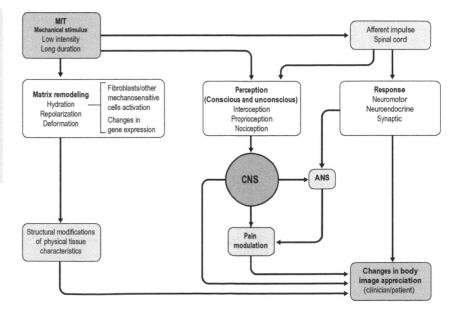

	Main indications	Main contraindications

Table 41.1
MIT indications and contraindications
	• Patients with dysfunctions that are:
	   ◦ orthopedic
	   ◦ neuroorthopedic
	   ◦ post-traumatic
	   ◦ degenerative
	
	• Diseases of the nervous system (central and peripheral)
	
	• Pelvic floor disorders
	
	• Circulatory diseases
	
	• TMJ dysfunction
	
	• Sports injuries
	
	• Respiratory disorders
		• Aneurysms
		
		• Systemic diseases
		
		• Inflammatory soft tissue process in the acute phase
		
		• Acute circulatory deficiency
		
		• Advanced diabetes
		
		• Anticoagulant therapy
		
		• General contraindications to any manual therapy procedure

information through the matrix (Pilat, 2003). If proper fascial dynamics (gliding between endofascial fibers and interfascial planes) are impaired then the optimal body behavior may be affected. This is also related to the proper exchange of fluids (Schleip et al., 2012).

Syndrome formation

'The capacity of the various collagen layers to slide over each other may be altered in cases of over-use syndrome, trauma or surgery' (Stecco, 2008). Thus, the body may develop fascial entrapments that redirect and distort biomechanical movement patterns and facilitate the creation of dysfunctions. Purslow (2010) says that the ECM is continually remodeled and could be mechanically adapted. The reduction of mobility can also alter the quality of blood circulation, which becomes slow and heavy, leading in extreme cases to ischemia and deterioration of the quality of muscular fibers. Excessive stimulation of the production of collagen fibers leads to the development of fibrosis in the myofascial system. The result is loss of matrix quality and consequently formation of entrapment areas (the areas with alteration of the physiological movement as regards its amplitude, speed, resistance, and coordination) (Pilat, 2009) (see Fig. 41.3).

These fascial entrapments promote the formation of compensatory (substitute) movement patterns. Regardless of the cause of the entrapment, if they persist for long periods of time, they eventually lead to excess load and ultimately dysfunction (Pilat, 2003).

These changes influence mostly the loose connective tissue structures and affect the specialized structures (dense regular and irregular connective tissue), producing excessive density and fiber reorientation. The specialized structures are tendons, ligaments, and the articular capsules. Short-term changes will affect the local function and the long-term changes, which may potentially result in global dysfunction patterns.

Fascial entrapment areas

According to Pilat (2015), the most common areas vulnerable to fascial entrapment formation are:

• Bonding areas between fascial structures in places of extensive load (e.g., the bicipital aponeurosis that is not only a structure that protects the neurovascular bundle, but is also a dynamic stabilizer of the biceps' tendon in its lower insertion) (Eames et al., 2007).

• Areas with excessive friction (tendons with tendinous sheaths reinforced by the retinacula). An increase in the compression level between tendon and retinacula leads to fibrocartilaginous changes (Benjamin, 1995).

• Areas with insertion of numerous fascial structures with great fibrous density (i.e., scapular spine). Those regions mechanically operate as areas of movement links and distribution. When the entrapment occurs it may create a change in the local movement and/or a referred compensation process (Fernández-de-las-Peñas & Pilat, 2012).

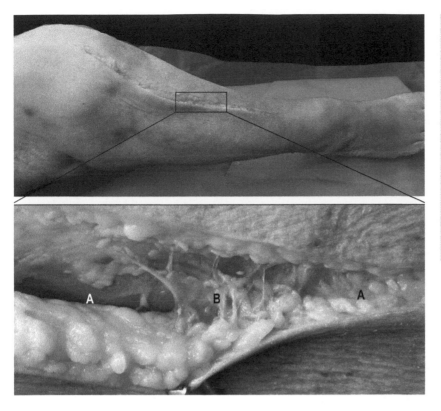

Figure 41.3
Fascial entrapments on the lateral aspect of the leg in an unembalmed cadaver dissection.
Top: anterolateral aspect of the left leg.
Bottom: close-up view of fascial entrapments between the superficial and deep fascia layers.
A Normal relationship between both layers; **B** Area of entrapments

- Areas with prolonged and/or repeated hypomobility (e.g., as a result of adjusting to poor posture).

- Body segments affected by traumatic or surgical processes.

- Structures involved in the protection of the neurovascular continuum (e.g., the popliteal fossa).

Assessment process

A suggested clinical evaluation protocol is summarized in Figure 41.4. Special attention should be addressed to global functional tests when the patient performs integrated movements, which are often similar to everyday activities. MIT is a patient-oriented therapy, so the patient's personal interpretation of the assessment is very important.

Electromyography (EMG) (Bertolucci, 2008) and sonoelastography (Martinez & Galán-del-Río, 2013) are two of the main methods of obtaining an objective assessment that allows us to observe tissue changes in real time.

Principles of MIT application mechanisms (Pilat, 2014)

Fascia is a mechanosensory system, as evidenced by a variety of processes (Chiquet et al., 2003), and it has three properties that are sensitive to mechanical forces. Each of these operates at a different level, potentially influencing the others:

- *Mechanotransduction:* This is a process by which mechanical input is converted into a biochemical response (Ingber, 2003).

- *Piezoelectricity:* Because collagen is a semiconductor it is suggested that it is capable of forming an integrated electronic network that enables the interconnection of fascial system components (Ahn & Grodzinsky, 2009).

- *Viscoelasticity:* This is a property of fascia that describes its characteristics of viscosity and elasticity (Chaudhry et al., 2007).

These three mechanisms can act at different times, can complement each other, and the system can

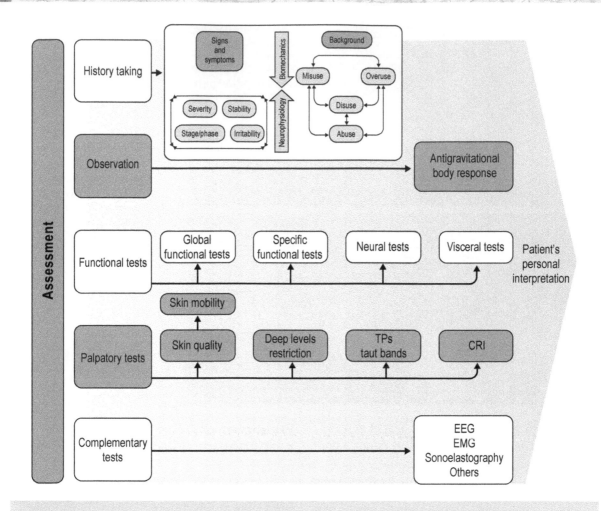

Figure 41.4

Assessment protocol. EEG = electroencephalogram; EMG = electromyography; TPs = trigger points. Reprinted with permission from Pilat A., 2014. Myofascial induction approaches. In: Chaitow L. *Fascial Dysfunction: Manual Therapy Approaches*, Handspring.

switch between them at any phase of clinical application (Vaticón, 2009).

Mechanical characteristics of MIT application

- Gentle force application.

- It never forces the articular range of motion (ROM).

- It follows the facilitated movement.

- Through the mechanoreceptors, the fascial system is in a continuous process of internal communication (Vaticón, 2009):

- somato–somatic
- somato–visceral
- viscero–visceral
- viscero–somatic.

Definition of the myofascial induction therapy process

Myofascial induction therapy application is an ensemble of procedures focusing on optimizing function and balance within the fascial system. The approach looks for local corrections, recovery of global dynamics, and painless body performance. The treatment protocol is divided into two phases: superficial (stroke) technique applications and subsequently deep procedures. The myofascial induction process may be applied combined with other manual therapy strategies.

Clinical procedure principles (Pilat, 2003; Pilat, 2009; Pilat, 2014; Pilat, 2015)

- All procedures (protocols) must be individualized according to the treated dysfunction (pathology) and the patient's individual needs as regards age, physical and emotional conditions, cultural aspects, and gender. The choice of the specific technique also depends on the skills of the therapist.

- Biomechanically, the myofascial system responds to compression and traction forces. These are two mechanical strategies used when applying MIT.

- The direction of the releasing movement is toward facilitation. The clinician should refrain from performing movements in an arbitrary direction.

- The clinician chooses the body region affected by myofascial dysfunction that may be associated with pain and/or dysfunction (hypo- or hypermobility, incoordination, lack of strength, etc.). The body region should be identified during the initial assessment process discussed above.

- Each body region affected by dysfunction requires a specific procedure application (Pilat, 2003).

- The clinician tenses the tissue referred to as the first restriction barrier by applying a tridimensional, slow, and gradual compression or traction. The pressure is constant during the first 60–90 seconds, the time required for releasing the first restriction barrier (the beginning of the viscoelastic response).

- During the first phase of the application the therapist barely induces the tissue to move.

- Upon overcoming the first restriction barrier, the therapist accompanies the movement in the direction of the facilitation, pausing at each additional barrier.

- In each technique, one must overcome at least three to six consecutive barriers and the minimum time of application is three to five minutes.

- The tension on the tissue must be constant, but the pressure applied by the therapist may be modified after overcoming the first barrier. Pressure should be reduced when abundant activity and/or pain is perceived.

Examples of MIT application

Levator scapulae muscle fascia induction (Fig. 41.5)

The patient lies on the side that is not being treated. The clinician sits in a chair at the headboard of the table. With the fingertips of the ring, middle, and index fingers, the therapist 'embraces' the inferior angle of the scapula and pulls in a cranial direction. Next the therapist flexes the last phalanges of the index and middle fingers of the other hand, and applies contact halfway along the upper trapezius muscle. With the pads of these two fingers the therapist presses the trapezius muscle and presses the fingertips on the levator scapulae muscle insertion. This compression should be maintained for up to three minutes. This should be followed by a facilitating movement.

Thoracolumbar fascia-assisted induction (Fig. 41.6)

The patient is lying prone. The therapist leans over the patient so that he can contact, with his elbow, the lumbar paravertebral mass on the affected side (which is uppermost). Then, with the elbow, the

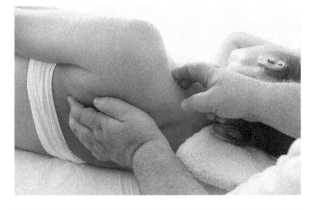

Figure 41.5
MIT application on the levator scapulae muscle

therapist performs a longitudinal stroke in a cranial direction, close to the spinous processes line. Simultaneously, the therapist must resist the flexion of the thigh and leg, actively conducted by the patient. The hip flexion should move forward with the same rate of progress as the motion made by the therapist's sliding elbow. The contraction that affects the patient inhibits defensive muscle tension. The maneuver is repeated three times on both sides.

Scientific evidence

This section focuses on scientific evidence relating to the results in this author's chapter on 'Myofascial induction approaches' in *Fascial Dysfunction: Manual Therapy Approaches* (Pilat, 2014). A growing number of articles relating to the clinical results of myofascial induction techniques have been published based on studies of patients with pain syndromes and healthy subjects. A number of studies have shown significant changes linked to responses of the autonomic nervous system (ANS).

Research related to pathology

- An objective model for evaluating the effect of application of myofascial induction techniques in muscular lesions with dynamic sonoelastography was created by Martínez Rodríguez & Galán-del-Río (2013).

- Leonard et al. (2009) reported that connective tissue manipulation improved peripheral circulation and enhanced wound-healing processes in 20 patients with diabetic foot ulcers.

- Tozzi (2012) investigated nonspecific low back pain in relation to kidney mobility. Using real-time ultrasound, this study demonstrated that 'osteopathic fascial manipulation decreased pain perception and improved renal mobility',

- Useros & Hernando (2008) concluded that myofascial induction has beneficial effects in patients with brain damage, with special emphasis on automatic posture control.

- In patients with unilateral spatial neglect (an alteration of the head's position with respect to the median line), Vaquero Rodríguez (2013) observed significant results for the sensitivity variable in the experimental group treated with myofascial induction techniques, compared to those treated with Bobath therapy.

- Fernández-Lao et al. (2011) applied myofascial release (MFR) techniques in breast cancer survivors. The authors observed that MFR led to an immediate increase in salivary flow rate, suggesting the parasympathetic effect of the intervention.

- Vasquez (2011) reported the effectiveness of myofascial induction techniques in treating swimmer's

Figure 41.6
MIT application on the thoracolumbar fascia

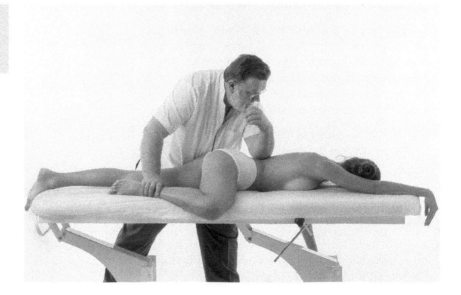

shoulder with respect to articular balance and pain.

- Arguisuelas-Martínez (2010) demonstrated the effects of lumbar spine manipulation and thoracolumbar myofascial induction techniques on the spinae erector activation pattern.

- In a double-blind study, Urresti-López (2011) applied the suboccipital induction technique to 26 subjects with chronic neck pain. Electroencephalogram (EEG) changes were observed in the latency reduction in the experimental group as compared to the control group. This result suggests that improvements in cognitive processes including attention, memory activation, and associative states are associated with the P300 wave. Lack of changes in other EEG parameters discarded the influence of vascular modifications.

- Heredia-Rizo et al. (2013) demonstrated that application of suboccipital muscle inhibition technique immediately improved head position. Additionally, it immediately decreased the mechanosensitivity of the greater occipital nerve.

- A comparative study was performed by Ramos-González et al. (2012) on the effectiveness of MFR and physiotherapy for venous insufficiency in postmenopausal women. The control and experimental group patients received kinesiotherapy treatment. The experimental group patients also received MFR treatments. The combination of MFR and kinesiotherapy improved the venous return, relieved pain, and improved the quality of life in postmenopausal women with venous insufficiency.

- Ajimsha et al. (2012) presented evidence that MFR is more effective than a control intervention for lateral epicondylitis in computer professionals.

- In a study performed with 74 fibromyalgia patients (analyzing experimental and placebo groups), Castro-Sánchez et al. (2011) state that MFR can improve pain, anxiety, quality of sleep, depression, and quality of life in patients with fibromyalgia.

- In a study performed with 86 fibromyalgia patients, Castro-Sánchez et al. (2010) observed that MFR improved pain, sensory, and affective dimensions without change in postural stability as compared to a placebo group. The authors suggested that lack of a postural stability test with a higher level of difficulty might have an effect on the result. They concluded that MFR techniques can be a complementary therapy for fibromyalgia syndrome.

Clinical research in healthy subjects

- Fernández-Pérez et al. (2013) observed major immunological modulations with an increased B lymphocyte count 20 minutes after the craniocervical application of MIT.

- Toro (2009) reported the application of a single session of manual therapy (including myofascial induction techniques) produced an immediate increase in heart-rate variability and a decrease in tension, anger status, and perceived pain in patients with chronic tension-type headache.

- Arroyo-Morales et al. (2008) reported that the heart-rate variability and blood pressure recovery after a physically stressful situation were improved by myofascial release as compared to sham electrotherapy treatment.

- Henley et al. (2008) demonstrated quantitatively that cervical myofascial release shifts sympathovagal balance from the sympathetic to the parasympathetic nervous system.

- In a study involving 41 healthy males randomly assigned to experimental or control groups, Fernández-Pérez (2008) reported significantly decreased anxiety levels in healthy, young adults after the application of myofascial induction treatment. Additionally, significantly lower systolic blood pressure values were observed, as compared to baseline levels.

Conclusion

The application of MIT may be of benefit in the treatment of musculoskeletal dysfunctions. We suggest that MIT be included in the therapeutic process. Despite the fact that research related to the scientific basis of MIT is growing, clinical evidence remains limited and requires unified research criteria including:

- more objective evaluation processes

- classification of strategies (local versus global approach)

- unification of parameters as to force, timing, intensity, and frequency of application

- identification and analysis of responses in different body systems

- identification and classification of non-responders

- analysis of long-term results.

One factor is the difficulty of quantifying treatment outcomes and isolating them from other collateral phenomena. The development of new assessment methods (e.g., sonoelastography) will help in this challenge.

Clinicians familiar with other myofascial therapy approaches (e.g., myofascial release, according to R. Ward [2003], originated from the concept of A. T. Still, and also widely described by C. Manheim [2008] and J. F. Barnes [1990] and others) will find similarities with myofascial induction, each with different nuances, based on a similar clinical reasoning concept that allows them to complement each other.

References

Ahn, A. C., Grodzinsky, A. J. 2009 Relevance of collagen piezoelectricity to 'Wolff's Law.' *Medi Eng Phys* 31:733–741.

Ajimsha, M. S., Chithra, S., Thulasyammal, R. P. et al. 2012 Effectiveness of myofascial release in the management of lateral epicondylitis in computer professionals. *Arch of Phys Med Rehabil* 93:604–609.

Arguisuelas Martínez, M. D. 2010 Effects of lumbar spine manipulation and thoracolumbar myofascial induction technique on the spinae erector activation pattern. *Fisioterapia* 32:250–255

Arroyo-Morales, M., Olea, N., Martínez, M. et al. 2008 Psychophysiological effects of massage-myofascial release after exercise. *J Altern Complement Med* 14:1223–1229.

Barnes, J. 1990 *Myofascial Release.* MFR Seminars: Paoli.

Benjamin, M. 1995 Fibrocartilage associated with human tendons and their pulleys. *J Anat* 187:625–633.

Bertolucci, F. 2008 Muscle repositioning: a new verifiable approach to neuro-myofascial release? *J Bodyw Mov Ther* 12:213–224.

Castro-Sánchez, A. M., Matarán-Peñarrocha, G. A., Arroyo-Morales, M., et al. 2011 Effects of myofascial release techniques on pain, physical function, and postural stability in patients with fibromyalgia: a randomized controlled trial. *Clin Rehabil* 25:800–813.

Castro-Sánchez, A. M., Matarán-Peñarrocha, G. A., Granero-Molina, J., et al. 2010 Benefits of massagemyofascial release therapy on pain, anxiety, quality of sleep, depression, and quality of life in patients with fibromyalgia. *Evid Based Complement Alternat Med* Published online December 28, 2010. http://www.ncbi.nlm.nih.gov/pmc/articles/PMC3018656/ [accessed March 11, 2016].

Chaudhry, H., Huang, C., Schleip, R. et al. 2007 Viscoelastic behavior of human fasciae under extension in manual therapy. *J Bodyw Mov Ther* 11:159–167.

Chiquet, M., Renedo, A. S., Huber, F. et al. 2003 How do fibroblasts translate mechanical signals into changes in extracellular matrix production? *Matrix Biol* 22:73–80.

Chou, R., Shekelle, P. 2010 Will this patient develop persistent disabling low back pain? *JAMA* 303:1295–1302.

Corey, S. M. 2011 Sensory innervation of the nonspecialized connective tissues in the low back of the rat. *Cells Tissues Organs* 194:521–530.

Eames, M. H., Bain, G. I., Fogg, Q. A. et al. 2007 Distal biceps tendon anatomy: a cadaveric study. *J Bone Joint Surg Am* 89:1044–1049.

Fernández-de-las-Peñas, C., Pilat, A. 2012. Chapter 11.1 Soft tissue manipulation approaches to chronic pelvic pain (external). In: Chaitow L, Lovegrove Jones R. (eds) *Chronic Pelvic Pain and Dysfunction: Practical Physical Medicine.* Elsevier: Edinburgh.

Fernández-Lao, C., Cantarero-Villanueva, I., César Fernández-de-las-Peñas, C. et al. 2011 Widespread mechanical pain hypersensitivity as a sign of central sensitization after breast cancer surgery. *Pain Med* 12:72–78.

Fernández-Pérez, A. M., Peralta-Ramírez, M. I., Pilat, A. et al. 2008 Effects of myofascial induction techniques on physiologic and psychologic parameters: a randomized controlled trial. *J Altern Complement Med* 14:807–811.

Fernández-Pérez, A. M., Peralta-Ramírez, M. I., Pilat, A. et al. 2013 Can myofascial techniques modify immunological parameters? *J Altern Complement Med* 19:24–28.

Gillies, A. & Lieber, R. 2011 Structure and function of the skeletal muscle extracellular matrix. *Muscle Nerve* 44:318–331.

Haouzi, P., Hill, J. M., Lewis, B. K. et al. 1999 Responses of group III and IV muscle afferents to distension of the peripheral vascular bed. *J Appl Physiol* 87:545–553.

Henley, C. E., Ivins, D., Mills, M. et al. 2008 Osteopathic manipulative treatment and its relationship to autonomic nervous system activity as demonstrated by heart rate variability. *Osteopath Med Prim Care.* 2:7.

Heredia-Rizo, A. M., Oliva-Pascual-Vaca, A., Rodríguez-Blanco, C. et al. 2013 Immediate changes in masticatory mechanosensitivity, mouth opening, and head posture after myofascial techniques in pain-free healthy participants. *J Manip Physiol Ther* 36:310–318.

Huijing, P. A 2007 Epimuscular myofascial force transmission between antagonistic and synergistic muscles can explain movement limitation in spastic paresis. *J Electromyography Kinesiol* 17:708–724.

Huxley, A. F., Simmons, R. M. 1971 Proposed mechanism of force generation in striated muscle. *Nature* 233:533–538.

Ingber, D. E. 2003 Mechanobiology and diseases of mechanotransduction. *Ann Med* 35:564–577.

Kaufman M. P., Hayes S. G., Adreani C. M. et al. 2002 Discharge properties of group III and IV muscle afferents. *Adv Exp Med Biol* 508:25–32.

Kumka, M., Bonar, B. 2012 Fascia: a morphological description and classification system based on a literature review. *J Can Chiropr Assoc* 56:179–191.

Lancerotto, L., Stecco, C., Macchi, V. et al. 2011 Layers of the abdominal wall: anatomical investigation of subcutaneous tissue and superficial fascia. *Surg Radiol Anat* 33:835–842.

Langevin, H. M. 2011 Fibroblast cytoskeletal remodeling contributes to connective tissue tension. *J Cell Physiol* 226:1166–1175.

Langevin, H. 2014 Fascia science and clinical applications: response. Langevin's response to Stecco's fascial nomenclature editorial. *J Bodyw Mov Ther* 18:444.

Langevin, H. M., Huijing, P. A. 2009 Communicating about fascia: history, pitfalls, and recommendations. *Int J Ther Massage Bodywork* 2:3–8.

Leonard, J. H. et al. 2009 Physiological effects of connective tissue manipulation on diabetic foot ulcer. In: Huijing, P. A., Hollander, P., Findley, T. W., Schleip, R. (eds) *Fascia Research II: Basic Science and Implications for Conventional and Complementary Health Care.* Elsevier GmbH: Munich, p. 95.

Lin, Y.-W., Cheng, C. M., LeDuc, F. R. et al. 2009 Understanding sensory nerve mechanotransduction through localized elastomeric matrix control. *PLOS One* 4:e4293.

Manheim, C. 2008 *The Myofascial Release Manual.* 2008, Slack Incorporation.

Martínez Rodríguez, R., Galán-del-Río, F. 2013 Mechanistic basis of manual therapy in myofascial injuries. Sonoelastographic evolution control. *J Bodyw Mov Ther* 17:221–234.

Pilat, A. 2003 *Inducción Miofascial.* Madrid: MacGraw-Hill.

Pilat, A. 2009 Myofascial induction approaches for headache. In: Fernández-de-las-Peñas C, Arendt-Nielsen L., Gerwin R. D. *Tension Type and Cervicogenic Headache: Pathophysiology, Diagnosis and Treatment.* Jones & Bartlett Publishers: Boston.

Pilat, A. 2014 Myofascial induction approaches. In: Chaitow L. (ed) *Fascial Dysfunction: Manual Therapy Approaches,* Handspring.

Pilat, A. 2015 Chapter 63 Myofascial induction approaches. In: Fernández de las Peñas C., Cleland J. A., Dommerholt J. (eds), *Manual Therapy for Musculoskeletal Pain Syndromes of the Upper and Lower Quadrants: An Evidence and Clinical Informed Approach.* Elsevier: London.

Purslow, P. P. 2010 Muscle fascia and force transmission. *J Bodyw Mov Ther* 14:411–417.

Ramos-González, E., Moreno-Lorenzo, C., Matara'Penarrocha, G. A., Guisado-Barrilao, R., Aguilar-Ferrándiz, M. E., Castro-Sánchez, A. M. 2012 Comparative study on the effectiveness of myofascial release manual therapy and physical therapy for venous insufficiency in postmenopausal women. *Complement Ther Med* 20:291–298.

Remvig L., Ellis R. M., Patijn J. 2008 Myofascial release: an evidence-based treatment approach? *Int Musculoskelet Med* 30:29–35.

Schleip, R., Jäger, H., Klingler, W. 2012 What is 'fascia'? A review of different nomenclatures. *J Bodyw Mov Ther* 16:496–502.

Stecco, C. 2008 The expansions of the pectoral girdle muscles onto the brachial fascia: morphological aspects and spatial disposition. *Cells Tissues Organs* 188:320–329.

Stecco, C. 2014 Why are there so many discussions about the nomenclature of fasciae? *J Bodyw Mov Ther* 18:441–442.

Swanson, R. L. 2013 Biotensegrity: a unifying theory of biological architecture with applications to osteopathic practice, education, and research. *J Am Osteopath Assoc* 113:34–52.

Taguchi, T., Hoheisel, U., Mense, S. 2009 Dorsal horn neurons having input from low back structures in rats. *Pain* 138:119–129.

Tesarz, J., 2011 Sensory innervation of the thoracolumbar fascia in rats and humans. *Neuroscience* 194:302–308

Toro, C. 2009 Short-term effects of manual therapy on heart rate variability, mood state, and pressure pain sensitivity in patients with chronic tension-type headache: a pilot study. *J Manip Physiol Ther* 32:527–535.

Tozzi, P. 2012 Low back pain and kidney mobility: local osteopathic fascial manipulation decreases pain perception and improves renal mobility. *J Bodyw Mov Ther* 16:381–391.

Urresti-López, F. J. 2011 Miodural bridge stimulation via suboccipital inhibition technique modifies the electroencephalogram significantly in reaction times producing cognitive changes that do not occur in the control group. D.O. Tesis para la obtención del diploma en osteopatía. SEFO-EOM.

Useros, A. I., Hernando, A. 2008 Liberación miofascial aplicada en un paciente adulto con daño cerebral. *Biociencias* 6:1–7.

van der Wal, J. C. 2009 The architecture of connective tissue as parameter for propioception: an often overlooked functional parameter as to proprioception in the locomotor apparatus. *Int J Ther Massage Bodywork* 2:9–23.

Vaquero Rodríguez, A. 2013 Influence of myofascial therapy applied to the cervical region of patients suffering from unilateral spatial neglect and head deviation with respect to the median line. In: Pons J. L., Torricelli D., Pajaro M. (eds) *Covering Clinical and Engineering Research on Neurorehabilitation. Volume I.* Springer: Berlin, Heidelberg, 371–374.

Vasquez, C. 2011 Effectiveness of the myofascial induction technique in the swimmer's shoulder with respect to the articular balance and pain. *Cuestiones de Fisioterapia.* 40:177–184.

Vaticón, D. 2009 Sensibilidad myofascial: el sistema craneosacro como la unidad biodinámica, *Libro de Ponencias XIX Jornadas de Fisioterapia.* 24–30, EUF ONCE, Universidad Autónoma de Madrid: Madrid.

Ward, R. 2003 *Foundations for Osteopathic Medicine.* 2nd ed. Lippincott, Williams & Wilkins: Hagerstown, MD.

Yucesoy, C. 2010 Epimuscular myofascial force transmission implies novel principles for muscular mechanics. *Exerc Sport Sci Rev* 38:128–134.

STRAIN AND COUNTERSTRAIN IN RELATION TO FASCIA

John C. Glover, William H. Devine

Overview

Strain and counterstrain, typically shortened to counterstrain (CS), is an osteopathic manipulative model of fairly recent origin. It is taught in osteopathic programs throughout the world and is classified as a passive, indirect model. In general, it is a positional release model that shares some characteristics with other models. Due to the gentle forces used to affect a response it is well tolerated by the entire spectrum of patients. It is effective for treatment of acute as well as chronic problems and can be applied from the toes to the cranium and everything in between. It is an easy technique to learn and is very helpful in developing tissue handling skills, especially for the subtle motions palpated in myofascial, cranial, and visceral models. While CS is easy to apply, it requires a keen ability to observe and palpate whole body inter-relationships, understand functional patterns, and integrate anatomical details in order to apply the model efficiently in a busy practice.

Introduction

CS was developed by Lawrence H. Jones DO, FAAO over a period of about 19 years, beginning in 1955. When he graduated from the College of Osteopathic Physicians and Surgeons (Los Angeles) in the 1930s the teaching of osteopathic manipulative models was restricted to only two methods: soft tissue manipulation, referred to as myofascial in some schools, and high-velocity/low-amplitude thrust techniques. The cranial concept was not taught to osteopathic students at that time. Jones's goal was to start a general practice that would involve utilizing osteopathic manipulative treatment (OMT) on a regular basis. He had no intention of developing a new osteopathic manipulative model; it simply evolved out of a need to treat a patient's complaint.

A patient presented to his office in rural Oregon with a complaint of psoitis of two months' duration. He treated the patient using the manipulative approaches he had learned in school that had served him well over the years. This time, however, they failed to produce the desired result. In an effort to address the patient's request to find a comfortable position for sleeping, Jones experimented with a variety of ways to position the patient until he found one that resolved the discomfort. He let the patient stay in his position of comfort while he saw two patients and when he slowly returned him to an upright position both he and the patient were surprised to find the pain had resolved spontaneously. After this success he experimented with whole body positioning for a while, but changed to applying specific local positioning of diagnosed traditional segmental dysfunctions because whole body positioning was too time-consuming. With further evolution of the model Jones correlated specific locations of discrete areas of tenderness (counterstrain points) with specific segmental somatic dysfunctions. He originally termed the discrete areas of tenderness trigger points after the work of Janet Travell MD, but on closer evaluation realized the two points were not the same. Initially only posterior counterstrain points were identified and later Jones found anterior counterstrain points that increased the efficacy of his treatment approach. Over 19 years Jones mapped the location of counterstrain points associated with specific somatic dysfunctions of the spine, pelvis, ribs, lower extremities, upper extremities, and the cranium. He published the first paper on the new model (Jones, 1964). Later, his Fellowship in the American Academy of Osteopathy (FAAO) thesis evolved into a textbook that was published by the American Academy of Osteopathy (Jones, 1981). He continued to identify new tender points throughout his practice life, but never felt he had identified them all. In fact, he encouraged his students to continue looking and share newly identified counterstrain points with colleagues (Fig. 42.1).

Jones knew Harold Hoover DO and was familiar with his functional work, using indirect applications of force to treat somatic dysfunction in different regions of the body (Jones, 1981), and integrated this concept as part of his model but in a different way. Later, Stanley Schiowitz DO, FAAO utilized indirect positioning combined with a facilitating force for treatment in his facilitated positional release model. Early in his effort to rediscover A. T. Still's techniques of exaggeration of the somatic dysfunction, Richard Van Buskirk DO, PhD, FAAO utilized an indirect starting position that is essentially the same as the CS position for that dysfunction as a monitor. He would identify an associated counterstrain point to monitor the effectiveness of his indirect positioning, and then apply an activating force before beginning an arc of motion from the indirect position, past neutral, and through the restrictive barrier while maintaining the force.

Consideration of neuromusculoskeletal reflexes and neurophysiology came later for Jones as he was asked how his model worked. The work of Irvin M. Korr PhD and others are mentioned as the first scientific explanation of the mechanism for CS, and much more has been published since (Jones, 1981; Korr, 1975). For example, Meltzer and Standley (2007) published an in vitro study of fibroblasts, which demonstrated the effect of strain on tissue and then response to the release of strain. Demonstrations of the chemical

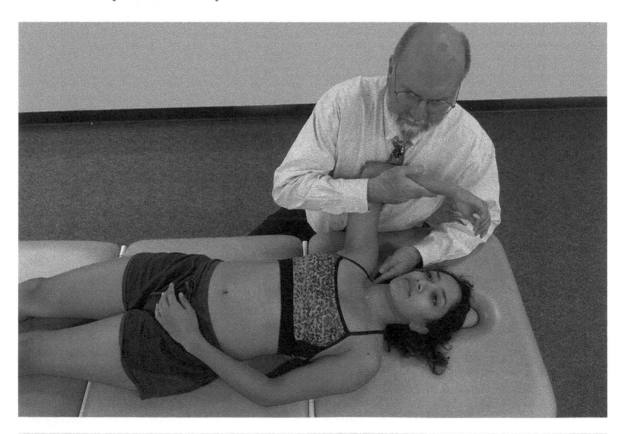

Figure 42.1
Treatment for a supraspinatus counterstrain point

changes, as well as other physiologic effects at the cellular level of strained tissue are important to a greater understanding of the role of fascia in somatic dysfunction (Meltzer & Standley, 2007).

Jones encouraged the modifications some of his students made to his model. Harmon Myers DO studied Travell's work on myofascial pain syndromes and combined it with Jones's work to develop a very effective integrated approach (Myers et al., 2012). His innovation uses myofascial patterns to help find the significant counterstrain points and treat them, using the application of functional anatomy with CS. Others have followed, using the mechanoreceptors in the fascia as well as joint, ligament, and tendon to guide treatment (Myers et al., 2012).

Aims and objectives

The aim of CS is restoration of maximal tissue function to enable the individual to find and maintain health. This is accomplished by treating aberrant neural function that affects motion through myofascial tissue, fluid dynamics by means of blood and lymphatic flow, and interactions between somatic structures and the viscera. When the neural component of a somatic dysfunction is addressed there is the potential to affect any tissue or structure related neurologically. Neural dysfunction may express in a variety of ways. The key to effective and efficient application of CS is identification of the most significant counterstrain points, not just a point that is somewhat tender. Many counterstrain points may exhibit some level of tenderness, but may not represent a significant somatic dysfunction. When learning the CS model, subclinical counterstrain points may be identified and used to practice accurate positioning, but efficiency in using the model comes by learning to identify the most significant counterstrain points.

Indications and contraindications

Indications

Indications for the application of CS are many. Most applications by the experienced practitioner will be for acute, painful somatic dysfunctions often with tissue swelling and associated alteration of a proprioceptive reflex and increased nociceptive reflex.

Pain and spasm will be present in acute situations, often with facial distortion, inflammation, and congestion. The CS treatment position will often rebalance the mechanoreceptors, decrease the protective reflexes, and facilitate the removal of inflammatory elements from the tissues. One of the challenges of treating acute somatic dysfunction is patient intolerance of movement of the affected tissues. The indirect positioning used with CS is typically well tolerated.

Chronic somatic dysfunctions are often initially treated with CS as an adjunct with other techniques such as post isometric muscle energy or gentle thrust techniques. Presence of a counterstrain point may interfere with effective resolution of spinal dysfunction treated with thrust techniques in the acute phase and often is the reason patients find thrust techniques painful. If a tense, rubber-band-like yielding of the restrictive barrier is palpated when evaluating, as opposed to a rigid feeling, it identifies the presence of a counterstrain point that needs to be treated with CS. Using CS first may eliminate the need to use thrust techniques or make it easier if an articular bind is still present.

The effect of using CS with both acute and chronic problems is reduction of analgesia and tissue healing as well as restoration of function of a facilitated segment or injured tissue. The effective treatment of a counterstrain point is diagnostic and often identifies the related structures involved by the location of the counterstrain point and the position of comfort used for treatment. Use of CS on a hypershortened muscle will usually restore normal resting length and reduce inflammatory elements and abnormal neuroelectrical and neurochemical changes. CS can be used on somatic dysfunction in any area of the body with great safety.

CS is indicated in the treatment of somatic dysfunction of essentially any patient population, the requirements being the presence of a significant counterstrain point and the ability of the patient to voluntarily relax. The model has been successfully applied in children, adolescents, and adults including the geriatric population, and in ambulatory as well as hospitalized patients, including those in the intensive care unit and pregnant patients. Of all these groups, children are the most challenging due to the difficulty of requiring a child to remain passive for extended periods.

Contraindications

Absolute

Absolute contraindications for CS are rare. As with all manipulative models, lack of patient consent is an absolute contraindication. In addition, positioning that directly affects the site of an unstable fracture is another absolute contraindication. There should not be any increase in the nociceptive reflex, increased spasm, or pain while in the treatment position. If any of these are present, the technique will not be effective and may be an indication of a missed pathology. In these cases, treatment should be stopped and additional history, physical examination, and possibly imaging studies carried out before proceeding.

Relative

There are a number of relative contraindications for CS. One group that does not benefit from CS is patients who cannot relax voluntarily. Although some patients have a problem voluntarily letting muscles relax, usually a little teaching and encouragement from the practitioner allows most to learn to become passive. Pathological conditions that include spastic contractions (therefore unable to be controlled by the patient) have not responded well to this treatment model. Very weak or gravely ill patients require caution when considering CS as a treatment – a gravely ill patient being an individual who is close to death. The concern is that if a severe treatment reaction were to occur it may contribute to a patient's demise. Pregnant patients, especially in the third trimester, can be a challenge to position. Any position that puts too much pressure on the growing uterus or compromises the major blood vessels should be avoided. Another population in which positioning may cause a problem is patients with severe osteoporosis or diseases of lost bone matrix, due to the possibility of causing a pathological fracture. Consideration of the benefit gained versus the possibility of a pathological fracture must be accessed in these individuals. Patient populations in which specific positioning may also be problematic include rheumatoid arthritis patients, Down syndrome patients, and

degenerative-joint-disease patients where cervical rotation associated with motion, especially about the dens, may be problematic.

Patients with cervical vertebral artery disease may require caution in treating with the extension positions used for posterior cervical counterstrain points. The concern is if the positioning either compromises the vertebral artery by occluding it or produces tearing due to the resulting tension on the vessel. Careful observation for altered eye motions (strabismus or nystagmus) if the patient reports dizziness or neurological symptoms is important as these may be indications of neurological compromise and the patient should be returned to a neutral position without hesitation. Hyper-rotation and hyperextension are the primary motions that may cause problems in patients where normal joint architecture is not present. Another area of caution is in those patients who have ligamentous damage where the positioning puts additional stress on a damaged ligament. Traumatic knee injuries that may result in a partial tear of a cruciate ligament must be thoroughly evaluated prior to applying the hyperextension force used to treat counterstrain anterior and posterior cruciate ligament counterstrain points (Rennie et al., 2012).

Post-treatment reaction

A small percentage of patients may experience a post-treatment flare-up of pain or hyperalgesia, primarily after the initial visit. This is thought to be due to the release of local inflammatory agents from the original injury, including bradykinins, cytokines, lactic acid, and other compounds (Meltzer & Standley, 2007). The phenomenon occurs in the antagonist muscle and related fascia and can start several hours after treatment, but most typically presents the following morning. Most of these patients experience the reaction as a generalized flulike feeling, typically lasting one to two days and very rarely up to five days. Recommending the patient stays well hydrated after treatment decreases or eliminates the reaction. Typically treatment reactions do not recur after subsequent treatment using CS. The response may also be due to incomplete washout of the inflammatory products following the initial injury due to decreased circulation through the hypertonic myofascial tissue and subsequent release resulting from relaxation of the tissue following effective treatment. The effect is usually well tolerated and self-limited. Improved function of the affected tissues usually follows. If not, the possibility of missed pathology should be considered.

Methods of assessment

Basic counterstrain:

On its most basic level CS is about finding a significant counterstrain point and positioning the patient in a way that produces a spontaneous release before slowly returning the patient to a stable position. The resulting changes may affect pain, motion, fluid dynamics, and/or organ function; in essence any tissue under control of the neural elements associated with the counterstrain point. For many people CS is nothing more than finding an area of tender tissue and mimicking a position pictured in a CS text. While this simplistic approach may provide benefit to a patient, it does not come close to achieving the potential of the model to optimize body function. Initially students have difficulty palpating the associated myofascial changes that allow greater efficiency in utilizing the model.

Basic steps (Fig. 42.2)

1. Find a significant counterstrain point.
2. Position the patient in a position of comfort that eliminates tenderness.
3. Maintain the position with the patient passive for 90 seconds.
4. Slowly return the patient to the starting or neutral position.
5. Recheck the tenderness of the counterstrain point.

Note: In order to accomplish the five steps, a means of communication to ascertain the tenderness level (usually a 0–10 tenderness scale) must be established with the patient and the counterstrain points must be continuously monitored for changes in tenderness and myofascial tension.

Jones's maps of counterstrain points throughout the body provide a starting point of where to look for significant counterstrain points. Then, if the patient is placed in a position approximating those illustrated in texts, it usually only requires fine tuning to eliminate the tenderness. The tenderness elicited by pressing the counterstrain point was the key element, but success in identifying a truly significant counterstrain point was tied to anatomical location, the amount of pressure used, the vector used to press, and the ability of the patient to perceive tenderness. An advancement of the ability to find a counterstrain point comes with the ability to palpate tissue tension differences in the myofascial tissues that are unrelated to the patient's ability to perceive tenderness and tied to the palpatory ability of the practitioner, which is more reliable.

Palpation of counterstrain points

Traditional osteopathic structural examination has focused on TART findings: tissue texture abnormalities, asymmetry, restriction of motion, and tenderness or change of sensation as evidence of the presence of somatic dysfunction. CS evaluation is focused on identification of significant counterstrain points that are linked to functional changes and have a neural component. The better the ability to find which counterstrain points are related to the key dysfunction, the more effective the treatment will be in bringing the patient to maximal functioning.

The art of palpation of counterstrain points is learned, as with any other psychomotor skill in manual treatment, by repeated hands-on experience. It is easier to learn on a patient with a symptomatic somatic dysfunction enhanced by a detailed history of the original injury. The patient will often relate a body position that gives comfort or ease of symptoms and a position of activity that will make symptoms worsen, which adds context to the palpatory experience. Some practitioners of CS feel counterstrain points are located only in muscle tissue, but most who use the model extensively feel the counterstrain points are located in connective tissue, including fascia, tendons, and ligaments, in addition to muscle.

On the initial visit, it is helpful to observe the patient come into the examination room, sit down, and get up onto the examination table. Complete attention to body movement or guarding of motion may provide valuable clues to identify the location of a counterstrain point in a particular muscle group or region. Body position at rest should be noted and may be exaggerated to be used as a possible treatment position with a corresponding counterstrain point. Once an area of potential dysfunction is determined, then specific tissue locations are evaluated for the presence of tenderness and tissue texture abnormalities – typically increased tension. The amount of pressure used to elicit tenderness of a counterstrain point is approximately that which is needed to blanch the nail bed of the diagnosing finger, and it does not radiate. The same pressure will not produce tenderness in

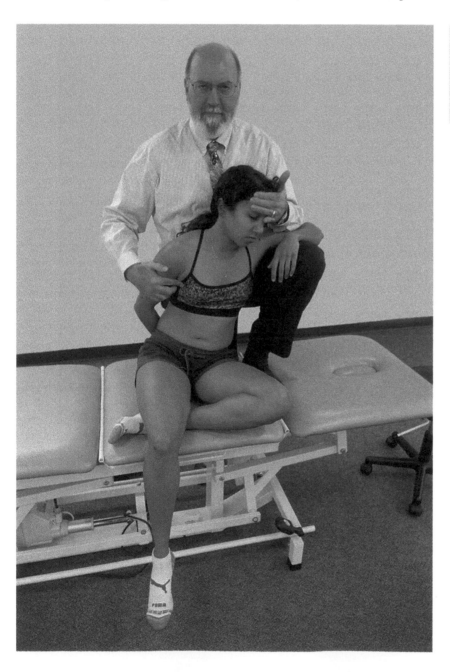

Figure 42.2
Applying the basic steps to treatment of an anterior third rib counterstrain point

healthy tissue. This pressure is about 4 kg/cm² (Travell & Simons, 1992), but the pressure needed to elicit tenderness varies with the depth of the counterstrain point from the body surface and the tissues over it.

Learning the location of the counterstrain points is tedious for some, but like any system of diagnosis or treatment, time spent using the model makes remembering the location of the counterstrain points easier. Using the historical clues from a patient in addition to their body habitus and functional evaluation also makes it quicker to locate the counterstrain points. Experience in palpating counterstrain points provides the practitioner with the opportunity to use palpation of the myofascial tissue tension of the counterstrain point to identify not only a counterstrain point but also the severity of the dysfunction. The experienced palpater feels the myofascial tension in the tissue surrounding the counterstrain point, uses it to locate the center of the counterstrain point, and can do so without eliciting tenderness. The practitioner chooses when to test the counterstrain point and may announce the presence of the counterstrain point to the patient before pressure is applied, which identifies the skill of the practitioner to the patient.

If the counterstrain point radiates pain with localized pressure, is has become a myofascial trigger point. This may require additional measures and time to treat, but CS will still be effective in most cases. Travell & Simons (1992) cataloged myofascial trigger points as part of their work on myofascial pain syndromes. Links between Travell's myofascial trigger points and specific counterstrain points have been observed for many years and have recently been tabulated (Myers et al., 2012).

Jones originally identified and taught about 150 counterstrain points, but currently practitioners have increased that number to over 300 counterstrain points. The points have been found in muscle, ligament, tendon, and fascia. The largest increase in new counterstrain points has come by identifying counterstrain points associated with lymphatic congestion and visceral dysfunction. These two new groups of counterstrain points typically require much less time in the treatment position, often only 10 to 20 seconds.

Methods of intervention

Counterstrain points are located in hyperirritated, facilitated muscle and connective tissue. Care must be used in positioning the patient. The passive movement of the patient into the treatment position should be slow, with attention given to the continuous response of the tissue as tension of the counterstrain point changes. If the patient is significantly larger than the practitioner, the patient can actively be guided to move themselves into the approximate treatment position before becoming passive, at which point the position is fine-tuned by the practitioner. Careful monitoring of the counterstrain point during positioning will guide the practitioner to the ideal treatment position. If the patient is moved in a direction away from the ideal treatment position, the tension of the myofascial tissue of the counterstrain point will increase, whereas if they are moved toward the ideal treatment position, the tension will decrease. Continuous monitoring of the counterstrain point while in the treatment position will provide immediate feedback as to the state of release and will identify the end point of treatment.

The myofascial changes of the counterstrain point and surrounding tissue are not uniform with all counterstrain points. Some counterstrain points in the ideal treatment position produce a reduction of tenderness but little change in the surrounding myofascial tissue. Other counterstrain points exhibit a great deal of myofascial change. In Glover's experience, the greater the myofascial changes palpated during time in the treatment position, the greater the functional changes and the longer the resolution of the somatic dysfunction following treatment. In these cases, the initial response of the surrounding myofascial tissue when put in the ideal treatment position is a random motion in multiple planes, which then eventually changes to a repeating pattern of symmetrical motion when treatment is complete. The symmetrical pattern may be flexion/extension, internal/external rotation, expansion/contraction, or any repeating pattern. The time it takes to occur may be as little as 10 seconds or greater than 120 seconds, but commonly is close to 90 seconds.

Several actions may improve the time needed to reach the ideal treatment position. Devine has found that adding a gentle fascial traction into the counterstrain point improves the effectiveness of the positioning and extent of the resolution of function to the associated myofascial structures.

When the positional release is complete the patient can be moved back into a neutral biomechanical position and the counterstrain point is rechecked to see what, if any, tenderness remains. It is important to note that while the patient can assist the practitioner to get into the treatment position, if necessary, the patient must remain passive throughout the 90 seconds of treatment and the slow return to a neutral position. Failure to remain passive often decreases the beneficial effects of the treatment. The first few degrees of motion out of the treatment position are the most important because the objective is to avoid activation of the fast-twitch receptors in the muscle spindles (Nagrale et al., 2010).

Once the patient has been returned to a neutral position it is important to recheck the counterstrain point. It is not unusual to have a little residual tenderness present, a 1 or 2 on the 10-point scale, but tenderness greater than 3 indicates an ineffective treatment and the reason needs to be identified. Retreatment may be necessary or the identification of a more significant counterstrain point or visceral connection ascertained.

Considerations on intervention of treatment

Causative factors and mechanism of injury are unique to each patient. Therefore, the exact treatment position needed for effective treatment with CS will vary from one individual to another and is identified by the tissue response during positioning. The illustrated treatment positions in counterstrain texts are starting points that then need to be fine-tuned to the individual patient. Some general guidelines regarding counterstrain points are useful to keep in mind:

1. Scan for both anterior and posterior counterstrain points within a region before determining the most significant counterstrain point.

2. If there are multiple counterstrain points within a region, typically the one most tender is the most significant and should be treated first.

3. If there is a row of counterstrain points of equal tenderness within a region, treat the one in the middle.

4. Anterior counterstrain points typically require flexion.

5. Posterior counterstrain points typically require extension.

6. Midline counterstrain points typically require primarily flexion or extension.

7. The more lateral the counterstrain point, the more side-bending and rotation is typically required.

8. The goal is for complete reduction of tenderness, but a minimum reduction of 70% (3 on a 10-point scale) is required before treatment will be effective.

9. Use both tenderness and tissue texture changes to find the ideal treatment position.

10. The appearance of a therapeutic pulse at the counterstrain point while positioning or treating indicates myofascial relaxation and increased blood flow, which typically results in very effective treatment.

CS can be used in conditions associated with fused or nonmoving segments that exhibit somatic dysfunction or facilitation. The application of direct or indirect myofascial release to the dysfunctional myofascial tissue will treat the counterstrain point. Cervical stenosis, cervical fusion, lumbar stenosis, post lumbar and cervical laminectomy patients benefit by applying a 'strain' (direct myofascial tension) on the tissue and associated reciprocal tissue or muscle while monitoring the counterstrain point. The forces should be gentle, still providing 'strain' on the reflex opposite fascial tissues including fascial mechanoreceptors to reduce the activity of the counterstrain point (Myers et al., 2012). An example of the application of this modification involved a case of C5–C6 fusion with an associated left AC5 counterstrain point that was still symptomatic months after the surgery. Direct myofascial tension applied to the right posterior lateral fascia was used to produce a 'strain' into the tissue of the left AC5 tender point and resulted in effective treatment.

Physiological mechanisms

The mechanisms explaining the effects of CS are still under investigation and therefore are for the most part still theoretical and speculative. The initial explanation was provided years after Jones presented his original concept of the tender point and treatment by positioning. The first explanation was based on Korr's work on muscle spindles and somatic dysfunction, in which aberrant afferent input to the spinal cord from muscle spindles was considered the major progenitor in spinal facilitation with altered motor and sympathetic output causing musculoskeletal somatic dysfunction and its associated palpable changes (Korr, 1975). This explanation was used for other models of OMT at the time, with the somatic dysfunction as an aberration of neuromuscular function. CS, as well as other indirect methods, later was considered an afferent reduction technique (Johnston & Friedman, 1994). It was hypothesized that the communication pathways in the spinal cord at the level of the somatic dysfunction are influenced, and are modulating motor activity and output, through the silencing or reduction in activity of the muscle spindles associated with the somatic dysfunctions from the passive shortening of the involved myofascial tissues. Myofascial tissues have mechanoreceptors involved with the regenerative feedback of reflex. The alteration of action potential between the intra- and extrafusal muscle fiber activity that creates the aberrant input into the cord, causing the facilitation and alteration in motor output, is reduced (Korr, 1975; Johnson et al., 1994; Fossum & Fryer, 2009).

Recently, research has changed the emphasis from proprioceptors to nociceptors as the source of the aberrant afferent input into the cord, linked with facilitation or sensitization (Van Buskirk, 1990; Howell & Willard, 2005). There seems to be more research supportive of the notion that nociception alters motor output and control (Nijs et al., 2011), and models of somatic dysfunction have emerged that emphasize the nociceptive-driven disturbance to proprioception and motor control (Fossum & Fryer, 2009; Myers et al., 2012). This hypothesis closely matches current CS theories. Jones referred to the somatic dysfunction as an 'ongoing noxious process' (Jones et al., 1995). Many clinical trials seem to give supporting evidence

that CS reduces pain and increases muscle strength in symptomatic individuals (Myers et al., 2012).

There may also be some cellular-mediated events associated with the application of CS and its pain-alleviating effects. Research done by Meltzer & Standley (2007) involved modeling repetitive motion strain (RMS) on human fibroblasts in a laboratory model. Researchers were able to show that RMS significantly increased secretion of pro-inflammatory cytokines such as interleukin-6 (IL-6) and cell proliferation. Modeling a CS technique on fibroblasts subjected to RMS, they showed decreased IL-6 levels, suggesting an anti-inflammatory effect (Meltzer & Standley, 2007). Mechanically influencing fibroblasts in connective tissue may also have circulatory effects (Langevin, 2007), improving extracellular or local fluid dynamics, which could be beneficial in altering the tissue environment of the peripheral nociceptors as well as positively contributing to tissue healing after injury (Fryer & Fossum, 2009; Wong, 2012).

According to Van Buskirk the active ingredients accounting for the effects of CS are most likely multifaceted (Myers et al., 2012). Reducing nociception through both cellular- and receptor-mediated responses, as well as decreasing muscle spindle activity, may be two of the principal mechanisms through which CS results in pain reduction and improved motor function. It has been well established that nonopioid descending inhibitory pathways from the periaqueductal grey region (PAG) contribute to the hypoalgesic effects of manual treatment (Skyba et al., 2003; Hoeger-Bement & Sluka, 2007). It has been suggested that this hypoalgesic effect is segmentally organized and probably results from large-diameter afferent stimulation (Sluka et al. 2002). This is indirectly supported through the demonstration that low-threshold mechanoreceptors from joints and muscles project to neurons in the PAG (Yezierski, 1991).

Counterstrain points

Presently the most tenable hypothesis to describe the development of somatic dysfunction is the nociceptive model elaborated on by various authors (Van Buskirk, 1990; Howell & Willard, 2005; O'Connell, 2000;

Tozzi, 2015). Some newer concepts relating to the role of fascia in somatic dysfunction have been proposed (Tozzi, 2015). Briefly, the nociceptive theory of somatic dysfunction proposes that dysfunction develops from the ongoing cascade of events resulting from primary tissue injury in somatic tissues with peripheral and subsequent central sensitization (Fossum & Fryer, 2009). The original notion of Jones, based on Korr's paper (1975), is giving way to in vitro and in vivo clinical research. Although the altered mediation of central pain pathways as seen with central sensitization may cause generalized mechanical hyperalgesia in patients with musculoskeletal and visceral disorders (O'Neill et al., 2007), the potential relationship of this to the development of specific counterstrain points remains unclear. The fascia contains many of the tender points not previously described by Jones. He predicted that investigation of this system would advance together with changes in location and nomenclature. Jones described the original tender points as 'definitely specific manifestations of specific lesions' (Jones, 1964), and that the diagnosed tender point may be considered a palpable reference point for somatic dysfunction and does not represent the somatic dysfunction itself. Type II vertebral somatic dysfunctions are often, but not always, associated with the counterstrain point. Integration with clinical applications is changing CS theory and concepts.

The principles for the application of fascial forces to treat a counterstrain point are theorized in a paper by Tozzi on the neurofasciagenic aspects of somatic dysfunction (Tozzi, 2015). Additional ideas about somatic dysfunction and the important role of fascia are theorized in a paper by O'Connell exploring the piezoelectric effect in relation to the facilitated segment (O'Connell, 2000). Clinical correlation of pelvic diagnoses with specific counterstrain points have also been noted (Klock, 2012).

Clinical case

A brief case history utilizing CS for treatment of viscerosomatic reflex pain with viscerovisceral reflex somatic dysfunction

A 35-year-old multiparous, moderately obese female with postoperative paralytic ileus after a laparoscopic gall bladder surgery for cholecystitis with cholelithiasis was evaluated. The patient had abdominal distention and absence of bowel sounds with upper abdominal and periumbilical pain. The patient was not septic, the lungs were clear, and the patient was afebrile.

Prior to surgery the patient had Chapman's points positive for gall bladder inflammation, as well as positive imaging studies with typical clinical signs and symptoms of cholecystitis. Her health had been good prior to developing symptoms. Osteopathic structural examination demonstrated tissue texture changes in the right subscapular regions as well as the upper right quadrant of the abdomen. Counterstrain points were present over the anterior right thoracic region (AT7 and AT8 on the right).

The head of the hospital bed was elevated to 45 degrees in order to facilitate positioning of the patient. The lower extremities were slowly flexed, with both knees together, toward a counterstrain point that was superior and lateral to the umbilicus until the tenderness was eliminated. Gentle myofascial traction was given toward the counterstrain point in addition to the positioning. The abdominal pain was relieved completely, and the patient held in the treatment position for 90 seconds. The patient's legs were slowly replaced to normal position, the head of the bed lowered to 30 degrees and the foot of the bed elevated to 20 degrees. Flatus and bowel activity started about 3 minutes after the treatment. The patient then had a bowel movement later that day.

The surgical wound that cut through muscle and fascia along with the sutures used to close the wound caused nociceptive reflex activity, resulting in a somatovisceral reflex. Hyperinflation of the abdominal cavity during the surgical procedure mechanically strained the tissues and added to the viscerovisceral reflex activity. The instrumentation used during the surgery caused strain of the thoracic and abdominal tissues, resulting in viscerovisceral reflex spasticity. Both problems resulted in decreased peristaltic activity (inhibitory reflex) of the intestines and produced the ileus.

References and further reading

Fossum C., Fryer G. 2009 Cervical joint manipulation procedures applied to patients with headache. In: Fernández-de-las-Peñas C. et al. *Tension-Type and Cervicogenic Headache: Pathophysiology, Diagnosis and Management*. Boston: Bartlett & Jones.

Fryer G., Fossum C. 2009 Therapeutic mechanisms underlying muscle energy techniques. In: Fernández-de-las-Peñas C. et al. *Tension-Type and Cervicogenic Headache: Pathophysiology, Diagnosis and Management*. Boston: Bartlett & Jones.

Hoeger-Bement M. K., Sluka K. A. 2007 Pain: perception and mechanisms. In: Magee D. J. et al. (eds). *Scientific Foundations and Principles and Practice in Musculoskeletal Rehabilitation*. St Louis: Saunders Elsevier.

Howell J. N., Willard F. H. 2005 Nociception: new understandings and their possible relation to somatic dysfunction and its treatment. *Ohio Res Clin Rev* 15:12–15.

Howell J. N., Cabell K. S., Chila A. G., Eland D. C. 2006 Stretch reflex and Hoffman reflex responses to osteopathic manipulative treatment in subjects with Achilles tendonitis. *J Am Osteopath Assoc* 106:537–545.

Johnson W. L. Friedman H. D., Eland D. C. 2005 *Functional Methods: Manual for Palpatory Skill Development in Osteopathic Examination and Manipulation for Motor Function*. 2nd Ed. Indianapolis, IN: American Academy of Osteopathy.

Jones L. H. 1964 Spontaneous release by positioning. *The D.O.* 4:109–116.

Jones L. H. 1981 *Strain and Counterstrain*. Newark, OH: American Academy of Osteopathy.

Jones L. H., Kusunose R. S., Goering E. K. 1995 *Jones Strain-Counterstrain*. Boise, ID: Jones Strain-CounterStrain Inc.

Klock G. B. 2012 A logical approach to complicated sacral and innominate dysfunction. *J Am Osteopath Assoc* 22:21–35.

Korr I. M. 1975 Proprioceptors and somatic dysfunction. *J Am Osteopath Assoc* 74:638–50.

Langevin H. M. 2007 Potential role of fascia in chronic musculoskeletal pain. In: Audette J. F., Bailey A. *Integrative Pain Medicine*. Boston: Humana Press.

Meltzer K. R, Standley P. R. 2007 Modeled repetitive motion strain and indirect osteopathic manipulative techniques in regulation of human fibroblast proliferation and interleukin secretion. *J Am Osteopath Assoc* 107:527–536.

Myers H. L, Devine W. H, Fossum C., Glover J. C., Kuchera M., Kusunose R. S., Van Buskirk R. L. 2012 *Compendium Edition*: Clinical Applications of Counterstrain. 2nd Ed. Tucson, AZ: Tucson Osteopathic Medical Foundation Osteopathic Press.

Nagrale A. V., Glynn P., Joshi A., Ramteke G. 2010 The efficacy of an integrated neuromuscular inhibition technique on upper trapezius trigger points in subjects with nonspecific neck pain: a randomized controlled trial. *J Man Manip Ther* 18:37–43.

Nijs J., Paul van Wilgen C., Van Oosterwijck J., van Ittersum M., Meeus M. 2011 How to explain central sensitization to patients with 'unexplained' chronic musculoskeletal pain: practice guidelines. *Man Ther* 16:413–418.

O'Connell J. *Biomechanical Fascial Application and Release*. Indianapolis, IN: American Academy of Osteopathy, 2000.

O'Neill S., Manniche C., Graven-Nielsen T., Arendt-Nielsen L. 2007 Generalized deep-tissue hyperalgesia in patients with chronic low-back pain. *Eur J Pain* 11:415–420.

Rennie P. R., Glover J.C., Carvalho C. M., Key L. S. 2012 *Counterstrain and Exercise*: An Integrated Approach. 3rd Ed. Indianapolis, IN: Rennie-Max Publisher.

Skyba D. A., Rhadakrishnan R., Rohlwing J. J. et al. 2003 Joint manipulation reduces hyperalgesia by activation of monoamine receptors but not opioid or GABA receptors in the spinal cord. *Pain* 106:159–168.

Sluka K. A., Hoeger M. K., Skyba D. A. 2002 Basic science mechanisms of non-pharmacological treatments of pain. In: Giamberardino M. (ed). *Pain: An Updated Review*. Seattle: IASP Press.

Snider K. T., Glover J. C., Rennie P. R., Ferrill H. C., Morris W. F., Johnson J. C. 2013 Frequency of counterstrain tender points in osteopathic medical students. *J Am Osteopath Assoc* 113:690–702.

Tozzi P. 2015 A unifying neuro-fasciagenic model of somatic dysfunction – underlying mechanisms and treatment – Part 1. *J Bodyw Mov Ther* 19:310–326.

Travell J. G., Simons D. G. 1992 *Myofascial Pain and Dysfunction: The Trigger Point Manual*. Vols 1 & 2. Philadelphia, PA: Williams and Wilkins.

Van Buskirk R. L. 1990 Nociceptive reflexes and the somatic dysfunction: a model. *J Am Osteopath Assoc* 90:792.

Wong C. K. 2012 Strain Counterstrain: current concepts and evidence. *Man Ther* 17:2–8.

Yezierski R. P. 1991 Somatosensory input to the periaqueductal grey: a spinal relay to a descending control center. In: Depaulis A., Bandler R. (eds). *The Midbrain Periaqueductal Grey Matter*. New York, NY: Plenum Press, pp. 356–386.

LONG LEVERAGE: A 'NEW' THERAPEUTICAL APPROACH TO FASCIA

Francisco Toscano-Jimenez, Cristina Gioja

'It is a question to apply all the science within and under the application of the principles of Osteopathy, as it is those which differentiate it from other forms of therapy.'

J. M. Littlejohn

Osteopathy in its original sense was considered and regarded as a set of therapeutical principles rather than just slick maneuvers of a manual therapy. It's curious to define, or shall we say redefine, the actual word 'osteopathy.' This word does not refer to the scope of treatment but indicates a certain meticulous affinity to anatomy. A. T. Still developed the word 'osteopathy' from the Greek words 'οστεον' and 'παθος,' which refer respectively to bones and to a certain empathy or sympathy toward an incoming experience.

Here we observe that osteopathy defines a therapeutical approach that values the role of the osseous structures as a medium through which the mechanical organic adjustment of the body is performed. The purpose of this article is to elaborate on the concept of 'body adjustment' (BA) as a method of treatment of the whole body and particularly in the field of fascia by using long leverage techniques.

Osteopathic theory and fascia

From the terminological point of view, the term 'fascia' is used as an umbrella term to describe different forms of connective tissue.[1–4] This connective tissue is omnipresent and continuous throughout the body from the most outer surface down to cellular level, taking on many different arrangements and densities depending on anatomy and function. When defining fascia, Stecco[3] describes it as an extended membranous substance that connects and coordinates all the tissues and structures of the body together. It shows a variety of functions in coordination, proprioception, support, and fluid dynamics as well as in the mechanical coordination of motor patterns in the musculoskeletal field and in neuro–hormonal–immune processes.

From an embryological point of view, the fascia derives from the mesenchyme – a subdivision of the primitive mesoderm of the embryonic germinal layer.[5] From this germinal layer tissues like tendons, ligaments, bone, bone marrow, muscle, blood, lymph, and vessels form.[6,7,1,2] It consequently creates an important relationship between soft tissues, the hard tissues, and the circulatory system. Fascia as a metabolic tissue depends for its health on nutritive sources provided by its close association to the neural and vascular supplies. At the same time, it acts as an important medium involved in the general nutrition and drainage of the body.[4,8]

These aspects were introduced by Still in the early 1900s. Still described fascia as a very complex system, emphasizing that:

'here we find cells, glands, blood and other vessels, with nerves running to and from every part. Here we could spend an eternity with our present mental capacity, before we could comprehend even a superficial knowledge of the powers and uses of the fascia in the laboratory of animal life.'[9 p.165]

A. T. Still described the relationships between the fluids systems – in particular the lymphatic system – and the musculoskeletal system, the nerves, and the fascia, finding the greatest causes for disease in the stagnant conditions of their circulation and in the modifications of the chemical composition of fascia itself. H. Magoun[10,11] extended this concept by describing the relationship between changes of the fiber organization and resistance of fascia to mechanical stressors.

The various components and arrangements of fibers give fascia a unique ability to react to the forces to which it is exposed, providing a fundamental functionality in the maintenance of erect posture and locomotion. The body's mechanical balance is not static, but continuously in a dynamic equilibrium in the attempt to preserve our antigravity posture. Osteopathic dysfunctions limit or reduce this ability by discontinuing unity and integrative function of the spine. Hence, the basic aspect of osteopathic dysfunction is related to failure of the ability to maintain the proper position under gravity.

This connective tissue shapes, forms, and differentiates tissues, viscera, and systems from one another and acts as a medium between the compartments of anatomy. Through its role in sheathing and investing the various tissues, it has an important function in relation to the vascular and neural conduit pathways in lymphatic circulation and in immune defense.

The different layers of tissues are closely connected to each other by several structures that, together with a rich vascularization and innervation, contribute to maintain the integrity of the tissues in a unit. The coordinative function of fascia is also evidenced by the fact that all the muscles and fibers are attached to fascial membrane, which constitutes a coordinating element of groups of soft and hard tissues.

A further interesting point is the association of fascia to the osseous structures and consequently its direct influence on the mechanics of the spine. There is always a direct or indirect attachment to the osseous framework of the body, therefore creating an important correlation from an osteopathic perspective. This aspect is of maximum importance in osteopathic therapeutics, in the attempt to correct the body posture, according to the mechanical theory of gravity lines proposed by Littlejohn and Wernham.

Mechanical laws and mechanical theory are an important underlying factor in the altered physiology of the body and often play a key part in the etiology of conditions encountered in clinical practice.[12,13,14,11,15]

Structures and gravity

Considering the body from the standpoint of its mechanics, it can be seen as an assembly of parts and materials composed, connected, and coordinated together by elastic elements that are able to sustain loads and react to forces to which the body is exposed. The body is constantly subjected to tension, compression, and torsion forces and its behavior may be explained according to physical laws.[16]

The inevitable force of gravity has allowed the body to develop into a unique system of spinal arch arrangements and cavities. These specific arrangements enable the body to respond efficiently to mechanical, fluid, and gaseous forces during the interplay of cavity pressure differentials.

The complexities of the human structure express the complexity of life under the constant compressive nature of gravity. As noted by Fryette,[17] gravity is the natural force that exerts a constant load on the body, attracting it toward its point of application and determining the need of a continuous adaptation to maintain the erect position.

His famous quotation 'gravity kills the patient' expresses the idea that if the structure of the spine is not able to counterbalance gravity via a specific pulling reaction, the structure is unable to support itself. In the human body, the forces that oppose gravity are represented by extension forces, through muscles and their fasciae, and by the cavity pressure interplay. Several types of internal and external forces act continually on the erect posture. These forces, exerted by the pressure of fluids and gases, are balanced against forces of compression and tension acting on the spine. All these forces are capable of various distortional effects depending on their resistance and the elasticity of the tissues.

In general, all physiological processes active in maintaining this equilibrium are associated with the coordinating function of the nervous system, so that postural integrity can only be assured as long as the body is in an equilibrated relationship to all the forces to which it is exposed. When analyzing posture or movement there is an underlying coordinated orchestra of stimulatory or inhibitory impulses that equilibrate optimal statics or dynamics.

As described by Selye[18] and Cannon,[19] the body functions in an interplay of forces in response to changing circumstances, all acting continuously in order to maintain equilibrium and homeostasis.

Therefore, a treatment approach was developed by Littlejohn based on integration not only of the different anatomical structures, but also their physiological interrelations.

The mechanical role of fascia

Purslow and Delage describe an important correlation between muscle fascia and the function of muscle in respect of force transmission and mechanics.[20]

One important function of fascia is its role in providing pliability and tensile strength to the body. The organization of fibers in fascia follows a different pattern depending on the particular area of the body and adapting to the specific needs of the organism.[21,8] The simplest form of organization of collagen fibers is into a *crimped structure,* which offers the best response to a longitudinal traction force. It is thought that continued traction forces applied to the fibers will eventually result into a change of the collagen arrangement, deforming it into an uncrimped structure. This simple structure arrangement is not efficient enough to cope with multidirectional forces, so that in areas that are subjected to a variety of forces the organization of the collagen shows several degrees of directions in order to cope adequately and provide the resistance to *strain.*

The behavior of fascia to resist different types of forces depends on the amount, density, and directional alignment of the collagen fibers. Another important component of fascia is represented by the elastic fibers, which are distributed in a conformation known as 'random coil'. This apparent disorganization is the key to the elastic capacity of fascial membranes. This typical coordinated distribution of fibers can be subjected to different types of forces from various directions. The elastic component gives fascia another important characteristic. It provides the elastic recoil mechanism of the tissues. This mechanism gives the soft tissue the capacity to store potential kinetic energy. This is observed in tendons and ligaments during locomotion. The balance between collagen and elastic elements determines the degree of strength, plasticity, and flexibility of the fascial tissue. Furthermore, the organization of the layers of fascia is directly linked with the particular characteristics of the tissues in the specific areas of the body.

It is here that the connective tissue becomes clinically relevant as it is exposed to the various forms of mechanical forces that it has to withstand.

The fact that connective tissue and fascia are richly innervated[22,23,2,24] makes this tissue highly susceptible to neural irritation caused by excessive and continuous mechanical loading and chemical alterations.

The properties of fascia in mechanical resistance, may be altered by *densification,* a process induced by mechanical forces, chemical agents, or physical factors, as seen in the osteopathic dysfunctions.

Littlejohn and Burns studied exhaustively the effects of osteopathic dysfunctions on joints and the associated tissues and nerves in correlation to compensatory effects on the spine. It was L. Burns, in particular, who offered a complete description of the chemical and physical changes associated with dysfunctions, from local inflammatory conditions to changes in the pH level of tissues, to fibrosis and permanent rigidity.[25,26]

When a normal force is applied to a tissue in a rhythmical way it provides a positive stimulus promoting the activity of the tissue itself via its circulation and drainage. If an abnormal force is applied, or if the force is applied in a permanent arrhythmical way that may lead to progressive deformation of the fibers of the fascia, that in turn will create an adaptive response by modifying their spatial organization. The resulting effect is that the tissues organize themselves in a permanent conformation, depending on the direction and type of forces applied, consequently reducing mobility, contractility, and the capacity to resist other vectors of forces.

Furthermore, the organization of collagen shows a high level of complexity, being distributed and organized in wavelike and parallel fiber arrangements. The first arrangement is able to influence the nerve endings and the second one the muscular tissues.

Consequently, changes in the conformation have an effect on muscle chains, on the spinal arches, and on the nerves, influencing the mechanical behavior of the body and its resistance to gravity.

Given all these mechanophysiological correlations of fascial tissues, the treatment approach is concerned with affecting the connective tissue at the biochemical level in the extracellular medium as well as the mechanical aspect of the forces to which the body is exposed.

The physiological physics of gravity lines and fascia

Every individual needs to adjust to gravity by developing and maintaining a particular musculoskeletal organization in different planes in space. As evidenced by Hoover and Nelson,[27] the body has its own particular pattern of response to gravity, which is influenced by several factors. Considering the mechanics of the body, the ability of a structure to cope with the forces imposed on it depends on its physical characteristics and its mobility.

In his paper about the effects of gravity, Cathie[28] examined the relationship between postural defects and changes in soft tissues, proving that muscular and fascial pull forces may determine permanent alterations in the curves of the spine. Particularly, thick fascia is more associated with postural muscles and plays a major role both in the maintenance of posture and in the establishment of dysfunctions. As observed by Cathie, changes in the tonic state of fascia and muscles determine a consequent structural alteration in the arches and joints, which in turn reduces the capacity of the whole body to adapt under the load of compressive forces.

The mechanical theory proposed by Littlejohn and Wernham describes body unity using a set of parallel and nonparallel lines that are the results of forces applied to the body itself. The central gravity line

(CGL), the anteroposterior line (AP), and the posteroanterior line (PA) (Fig. 43.1) are expressions of our

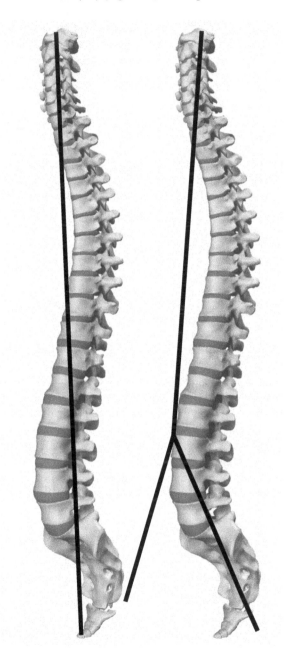

Figure 43.1
Left: anteroposterior gravity line (AP). Right: posteroanterior gravity line (PA)

ability to resist gravity, preserve equilibrium, and harmonize the internal and external forces in order to maintain homeostasis. According to Littlejohn and Wernham's theory, the CGL is a vertical line that starts between the occipital condyles at the odontoid process, passes downward through the body of L3 and the anterior sacral promontory, and finally reaches the ankles. L3 is indicated as the mechano-physiological 'center of gravity' of the body. The AP line is an oblique line passing from the anterior margin of the foramen magnum to the tip of the coccyx. The PA line is an oblique line that follows the opposite route, that is, from the posterior margin of foramen magnum to the hips, bifurcating in front of the articulation L2–L3.

These lines have a particular function, and are represented in a combined form as seen in the polygons of forces model, by Wernham.[29] The polygons of forces represent a mechanophysiological model of body unity, in which integrity of the arches is associated with a perfect physiological balance of vital forces (Fig. 43.2).

Given these considerations, the physiological integrity of the body and its parts are closely related to the center of gravity as the center of structure and function of the body, thus creating a hypothetical center of balance between internal forces, gravity, and environmental factors.[29,30]

These mechanophysiological correlations result in links between the structural integrity, rhythmic physiological activities, and the nutritive and trophic conditions of the tissues of the body. The vital actions of the blood and the nervous force represent the two great regulating factors that come into a direct association with postural integrity.

Hence, the balanced and integrated body stands in a unique relationship between a 'center of balance' from a physiological point of view and a 'center of gravity' from a mechanical point of view.

However, in most cases, the final posture is the effect of a series of compensatory patterns caused by factors that reorganized the spinal column into alterations of its lateral and anterior–posterior curvatures.

In his research on mechanics, Wernham described a common particular pattern found in patients,

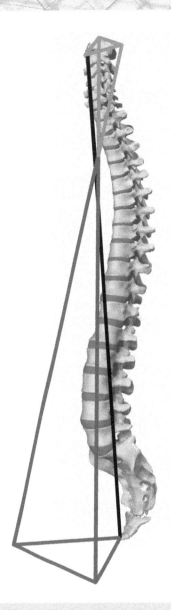

Figure 43.2
Polygons of forces model

characterized by a sacral and pelvic torsion followed by a succession of several small lateral curvatures with opposite convexities. This common compensatory pattern was named the 'Universal Lesion Pattern.' Similar compensatory patterns were also found by Zink and Schamberger.[31] These postural conditions are common. It means that under gravity the body is in a perpetual state of structural compensation, realized through changes in the pelvis and the arches of the spine.

In order to guarantee solid support for the erect body, stabilization during locomotion, and the preservation of the cavity pressure interplay, all the gravity lines have to cross the spine and the hips at specific 'resistance points' that work as 'solid anchors' for the lines themselves. In this way, the spinal structures are also able to dissipate the entering forces, preventing damage and irritation of the spine and contributing to the maintenance of the rhythmical mobility of muscles, ligaments, and fascia.

Misplacement of these lines allows abnormal force vectors to enter the body at different planes, causing weight to fall on structures, tissues, and organs of the body that do not have a weight-bearing function. This will lead to permanent alterations in their tension and fiber organization, will reduce mobility, and will set up a vicious circle of compensatory patterns. Furthermore, the changes in the spinal arches modify the pressure of cavities and the fluid circulation, predisposing the body to disease. This is particularly important in the abdominal field, where the organs are suspended and maintained in their position by the cavity pressure differentials and the vascular and fascial apparatus. These osteopathic considerations offer a new therapeutical perspective.

Osteopathic therapeutics and body adjustment

The concept of 'body adjustment' was the very basis of Littlejohn's continuous study of osteopathy. He emphasized that osteopathy must be applied within and under its principles, as these principles characterize it and differentiate it from other sciences and therapies.

It was these fundamental laws of osteopathy that caused Littlejohn use the word 'adjustment' in a very particular way. He described the adjustment of the body to itself, to its parts, and to its environment as the rational means to establish optimal conditions for health.[14]

The therapeutical aim is the reintegration of the body in relation to its structure, function, and environment without confining the osteopathic

principles to either forms of application or isolated treatment of any tissue or parts of the body.

According to Wernham,[30] osteopathic treatment was based on facilitating the body to return to the body itself, thus clearly highlighting the natural and innate capacities of the body. These self-regulating and self-adjusting capacities of the body are seen as the integral characteristic of the human organism.

In early osteopathic history, treatment was always based on the original concept of body unity. When looking at these developments in osteopathy the treatment was not directed to a particular tissue but to the patient, therefore bringing in a series of factors important in the etiological development of the presenting symptoms. In other words, the aim of the work is to focus on the patient as an organism in order to readjust the condition through the concepts of physiological physics.

Littlejohn and Wernham describe mechanics as the interface between structure and function, and therefore elemental as the basis of osteopathic therapeutics.

Body adjustment is an analysis and treatment based on evaluation of the organization of the body in relation to the center of gravity line over a base support. In other words, it is a postural analysis in order to correlate the individual's body mechanics in health or ill-health, therefore creating a mechanophysiological relationship for the patient. This evaluation of body mechanics and mechanical forces on the body has become a fundamental osteopathic criterion.

The method is characterized as an articulatory technique employing long leverages in order to deal with all tissues conjointly.

The use of long levers is a mechanical practical approach as it facilitates leverages and application of fulcra throughout the body. It consequently brings into play every muscular, ligamentous, and fascial insertion in the spine and pelvis, with special emphasis only where it is necessary.

The upper and lower extremities, due to the rotating nature of the articular movement, are used as efficient levers in order to diagnose and treat the body's mechanophysiological alterations. This method is deliberately routine in order to ensure a fine differentiation between the diagnostic value of the articulation and its therapeutical application.

Rhythmic articulatory technique mimics the natural movements of the body, taking into account all planes and axes of movement and consequently addressing the local arthrokinematic functions.

Most importantly, the use of long leverages allows efficient access to the lines of forces, as seen in Littlejohn and Wernham's polygons of forces model. The anterior and posterior gravity lines and the polygons they form move around the center of gravity as the axis of movement. It leads to body adjustment occurring through the body lines and triangles rather than through the spinal column. Individual groups of vertebrae function not in relation to the spinal column but in relation to the lines and triangles.[29]

Consequently, the adjustment of the body is closely related to the forces acting on the body rather than just to the structures involved.

This correlates the tangible with the intangible and the visible with the invisible.

Upper and lower extremities are not treated separately from the body as they are embryological outgrowths from the axial skeleton and have direct relationship via somatic structures and neurovascular pathways. The use of these leverages not only has a local adjustive effect on the spinal segments at which the force vector is focused but also influences the vascular system. The circulation of arterial, venous blood and lymph may be stimulated via the treatment of their corresponding spinal centers.

The therapeutical benefit of using the long lever avoids high-velocity forces being transmitted to articular and periarticular structures, thereby preventing unnecessary trauma to the adjacent tissues.

From a clinical view, the action is directed conjointly to all body tissues, as it is not possible to adjust the abnormal to the normal, meaning that local treatment will remain local without general or permanent effects if the underlying field of physiology is not addressed.

Arches of the spine and muscular chains

The spinal column is described from a structural perspective as a vertical organization composed of a series of arches. There are anterior–convex cervical and lumbar arches and two posterior–convex thoracic and sacral arches. From a developmental perspective there is a differentiation between the primary posterior convex arches, associated with the primary foetal curve, and the anterior convex arches, related to movements and the primitive reflexes of intrauterine and early life. The primary curves are related to forces of flexion, whereas the secondary curves are related to extension forces. The lordotic arches develop during the demands of the body to establish a sense of midline during the process of acquiring the ability to sit and stand.

The arrangement of the arches of the vertical structure outlined below allows the radial downward force of compression forces to be converted into a postural stress, creating interplay between compression and tension forces through the vertebral column. The arrangement of the arches of the spinal column is an extremely efficient design that allows the maintenance of the spinal structure without compromising the ability of movement.

From the structural perspective the integrity of the arches is related to their relationship with the intra-arch points known as *keystones*. In the vertebral column the areas of the second and third cervical, the dorsal area between the fourth and sixth (depending on stage of development and ossification) and the second and third lumbar vertebrae act as integral keystones for the maintenance of the arches. This arrangement is only able to provide the structural and functional relationship if the elasticity of the associated soft tissues is intact. Here it is important to differentiate between the function of the active and passive tissues. The active tissues are represented by the muscular and fascial tissues with their associated nerve supply and the passive structural elements refer to the ligamentous tissues. It is here, from a structural perspective, that there is an important relationship between these associated soft tissues and the important keystones of the arches.

An important value of the function of the vertebral column is associated with other inter-arch points, also known as *pivots*. These pivots are key vertebrae from a functional perspective, acting as link vertebrae between the arches in order to accommodate, regulate, and modulate function. These pivot points in the spine are associated with the fifth cervical, ninth thoracic, and fifth lumbar vertebrae (Fig. 43.3).[29]

When evaluating the vertebral column in locomotion there is an important relationship between the coordination of the shoulder and pelvic girdles, creating at the articulation between the second and third lumbar vertebrae a crossover point between opposite sides. Anterior and posterior crossed muscular chains meet in an area associated with L3 where there is a convergence of torsional forces and extensory forces, as marked by a dense fascial and muscular arrangement (Fig. 43.4).

In mechanical theory, the articulation of L2–L3 is related to the passage of the PA line, which coordinates mobility and motility through the physiological forces and is associated with the gravitational stability of the spine. The AP line also represents the effects of the forces of extension by providing an anterior and superior support mechanism for the body. Here the important role of T11 and T12 as the *inter-current point* of that line provides mechanical resistance to the loss of integrity of the arches of the vertebral column. The connection between the crossed chains and L3 shows a close connection of fascia and muscles in relation to the arches of the spine.

According to Littlejohn and Wernham's model, the central gravity line passes through the vertebral body of L3, emphasizing the particular function of this vertebra as a solid point in the maintenance of equilibrium and in motor organization. In Wernham's mechanical theory the pelvis and the legs are described as being in 'suspension' off the center of gravity point at L3. Based on its anatomical and functional characteristics, L3 presents itself as a very particular vertebra interpreted as the central point of the whole body. The application of long leverage via the extremities is therefore able to affect the spine, the soft tissues, and all the relevant mechanical behaviour of the body as a unit.

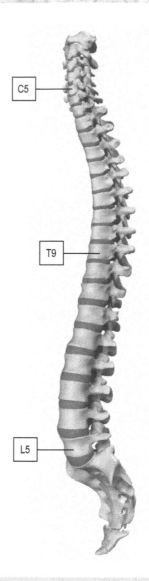

Figure 43.3
The pivots of the spine. T9 is also a keystone

The cross-pattern movement of both girdles can be associated with the cross-muscular chains that regulate and coordinate torsional movements between the upper and lower half of the body. This torsional movement of the upper and lower girdles accentuates from a functional point of view in the lower dorsal spine at the level of T11 and T12. This in turn creates an important correlation between L3 from a struc-

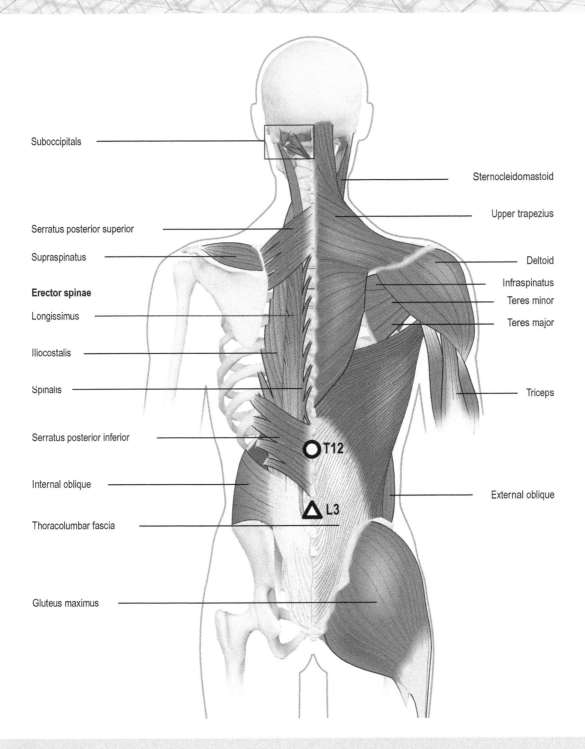

Figure 43.4
T12 and L3 and their relationship with the muscles and fascia of the back

tural perspective in relation to the center of gravity line and T11 and T12 from a functional point of view and their common association with the thoracolumbar fascia as the soft tissue mechanism active as the extensor force of the column. Consequently, these observations indicate significant associations between the extensor forces and the AP gravity line with its important correlation to T11 and T12 as the inter-current area and point of crossover through the vertebral column. This important vertebral level plays a fundamental role in the maintenance of anteroposterior arch integrity and as a center of torsion in trunk movements.

In the body adjustment approach, the mechanical correction passes through the harmonization of soft tissues, including the muscular chains, in relation to the arches of the spine. However, as observed by Littlejohn, adjustment is not only based on mechanical corrections but it is also an organic treatment to normalize the relationship of the arches with the associated soft tissues and nervous activity. It is evident, therefore, that osteopathic treatment also has an effect on visceral life, assisting nutrition, motility, and circulation.

In view of the observations above, the therapeutical effects of body adjustment on fascia can be said to be due to three main factors:

- The correction of posture, accompanied by removal of abnormal forces, restoring the capacity of fascia for a normal resistance and elastic recoil.

- The stimulation of a normal blood and lymphatic circulation, in order to guarantee a normal physiology of tissues.

- The reintegration of the autonomic nerves' control of fascia via the correction of osteopathic dysfunctions.

These factors guarantee therapeutical power by the reorganization of myofascial tension and metabolism.

Myofascial treatment: a new perspective

Classical myofascial treatment is based on the application of local or segmental techniques, aimed at restoring a normal elastic response of tissues, circulation,

and drainage. Myofascial treatment may significantly reduce pain, promote physical function, and help in restoring circulation, but for our purposes the main aspect is to define the effects on the posture of the body. In order to maximize the benefit on general posture, every fascial therapy has to consider the close relationship of fascia with all the soft and hard tissues of the body.

The treatment of fascia, the ubiquitous membrane linking all the tissues and structures of the body, has to respect and follow the intrinsic basic unity of the body as a mechanophysiological system, in which nerves; blood and lymphatic vessels; and soft and hard tissues are inseparable and work together in a conjoint system.

Restriction of mobility in any part of the body will affect the whole system, leading to compensations throughout. Therefore, a definitive treatment approach must be chosen that considers the general antigravity arrangement of the spine, as suggested in the mechanical models of Littlejohn and Wernham.

A local treatment of fascia may relieve pain and restore mobility and a proper blood supply, but the definitive integration of the dysfunctional areas with the whole system is obtained only with a total adjustment of the body, that is, removing the abnormal vectors of forces that alter the mechanical stability of the body and promoting the process of integration.

Technique applied to fascia must follow the natural integration of the bodily parts, working on the relationship between tissues, bones, blood vessels, and nerves conjointly and at the same time, in order to change the mechanics of the body.

The method we propose consists of the application of a rhythmical routine based on long leverage techniques. The body adjustment routine primarily addresses the forces that act upon the connective tissues. This treatment method reintegrates the body from a biomechanical point of view by improving postural relationships via the functioning of the spinal arches and the integrity of pelvic mechanics, thus affecting the tissues' responses to forces. Therefore, evaluation of mechanical factors is of importance and must be addressed in treatment if the causative factor beyond the local tissue condition is also to be considered.

Furthermore, body adjustment addresses the physiological forces that regulate homeostasis and normalize nervous activity and the circulation of fluids. This osteopathic perspective implements a series of aspects that must be considered in order to address the etiological factors of the osteopathic dysfunction. The consideration of the underlying mechanophysiological relationships ensures a more comprehensive evaluation of the body.

In the body adjustment approach, fascia is treated both directly and indirectly – directly by correcting the passage and distribution of mechanical forces, and indirectly through the reaction on circulation and on nervous activity. By normalizing the vector of forces acting through the body and correcting the relationship between the spinal arches a more adequate tension mechanism of fascia and muscles is restored. This will consequently improve their rhythmical contractility, allowing for normal motility. As Schleip[32,1] showed, fascia has intrinsic contractility, which is in part regulated by the autonomic nervous system. The balance between the sympathetic and the parasympathetic nervous systems regulates the diameter of blood and lymphatic vessels, therefore contributing to the distribution of fluids throughout the body and normalizing the circulation of fascia.

Rebalancing the nervous activity contributes to normal rhythmical fascial activity, which in turn is fundamental for proprioception, coordination of motor patterns, and lymphatic circulation.

In one way, body adjustment can be defined as a general treatment, but the word 'general' should not be confused with 'vague'.

In principle and in practice, the concept of general treatment should not be considered to be synonymous with unspecific treatment and local treatment with specificity.

The term 'general' in this context refers to analysing the presenting condition of the patient as a whole, considering his or her mechanophysiological state according to Wernham. All treatment must be specific to the demand of the organic unity of the body and the requirements of the particular individual.

Conclusion

The practice of osteopathy is based on solid mechanical and physiological principles according to the laws of physics, so that the treatment of fascia is a part of body adjustment as it is a complete approach involving all tissues and organs in a natural way. The method considered approaches the body as a whole and therefore avoids isolating parts and treating them out of the context of their physiological relationships. It is through the use of long leverages that the treatment of the body can follow and appeal to the laws of the natural 'physiological physics' of the body as a unit. Our principles of treatment are based, according to A. T Still, on the most important step of osteopathic therapeutics, *to believe in our own body and stimulate its inherent resources for balance and health.*

References

1. **Schleip R., 2012** Fascia as an organ of communication. In: Schleip R., Findley T. W., Chaitow L., Huijing P. A. (eds) *Fascia: The Tensional Network of the Human Body*, Churchill Livingstone, Edinburgh, pp. 77–79.

2. **Snyder G. E. 1954.** Embryology and physiology of fascia. Reprinted in AAO Year Book of selected osteopathic papers, 1970, Oct:147–158.

3. **Stecco C., Macchi V., Porzionato A., Stecco A. et al. 2010.** The ankle retinacula, morphological evidence of the proprioceptive role of the fascial system. *Cells Tissues Organs* 192:200–210.

4. **Willard F. 2007.** Fascial continuity: four fascial layers of the body. Extract from the First International Fascia Research Congress, Boston.

5. **Blechschmidt E. 2004.** *The Ontogenetic Basis of Human Anatomy: A Biodynamic Approach to Development from Conception to Birth.* North Atlantic Books, Berkeley, MA.

6. **Huber G. C. 1930.** *Piersol's Human Anatomy*, IX edition, Lippincott, Philadelphia, PA.

7. **Schleip R. 2003.** Fascial plasticity – a new neurobiological explanation. *J Bodyw Mov Ther*:11–19;7:104–116.

8. **Willard F. H. 2012.** Somatic fascia. In: Schleip R., Findley T. W., Chaitow L., Huijing P. A. (eds) *Fascia: The Tensional Network of the Human Body*, Churchill Livingstone, Edinburgh, pp. 11–17.

9. **Still A. T. 1899.** *Philosophy of Osteopathy*, Academy of Osteopathy, Kirksville, MO.

10. **Magoun H. I. 1970.** The myth of osteopathic lesion. AAO Year Book of selected osteopathic papers, Oct:142–143.

11. **Magoun H. I. 1954.** *Fascia in the writing of A. T. Still*. Reprinted in AAO Year Book of selected osteopathic papers, 1970, Oct:159–168.

12. **Goldthwait J. E., Thomas L. C. 1922.** *Body Mechanics in Health and Disease*, Houghton Mifflin Company, Cambridge.

13. **Ingber, D. E. 2008.** Tensegrity-based mechanosensing from macro to micro. *Prog Biophys Mol Bio* 97:163–179.

14. **Littlejohn J. M. 1907.** *Principles of Osteopathy*, American College of Osteopathic Medicine, Chicago, IL.

15. **Wernham J. 1956.** *Year Book*, JWCCO editions, Maidstone.

16. **Gordon J. E. 1978.** *Structures or Why Things Don't Fall Down*, Da Capo Press, New York, NY.

17. **Fryette H. 1954.** *Principles of the Osteopathic Technique*, AAO editions.

18. **Selye H. 1956.** *The Stress of Life*, McGraw-Hill, New York, NY.

19. **Cannon W. B. 1929.** *Bodily Changes in Pain, Hunger, Fear and Rage*, Appleton & Co, New York, NY.

20. **Purslow P., Delage J. P. 2012.** General anatomy of the muscle fascia. In: Schleip R., Findley T. W., Chaitow L., Huijing P. A. *Fascia: The Tensional Network of the Human Body*, Churchill Livingstone, Edinburgh, pp. 5–10).

21. **Schleip R., Muller D. G. 2013.** Training principles for fascial connective tissues: scientific foundation and suggested practical applications. *J Bodyw Mov Ther* 17:103–115.

22. **Juhan D. 1985.** *Job's body. A Handbook for Bodywork*, World of Books, UK.

23. **Langevin H., Yandow J. 2002.** Relationship of acupuncture points and meridians to connective tissue planes. *Anat Rec* 269:257–265.

24. **van der Wal J. C., 2012.** Proprioception. In: Schleip R., Findley T. W., Chaitow L., Huijing P. A. *Fascia: The Tensional Network of the Human Body*, Churchill Livingstone, Edinburgh. pp. 82–87.

25. **Burns, L. 1907.** *Studies in Osteopathic Science. Basic principles. Vol.1* The Occident Printery, Los Angeles, CA.

26. **Burns, L. 1917.** The effects of lumbar lesions. The A. T. Still Research Institute, Bulletin no. 5, Chicago.

27. **Hoover H. V., Nelson C. R. 1950.** Effects of gravitational forces on structure. Reprinted in AAO Year Book of selected osteopathic papers, 1970:116–124.

28. **Cathie A. G. 1949.** Soft tissue changes that may follow postural defects. *J Am Osteopath Assoc* 48:235–238.

29. **Wernham J. 1985.** *Mechanics of the Spine and Pelvis*, JWCCO editions, Maidstone.

30. **Wernham J. 1995.** *Lectures on Osteopathy*, Vol.1, JWCCO editions, Maidstone.

31. **Pope R. E. 2003.** The common compensatory pattern: its origin and relationship to the postural model. AAO 13:19–40.

32. **Schleip R., Klinger W., Lehmann-Horn F. 2006.** Active fascia contractility: fascia may be able to contract in a smooth muscle-like manner and thereby influence musculoskeletal dynamics. *Med Hypotheses* 65:273–277.

BALANCED LIGAMENTOUS TENSION TECHNIQUE (BLT)

Paolo Tozzi, Cristian Ciranna-Raab

Overview

Balanced ligamentous tension (BLT) technique is a traditional osteopathic approach addressing capsulo-ligamentous tissues under an uneven state of tension. Considering the structures being worked, BLT may fall within the concept of the osteopathic biomechanical model as it produces beneficial effects on posture, proprioception, motor control, and joint motion. However, if the underlying physiological mechanisms are taken into account, it may also belong to the neurological model as it induces various reflexes and responses from the functionally integrated unit of the neuromusculoskeletal system. What is certain is that BLT conceives each joint in the body as a balanced ligamentous articular mechanism that may be altered after injury, infection, or mechanical stress. The resulting articular strain is addressed in an indirect manner (i.e., by engaging the preferential joint vectors of motion and therefore by getting away from the barrier). Tissues are first disengaged from their protective position, and then brought into their dysfunctional pattern toward the direction of ease, up to the point where a ligamentous tensional compromise is achieved and a release is felt. This process has been traditionally referred to as a *disengage–exaggerate–balance* procedure. Despite its original application being reserved for articular structures, it has also been applied to membranous, fascial, visceral, and fluid elements, showing equal efficacy when appropriately performed. In fact, regardless of the tissues being addressed, the principles of the approach remain the same: to acknowledge tissue motion, find a tensional compromise, and wait for a response from the inherent body potency. As such, BLT has proved effective in various clinical conditions, although further research is needed to explore the underlying mechanisms and to better define its limits, benefits, and contraindications. Nowadays it is still a commonly used technique in osteopathic practice, being mostly appreciated for its safe and non-invasive nature, beyond its efficacy and therapeutic properties.

Introduction

As suggested by the work of Blechschmidt & Gasser (2012), each constituent of the connective tissue in the body presents a functional and anatomical continuity, due to the common embryologic origin from the mesoderm. However, loading demands acting through and upon tissues may determine their differentiation into cartilage and bone – when resisting local compression is required – or into ligaments, fascia, and aponeurosis, when resisting tensional forces is needed. Consequently, the arrangement, length, and density of fibers are also dictated by local tensional demands. Nevertheless, although tissues seem to specialize in response to mechanical forces, their structural and functional interconnection is always maintained at each stage of embryological and foetal development. This requires an alternative architectural view of joint structures involved in transmission and conveying of mechanical forces from the traditional division of muscles, ligaments, and bones. In fact, there appears to exist an interrelationship and continuity of joint connective tissues, with tendons and aponeuroses merging with capsular and ligamentous elements, often relying on specialized fascial tissue to insert onto the skeleton (van der Wal, 2009). This whole-body connection between bones, ligaments, fascia, and muscles has been referred to as 'ectoskeleton' (Wood Jones, 1944). Ligaments, in particular, are suggested to be organized in series rather than in parallel with the corresponding muscular, tendinous, and fascial structures, thus acting as active (rather than simply passive) elements for transmission of forces into the joint complex. In contrast with the traditional view, where ligaments are seen as passive and fixed structures that just limit motion at the very end of its range, the proposed arrangement in series instead allows ligaments to be under tension throughout the range of a given joint motion, thus providing proprioceptive inputs and motor control at every degree of movement. From an anatomical perspective, this shows an interconnected structural network, indicating a 'fascio–musculo–ligamento–capsulo–articular' continuity, as has also been proposed in the spine with the so-called 'ligamentous complex system' (Willard, 1997). Ligaments of the lumbar spine and sacrum have been described as a continuous connective tissue stocking, extending from the posterior thoracolumbar fascia to the anterior longitudinal ligament, including, from superficial to deep, the supraspinous, interspinous, and flavum ligaments. While posteriorly the multifidus muscle is anchored to the supraspinous ligament, and the abdominal muscles to the thoracolumbar fascia, anteriorly the ligamentum flavum extends to the facet joint capsules. Therefore, the ligamentous complex guarantees an anatomical interconnection between myofascial planes and osteoarticular structures, possibly acting as force transducers by translating the tension of the thoracolumbar fascia, developed in the extremities and torso, into the lumbar spine. From a physiological view, this mechanism can be plausibly applied to most joints in the body, revealing an integrated, multistructured, multifunctional unit, whose elements cooperate to coordinate muscle force, to control gross and fine motion, to minimize stress on bony and cartilaginous structures, and to reduce general energy expenditure. The idea clearly emerges that ligamentous structures do not work in an isolated manner, but are integrated into a more complex 'connective tissue system' instead, playing different functional roles (Box. 44.1).

In light of the above considerations, the key concept of BLT that every joint in normal condition is a reciprocal tension mechanism, in a balanced state of tension of its capsular and ligamentous elements, can be easily understood. 'In normal movements, as the joint changes position the relationships between the ligaments also change, but the total tension within

---

Box 44.1

Possible functional roles of the 'connective tissue complex'

- Joint stability

- Proprioception

- Nociception

- General movement coordination

- Distribution of mechanical forces

- Gross and fine motor control

- Hydraulic pumping during contraction and relaxation phases

- Stress reduction on cartilaginous and osseous structures

- Energy saving

---

the articular mechanism does not' (Carreiro, 2009a). Similarly, this principle can be applied in a clinical context, especially when proprioception as well as muscle response during joint motion and position are compromised and need to be addressed. In this sense, BLT belongs primarily to the osteopathic biomechanical model. This model looks at the body as an integration of somatic components, mainly from the musculoskeletal system (DeStefano, 2011a): bones, capsules, ligaments, tendons, aponeurosis, muscles, fascia. They are all in a constantly static and dynamic balance for giving and maintaining a body posture monitored and influenced by proprioceptive information. Any mechanical stress or articular strain would affect this dynamic equilibrium, leading to a general increase in energy expenditure, altered proprioception, postural unbalance, musculoskeletal pain, impediment of neurovascular function, changes in articular mechanics, and ligamentous tension in particular (Hruby, 1992). Therefore, when an injury or any articular disturbance occurs, the physiological and tensional ligamentous balance may be compromised. Consequently, the joint or tissue, when taken beyond its physiological barrier, remains dysfunctional, failing to return to its normal position, therefore shifting its balance point. This change may produce proximal and distal effects that include various types of compensatory patterns and dysfunctional complexities (Kuchera & Kuchera, 1994): first degree, when a local osteopathic lesion may take place and produce symptoms (an anterior talus following an inversion ankle injury); second degree, when mechanically or functionally related structures become involved and symptomatic (a secondary posterior ileum causing sacroiliac pain following the ankle strain); and third degree, when global effects are produced and distant symptoms from the original site of dysfunction are caused (neutral, sidebent, and rotated (NSR) group lesions in the spine and sphenobasilar synchondrosis (SBS) functional asymmetry following the previous changes).

BLT aims to restore the tensional and functional equilibrium, by looking for and maintaining a balanced tensional point within the tissues involved, from which the inherent body potency may find its way to correction. this approach, also known as 'ligamentous articular strain' (LAS), has been reportedly developed by A. T. Still, founder of osteopathy, and then greatly expanded by R. and H. Lippincott, R. Becker and A. Wales (Crow, 2011). However, the major contribution to its development came from W. G. Sutherland, the 'father of cranial osteopathy'. In *Contributions of Thought*, Sutherland (1998a) describes the BLT approach as an application of cranial treatment principles to the rest of the body and extremities. BLT techniques were originally published in the 1949 *Yearbook of the Academy of Applied Osteopathy* (Lippincott, 1949). Although originally conceived as an indirect manipulative intervention addressed to articular strains, it has also been applied to membranous torsions (falx, tentorium, interosseous membranes) and referred to as 'balanced membranous tension technique'. Likewise, when applied to fascial dysfunctions it became 'balanced fascial tension technique' (Moeckel & Mitha, 2008), keeping always the same concept and principles even when addressing body fluids (cerebrospinal, synovial, lymphatic, arterovenous, interstitial) or visceral capsules and ligaments. In these cases, it was respectively named 'balanced fluid and visceral tension technique'.

Aims, indications, evidences

BLT is a noninvasive, safe, and fairly common technique amongst the osteopathic profession (Sleszynski & Glonek, 2005). Because of its gentle application,

it is usually perceived as a pleasant and relaxing technique by the patient, although it requires a discrete amount of palpatory skill and experience from the practitioner. BLT is often chosen when clinical assessment finds any sign of:

- *Articular strain:* loss of function, pain, restriction of joint mobility, joint laxity
- *Muscular involvement:* muscle stiffness or spasm, altered myofascial tissue motility
- *Impairment of fluid dynamics:* impeded arterial supply, venous and lymphatic drainage, synovial or cerebrospinal fluid circulation
- *Altered neurological control:* including sensation or proprioception, deficiencies in fine and gross motor control.

Most of the time these changes are the result of inflammation, infection, macrotrauma, or repetitive microtraumatic events following positions and activities related to work, sport, or hobbies. However, they might be also caused by compensatory patterns generated by primary lesions found elsewhere in the body. In any case, the resulting articular strain may alter joint position and body posture, at both a local and global level, predisposing the body to reoccurrence of injuries and the establishment of chronic dysfunctional patterns.

Consequently, the clinical aims of applying BLT are generally to:

- correct articular strain
- release capsular and ligamentous tension
- normalize joint dysfunction, including acute articular ones
- balance autonomic activity
- promote synovial fluid circulation
- relieve vascular congestion
- release nerve entrapment.

If we consider the secondary effects of its application, BLT may be viewed as falling under the concept of the respiratory–circulatory osteopathic model. In fact, the latter emphasizes the importance of ensuring free circulation of body fluids, as well as their oxygenation through an efficient respiratory system. Any disturbance of gaseous cellular exchange, or of arterial supply and venolymphatic (as well as synovial, interstitial, and cerebrospinal) drainage represents a threat to the homeostatic potential of the body (Degenhardt & Kuchera, 1996). Areas of edema and congestion are of primary interest for this model. However, the opening of connective tissue pathways to restore a normal tissue tension is crucial for bringing fluid motion back to normal (Zink, 1977). This is why BLT could be considered from a respiratory–circulatory perspective, since it restores normal pressures within and between tissue layers by balancing intrinsic tensional forces, thus exerting a beneficial impact on fluid dynamics. This would promote the removal of inflammatory mediators, possibly reducing symptoms and pain, together with resetting aberrant neural reflexes in the area; it would also help in reducing edema or congestion, promoting tissue repair and function; finally, it would improve joint motion and restore a normal tension in the surrounding myofascial structures. It is now easy to understand why BLT has been traditionally indicated for a variety of conditions (Box 44.2).

BLT has been demonstrated to be an effective integrative technique to the osteopathic treatment of:

- postinfective middle ear effusion (Steele et al., 2010), colonic inertia (Cohen-Lewe, 2013), and chronic neck and low back pain with a history of standard treatment failure (Gronemeyer et al., 2006)

- gastrointestinal disturbances in premature infants, contributing to reducing the length of stay in an intensive care unit (Pizzolorusso et al., 2011), as well as in the management of hospitalized premature infants with nipple-feeding dysfunction (Lund et al., 2011)

- hospitalized patients with chronic cardiovascular disease (Kaufman, 2011), as well as in the management of subjects at high risk of cardiovascular events (Cerritelli et al., 2011)

- patients with coronary artery bypass graft, promoting beneficial hemodynamic effects on patient recovery (O-Yurvati et al., 2005)

> **Box 44.2**
>
> ## Indications for BLT
>
> - Joint injury, articular and myofascial dysfunctions (Speece & Crow, 2009a)
>
> - Chronic pelvic pain in women (Tettambel, 2005)
>
> - Coccydynia (Fraix & Seffinger, 2011)
>
> - Tenosynovitis and plantar fasciitis (Modi & Shah, 2005)
>
> - Foot-drop symptoms, when applied to the fibular head and interosseous membrane (Kuchera, 2011a)
>
> - Lymphatic congestion and local edema (Kuchera, 2011b; Nicholas & Nicholas, 2008)
>
> - Osteoporosis, headache, and acute asthma (DiGiovanna et al., 2005)
>
> - Brachial plexus injuries and Erb's palsy, suckling dysfunctions, migraine and sinusitis (Carreiro, 2009b), as well as sensory integration disorders (Moeckel & Mitha, 2008) in infants and children
>
> - Chronic low back pain, for which BLT is one of the 14 most commonly used techniques (Licciardone et al., 2008)

- hospitalized patients in general, producing a reduction of anxiety and pain (Pomykala et al., 2008).

BLT has also been shown to be a useful integrative technique in osteopathic treatment for migraine headache, at a lower cost than that provided by allopathic intervention (Schabert & Crow, 2009). Finally, it has been shown to be an effective technique in animal practice too, producing significant changes in dogs with knock-knee (Accorsi et al., 2012a) as well as having immediate anti-inflammatory effects when applied to dogs with polyarthritis (Accorsi et al., 2012b).

However, as recently found mainly in pediatric osteopathic research (Posadzki et al., 2013), most of these studies show various methodological limits to a certain extent, including the common recruitment of small population samples; the generally poor control of the variables, bias, or of the placebo effect; a very short or even absent follow-up; and infrequent use of blind studies for subjects, although blind studies were occasionally applied to examiners.

BLT is relatively counterindicated in cases of bone fracture, joint dislocation and gross instability, infection, malignancy, severe osteoporosis, and open wound (Nicholas & Nicholas, 2008). As for most of the indirect techniques when applied at a local site, the absolute contraindications are recent closed head injury, acute vascular accident, bleeding or aneurysm, and acute visceral infections (WHO, 2010).

Treatment protocol

BLT is primarily an indirect technique, safe and non-invasive in its application, usually associated with light touch and patient cooperation. According to Crow (2005), the amount of force used in BLT is generally 1–3 lbs, whereas LAS techniques may require up to 40 lbs. However, the practitioner should always remain within tissue-permitted motion and respect elastic limits, and avoid applying too much pressure that would cause patient discomfort and guarding. During the entire performance of the technique, it is crucial that the practitioner remains in a constantly active, perceptive state, looking for diagnostic clues as the patient responds to treatment. The anatomical visualization of the body region being approached may also reinforce the procedure and its therapeutic effect. BLT is generally simplified into three main steps: disengage–exaggerate–balance. However, its procedure can be better expanded in seven phases:

1. *Functional diagnosis:* should be based upon an accurate assessment of the involved structures, aiming to locate the main features of somatic dysfunction: restriction of motion, positional asymmetry, tissue texture change, and tenderness (DeStefano, 2011b). When an articular strain occurs, even if it doesn't cause any ligamentous disruption, an unbalanced tension may take place in the capsuloligamentous complex around and within the joint involved. This causes a tendency for easier movement to occur toward the direction of the strain, that means toward the 'shortened'

ligamentous complex. Conversely, a reduced range of motion is perceived when the joint is tested in the opposite directions. At the end of the evaluation, the practitioner should have identified the dysfunctional joint vectors to address during the maneuver.

2. *Disengagement:* either traction or compression may be used at this stage (although the second is more commonly applied) to initially disengage the joint involved and allow motion to occur with least resistance. 'This is similar to pushing in the clutch on a car to shift gears' (Speece & Crow, 2009b). This force helps the practitioner to feel the inherent tissue motion while seeking a neutral point.

3. *Exaggeration:* the joint is taken in the direction of ease that normally matches the vectors of the articular strain. The position of relative freedom is exaggerated, allowing the expression of strained tissues only up to the point where all forces (torsion, shear ...) balance each other out to a neutral point. This is probably the most crucial phase of the procedure, since ligaments, membranes, and fascia are engaged toward a position of ease and of least resistance, or are simply matched in their tone. This requires good palpatory skills and a consistent perceptive state to feel for any diagnostic clue and position the joint accordingly. It is fundamental to constantly visualize the anatomy of the area being worked, while sensing the motion expressed from surrounding tissues. However, the practitioner should always remain within the articular field of permitted motion and never exaggerate the strain beyond the balance point (Moeckel & Mitha, 2008).

4. *Balance:* once all connective tissue tensions are equally balanced in every direction, and all the vectors of joint motion are in a state of balance, there should be a sense of poise in a neutral field. 'The articulation is carried in the direction of the lesion position as far as is necessary to cause tension of the weakened elements of the ligamentous structure to be equal to or slightly in excess of the tension of those that are not strained. This is the point of balanced tension.' (Lippincott, 1949). This is the state in which there is minimum resistance to the self-correcting intelligence of tissues.

5. *Holding:* The balance point is held, allowing 'physiologic function within to manifest its own unerring potency' (Becker, 1990). At this phase, tissues being held in a balance state may require further minor changes, or accessory motions that the practitioner must acknowledge, add, and keep (refining stage). If the practitioner does not accomplish this appropriately, the release may take longer to occur (or it may not happen at all), since tissues will have to find balance by their own intrinsic potency. Certainly, the ability to recognize and to accommodate such extra tissue requests may be what makes of an osteopath an experienced practitioner when it comes to applying BLT technique. Once the final balance point is gained, it is held. Right at this phase, the tensional and neurological information are elaborated until a still point takes place before corrective changes occur. However, the practitioner should bear in mind that too firm a hold may prevent the change from happening. Since ligaments are not under voluntary control, Sutherland recommended using the inherent forces of the body to promote tissue release. These forces are traditionally distinguished into voluntary and involuntary. The former are various types of patient cooperation that may be requested as an 'enhancing maneuver' to the technique, such as forced respiration, specific body positioning, or selected muscle group contraction (Kimberly, 1980). The involuntary forces are instead intrinsic homeostatic potencies present in the natural rhythmic activities of living tissues. Such rhythms as the craniosacral or fascial ones are not under the direct control of the patient, yet can be engaged by the practitioner to reinforce the therapeutic effect of the maneuver. Regardless of the assisting force being employed, the general concept is to apply it in the most appropriate modality and direction in order to exaggerate dysfunctional tissue vectors. For instance, having located a balance point for a T2 in ERS-Left, the patient can be asked to hold his or her breath in inhalation and to slowly drop the left arm down toward the left foot. Obviously these motions need to be constantly monitored by the practitioner, who will ensure that they are performed according to tissue needs. The aim would be to exaggerate the dysfunctional vectors, so as to reduce their allostatic influence, and finally to overcome 'the resistance of the defense mechanism of the body to the release of the lesion' (Lippincott, 1949).

6. *Releasing:* a release is felt and the joint is brought back into its normal position by the restored balanced ligamentous tension itself. A sense of melting, softening, and of fluid reorganization within tissues may be perceived together with warmth, expansion, and a restoration of joint midline. If a release is not achieved, the exact balance point may have not been adequately identified. If this is the case, the procedure should be repeated from the balance phase.

7. *Reassessment:* the joint is reassessed in all planes of motion. A positional and functional symmetry should be found, together with a freedom of motion.

The same procedure can be applied to membranous structures as well as to fascial tissues and visceral ligaments showing some features of strain or dysfunction. In any case, the practitioner chooses the most appropriate hold after having assessed the lesional pattern. He or she then disengages, exaggerates, balances and holds the membranous/fascial/visceral tensions up to when they yield, asking for patient cooperation when needed. In addition, by focusing the intention on the appropriate tissue depth, this approach can also be addressed specifically to fluid elements that have undergone some sort of trauma. Consequently, their physiological balance point may be disrupted or shifted elsewhere, altering fluid circulation, its related function, the chemical milieu and the surrounding tissue tension. According to the level being involved, the practitioner may connect to the cerebrospinal, lymphatic, interstitial, or arterovenous field in order to guide fluids towards a neutral point. Regardless of the tissue being compromised, the point of balanced tension is a sensation of contrast between freedom and restriction of mobility (Magoun, 1976a).

Furthermore, the osteopath should be aware that the point of BLT may also be located to support the application of high-velocity thrust to the joint involved, as suggested in the following analogy attributed to A. T. Still: 'If you had a horse tied to a post and you wanted to untie him, you wouldn't first frighten him so that he would pull back on the rope to hold it tight during the untying operation, would you?' (Fryette, 1954).

Mechanisms

As presented in the introduction to this chapter, the latest research suggests that muscles, capsules, ligaments, and related fascial structures may work together as a functional unit. It is then plausible that when muscle contraction occurs, ligaments and fascia are automatically engaged, working as a connective tissue complex, assisting in joint stabilization, regardless of the articular position or phase of muscle contraction (Libbey, 2012). Furthermore, from a physiological point of view, afferent mechanoreceptors in ligaments seem to be capable of eliciting a ligamentomuscular reflex that may exert inhibitory effects on related joint muscles (Solomonow, 2009). Articular strains may alter this normal proprioceptive role of the capsuloligamentous complex, leading to an impaired reflex muscular activation. This may in turn change the load on ligaments themselves. As a result, corrupted mechanoreceptor signals may produce higher stress, neural and connective tissue inflammation, and, over time, chronic pain (Panjabi, 2006). Nevertheless, this same reflex may play a therapeutic role during BLT application, by being employed during the disengagement and exaggeration phases, so as to produce an effect on the state of tension of the entire 'fascio–musculo–ligamento–capsulo–articular' complex. In this sense, Sutherland's words (1998b) are truly appropriate: 'The ligaments, not the muscles are the natural agencies for this purpose of correcting the relations and positions of joints'.

Initially, when BLT is applied, the strained joint receives a disengagement force: this may reduce or remove the collagen fibers 'crimping' (undulations present when not under tensile loading) around the joint, creating a temporary lengthening of collagenous structures (Threlkeld, 1992), and a consequent increase in proprioceptive information. Then, an exaggeration of dysfunctional pattern is pursued. This method of unloading tissues may decrease neural inputs together with reducing physical stress. According to Van Buskirk (1990), positioning a joint into ease may produce a modulation of muscle tone and tension in related fascial structures. In addition, the activation of mechanoreceptors in ligaments may affect both local blood supply and tissue viscosity, causing either local or systemic effects (Schleip, 2003). Moreover, the position of ease may quiet nociceptive input from the worked area to the possibly facilitated spinal level. The consequent reduction of peripheral biochemicals linked to nociception may dampen local edema and lower sympathetic drive, which may have previously encouraged local vasoconstriction and diminished lymphatic flow in the joint involved.

From this perspective, BLT might be considered as belonging to the neurological osteopathic model. According to this model the body is a complex neural network of central, peripheral, and autonomic components. They all need to be assessed to detect any sign of aberrant reflexes, caused by various types of sensitization, or spinal facilitation underlying somatic dysfunction (Van Buskirk, 1990). Manipulative treatment using this model includes techniques that reduce nociception, promote autonomic balance, and reset aberrant reflexes, as with BLT.

Subsequently, during BLT application, a position of balanced tension is achieved. At this stage, the neurological proprioceptive feedback from involved tissues may be kept at a low level while their involuntary motion quietens and generally passes through a still point. A complex interplay between different body rhythms and fluid dynamics may occur at this point, up to when a release is felt. Sutherland himself (1998a) referred to the cranial rhythmic impulse (CRI) as a tide propagating throughout the entire body, including fluids, so as to create an interstitial fluid flow bathing every cell, and this concept has been recently encouraged by research (Chikly & Quaghebeur, 2013). Through this tide, nutrients are carried to cells and wastes are removed away. This motion, referred to as the 'breath of life' (Becker, 1997), is recognized as essential for cellular respiration and metabolism (Magoun, 1976b). In case of dysfunction, the interstitial fluctuation would be impaired. Hence, the pain in the area may result from tissue hypoxia and a build-up of waste products, such as prostaglandins and nitrogenous waste. By appealing to the CRI during BLT application, fluid motion can be restored, function can be regained, and a balanced tissue tension can be re-established. 'If you recognized the real element, the breath of light in the fluctuation of the cerebrospinal fluid, I think you would begin to come closer to the success of Dr. Still in his knowledge of the human body'. (Sutherland, 1998c).

Cellular and fluid exchanges take place within and through the matrix. According to the tensegrity model, the whole body is a three-dimensional visco-elastic matrix, balanced by an integrated system of compressional–tensional forces in dynamic equilibrium. In this vision, bones are the nontouching rods that play the role of compression struts, embedded in a continuous connecting system (the tension system) that is the myofascial ligamentous continuum in the body (Levin, 1990). Such a system exhibits a balanced tension as well as a three-dimensional and dynamic ability to adapt to any force introduced anywhere in the system. Thanks to its hierarchical organization, any force applied can influence any part of the entire system, from cellular to the entire body and vice versa, through a nonlinear distribution of forces. Research has shown that changes in tissue structure may alter the arrangement of the cytoskeleton, which in turn can influence gene expression and cellular metabolism (Chen & Ingber, 1999). For instance, fibroblast strain may set in motion a cascade of events that attenuate proinflammatory effects, while at the same time stimulating anti-inflammatory signaling pathways (Tsuzaki et al., 2003), thus influencing pain perception. A brief, moderate amplitude (20–30% strain) stretching of connective tissue decreases both TGF-ß1 and collagen synthesis, preventing soft tissue adhesions (Bouffard et al., 2008). Therefore, beneficial, light, and balanced strain, such as that applied during a BLT session, may be sensed at the cellular level normalizing tissue structure and function. In this sense, 'BLT is perhaps one of the best examples of how the concept of tensegrity can be applied in treatment' (Parsons & Marcer, 2006). In addition, strain duration and direction seem to play a role in tissue response, as well as strain magnitude, since they both seem to differentially regulate cell growth, ion conductances, and gene expression, responding accordingly with differential stretch-activated calcium channel signaling (Kamkin et al., 2003).

Finally, during the BLT 'balance and hold' phase, the practitioner may request respiratory cooperation. Traditionally, respiration has been used in osteopathic practice to promote patient relaxation, or to divert the patient's attention, but it is also used for assessing and treating cranial, vertebral, appendicular, visceral, and soft tissue dysfunctions, especially in the case of acute presentations (Kimberly, 1949). Also, Sutherland proposed to use it as a specific tool to exaggerate dysfunction and induce correction, as clearly explained by Hoover (1945):

'A given lesion occurs at a certain point in the respiratory cycle and in a certain position. In correction, the related parts are moved to the point of release by slight exaggeration of the lesion as the patient breathes deeply. The release occurs in the position at which the insult to the joint took place and at the point in the respiratory cycle at which the lesion was produced. In that certain position and at that certain point the respiratory movement picks up the abnormally related parts and swings them into motion in unison with contiguous parts.'

Such respiratory contribution may play a role in myofascial relaxation and improvement in joint mobility. In fact, respiration seems to be synchronized with cerebral activity (Busek & Kemlink, 2005) and to produce an effect on myofascial tension (Cummings & Howell, 1990) even on nonrespiratory muscles (Kisselkova & Georgiev, 1979). This makes plausible the influence of respiration on the musculoskeletal system.

Clinical cases

The following case examples represent common clinical presentations. The authors consider these presentations appropriate for a BLT approach.

Clinical case 1: postural repetitive stress

A 43-year-old female secretary presents with cervicogenic headaches (occipital to frontal–bilateral) associated with a slight degree of occasional vertigo and nausea during acute phases, which occur four to six times a month. The patient controls the headaches generally with nonsteroidal anti-inflammatory drugs, and is conscious that the headaches are mainly caused by her sitting working posture and her sedentary life. Osteopathic assessment reveals somatic dysfunction at the cervicodorsal and suboccipital regions, which could explain her symptoms.

Suggested treatment protocol using the BLT approach

The BLT approach should address spinal (thoracic and cervical) mechanics, the upper ribs in order to open her thoracic outlet and increase drainage, and finally the shoulder girdle, which in most patients of this category appears closed and restricted, affecting the mechanics of the head and neck and drainage from the head (Fig. 44.1).

Clinical case 2: sport-related injury and biomechanical adaptation

A 25-year-old amateur soccer player is presenting with repetitive left ankle sprains. He has been treated with rest, ice, and nonsteroidal anti-inflammatory drugs, but since the last acute episode, pain is recurrently felt in the ankle region and lower back during physical activity, which does not allow him to train regularly.

Suggested treatment protocol using the BLT approach

The BLT approach will consider the ligamentous system of the ankle, but inevitably look also at the fibular mechanics; its interosseous membrane; the knee, hip, and pelvis; and the lumbar spine. In light of the repetitive strains, some degree of adaptation involving the whole lower extremity and the pelvis will be clinically relevant. Certainly, specific adjustment of the joints involved might play a fundamental role in the treatment plan, but adaptive responses in the whole ligamentous apparatus will be worth considering (Fig. 44.2).

Clinical case 3: pediatric dysfunction

A three-month-old healthy infant presents with torticollis and a positional plagiocephaly (flat right occiput). Literature (Rogers et al, 2009) has shown the association of positional plagiocephalies and

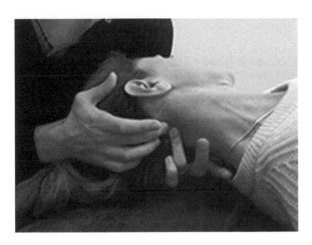

Figure 44.1

Showing the typical contact for a suboccipital BLT technique in an adult, addressing ligamentous articular strain in the suboccipital region. The technique is performed with the patient supine, the head turned in a neutral position and the middle fingers of both hands placed over the suboccipital musculature, creating a lever between the occiput and the first cervical vertebrae. In order to address the different levels, the motion induced through a light movement of the hand can be directed either through flexion and extension for the C0–C1 complex or in rotation for the C1–C2 area

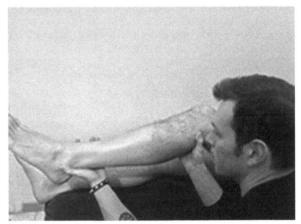

Figure 44.2

Showing the classical hand-hold for the membranous release between the fibula and the tibia. The patient lies supine and the whole weight of the lower leg is taken by the therapist, contacting with the right hand proximally the fibula head and distally the malleoli. Light antagonistic rotational movements of the hands in internal and external rotation will address the membranous tensions

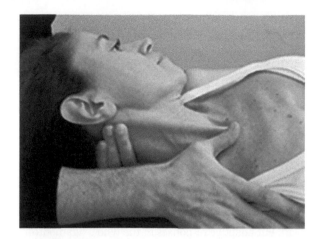

Figure 44.3
Showing the contact at the origin and insertion sites of the sternocleidomastoid muscle (for demonstration purposes the subject shown in the picture is an adult). A slight rotation and side-bending of the head away from the dysfunctional side will engage the muscular tissues and the therapist will address the tissue response by holding the clavicle down and balancing the muscular parts by rotating and side-bending toward the lesion

torticollis, which is a good example of where the BLT approach could be used in order to normalize what W. G. Sutherland called reciprocal tensions. Considering the state of the tissues in an infant, not yet well defined, and mainly consisting of fascial and collagen structures, different regions should be considered while treating the patient.

Suggested treatment protocol using the BLT approach

A possible treatment approach would be to address the suboccipital region, the mandible, and the shoulder girdle with special attention to the clavicle for its insertional importance, besides physiotherapy and specific postural exercises that should be performed regularly (Fig. 44.3).

References

Accorsi, A., Barlafante, G., Cerritelli, F., et al., 2012a. Osteopathic manipulative treatment for knock knee: a case finding. In: Proceedings of the First International Congress of Osteopathy in Animal Practice, Rome, Italy. p. 11. Available at: www.congressodiosteopatia.it/congresso_osteopatia_veterinaria/pdf/atti-congresso.pdf [accessed April 16, 2016].

Accorsi, A., Lucci, C., Pizzolorusso, G., et al., 2012b. Case-report: impact of OMT on biochemical mediators of inflammation. In: Proceedings of the First International Congress of Osteopathy in Animal Practice, Rome, Italy. pp. 10–11. Available at: www.congressodiosteopatia.it/congresso_osteopatia_veterinaria/pdf/atti-congresso.pdf [accessed April 16, 2016].

Becker, R. E., 1990. Foreword. In: Sutherland W. G. *Teachings in the Science of Osteopathy.* Sutherland Cranial Teaching Foundation, Fort Worth, TX.

Becker, R. E., 1997. *Biokinetics and Biodynamics of Human Differentiation: Principles and Applications..* Brooks, R. E. (ed.), Rudra Press, Portland, OR.

Blechschmidt, E., Gasser, R. F., 2012. *Biokinetics and Biodynamics of Human Differentiation: Principles and Applications.* North Atlantic Books, Berkeley.

Bouffard, N. A., Cutroneo, K. R., Badger, G. J., et al., 2008. Tissue stretch decreases soluble TGF β1 and Type-1 pro-collagen in mouse subcutaneous connective tissue: evidence from ex vivo and in vivo models. *J Cell Physiol* 214:389–395.

Busek, P., Kemlink, D., 2005. The influence of the respiratory cycle on the EEG. *Physiol Res* 54: 327–333.

Carreiro, J. E., 2009a. *Pediatric Manual Medicine: An Osteopathic Approach.* Churchill Livingstone Elsevier, Edinburgh. p. 5.

Carreiro, J. E., 2009b. *Pediatric Manual Medicine: An Osteopathic Approach.* Churchill Livingstone Elsevier, Edinburgh.

Cerritelli, F., Carinci, F., Pizzolorusso, G., et al., 2011. Osteopathic manipulation as a complementary treatment for the prevention of cardiac complications: 12-months follow-up of intima media and blood pressure on a cohort affected by hypertension. *J Bodyw Mov Ther*:68–74.

Chen, C. S., Ingber, D. E., 1999. Tensegrity and mechanoregulation: from skeleton to cytoskeleton. *J Osteoarthritis Res Soc Int* 7:81–94.

Chikly, B., Quaghebeur, J., 2013. Reassessing cerebrospinal fluid (CSF) hydrodynamics: a literature review presenting a novel hypothesis for CSF physiology. *J Bodyw Mov Ther* 17:344–354.

Cohen-Lewe, A., 2013. Osteopathic manipulative treatment for colonic inertia. *J Am Osteopath Assoc* 113:216–220.

Crow, W. M. T., 2005. Ligamentous articular strain and balanced ligamentous tension technique. In: DiGiovanna, E. L., Schiowitz, S., Dowling, D. J. (eds), *An Osteopathic Approach to Diagnosis and Treatment.* 3rd Edn., Lippincott Williams & Wilkins, Philadelphia, PA. p. 103.

Crow, W. M. T., 2011. Balanced ligamentous tension and ligamentous articular strain. In: Chila, A. G. (ed.), *Foundations of Osteopathic Medicine.* 3rd Edn., Lippincott Williams & Wilkins, Philadelphia, PA. Ch 52A.

Cummings, J., Howell, J. 1990. The role of respiration in the tension production of myofascial tissues. *J Am Osteopath Assoc* 90:842.

Degenhardt, B. F., Kuchera, M. L., 1996. Update on osteopathic medical concepts and the lymphatic system. *J Am Osteopath Assoc* 96:97–100.

DeStefano, L. A., 2011a. *Greenman's Principles of Manual Medicine.* 4th Edn., Williams and Wilkins, Baltimore, MD. p. 48.

DeStefano, L. A., 2011b. *Greenman's Principles of Manual Medicine.* 4th Edn., Williams and Wilkins, Baltimore, MD. pp. 11–12.

DiGiovanna, E. L., Schiowitz, S., Dowling, D. J. (eds), 2005. *An Osteopathic Approach to Diagnosis and Treatment.* 3rd Edn., Lippincott Williams & Wilkins, Philadelphia, PA. pp. 229; 581; 620.

Fraix, M.P., Seffinger, M.A., 2011. Acute low back pain. In: Chila, A. G. (ed.), *Foundations of Osteopathic Medicine.* 3rd Edn., Lippincott Williams & Wilkins, Philadelphia, PA. Ch. 69.

Fryette, H. H., 1954. *Principles of Osteopathic Technique.* Academy of Applied Osteopathy, Carmel, CA. p. 62.

Gronemeyer, J., Audette, J. F., Drexler, J. H., et al., 2006. Retrospective outcome analysis of osteopathic manipulation in a treatment failure setting. In: 50th Annual AOA Research Conferencwe – Abstracts. *J Am Osteopath Assoc* 106:471–510. C39.

Hoover, H. V., 1945. Use of respiratory movement as an aid in correction of osteopathic spinal lesions. *J Am Osteopath Assoc* 45:109–111.

Hruby, R. J., 1992. Pathophysiologic models and the selection of osteopathic manipulative techniques, *J Osteopath Med* 6:25–30.

Kamkin, A., Kiseleva, I., Isenberg, G., 2003. Activation and inactivation of a non-selective cation conductance by local mechanical deformation of acutely isolated cardiac fibroblasts. *Cardiovasc Res* 57:793–803.

Kaufman, B., 2011. Adult with chronic cardiovascular disease. In: Chila, A.G. (ed.), *Foundations of Osteopathic Medicine.* 3rd Edn., Lippincott Williams & Wilkins, Philadelphia, PA. Ch. 55.

Kimberly, P. E., 1949. The application of the respiratory principle to osteopathic manipulative procedures. *J Am Osteopath Assoc* 48:331–334. Reprinted 2001, *J Am Osteopath Assoc* 101:410–413.

Kimberly, P. E., 1980. Formulating a prescription for osteopathic manipulative treatment. *J Am Osteopath Assoc* 79:506–513.

Kisselkova, H., Georgiev, V., 1979. Effects of training on post-exercise limb muscle EMG synchronous to respiration. *J Appl Physiol Respir Environ Exerc Physiol* 46:1093–1095.

Kuchera, M. L., Kuchera, W. A., 1994. *Osteopathic Principles in Practice.* Greyden Press, Columbus, OH. pp. 298–300.

Kuchera, M. L., 2011a. Lower extremities. In: Chila, A. G. (ed.), *Foundations of Osteopathic Medicine.* 3rd Edn., Lippincott Williams & Wilkins, Philadelphia, PA Ch. 42.

Kuchera, M. L., 2011b. Lymphatics approach. In: Chila, A. G. (ed.), *Foundations of Osteopathic Medicine.* 3rd Edn., Lippincott Williams & Wilkins, Philadelphia, PA Ch. 51.

Levin, S. M., 1990. The myofascial skeletal truss: a system science analysis. In: Barnes, J. F. (ed.), *Myofascial Release.* Rehabilitation Services Inc., Paoli, PA.

Libbey, R., 2012. Ligamentous articular strain technique – a manual treatment approach for ligamentous articular injuries and the whole body. *J Prolother* 4:e886–e890.

Licciardone, J. C., King, H. H., Hensel, K. L., et al., 2008. Osteopathic health outcomes in chronic low back pain: the osteopathic trial. *Osteopath Med Prim Care* 2:5.

Lippincott, H. A., 1949. The osteopathic technique of Wm G. Sutherland DO. In: *Yearbook of the Academy of Applied Osteopathy.* Reprint: American Academy of Osteopathy, Indianapolis, IN.

Lund, G. C., Edwards, G., Medlin, B., et al., 2011. Osteopathic manipulative treatment for the treatment of hospitalized premature infants with nipple feeding dysfunction. *J Am Osteopath Assoc* 111:44–48.

Magoun, H. I., 1976a. *Osteopathy in the Cranial Field.* 3rd Edn. Northwest Printing, Boise, ID. Ch. 5.

Magoun, H. I., 1976b. *Osteopathy in the Cranial Field.* 3rd Edn. Northwest Printing, Boise, ID. Ch. 2.

Modi, R. G., Shah, N. A., 2005. *Complex Review: Clinical Anatomy and Osteopathic Manipulative Medicine.* Blackwell, Malden, MA. Ch. 9–10.

Moeckel, E., Mitha, N., 2008. *Textbook of Pediatric Osteopathy.* Churchill Livingstone, Edinburgh. Ch. 8.

Nicholas, A., Nicholas, E., 2008. *Atlas of Osteopathic Techniques.* 2nd Edn., Lippincott Williams & Wilkins, Philadelphia, PA Ch. 14–16.

O-Yurvati, A. H., Carnes, M. S., Clearfield, M. B., et al., 2005. Hemodynamic effects of osteopathic manipulative treatment immediately after coronary artery bypass graft surgery. *J Am Osteopath Assoc* 105:475–481.

Panjabi, M. M., 2006. A hypothesis of chronic back pain: ligament subfailure injuries lead to muscle control dysfunction. *Eur Spine J* 15:668–676.

Parsons, J., Marcer, N., 2006. *Osteopathy: Models for Diagnosis, Treatment and Practice.* Elsevier Churchill Livingstone, Edinburgh. p. 221.

Pizzolorusso, G., Turi, P., Barlafante, G. et al., 2011. Effect of osteopathic manipulative treatment on gastrointestinal function and length of stay of preterm infants: an exploratory study. *Chiropr Man Therap* 19:15.

Pomykala, M., McElhinney, B., Beck, B. L., et al., 2008. Patient perception of osteopathic manipulative treatment in a hospitalized setting: a survey-based study. *J Am Osteopath Assoc* 108:665–668.

Posadzki, P., Lee, M. S., Ernst, E., 2013. Osteopathic manipulative treatment for pediatric conditions: a systematic review. *Pediatrics* 132:140–152.

Rogers, G. F., Oh, A. K., Mulliken, J. B., 2009. The role of congenital muscular torticollis in the development of deformational plagiocephaly. *Plast Reconstr Surg* 123:643–652.

Schabert, E, Crow, W. T., 2009. Impact of osteopathic manipulative treatment on cost of care for patients with migraine headache: a retrospective review of patient records. *J Am Osteopath Assoc* 109: 403–407.

Schleip, R., 2003. Fascial plasticity – a new neurobiological explanation. Part 1. *J Bodyw Mov Ther* 7:11–19.

Sleszynski, S. L., Glonek, T., 2005. Outpatient osteopathic SOAP note form: preliminary results in osteopathic outcomes-based research. *J Am Osteopath Assoc* 105:181–205.

Solomonow, M., 2009. Ligaments: a source of musculoskeletal disorders. *J Bodyw Mov Ther* 13:136–154.

Speece, C., Crow, T., 2009a. *Ligamentous Articular Strain: Osteopathic Manipulative Techniques for the Body.* Eastland Press, Seattle, WA.

Speece, C., Crow, T., 2009b. *Ligamentous Articular Strain: Osteopathic Manipulative Techniques for the Body.* Eastland Press, Seattle, WA. p.24.

Steele, K. M., Viola, J., Burns, E. et al., 2010. Brief report of a clinical trial on the duration of middle ear effusion in young children using a standardized osteopathic manipulative medicine protocol. *J Am Osteopath Assoc* 110:278–284.

Sutherland, W. G., 1998a. Contributions of thought. In: Sutherland, A. S., Wales, A. L. (eds.), *The Collected Writings of William Garner Sutherland, D.O.* 2nd Edn., The Sutherland Cranial Teaching Foundation, Yakima, WA.

Sutherland, W. G., 1998b. Contributions of thought. In: Sutherland, A. S., Wales, A. L. (eds.), *The Collected Writings of William Garner Sutherland, D.O.* 2nd Edn. The Sutherland Cranial Teaching Foundation, Yakima, WA. p. 160.

Sutherland, W. G., 1998c. Contributions of thought. In: Sutherland, A. S., Wales, A. L. (eds.), *The Collected Writings of William Garner Sutherland, D.O.* 2nd Edn. The Sutherland Cranial Teaching Foundation, Yakima, WA. p. 291.

Tettambel, M. A., 2005. An osteopathic approach to treating women with chronic pelvic pain. *J Am Osteopath Assoc* 105:S20–22.

Threlkeld, J., 1992. The effects of manual therapy on connective tissue. *Phys Ther* 72:893–902.

Tsuzaki, M., Bynum, D., Almekinders, L., et al., 2003. ATP modulates load-inducible IL-1beta, COX 2, and MMP-3 gene expression in human tendon cells. *J Cell Biochem* 89:556–562.

Van Buskirk, R. L 1990 Nociceptive reflexes and the somatic dysfunction: a model. *J Am Osteopath Assoc* 90:792–805.

van der Wal, J., 2009. The architecture of the connective tissue in the musculoskeletal system – an often overlooked functional parameter as to proprioception in the locomotor apparatus. *Int J Ther Massage Bodywork* 2:9–23.

Willard, F. H., 1997. The muscular, ligamentous and neural structure of the low back and its relation to back pain. In: Vleeming, A., Mooney, V., Snijders, C. J., et al. (eds), *Movement, Stability and Low Back Pain: The Essential Role of the Pelvis.* Churchill Livingstone, Edinburgh.

Wood Jones, F., 1944. *Structure and Function as Seen in the Foot.* Baillière, Tindall and Cox, London.

World Health Organization (WHO), 2010. Safety issues. In: Benchmarks for training in osteopathy, WHO, Geneva, Switzerland. pp. 17.

Zink, J. G., 1977. Respiratory and circulatory care: the conceptual model. *Osteopath Ann* 5:108-112.

FASCIAL MANIPULATION® AND THE BIOMECHANICAL MODEL OF THE HUMAN FASCIAL SYSTEM

Julie A. Day, Carla Stecco, Antonio Stecco

Overview

Fascial Manipulation® is a manual method for the treatment of musculoskeletal and visceral fasciae dysfunctions. This chapter focuses on the biomechanical model applied in the interpretation of musculoskeletal fascial dysfunctions. There is growing consensus that efficient activity of joints, muscles, tendons, and internal organs requires a normal, functioning fascial system. This interpretative model, developed by physiotherapist Luigi Stecco, incorporates the fascial system as an active component of the musculoskeletal system. It represents a simplification of fascial complexity, a type of beginner's guide to the human fascial system. Nevertheless, it is the basis for a variety of research projects in the fields of anatomy, physiology, and clinical studies.

Introduction

The three-dimensional structure of the fascial system and its extensiveness throughout the entire body makes clinical interpretation of dysfunction particularly complex. While numerous studies implicate fascia as the tissue primarily involved in myofascial pain, fascial continuity is not always addressed from an anatomical and functional perspective. Taking into account the relationship between deep fascia, muscles, and the peripheral nervous system, Luigi Stecco has drawn on his clinical experience to develop a biomechanical model to assist therapists in the interpretation of fascial dysfunctions. This model is applied in the manual method known as Fascial Manipulation®.

History

A physiotherapist since 1973, Luigi Stecco has always divided his time between study and clinical practice.

To elaborate his model for the interpretation of fascial dysfunctions, Stecco compared numerous anatomy texts, gleaning from them what little information was available about fascial anatomy at the time. Comparing myofascial trigger points and acupuncture theory, he also explored musculoskeletal system development in different species, from the simpler forms of life to human embryology.

He reached the conclusion that to understand the human fascial system as an integral part of the musculoskeletal system it was necessary to break away from standardized teachings. Considering movement only in terms of muscles with origins and insertions that move bones was no longer a valid option.

His theories were first published in Italian in 1990 (Stecco, 1990). The first English translation of one of his texts was published in 2004 (Stecco, 2004).

Clinically, Stecco recorded pain patterns correlated with movement impairments and developed palpatory tests to identify altered deep fascia in specific areas (Stecco & Stecco, 2009).

Anatomical and histological studies based on Stecco's theories have subsequently led to a better understanding of the characteristics of deep fascia and its regional differences.

Anatomical studies

Dissections of unembalmed cadavers have demonstrated that biarticular muscles extend important myotendinous expansions of their deep fascia well beyond any bony insertion of the same muscle, forming a continuum between deep fascia in contiguous segments. In the upper limb, for example, apart from the well-known lacertus fibrosus (biceps brachialis' myotendinous expansion onto the antebrachial fascia), the latissimus dorsi, deltoid, triceps brachialis, and extensor carpi ulnaris are other examples of muscles that extend myotendinous expansions onto the deep fascia of neighboring segments (Stecco, et al., 2007a).

Deep fasciae of the limbs, the thoracolumbar fascia, and the abdominis rectus sheath have aponeurotic-type features. Aponeurotic-type fasciae have a strong resistance to traction even when tensioned in different directions, and they exhibit minimal adaptation to stretch (Stecco et al., 2009b).

The superficial trunk muscles, pectoralis major, latissimus dorsi, deltoid, and gluteus maximus muscles have developed within the superficial layer of deep fascia and are segmented by numerous intermuscular septa. Deep fascia in these areas could be considered a type of epimysial fascia (Stecco et al. 2009a).

Histological studies

Histological studies have shown that fiber content of deep fascia consists of undulated collagen fibers and elastic fibers, with their relative percentages varying from region to region. Aponeurotic-type fasciae consist of two to three sublayers of parallel collagen fiber bundles. Fiber bundles within adjacent sublayers are orientated in different directions, forming angles between 75°–80° (Stecco et al., 2008). Each sublayer has a mean thickness of $277\,\mu m$ ($\pm$ SD 86.1 μm) and sublayers are separated by a thin layer of loose connective tissue (mean thickness $43 \pm 12\,\mu m$), permitting individual sublayers to slide independently (Benetazzo et al., 2011).

Hyaluronic acid (HA) is a primary element of the extracellular matrix (ECM) of loose connective tissue and its concentration determines the density of these sublayers. HA is thermosensitive, readily responding to local increases in temperature (Stecco et al., 2011). This aspect and its physiological implications will be discussed later in this chapter (see the section on 'Possible physiological mechanisms').

Lastly, deep fascia is well innervated with mechanoreceptors and free nerve endings. Furthermore, the capsules of Pacini and Ruffini corpuscles, muscle spindles, and Golgi tendon organs are continuous with epimysium and perimysium (Stecco et al., 2007b), suggesting that deep fascia has the potential to affect proprioception and motor control (Stecco et al., 2010).

The biomechanical model

The scope of Stecco's biomechanical model is to simplify analysis of the fascial system while introducing its functional role within the musculoskeletal system. Originally orientated toward the relationship between acupuncture meridians and fascial continuity, Stecco later realized that by dividing the body into 14 segments (Fig. 45.1) he could distinguish what he called six myofascial units (MFU) for each segment (Stecco, 2004).

He reasoned that:

- The motor cortex does not plan or execute movement in terms of muscles with origins and insertions, but mostly in terms of direction, angles and intention of movement.

- Each joint is moved by a varying combination of motor units being activated within monoarticular and biarticular muscles.

Therefore, each MFU consists of:

- motor units that activate muscle fibers pertaining to biarticular and monoarticular muscles that work together to move a body segment in a specific direction

- the joint that is part of each MFU (where movement occurs)

- the nerve (afferents, efferents) and vascular components

- the fascia that connects all these components together.

The majority of our daily activities consist of rapid, selective activation of motor units within muscles in different segments, rather than the activation of entire muscles. Motor units activate muscle fibers that are not always adjacent to one another and can even be located in different muscles. Changing degrees of force and precision during any given movement govern motor unit activation. The intramuscular fascial components (epimysium, perimysium, endomysium) form a type of fascial skeleton that unites nonadjacent muscle fibers.

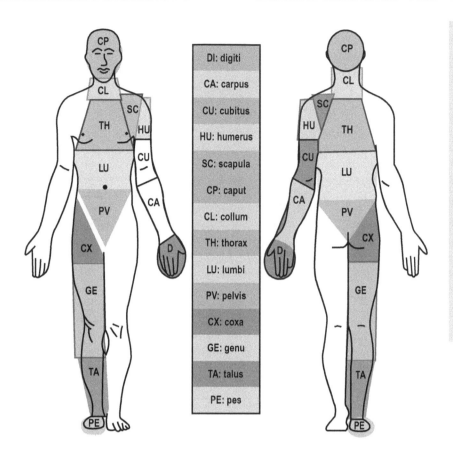

DI: digiti	
CA: carpus	
CU: cubitus	
HU: humerus	
SC: scapula	
CP: caput	
CL: collum	
TH: thorax	
LU: lumbi	
PV: pelvis	
CX: coxa	
GE: genu	
TA: talus	
PE: pes	

Figure 45.1

Fourteen body segments. As each segment comprises joint(s), portions of muscles that move the joint(s), and the fascia surrounding these muscle fibers, Luigi Stecco chose to use Latin terms to describe these segments. Reproduced with permission from Chapter 9 of *Fascial Dysfunction – Manual Therapy Approaches*, edited by Leon Chaitow, 2014, Handspring Publishing

By studying muscle conformation and their tensional vectors, Stecco realized that whenever muscle fibers within a MFU are activated to bring about movement, tension could be conveyed via this intramuscular fascial skeleton to a specific location on the deep fascia. He called these small focal areas on the deep fascia 'centers of coordination' (CC) and was able to map a CC for each MFU. CCs form within the deep fascia because, partially, it:

- inserts onto bone

- is free to glide over the muscle

- is tensioned, both by insertions of muscle into fascia and of fascia onto muscle.

Stecco reasoned that the interpretation of movement impairment could be simplified by considering movements on the three planes (sagittal, horizontal, and frontal), and promptly designated new terms to describe movement solely in terms of direction (Table 45.1).

MFUs that work in a specific direction on a spatial plane connect to one another via their biarticular muscle component and the associated myotendinous expansions that extend from one segment to the next.

Sagittal plane	Frontal plane	Horizontal plane
Antemotion – all forward movements	Lateromotion – all outward movements	Extrarotation – all outward rotatory movements
Retromotion – all backward movements	Mediomotion – all movements towards the midline	Intrarotation – all inward rotatory movements

Table 45.1

New terms used by Luigi Stecco to describe movement on spatial planes

These connections between unidirectional MFUs form the myofascial sequences (MF sequences). Given that the majority of our activities are multisegmental, MF sequences help to coordinate the various body segments during movement.

Normally, the continuous flux of muscle fibers contracting and relaxing during movement stimulates muscle spindles, Golgi tendon organs, and other mechanoreceptors embedded within muscular fascia to provide accurate feedback and assist regulation between agonist and antagonist MFUs and their respective sequences.

Stecco identified other areas he called 'centers of fusion' (CF), where tensional vectors from several MFUs converge. Mostly located over retinacular structures, CFs are involved in coordinating the transition of movement from one plane to another.

If the deep fascia that envelops, divides, and unites muscle fibers of an MFU is gliding correctly, then activation of embedded receptors provides accurate topographical feedback to the central nervous system (CNS) and movement is harmonious, coordinated, and effective. Lack of gliding within the deep fascia around CCs and CFs could potentially alter afferent information, either modifying muscle fiber recruitment or disrupting fiber activation altogether. Consequently, unaligned tension on the joint of the MFU initially causes adaptation and, if uncorrected, triggers pain in a specific region around the joint. Stecco calls these regions 'centers of perception' (CP) because this is where movement occurring at the joint is perceived. Characteristically, the CC of a MFU is at a distance from its respective CP.

In summary, MFUs and MF sequences are functional concepts that have an anatomical substratum of fascial continuity via:

- continuity of fascia with mechanoreceptors
- muscular insertions onto fascia
- myotendinous expansions of muscular fascia from one segment to another.

Instead of considering muscles as individual entities, these concepts introduce a functional interpretation of myofascial-skeletal physiology.

Aims and objectives of the Fascial Manipulation® method

The Fascial Manipulation® method for musculoskeletal dysfunctions aims to restore coordination and harmony of movement by normalizing the deep fascia in key areas (CCs and CFs). As deep fascia lies below the hypodermis, manual therapists are able to palpably perceive lack of gliding in this tissue.

Stecco calls these alterations 'densifications.' Densification is due to increased viscosity of loose connective tissue within fascia. It indicates an altered chemical state of the tissue's ECM and potentially signifies dysfunction within corresponding MFUs. Densification can lead to fascial fibrosis, an alteration of the collagen fibrous bundles (Pavan, et al., 2014).

Therefore, in reference to the biomechanical model, therapists analyze the spread of tension in each individual case, in order to identify the correct combination of CC/CFs that require treatment.

Modality of assessment

Stecco has devised a particular assessment chart for Fascial Manipulation® (Stecco & Stecco, 2009), where therapists use abbreviations to annotate information, including the patient's history and their presenting symptoms.

When acquiring the patient's history, therapists focus on the sequence of traumatic events or, in the absence of trauma, the development of pain and limitation. A previous problem that is no longer causing pain or limitation can frequently be the cause of a presenting acute pain, because the fascia often responds to trauma by developing a 'densification'. Once established, this localized lack of glide may be neutralized via compensatory tension along an MF sequence. Therefore, chronology can help the therapist to understand where and when musculoskeletal dysfunctions have developed and how they have progressed.

Even minor painful areas are useful in indicating a disturbed sequence or plane. Information such as paresthesia or pain in the extremities, traumas with a nonphysiological healing time, and/or the presence of scarring are also considered.

An accurate compilation of the assessment chart helps therapists to select the correct combination of CC/CFs to treat. The chart also provides concise documentation of treatment sessions.

The therapist formulates a preliminary hypothesis by considering:

- On which plane have the various compensations developed?

- What was the initial trauma or dysfunction that determined these compensations?

- Do these compensations ascend or descend along an MF sequence?

- Are there any hidden compensatory strategies?

For example, if all of the concomitant symptoms are distributed in:

- the lateral and/or medial part of the body, then a disturbance on the frontal plane may be hypothesized

- in the anterior and/or posterior region, then a sagittal plane dysfunction may be hypothesized, and so forth.

The assessment process involves movement and palpation assessments. Based on their hypothesis, therapists examine a maximum of three body segments, using codified movement tests to identify any faulty or painful movements on the three spatial planes. Following palpation of selected segments, a treatment plan is carried out and retesting of movement is performed immediately after treatment to evaluate outcome.

Principles and method of application

During palpation assessment, the most indicated areas for treatment are CCs and CFs that are painful, densified, and produce referral of pain. The sum of the densified areas in different segments indicates the most compromised plane of movement. Therapists treat only densified areas and in a balanced combination (e.g., on one plane – sagittal, horizontal, or frontal).

Treatment involves a deep, kneading massage over selected CC/CFs, using knuckles, elbows (Fig. 45.2) and sometimes fingertips to apply pressure while maintaining a tangential oscillatory movement. The application of a three-dimensional mathematical model to explore the relationship between different manual therapy motions on fascial layers suggests that tangential, oscillatory movement and

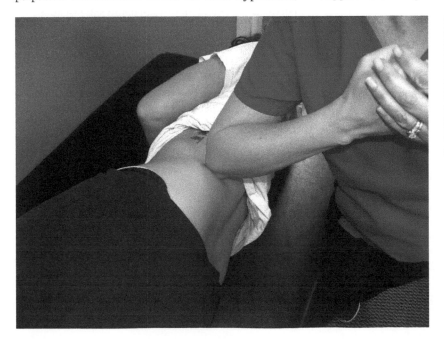

Figure 45.2
Example of treatment using the elbow on the center of coordination (CC) for the lateromotion myofascial unit (MFU) in the lumbar segment

Table 45.2
Relative contraindications and adaptations for Fascial Manipulation® treatment

Condition	Adaptations for treatment
Acute edema or tendinitis	Work above or below the inflamed/swollen area
Lymphedema	The superficial fascia technique is more indicated
Recent trauma without diagnosis	Consider red flags
Oncological patient	Consult with oncologist for approval prior to treatment
Severe bleeding disorder	Use a lighter pressure
Corticosteroid therapy	Be aware that post-treatment reactions can be dampened
Severe immunodeficiency	Use lighter pressure to avoid overstressing the system

perpendicular vibration may increase the action of the treatment in the ECM (Roman et al., 2013).

Treatment is carried out over each densified area for several minutes. Friction against the fascia produces heat, which is necessary to modify the consistency of the ECM and initiate the process required for healing. In one study of the application of Fascial Manipulation® in 40 subjects (Ercole et al., 2010) an average of 3.24 minutes was required for palpable changes to occur in densified tissues. These changes have also been documented by ultrasound and elastography (Luomala et al., 2014).

Indications and contraindications

The key indication for the Fascial Manipulation® method is pain or lack of mobility within the fascial network due to impairment of its sliding system. This can include musculoskeletal problems such as temporomandibular joint dysfunctions, myotensive headaches, acute torticollis, whiplash-associated disorders, low back pain due to lumbar discopathy or lumbar facet pain, piriformis syndrome, coccydynia, patellar femoral misalignment, chronic ankle sprain sequels, post-fracture stiffness, plantar fasciitis, rotator cuff tendinitis, epicondylitis, and carpal tunnel syndrome.

Fever is a contraindication to treatment as the body is already in an inflamed state and treatment creates ulterior, although localized, inflammation. Skin lesions in the region of the CC/CF are a limitation to treatment. Furthermore, therapists should avoid applying this approach in an area with recent history of deep vein thrombosis. Some relative contraindications necessitate appropriate therapeutic adaptations (Table 45.2).

Possible physiological mechanisms

The physiological mechanisms involved in this treatment modality are related to the histological structure of deep fascia. With collagen fibers organized in multiple layers, each sublayer being orientated in a different direction, a thin film of loose connective tissue separates each sublayer, ensuring interlayer gliding. The ECM of loose connective tissue, and between the collagen fibers of epimysial fascia, is rich in hyaluronic acid (HA) (Stecco et al., 2011). HA is a hydrating, space-filling polymer that acts as a lubricant, allowing fascia to slide smoothly over muscle fibers and tendons. However, aggregation of HA, which occurs in pathological conditions, reduces its lubricating properties by increasing viscosity. Such aggregation tends to occur particularly on thin, flat surfaces, such as fascial sheaths or sublayers. The presence of lactic acid, which lowers the pH of the tissue, can facilitate this phenomenon. Deep manual friction is one method that can increase tissue temperature and produce local alkalinization, reversing HA aggregation by setting off a self-resolving inflammatory reaction, which is a particular characteristic of the HA molecule. This provides the physiological and biochemical explanation for perceivable changes in altered deep fascia during manual treatment (Stecco et al., 2013).

References

Benetazzo L., Bizzego A., De Caro R., Frigo G., Guidolin D., Stecco C. 2011. 3D reconstruction of the crural and thoracolumbar fasciae. *Surg Radiol Anat.* 33(10):855-862.

Ercole B., Stecco A., Day J. A. D., Stecco C. 2010. How much time is required to modify a fascial fibrosis? *J Bodyw Mov Ther.* 14(4):318-325.

Luomala T., Pihlman M., Heiskanen J., Stecco C. 2014. Case study: could ultrasound and elastography visualized densified areas inside the deep fascia? *J Bodyw Mov Ther.* 18(3):462-468.

Pavan P. G., Stecco A., Stern R., Stecco C. 2014. Painful connections: densification versus fibrosis of fascia. *Curr Pain Headache Rep.* 18(8):441.

Roman M., Chaudhry H., Bukiet B., Stecco A., Findley T. W., 2013. Mathematical analysis of the flow of hyaluronic acid around fascia during manual therapy motions. *J Am Osteopath Assoc.* 113(8):600-610.

Stecco L. 1990. *Il Dolore e le sequenze neuro-mio-fasciali.* Palermo: IPSA.

Stecco L. 2004. *Fascial Manipulation for Musculoskeletal Pain.* **Padova: Piccin.**

Stecco C., Gagey O., Belloni A., Pozzuoli A., Porzionato A., Macchi V., Aldegheri R., De Caro R., Delmas, V. 2007b. Anatomy of the deep fascia of the upper limb. Second part: study of innervation. *Morphologie.* 91(292):38-43.

Stecco C., Gagey O., Macchi V., Porzionato A., De Caro R., Aldegheri R., Delmas V. 2007a. Tendinous muscular insertions onto the deep fascia of the upper limb. First part: anatomical study. *Morphologie.* 91(292): 29-37.

Stecco A., Gesi M., Stecco C., Stern R. 2013. Fascial components of the myofascial pain syndrome. *Curr Pain Headache Rep.* 17(8):352.

Stecco A., Macchi V., Masiero S., Porzionato A., Tiengo C., Stecco C., Delmas V., De Caro R. 2009a. Pectoral and femoral fasciae: common aspects and regional specializations. *Surg Radiol Anat.* 31(1):35-42.

Stecco C., Macchi V., Porzionato A., Morra A., Parenti A., Stecco A., Delmas V., De Caro R. 2010. The ankle retinacula: morphological evidence of the proprioceptive role of the fascial system. *Cells Tissues Organs.* 192 (3):200-210.

Stecco C., Pavan P. G., Porzionato A., Macchi V., Lancerotto L., Carniel E. L., Natali A. N., De Caro R. 2009b. Mechanics of crural fascia: from anatomy to constitutive modelling. *Surg Radiol Anat.* 31(7): 523-529.

Stecco C., Porzionato A., Lancerotto L., Stecco A., Macchi V., Day J. A., De Caro R. J. 2008. Histological study of the deep fasciae of the limbs. *J Bodyw Mov Ther.* 12 (3):225-230.

Stecco L., Stecco C. 2009. *Fascial Manipulation: Practical Part.* Padova: Piccin.

Stecco C., Stern R., Porzionato A., Macchi V., Masiero S., Stecco A., De Caro R. 2011. Hyaluronan within fascia in the etiology of myofascial pain. *Surg Radiol Anat.* 33(10):891–896.

CLINICAL INTEGRATION OF FASCIAL APPROACHES

Christian Fossum

'How many times must I tell you neither osteopathy nor its application to the patient can be passed around on a platter. It cannot be given to you with the "How to Use" instruction card attached to the handle. Its application to the patient must be given by reason and not by rule; you delve and dig for it yourself, or you do not get it at all'.

H. H. Gravett (1954)

'A senior colleague with whom I discussed the first draft of this editorial commented: "It's as a patient that I never want to meet such a person as a "doc-in-a-box". Indeed it is my biggest fear about the long-term consequences of QOF (quality outcomes framework): that it produces doctors who don't think, and in the end who can't think'.

D. Mant (2009)

Introduction

The past decade has seen a renewed interest from basic scientists and clinicians coming together to debate the known, the speculative, and the unknown in the current knowledge and understanding of the connective tissue or the fascia of the human body. The possible implications of this tissue complex in surgery, medicine, manipulative and body-based practices, sports, and fitness have been widely discussed (Findley & Schleip, 2007; Hujing et al., 2009; Schleip et al., 2012). In the manipulative and body-based practices, practical interest in the fascia dates back to the early days of the osteopathic profession and the preoccupations of A. T. Still (1828–1917) with this complex tissue of the body, which he considered the anatomical repository for the regulation of health (Still, 1899, 1902a; Lever, 2013). Limited by a nineteenth-century understanding of anatomy, physiology, and biochemistry, he did not detail the mechanics of this. At the time much of the knowledge concerning the structure and function of these tissues was as yet unknown, unexplained, or unexplored, so it should come as no surprise that Still's references to the fascia did not convey the intended idea to his listeners (Becker, 1947). More recently, several of his views have been reviewed and discussed in the context of history (Stark, 2006) and current knowledge. These include views on fascial coverings; fascia and sliding; fascia and fluid flow; fascia and respiration; and innervation of fascia (Findley & Shalwala, 2013). Central to Still's tenets was the integrity of the musculoskeletal system, the nervous system and the body fluids, all of which he considered to be of great importance in the maintenance and expression of function, health, and natural immunity (Deason, 1934; Korr, 1979). These considerations have for the past century served as a source of inspiration in the development of multiple metanarratives underpinning various manipulative approaches to the fascia.

The objective of this chapter is not to provide a state-of-the art review of current knowledge of the fascia based on research, nor does it seek to engage in the tension existing between clinical practice, experience, and evidence-based medicine. It is to outline a didactical, practical, and integrated approach to the fascial system based on the principles embraced by the osteopathic profession.

Principles and models of manipulative care

Osteopathy started on the premise that variations from the normal in the supporting structures of the body, including bones, ligaments, muscles, and fascia, and the related neural, vascular, and lymphatic elements, would lower the body's resistance to physical trauma, illness, and disease. Unlike the emerging etiological medicine of the nineteenth century, osteopathy did not limit itself to focusing on a single causality but viewed the patient from a multidimensional perspective, emphasizing the somatic component of disease. Combining functional thinking with manipulative skills, it constructed a concept centered on the role of the patient and his or her musculoskeletal system in healthful function, where the musculoskeletal system was seen as the interface between environmental factors and the internal physiology or milieu of the patient (Hoover, 1963). Practically, the somatic components were viewed as accessible, specific, responsive, and effective levers provided for and embodied in the manipulative care of patients, restoring the functional capacity of the organism (Korr, 1979). This thinking translated into a system of general practice that was person-focused or oriented and continuous rather than episodic, and that integrated a multidimensional understanding of illness, promoted health as a resource for living, and developed into a primary healthcare vision.

It may seem futile to abstract this philosophy of health care to a series of principles, but these may provide a rational starting point for discussing the models underpinning an integrated approach to the fascial system. They are:

- The body is a unit: the dynamic interaction between body, mind, and spirit.

- The reciprocal relationship between structure and function.

- The role of the body fluids in health and disease.

- The orchestrated and integrated function of the somatomotor, the autonomic and the neuroendocrine immune systems.

- The body is capable of self-regulation and self-healing in the face of dysfunction, illness, and disease.

From a clinical reasoning perspective, these principles alone do not inform the practical approaches to the problems presented by the patient, so they are seen in the context of the pathophysiological models used for problem-solving in osteopathic practice:

- the biomechanical–postural model

- the neurological–autonomic nervous system model

- the respiratory–circulatory model

- the metabolic model

- the behavioral model.

The common denominator through the models is the musculoskeletal system, which comprises approximately 60 per cent of the total body mass, and which is viewed in osteopathic theory and methods to be directly or indirectly involved with most pathophysiological processes occurring in the body. Through it we interact with our environment, and it functions by maintaining proper communication with and orchestrating its function with the somatomotor, autonomic, and neuroendocrine-immune systems. Thus, the musculoskeletal system is not just something we have, it is a large part of what we actually are, and it is by and through it that we recognize our existence in the world. Extending beyond the musculoskeletal system, the body is a living organism or system that has a remarkable capacity to rearrange itself through patterns of self-organization or adaptation, unless disturbances or forces acting upon it interfere with its continued existence, causing the system to become incoherent. Through this view, health therefore implies continual activity or change, reflecting the organism's creative responses to both internal and environmental challenges. These are multidimensional processes including the interaction between the body and the larger systems in which it is embedded, including the musculoskeletal system. Thus, health is a process, which depends on the body's flexibility or adaptability. Traditionally, osteopathy and osteopathic medicine have been an ecological way of uniting the internal biology and psychology, the external environment and the functioning patient into a unit that lives healthfully, if given the opportunity through successful adaptation. Figure 46.1 illustrates the pathophysiological models used for problem-solving in osteopathic practice.

Embodied in the osteopathic understanding of health and disease and its approach to patient-oriented care are the concepts of *integration* and *adaptation*. In its most naive forms, integration is the body as a unit, the dynamic interaction of body, mind, and spirit, and the aim of care is physiological and psychophysiological integration or 'giving the body back to itself' by improving exteroception and interoception. This is closely related to the orchestrated function of the somatomotor, the autonomic, and the neuroendocrine immune systems (Jänig 2014) (Fig. 46.2). Adaptation is the ability of the body to meet the demands of internal and external stress by having the reserves to make continuous short-term adjustments to the stress it is being subjected to (allostasis). The concept of adaptation extends the 'self' as a biological and psychophysiological entity into the environment and its ecology. Thus, addressing and targeting allostatic load, or the compounding effect of stress, which in traditional terms has been called the 'total osteopathic lesion' (the sum total of all mechanical, physiological, and psychological tensions) is essential to the management plan (Box 46.1).

Box 46.1

Total osteopathic lesion

The term 'total osteopathic lesion' shares similarities with other descriptive models, such as the general adaptation syndrome described by Selye in the 1950s, the biopsychosocial model described by Engel in the 1970s, and allostasis and allostatic load described by McEwen in the 1990s. It dates back to early osteopathic interpretations of 'adjustment,' or the adaptation of the patient to his or her structure, function, and environment through clinical intervention (Comstock, 1928).

To make this more understandable, this can be organized in a matrix where *principles* and *concepts* are interrelated and situated within the *salutogenic* framework (see Fig. 46.1). The salutogenic model of health, first proposed by Antonovsky (1987; 1996), deals with the individual's sense of coherence, and how culture, social forces, social positions, gender, ethnicity, genetics, and even plain luck influence one's life situation and sense of coherence. This emphasizes the role of culture in shaping life situations, giving rise to stressors and resources, contributing to life experiences of predictability, load balance, and meaningful

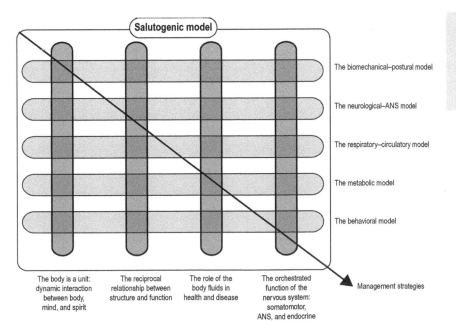

Figure 46.1

The osteopathic matrix. ANS = autonomic nervous system

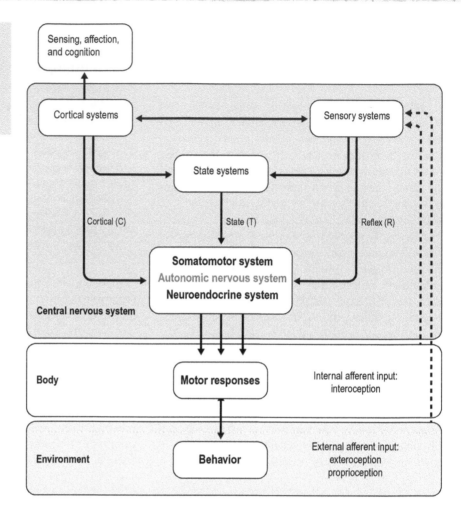

Figure 46.2
Functional organization of the nervous system to generate protective behavior

roles, facilitating the development of a sense of coherence, and shaping perceptions of health and well-being (Benz et al., 2014).

Moving back to patient management involving manipulative care, this should be more than a search-and-destroy mission for somatic dysfunction. Some rationale for therapy is required. The pathophysiologic or conceptual models described in the osteopathic literature serve as problem-solving tools allowing a multidimensional view of the patient and the clinical problem at hand, informing the appropriate course of action.

While the clinician may concentrate on the process using one model at a time, a therapeutic intervention and outcome will cross several models simultaneously. Each one of them helps specify the short- and long-term management goals and, based on this, combined with

the clinical presentation, the appropriate manipulative techniques are chosen to manage the case at hand. This modeling process, along with the knowledge of the principles of various types of manipulative techniques, can help to make the management of the somatic components of the presentation more effective, and identify additional strategies (nutritional, exercise, stress reduction, cognitive behavioral therapy, etc.).

The biomechanical–postural model

This model examines the interplay between local, regional, and global myofascial and articular biomechanical function, postural adaptation, and sensorimotor integration.

Through the lens of this model, the musculoskeletal system is the 'primary machinery of life', and the ability of the individual to repair damage and maintain healthy function is inextricably related to the biophysical efficiency of tissues and the related vascular, lymphatic, and neural processes. This model is not based on the premise of anatomical symmetry, but optimal organization of body mass and functions around an individual's central gravity line as a property of biomechanics and the physiology of postural control.

The respiratory–circulatory model

The physiological premise for this model is the efficiency of external respiration, the movement of body fluids, and, through this, the internal respiration throughout the body contributing to tissue repair and homeostasis. These principles are applied in treating the body using respiratory hydrodynamics, to achieve well-being.

The neurological model

Traditionally the autonomic nervous system and the spinal cord as 'organizer of disease processes' has been the central axis in this model, with its physiological and clinical expression through the considerations of viscerosomatic and somatovisceral reflex activity. A more contemporary view considers the integrated and orchestrated function of the somatomotor, autonomic, and neuroendocrine immune systems as central to health and well-being. This is also more aligned with physiological views from allostasis, allostatic load, and psychoneuroimmunology.

Discussion of the *metabolic model* and the *behavioral model* is beyond the scope of this chapter, and the reader is referred to other texts for information (Chila, 2011).

The models and the fascial system

Although the fasciae do not belong to a particular domain of body functions, three of the models discussed above are representative of the integrated view of the fascial system in this chapter:

- The fascia as an ectoskeleton: the biomechanical–postural model.
- The fascia as a hydrodynamic skeleton: the respiratory–circulatory model.
- The fascia as a receptoskeleton: the neurological model.

The fascia as an ectoskeleton

Myofascial and fascial continuity, and continuity through tendons and ligaments, blending with the periosteum, creates a 'bone–fascia–tendon system', a continuous soft-tissue skeleton that enables us to better understand the biomechanical functions of the fascia. The term 'ectoskeleton' was coined by Wood Jones in the early 1940s to capture the idea of this soft-tissue skeleton created by the compartment-forming fascia, complementing the bony skeleton, serving as a significant site of muscle attachment, and participating in myofascial force transmission. This ectoskeletal view, especially of the deep fascia, emphasizes the importance of tensile forces, both in force generation and force transmission, in biomechanical function. Furthermore, it is also important in the coordination of motion between various body segments, acting as a mechanical link. Thus, the model of the fascia as an 'ectoskeleton' gives anatomical and biomechanical plausibility to viewing the human body and its musculoskeletal system as a unit of function (Benjamin, 2009).

The fascia as a hydrodynamic skeleton

Based on the idea of natural immunity and resistance and the body being capable of self-regulation and self-healing, several generalizations were made in early osteopathy. One of them was pertaining to the role of the body fluids in health and disease, emphasizing the importance of tissue elimination by means of veins and the lymphatics, and unimpeded supply through the arterial end of the circulatory system. The fascia and the fascial system, and the role played by it in either aiding or obstructing elimination from cells and tissues, was given much attention (Deason, 1934), and it was viewed by Still as the anatomical repository for the regulation of health (Still, 1899, 1902a; Lever, 2013).

The role of the deep fascia and muscles in aiding venous and lymphatic return has been well described in the literature, and is based on a sound understanding of the anatomy of both the venous and the deep fascial system (Meissner et al., 2007; Benjamin, 2009). Vessels also travel in loose fibroelastic fascial tissue, and larger companion vessels are wrapped in protective sleeves by dense fascia (Becker, 1975), the fascia thus acting as vascular and lymphatic passageways. Altered tension through the fascia can either aid or obstruct movements of fluids.

Organization of the fascial system

In the integrated model of the fascia (the ectoskeleton, the hydrodynamic skeleton, and the receptoskeleton), the fascia can be illustrated through two main organizations:

• longitudinal organization

• horizontal organization.

The longitudinal organization can be viewed as a continuity from the cranial base to the pelvic floor, where the fascia is reciprocally structured as concentric rings (Willard et al., 2010). This is also continuous with the fascia of the upper and lower extremities. To illustrate this principle, the cervical region is a good example. A transverse cut through this region would show these concentric rings creating the vertebral compartment (the prevertebral fascia), the visceral compartment (the visceral fascia), the vascular compartment (the carotid sheath), and an external musculofascial collar (the superficial fascia) (Fig. 46.3). This organization creates compartments and fascial spaces for muscle, viscera, nerves, and vascular and lymphatic structures, and it maintains the mechanical, neural, and vascular integrity of the cervical region (Levitt, 1970; Hamilton, 1976; Parviz, 2011). Similar organizations, to a lesser extent, are found in the endothoracic, endoabdominal, and endopelvic regions (Willard et al., 2010).

This longitudinal organization is intersected with the horizontal organization, commonly referred to as the 'four diaphragms', terms that are somewhat misleading, as we are not talking about single structures horizontally dividing and creating borders for the body cavities. The term 'diaphragm' in this model is more a metaphor for an anatomical space with multiple structures rather than a single structure, and is associated with the transitional areas of the axial spine and pelvis. See Table 46.1 for an overview of the horizontal organization of the fascial system.

This modeling of fascial organization enables us to develop a practical approach to integrate the fascial system with musculoskeletal, respiratory, circulatory, and neural functions, as discussed later in this chapter. As for the specific anatomy of the longitudinally

Diaphragm	Anatomical space	Connecting tubes
Craniocervical diaphragm	The upper cervical spine, the cranial base, the suboccipital muscles*, and the intracranial fascia or membranes	Endocervical fascia
Cervicothoracic diaphragm	The upper thoracic vertebrae, upper ribs, sternum, shoulder girdle, and the fascia of the region (including the anterior cervical fascia, Sibson's fascia, axillary fascia, and clavipectoral fascia)	Endothoracic fascia
Thoracoabdominal diaphragm	The thoracolumbar junction, lower six ribs, xiphoid process, superior and inferior fascial coverings of the diaphragm, and the diaphragm	Endoabdominal fascia
Lumbosacral diaphragm	The pelvic girdle, fifth lumbar vertebrae, lumbopelvic muscles, and endopelvic fascia	Endopelvic fascia
* It is worth noting that the rectus capitis posterior minor muscles, the rectus capitis posterior major muscles, the obliquus capitis inferior muscles, and the nuchal ligament have connections and attachments to the spinal portion of the dura mater in the upper cervical region. These are commonly referred to as myodural bridges, and both anatomically and functionally contribute to the craniocervical diaphragm.		

Table 46.1
Overview of the horizontal organization of the fascial system

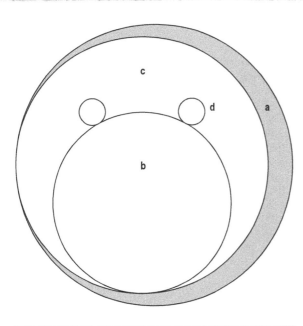

Figure 46.3
Schematic organization of cervical fascia as concentric cylinders or rings. **a** Musculofascial collar; **b** vertebral compartment: prevertebral fascia (perivertebral fascia); **c** visceral compartment: visceral fascia of the neck; **d** vascular compartment: carotid fascia

organized fascia, or the 'fascial tubes', there are plenty of variations in its descriptive anatomy. Even as early as 1838 it was noted by French anatomist Malgaigne that the fascia appeared in a new form under the pen of each author who attempted to describe it, an observation confirmed a century later when in 1941 Weintraub commented that precise descriptions and unions of the layers of the fascia were an expression of the individuality of the authors of the day and were different in each text (Levitt, 1970). As such, they are collectively 'tubes', referred to as the endocervical, endothoracic, endoabdominal, and endopelvic fascia, which of course are continuous with the fascia of the extremities.

Fascia, dysfunction, and the traditional osteopathic perspective

'Descriptions of fascia tend to be confusing because they are simply more obvious layers of the general connective-tissue packaging of the body; all connective tissue in the body is actually continuous with all other connective tissue ... Thus, in one sense, a fascia has no beginning and no end'. (Hollinshead , 1974)

Using anatomy texts as a map, thinking of them as explaining the territory, makes it relatively easy to try to associate fascial anatomy with the integrated functions of bones, joints, ligaments, muscles, viscera, vascular structures, lymphatics, and nerves. Although it is tempting to deduce clinical relevance from that, the seemingly chaotic and nonlinear organization of fascia, which enables its mobility and efficiency, makes it less likely to respond in such a predictable manner when considering its potential role in dysfunction. As a whole-body, continuous, three-dimensional viscoelastic matrix of structural support, it plays an active and modulating role in force generation and transmission, as well as mechanosensory fine-tuning (Klinger et al., 2014). Actively contributing to musculoskeletal dynamics, imbalance of these mechanisms may result in fascial dysfunction being a key contributor to pathomechanisms of several musculoskeletal pathologies and pain syndromes (Klinger et al., 2014), and it has been postulated that fascial tethering in the trunk and extremities may impact venous and lymphatic return by distorting anatomical relationships and influencing respiratory hydrodynamics (Becker, 1975; Zink, 1977; Mitchell, 1984).

The idea of dysfunctions amenable to manipulative intervention dates back to the beginning of osteopathy. A. T. Still, in expecting a 'masterful knowledge of anatomy and physiology' (Still, 1902b) from his osteopathic peers in understanding the complexity of the patient as a unit of functions in health and disease, wrote that:

'With a correct knowledge of the form and functions of the body and all its parts, we are then prepared to know what is meant by a variation in a bone, muscle, ligament, or fibre or any part of the body, from the least atom to the greatest bone or muscle. By our mechanical skill, preceded by our intelligence in anatomy, we can detect and adjust both hard and soft substances of the system. By our knowledge of physiology we can comprehend the requirements of the circulation of fluids of the

body as to time, speed, and quantity, in harmony with the demands of normal life'.
(Still, 1902c)

Unlike many modern descriptions of the 'manipulable lesion,'[1] the joint or the arthordial complex, is not the epicentre in this statement by Still where he enumerates the variant parts involved in affecting the function of the patient. Rather than viewing the 'lesions' as static structural abnormalities, administering manipulation to 'correct' such lesions based on the idea of specific anatomic malrelationship of bones and joints, the 'lesion' is considered to be a tissue unable to meet the demands made upon it for physiological action because it varied from the normal and so interfered with the ability of the patient to adapt (Hoover, 1963). This sentiment is echoed by Zink,[2] who defined the 'lesion' as blockage of the free flow of lymph and blood, or the inability of the tissues in a region to comply with the pattern of respiratory movement necessary for optimum efficiency (Mitchell, 1984). Thus a common denominator here may be the effect fascial tethering has on musculoskeletal dynamics, respiration, and tissue fluids.

Because the person is seen as a unit of functions, the symbiotic relationship between fascia with different densities (bones, muscles, ligaments, fascia, and fluids) extends to include the orchestrated action of the peripheral and central nervous system, including its mechanosensory and autonomic divisions, contributing to both exteroception and interoception, and through this the effector or motor sides of the somatosensory, the autonomic, and the neuroendocrine immune systems. The clinical approach becomes more person-centered and individualized rather than chasing 'somatic dysfunctions' where the assumption prevails that biological systems can be understood by dissecting out the minuscule components of dysfunctions and analyzing them in isolation.

---

[1] 'Osteopathic lesion', which later became the 'somatic dysfunction', defined as 'impaired or altered function of related components of the somatic (body framework) system including the skeletal arthordial, and myofascial structures, and their related vascular, lymphatic, and neural elements'.

[2] J. Gordon Zink DO, FAAO was an osteopathic physician who emphasized the role of respiratory–circulatory dynamics and its relationship to the body's biomechanical functions in the management of patients.

Box 46.2

A working description of dysfunction from a philosophical, practical view

Fascial dysfunction is the reversible loss of adaptability in tissues, making them less able to meet the compressional, tensional, and physiological demands placed upon the body. It affects biomechanical and postural, respiratory and circulatory, as well as mechanosensory and autonomic functions. This may affect the musculoskeletal and systemic capacity of the body.

Patterns

'Osteopathic lesion acts as a break of the stable equilibrium, which must exist in health, between the organism and its environment, both within and without'. (Atzen, 1913)

The human body being interpreted as a tensegrity structure where minor alterations may have an effect on the structure as a whole by changing the distribution of its stabilizing forces, compression, and tension, has proven beneficial to an expanded view of biomechanics (Levin, 2006). This also lends support to the concept of regional interdependence and pattern of dysfunctions. The underlying premise of this view is that seemingly unrelated dysfunctions or impairments in remote anatomical regions of the body may contribute to and be associated with the patient's presenting complaint (Sueki et al., 2013). The abnormal stress from a remote anatomical region to other parts of the body with development of subsequent dysfunctions may partly be explained by altered distribution of compression and tension throughout the body and partly through neurophysiologic responses where altered mechanosensory information facilitates changes in central patterns of motor responses involved in posture and movement (Sueki et al., 2013). The manifestation of subsequent dysfunctions depends on many variables such as the morphology of the individual, biomechanical properties of tissues, previous injuries and illnesses, existing dysfunctions, and neurophysiologic control, as well as behavioral and psychoemotional components. Patterns of dysfunctions are not static or constant, and may acclimatize or adapt to changing circumstances and demands placed on the body. They contribute to the increased allostatic load in the patient, and are not limited to the musculoskeletal and neurophysiological domains but as a part of the 'total lesion' may have visceral, systemic, and biopsychosocial effects (Fryette, 1954; Lewit, 2010; Chila, 2011; Sueki et al., 2013).

Torsioning of the fascial planes has been called the 'worst enemy of physiologic function' (TePoorten, 1989). Several 'universal patterns' or whole body torsions and deformations of tissue planes by tethering of the fascia have been described in the osteopathic profession, most notably from Neidner, Zink, and TePoorten (Cooper, 1977).

In addition to what has been described above as potential mechanisms, they are also considered to be caused by challenges to how individuals compensate and adapt to the gravitational force, or how the body is organized around its central gravity line in all three planes. When assessing and treating patterns of dysfunctions in patients, 'living pictures of the normal body' in a three-dimensional context are helpful.

However, the objective is not to restore symmetry of anatomy but to facilitate a more ideal physiological adaptation of the body around the central gravity line. This 'ideal pattern' should be better suited for posture, locomotion, and activities of daily life with less energy expenditure, and improved and more efficient respiratory hydrodynamics. This pattern is peculiar to the individual patient. Thus, the osteopathic treatment aims at improving the function of each person within his or her own pattern (Zink, 1977; Zink & Lawson, 1979).

Treatment considerations

There are several objectives when approaching the fascial system from a practical point of view. Decreasing the work of breathing by restoring full mobility and elasticity to the respiratory components of the body, progressively unblocking venous and lymphatic channels (starting centrally and working toward the distal vessels), and speeding up the flow rate returning the tissue fluids back to the cardiovascular system. Central to this is reducing the fascial tethering of the longitudinally organized fascia or fascial tubes. This can be done in a variety of ways. Treatment objectives are more important than methods and particular manipulative

Global approach	• Assessing and treating the transitional areas of the axial spine and pelvis, which include the horizontally layered myofascial structures
	• Addressing the lymphatic system from central towards distal or peripheral
	• Addressing local articular, fascial, fascial–ligamentous, and visceral dysfunction
Note: this is a more 'maximalist approach' to the fascial, fluid, and musculoskeletal system, where the body as a whole is treated to influence the parts	
Specific approach	• Using a selection of manual tests to highlight the areas of clinically significant dysfunctions, including traction and compression, assessment of ease–bind or tightness–looseness responses in tissues, motor responses to passive motion, and listening tests
	• This is a dynamic approach where patterns or layers of dysfunctions are prioritized and sequentially managed
Note: this is a more minimalist approach to the fascial, fluid, and musculoskeletal system, where the body as a whole is influenced by focusing on significant parts	

Table 46.2
Reducing the fascial tethering of the longitudinally organized fascia or fascial tube

approaches. Examples of different approaches are shown in Table 46.2.

Different practitioners may use different techniques according to their conceptual models and working definition of what constitutes a dysfunction. Most techniques addressing fascial dysfunctions are somewhat experimental in nature, guided by the appropriate responses in the anatomy and physiology of the individual. General guidelines on direct, indirect, and combined techniques are followed, and then adapted to the case at hand. A variety of long- and short-lever techniques, including high-velocity, low-amplitude HVLA, articulatory, muscle energy, counterstrain, functional techniques, ligamentous articular strain, balanced ligamentous tension, facilitated positional release, myofascial release, ligamentous-fascial release, Still techniques, and ventral techniques may be used to address fascial dysfunction and tethering.

The osteopathic treatment of the patient should not be a stereotypical routine or set of procedures applied to each patient. It is important though, irrespective of approach taken, that the patient is treated as an integrated unit of functions. When using a global approach, for instance, a few organizing principles can guide the manipulative management by sequencing the treatment:

1. The axial components associated with the horizontal organization of fascia are sequentially treated before the peripheral parts or the extremities. These are typically the transitional areas of the axial spine and pelvis, which in the activities of daily life are subjected to much physical stress and strain. It is not uncommon to start treating from below with the pelvis as the foundation on which the superstructures should be balanced.

2. Manual screening tests are used to assess for articular and myofascial dysfunction as well as fascial tethering in these regions, followed by the appropriate manipulative interventions.

3. The purpose of treatment is not to restore symmetry but to improve the adaptability and flexibility of the regions to meet the coordinated and functional requirements and demands of biomechanics, posture, respiration, and circulation.

There are several hypothesized benefits from treating the transitional areas of the axial spine and pelvis with the associated horizontal organization of fascia:

- Reducing articular dysfunction and myofascial tension may relieve structural distortion of lymph channels embedded in the fascial planes and traversing the horizontally organized myofascial structures that are parts of the 'diaphragms'.

- Reducing mechanical strain on the thoraco-abdominal pelvic cylinder, thus improving the respiratory function and efficiency of the respiratory diaphragm to give improved external respiration and internal respiration (tissue homeostasis: repair, adaptation, and maintenance).

- Improving the function of the transitional areas of the axial spine and pelvis may enable a better adaptation pattern of, and load transfer through, the spine and pelvis in all three planes.

- Facilitate movement in the spine and pelvis as an articulated whole.

- Improve the distribution of compression and tension through the longitudinally organized fascia of the body.

This sequencing treating the transitional areas of the axial spine and pelvis with associated diaphragms may then be followed by addressing the lymphatic system, from central to distal, augmenting fluid flow. This will also provide easy access to remaining significant visceral, fascial, and somatic dysfunctions, including in the extremities.

Conclusion

This chapter has provided a conceptual overview of traditional osteopathic perspectives addressing the fascia and fluid flow as an integrated part of musculoskeletal and systemic function. In osteopathy and osteopathic medicine, the fascia is not viewed as a tissue complex treated in isolation, but is considered to be a whole-body, continuous, three-dimensional viscoelastic matrix of structural support that is not separate from other functions.

References

Antonovsky A. (1987). *Unraveling the Mystery of Health*. New Jersey: Jossey-Bass.

Antonovsky A. (1996). *Health, Stress and Coping*. New Jersey: Jossey-Bass.

Atzen C. B. (1913). *JAOA*, July:684.

Becker A. (1947). The fascias. *Osteopathic Profession*, February; XIV(5).

Becker R. (1975). The meaning of fascia and fascial continuity. *Osteopathic Annals*, June.

Benjamin M. (2009). The fascia of the limbs and back – a review. *J Anat*, 214: 1–18.

Benz C., Bull T., Mittelmark M. et al. (2014). Culture in salutogenesis: the scholarship of Aaron Antonovsky. *Glob Health Promot*,21:16–23.

Chila A. G. (ed.) (2011). *Foundations of Osteopathic Medicine*. Philadelphia: Lippincott Williams & Wilkins.

Comstock E. S. (1928). The larger concept. *J Am Osteopath Assoc* February:463–464.

Cooper G. (1977). Some clinical consideration on fascia in diagnosis and treatment. In: *1977 Yearbook of the American Academy of Osteopathy*, Colorado Springs.

Deason W. J. (1934). Dr. Still – nonconformist. How the "Old Doctor" reached his conclusions on osteopathy. *The Osteopathic Profession*, August 1934.

Findley T. W., Schleip R, (eds) (2007). *Fascia Research, Basic Science and Implications for Conventional and Complementary Health Care*. Munich: Elsevier Urban & Fischer.

Findley T. W., Shalwala M. (2013). Fascia research congress evidence from the 100 year perspective of Andrew Taylor Still. *J Bodyw Mov Ther*. 17:356–364.

Fryette H. H. (1954). *Principles of Osteopathic Technique*. Carmel, CA: Academy of Applied Anatomy.

Gravett H. H. (1954.) The Gravett Papers. *Yearbook Academy of Applied Osteopathy*, California: Carmel, p. 36.

Hamilton W. J. (1976) *Textbook of Human Anatomy*. London: Macmillan.

Hollinshead W. H. 1974. *Textbook of Anatomy*. 3rd edition. Maryland: Harper & Row Publishers, pp. 14–15

Hoover H. (1963). A hopeful road ahead for osteopathy. *J Am Osteopath Assoc*, 62:32–45.

Hujing P. A., Hollander P., Findley T. W. Schleip R., (eds) (2009). *Fascia Research II*. Munich: Elsevier Urban & Fischer.

Jänig W. (2014). Sympathetic nervous system and inflammation: a conceptual view. *Auton Neurosci*, 182:4–14.

Klinger W., Velders M., Hoppe K. et al. (2014). Clinical relevance of fascial tissue and dysfunctions. *Curr Pain Headache Rep*, 18(8):439.

Korr I. M. (1979). *The Collected Papers of I. M. Korr*. Colorado: American Academy of Osteopathy.

Lever R. (2013). *At the still point of the turning world*. Edinburgh: Handspring Publishing.

Levin S. M. (2006). Tensegrity – the new biomechanics. In: Hutson M., Ellis R. (eds). *Textbook of Musculoskeletal Medicine*. Oxford: Oxford University Press.

Levitt G. (1970). Cervical fascia and deep neck infections. *Laryngoscope*, 80:409.

Lewit K. (2010). *Manipulative therapy: musculoskeletal medicine*. Edinburgh: Elsevier Churchill Livingstone.

Mant D. (2009). The problem with usual care. *Br J Gen Pract*, 58: 755–756.

Meissner M. H. Moneta G. Burnand K, et al. (2007). The hemodynamics and diagnosis of venous disease. *J Vasc Surg*, 46:4S–24S.

Mitchell F. L. Jr (1984). The respiratory–circulatory model: concepts and applications. In: Greenman P. E. (ed.) *Concepts and Mechanisms of Neuromuscular Functions*. Berlin: Springer Verlag.

Parviz J. et al (2011) *Surgical Anatomy of the Head and the Neck*. Harvard: Harvard University Press.

Schleip R., Findley T. W., Chaitow L., Huijing P. A. (eds) (2012). *Fascia: The Tensional Network of the Human Body*. Edinburgh: Churchill Livingstone Elsevier.

Stark J. (2006). *Still's Fascia*. Munich: Jolandos.

Still A. T. (1899). *Philosophy of Osteopathy*. Kirksville, MO: The Journal Printing Company.

Still A. T. (1902a). The *Philosophy and Mechanical Principles of Osteopathy*. Kirksville, MO: The Journal Printing Company.

Still A. T. (1902b). The *Philosophy and Mechanical Principles of Osteopathy*. Kirksville, MO: The Journal Printing Company. p. 18.

Still A. T. (1902c) The *Philosophy and Mechanical Principles of Osteopathy*. Kirksville, MO: The Journal Printing Company. pp. 20–21.

Sueki D. G., Cleland J. A., Robert S Wainner R. S. (2013). A regional interdependence model of musculoskeletal dysfunction: research, mechanisms, and clinical implications. *J Man Manip Ther*, 21:90–102.

TePoorten (1989). The common compensatory pattern. *The Journal of the New Zealand Register of Osteopaths*.

Willard F., Fossum C., Standley P. (2010). The fascial system. In: Chila A. G. (ed.). *Foundations of Osteopathic Medicine*. 3rd edition. Philadelphia: Lippincott Williams & Wilkins.

Zink J. G., Lawson W. B. (1979). An osteopathic structural examination and functional interpretation of the soma. *Osteopathic Annals*, 12 December;7.

Zink J. G. (1977). Respiratory and circulatory care: the conceptual model. *Osteopathic Annals*, March.

LYMPHO-FASCIA RELEASE AND VISCEROLYMPHATIC APPROACH TO FASCIA

Bruno Chikly

'Harmony only dwells where obstruction does not exist.'[1]

A. T. Still

Osteopathic lymphatic technique (OLT) and viscerolymphatic approach to fascia

Osteopaths, in clinical practice, often need to connect to the wholeness of their patient and find a way to quickly and elegantly assess the predicament that disturbs a specific structure. The treatment procedure in a mechanical model is often an approach that takes the tension of the tissue away.

> 'Dr. Andrew Taylor Still taught that technique, to be most effective, should be gentle, easy, and scientific.'[2]

Ideally, we should use the most efficient and least invasive techniques, with minimal force, to get to this result.

During the last 25 years, several techniques have emerged from the osteopathic model. Numerous well-known methods use a 'solid' model for the physical body, the musculoskeletal framework, and the fascia structure. Osteopathy also covers an entire domain of very different, gentle, 'fluid' techniques (e.g., cranial or lymphatic techniques) that were at one time considered to be more difficult to teach. These refined techniques allow practitioners to release restrictions in the body's fluid compartments to reinstate tissue health.

> '... exaggeration of the lesion ...This method is the more difficult of the two [exaggeration and direct methods] and for the instruction of students does not find favor with the author.'[3]

This eternal quest for the body's reinstatement of a more complete physical healing led to the development of a unified, noninvasive technique with great efficiency for the mechanical structures of the body, called lympho-fascia release (LFR). This approach brings together the advantages of the fluid techniques, using OLT, and the benefits of the solid model such as fascia approaches. The marriage of these two modalities can reduce restrictions with a touch that is gentle, efficient, and profound in its application.

> 'Somatic dysfunction is an 'impaired or altered function of related components of the somatic system: skeletal, arthrodial, and myofascial structures and related vascular, lymphatic, and neural elements.'[4]
> 'The presence of normal passive motion in one direction of one plane and resistance in the other is presumptive evidence of somatic dysfunctions.'[5]

As osteopaths, we are well versed in the fact that physical restrictions can result from accidents, surgeries, and other trauma and can manifest in the body as pain, edema, inflammation, spasms, loss of mobility, reduced range of motion, and fibrotic tissues. Some of these restrictions can form adhesions and can be very difficult to release.

> 'Somatic dysfunctions are accompanied by local inflammation and edema with modifications in blood and lymph flow.'[6,7]

A conventional approach is to look for these barriers in the body and break through them with a 'solid' model that usually involves some degree of force. Still, when we work only on the fascia fibers without moving the tissue fluid, we often have to use a certain stress on these fibers to get the results we want. Though this approach can lead to benefits for our patients, it can also result in moderate to significant side effects including pain, increased edema, inflammation, and eventually the stagnation of lymphatic interstitial fluid that could be associated with scar tissue. Further, some patients may not be able to receive such mechanical techniques if they present acute pathologies, recent surgeries or accidents, bleeding, or simply conditions that make it difficult to touch the client such as fibromyalgia. LFR enables us to softly engage the fascia and fluid simultaneously, releasing efficiently restrictions on the lymphatic interstitial fluid and fascia planes in one motion, avoiding most of the damaging side effects.

'In adjusting lesions it is obvious that a method which retraces the path of the lesion with a minimum of irritation is highly desirable.'[8]

So how does LFR work? Normally, when we perform OLT we connect with the fluid body and use a very exact stroke that will synchronize with the specific rhythm of lymph, its specific direction, and its specific depth within the relevant area. This stroke, being on the skin with a light pressure, will also naturally engage some of the fascia. By taking the soft touch of lymph drainage just a little deeper, practitioners are able to first engage the fascia then the lymphatic planes concurrently. With this approach, inspired by the osteopathic tradition of balanced ligamentous, the two systems work in tandem to maximize the body's response and improve patient outcomes.

'Dr. Sutherland recommended using the inherent forces within the body such as respiration, fluid mechanics, and postural changes to correct the strain. In general, the technique combines a fulcrum introduced by the physician with an activating force provided by the patient.'[9]
'These principles use the inherent forces of the body to make the reduction; they do not permit the well-known thrust method.'[10]

Essentially, the concept is quite simple. Balance membranous tension (BMT) and balance ligamentous

tension (BLT) were presented by W. G. Sutherland in 1942 and 1944, but this time the osteopath will bring the fascia to a point of balanced ease and then let the lymph and extracellular fluid move through relaxed fascia fibers.

'[Point of balance, neutral point, point of release]. It is the point in the range of motion where the articulation has been carried to the limit of its unrestricted motion and just into the range where tension or resistance is developing.'[10]

Basically, in the point of balance, the facial fibers are in the lowest tension possible within the tissue so we can send significant waves of fluid flow through the tissue. Then we send the lymphatic and interstitial fluids.

'Balance the membranes first. Do this in whatever fashion is least irritating to the tissues involved and which will give the operator the keenest possible perception of the tissue response.'[11]

The effects are instantaneous. The patient may feel a deep wave going through an area – releasing stagnation, inflammation, and especially deep chronic adhesion. When done correctly, LFR allows the body to create a single, powerful wave, called in physics a 'soliton', which can travel throughout the whole body (e.g., a healing 'tsunami').

A soliton is a nonlinear wave propagation discovered by the Scottish engineer John Scott Russell (1808–1882). The soliton wave is a dynamic balance between the wave's tendency to spread out (the dispersive effect) and the nonlinear motion (the superior part of the wave moves faster than the inferior parts).

The prime motto of an osteopath is to find the problem, 'fix it, and let it alone'. We need to put the tissue at zero pressure for it to reach a balance point. When the tissue is neutral in this way, the wave appears in response to that balance point and the fluid flows naturally, freely. We assist the wave but we don't create it or force it. We're not mechanical engineers doing something to the body, we're simply working with the body's own intrinsic intelligence and self-healing, self-regulatory mechanisms. That's where the profound impact of this technique lies. This wave, created with gentleness, will move through the body's restrictions.

Knowing the power of this wave, we no longer have to use a lot of force. Just by using the body's own internal forces, we are able to go deeper into the tissues and reach areas in the body that often cannot be addressed. Like this, we facilitate not only a local release but also a large number of releases all along the path of the wave as it travels through the body, interacting with other systems as it comes in contact with them.

There are numerous applications for LFR. It can be used very successfully for the treatment of chronic pain conditions because chronic pain is frequently an indication of congestion of the lymph associated with fascia restrictions. Because of its effectiveness in reducing scarring and inflammation, this approach also has positive implications for difficult cases including, for example, long-term fibrosis and fibromyalgia. In the case of a patient with fibromyalgia, LFR is an effective approach because it doesn't create additional inflammation within the body. In fact, LFR is such a gentle approach that it can be effective in treating different acute conditions and is also beneficial when working with the elderly and the young, or even our animal companions, all of whom may react negatively to a strong touch.

LFR is also very efficient at treating visceral or fascial dysfunctions. I don't use it as much for joints – I use other specific fluid articular techniques. A good patient assessment is essential to this technique. Osteopaths often concentrate on key lesions in the body to get a fast and durable improvement. If we only address secondary lesions in our treatment, the lymphatic 'wave' won't stay in place as well. Through proper assessment, we can listen to the body and find what condition the body is holding. We can then release the restrictions or lesions naturally and without a great deal of force.

Though this technique is relatively simple, it's also very specific in its application. Naturally, when you approach a patient with a soft, noninvasive touch you also have to be very precise with your assessment for the treatment to be successful. In OLT seminars, we work closely with therapists to help them develop the necessary skills for proper patient assessment. We spend a great deal of time learning specific techniques that allow therapists to work with the body's own consciousness, because without the ability to access the body correctly, this highly effective technique can miss the mark.

The real benefit of LFR is that, as osteopaths, we don't have to approach the body with the typical, strong 'no pain, no gain' approach and work through barriers. Instead, we can retrain our hands to start with the lightest touch possible and increase pressure from there as the body dictates. This allows us to release tension in a manner that's less stressful on our patients and on us. LFR and other light-touch applications can also prolong the amount of time for which a therapist can practice, because they're easier on the practitioner's hands and body than traditional manual techniques without compromising the effectiveness of the treatment. In this way, we can develop a new paradigm to healing: a 'less pain, more gain' approach for everyone involved.

LFR could seem counterintuitive at first because it's much less aggressive than some mechanical approaches, but it still has the same valuable effects on patients with far less impact on the osteopath's body. What's important to understand is that this type of specialization doesn't limit your practice, it gives more options while prolonging your ability to help others without hurting yourself in the process.

Sometimes releasing barriers in the body can feel like trying to open a strong safe. With the right key, the door will open easily, without force. LFR is one of those keys that can lead to a more fulfilling osteopathic practice.

> 'There is a definite difficult in the transition from art emphasis upon the nature and the direction of the bind...to an emphasis upon the nature and direction of the ease ... Both are extremely valuable ... It would seem to demand almost a year for the transition in order to preserve the old skills along with the new.'[12]

As with anything else, it takes some time and dedication to integrate this new tool, but you may end up using this approach for 95 percent of your fascial and viscerosomatic dysfunctions, and end up doing it for a long time because of the gentleness, precision, and long-term efficiency of LFR.

Visceral applications for osteopathic lymphatic technique

In this chapter we will elaborate a little more on the practical way to contact, assess, and treat the viscera using OLT.

Viscera need to be contacted with respect and non-invasiveness as they are very sensitive and can easily spasm or contract their ring muscles. Wait and let the information come to you rather than invading the visceral tissue. Be sure to be 'invited' by the organ. Very gently and gradually connect with the viscera, synchronizing with its quality and intrinsic movement.

Diagnosis

LFR diagnosis comprises:

- intraparenchymal (intrinsic) assessment of a visceral organ

- assessment of visceral ligaments

- assessment of visceral interfaces: the relationship between two organs.

In LFR the diagnosis can be made with ease. You may remember that one of the characteristics of a mechanical osteopathic lesion is the fact that there is a barrier in one direction of one plane and that, in three dimensions, in the opposite direction the tissue always presents the most 'ease.'

'The presence of normal passive motion in one direction of one plane and resistance in the other is presumptive evidence of somatic dysfunctions.'[5]

Therefore, the diagnosis of the osteopathic lesion will be done with ease and will have two outcomes:

1. The assessment will be often less invasive than when looking for a barrier. Even a slight position of the tissue against the barrier could possibly stimulate sympathetic activity and to some extent may 'retraumatize' some tissue.

2. The direction taken with ease for the diagnosis is also the start of the treatment. In the treatment we will take the tissue all the way to the maximum ease and stabilize it within the perfect point of balance.

Treatment

Different types of treatment are possible depending on the location, organ, pathology, and age of the patient, etc.

1. Open the surrounding nodes to facilitate lymphatic techniques.

2. Subacute condition: the basic lymphatic stroke of OLT is often used.

3. Chronic condition: LFR is often used.

Open the surrounding nodes

- Thoracic organs: we can open this group of nodes to facilitate lymphatic techniques including the cervical nodes, the axillary nodes, and the receptaculum chyli (cisterna chyli area).

- Abdominopelvic organs: we can add to the locations above the group of inguinal nodes.

- You can also repeat this procedure if needed after the treatment and 'rinse' the lymphatic flow.

In OLT we apply the basic lymphatic stroke

In the case of acute or subacute inflammation (e.g., acute or subacute laryngitis, sinusitis, appendicitis, etc.) the basic lymphatic stroke is the least invasive and most respectful technique to address these conditions.

The stroke used in OLT is osteopathic as it is very specific in its:

- *Rhythm:* the lymphatic rhythm defined by science or about 0.1Hz.

- *Direction:* toward the proper group of nodes.

- *Depth:* the specific layer of the lesion: skin, mucosa, muscle, fascia, viscera, dura, bone, and so on.

- *Quality:* the quality of the lymph flow and its potency provides various information about the health of the patient.

Many other techniques can be added, such as perceiving a slight lymphatic asynchrony between the left and right sides of the body, assessing if the local area is wet or dry as defined by Guyton (a wet area being an area with clinical or infraclinical fluid stagnation[13]), switching the lymph flow, creating a retrograde impulse, or using an extracellular fluid technique (EFT).

Lympho-fascia release

Lymphofascia release can be applied to chronic conditions as it addresses the stagnant fluid as well as the chronic adhesions present in many chronic dysfunctions. LFR can be applied within an organ (intraparenchymal) or between the organ and its ligamentous attachments, as well as between organs (at organ interfaces).

Clinical examples

Below are some simple clinical examples involving the trachea and lungs.

Box 47.3

Osteopathic lymphatic technique (OLT) and Lympho-Fascia Release

1. Open surrounding nodes

2. Assess and treat intraparenchymal areas

3. Assess and treat visceral ligamentous interfaces

4. Assess and treat intervisceral interfaces

   a. Subacute condition: often use the basic lymphatic stroke of OLT

   b. Chronic condition/scar: often use lympho-fascia release

---

Box 47.4

Trachea and bronchi

Open main surrounding nodes:

- Clavicles, axilla, receptaculum chyli

Intraparenchymal/intrinsic:

- LFR: look for cervical intratracheal lesion

Ligaments and interfaces:

- Trachea – esophagus

- Trachea – left then right bronchi

- Trachea – heart

- Interbronchial (bronchopericardial ligament)

- Bronchi – lung

- Left bronchi (hilum) – heart

Open main surrounding nodes

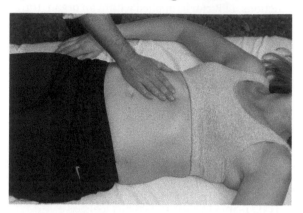

Figure 47.1

Open the supraclavicular group of nodes. This can be done facing the patient, as shown, or when standing at the head of the table. Synchronize with the specific rhythm, direction, depth, quality, and potency of the lymph flow as well as its slight lymphatic asynchrony. Image from LDV1 (Lymphatic Applications to Viscera 1) textbook, IH Publishing, 2010, reproduced with permission

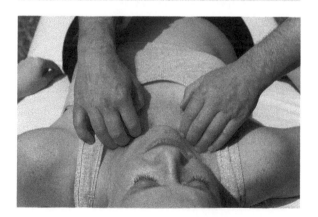

Figure 47.2

Open the clavicular nodes. This can be done facing the patient, as shown, or when standing at the head of the table. Synchronize with the specific rhythm, direction, depth, quality, and potency of the lymph flow as well as its slight lymphatic asynchrony. Image from LDV1 (Lymphatic Applications to Viscera 1) textbook, IH Publishing, 2010, reproduced with permission

Intraparenchymal/intrinsic assessment

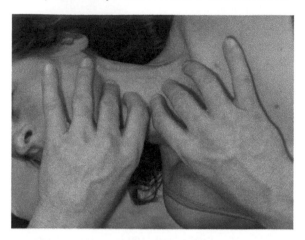

Figure 47.3

Assessing a cervical intratracheal lesion. In the case of a lesion you can apply LFR: bring the tissue to balance and send the lymph. Image from LDV1 (Lymphatic Applications to Viscera 1) textbook, IH Publishing, 2010, reproduced with permission

Ligaments and interfaces

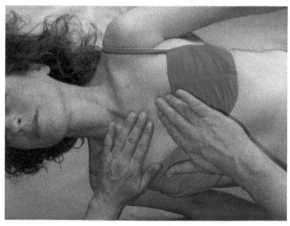

Figure 47.4

Assessing dysfunction between the thoracic trachea and the main bronchi. Apply LFR if needed. Image from LDV-TA (Lymphatic Applications to Viscera – Thorax/Abdomen) textbook, IH Publishing, 2010, reproduced with permission

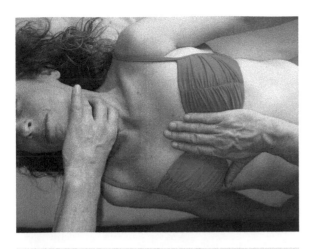

Figure 47.5

Assessing dysfunction between the cervical trachea and the heart pericardium (tracheopericardial ligament). Apply LFR if needed. Image from LDV1 (Lymphatic Applications to Viscera 1) textbook, IH Publishing, 2010, reproduced with permission

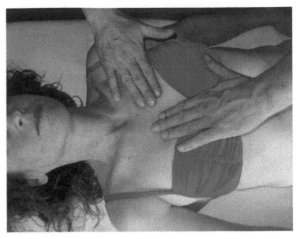

Figure 47.7

Assessing dysfunction between the main bronchi or main/secondary bronchi or between smaller bronchi. Apply LFR if needed. Image from LDV1 (Lymphatic Applications to Viscera 1) textbook, IH Publishing, 2010, reproduced with permission

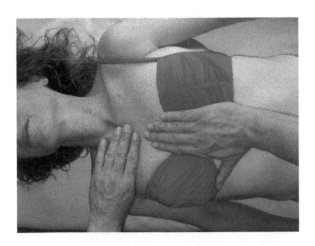

Figure 47.6

Assessing dysfunction between the thoracic trachea and the heart pericardium (tracheopericardial ligament). Apply LFR if needed. Image from LDV1 (Lymphatic Applications to Viscera 1) textbook, IH Publishing, 2010, reproduced with permission

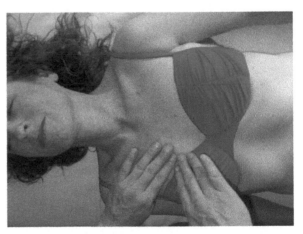

Figure 47.8

Assessing dysfunction between the lung and left or right bronchi. Apply LFR if needed. Image from LDV1 (Lymphatic Applications to Viscera 1) textbook, IH Publishing, 2010, reproduced with permission

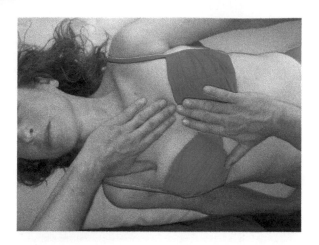

Figure 47.9

Assessing dysfunction between the heart pericardium and the left or right bronchi or secondary bronchi. Apply LFR if needed. Image from LDV1 (Lymphatic Applications to Viscera 1) textbook, IH Publishing, 2010, reproduced with permission

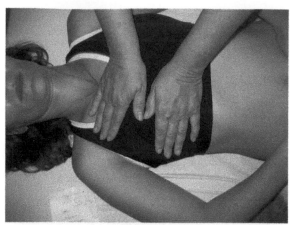

Figure 47.10

Assessing the parietal pleura. The parietal pleura can drain toward the cervical nodes, the internal mammary nodes, the parasternal or paraspinal nodes, the axillary nodes, or the receptaculum chyli. Apply LFR if needed. Image from LDV1 (Lymphatic Applications to Viscera 1) textbook, IH Publishing, 2010, reproduced with permission

Box 47.5

Anterior lungs

Open main surrounding nodes:

- Clavicles, axilla, receptaculum chyli

Intraparenchymal/intrinsic:

- LFR: look for intrapleural/intrapulmonary lesion

Ligaments and interfaces:

- Right lung: superior (horizontal) and inferior (oblique) fissures

- Left lung: oblique fissure

- Bronchopericardial membrane

- Interpulmonary ligament

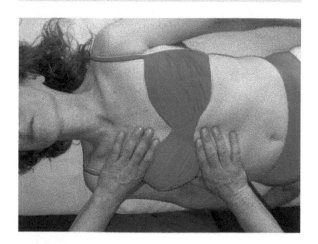

Figure 47.11

Assessing visceral pleural or intrapulmonary dysfunction. The visceral pleura as well as the pulmonary parenchyma usually drain toward the hilum of the lungs. Apply LFR if needed. Image from LDV1 (Lymphatic Applications to Viscera 1) textbook, IH Publishing, 2010, reproduced with permission

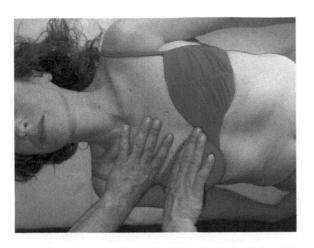

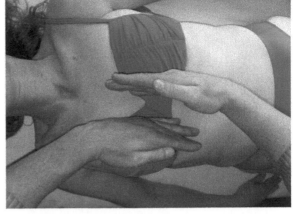

Figure 47.12

Assess dysfunction of the superior (horizontal) fissure of the anterior right lung (ribs 3–4). Apply LFR if needed. Image from LDV1 (Lymphatic Applications to Viscera 1) textbook, IH Publishing, 2010, reproduced with permission

Figure 47.14

Assessing dysfunction of the bronchopericardial membrane. Use two locations. This fascial structure is located anterior to the esophagus. Apply LFR if needed. Image from LDV1 (Lymphatic Applications to Viscera 1) textbook, IH Publishing, 2010, reproduced with permission

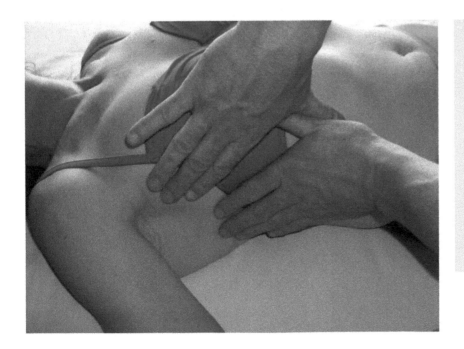

Figure 47.13

Assessing dysfunction of the inferior (oblique) fissure of the anterior right lung (ribs 5–6). The same procedure can be relevant to the anterior left lung. Apply LFR if needed. Image from LDV1 (Lymphatic Applications to Viscera 1) textbook, IH Publishing, 2010, reproduced with permission

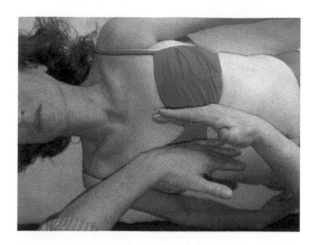

Figure 47.15
Assessing dysfunction of the interpulmonary ligament. The interpulmonary ligament usually connects the two pulmonary ligaments. Only one location is inferior (the lower part of the mediastinum). The placement of the hands is almost the same as for the lower location for the bronchopericardial membrane. This fascial structure is located posterior to the esophagus. Apply LFR if needed. Image from LDV1 (Lymphatic Applications to Viscera 1) textbook, IH Publishing, 2010, reproduced with permission

References

1. Still A. T. Philosophy of Osteopathy Kirksville, Mo: A. T. Still; 1899;197.

2. Lippincott H. A. Respiratory technique. *JAOA* 1948;31.

3. Ashmore E. F. *Osteopathic Mechanics: Review Questions for the Class of January, 1916.* Kirksville, MO: Journal Printing Co.; 1915.

4. American Association of Colleges of Osteopathic Medicine, Educational Council on Osteopathic Principles. *Glossary of Osteopathic Terminology.* American Association of Colleges of Osteopathic Medicine; 2009.

5. Kappler R. E., Jones, J. M., Kuchera W. A. Diagnosis and plan for manual treatment: a present prescription. In: Ward R. C. (ed.) *Foundations for Osteopathic Medicine.* 2nd edition. Baltimore, MD: William and Wilkins; 2003, p. 575.

6. Burns L. *Pathogenesis of Visceral Disease Following Vertebral Lesions.* Chicago: The American Osteopathic Association; 1948.

7. Korr I. M. Sustained sympathicotonia as a factor in disease. In: *The Collected Papers of Irvin M. Korr.* B. Peterson (ed). American Academy of Osteopathy, Colorado; 1978, p. 77–89.

8. McConnell C. Osteopathic studies, IV. *JAOA* 1931;31:206–212.

9. Carreiro J. E. Balanced ligamentous tension techniques. In: Ward R. C. (ed.) *Foundations for Osteopathic Medicine.* 2nd ed. Baltimore, MD: William and Wilkins; 2003, p. 917.

10. Lipincott R. C. Types of cranial treatment and their application. *J Osteop Cran Assoc.* Cranial Academy. Meridian Idaho. 1949;55–73.

11. Magoun H. I. *Osteopathy in the Cranial Field.* Denver, CO: Magoun H. I; 1951.

12. Bowles C. H. *A functional orientation for technic.* In: Academy of Applied Osteopathy, American Academy of Osteopathy (ed.) *Yearbook of the Academy of Applied Osteopathy.* 1956, p. 110.

13. Guyton A. C. and Hall J. E. *Textbook of Medical Physiology.* Philadelphia: Elsevier Saunders; 2007.

FASCIAL TREATMENT OF THE VASCULAR SYSTEM

Ralf Vogt

Introduction

The approach to treatment of vascular tissue is sometimes only possible by treating the surrounding fascial structures. Arteries and veins themselves are built of different tissue layers like the intima or inner layer, a layer consisting of smooth muscles (muscularis), and the outer layer or adventitia. This outer layer is tightly connected to vascular guiding connective tissue (Duivenvoorden et al., 2009). Any tension in the guiding fascia will have an influence on the vascular tube inside. But we should not forget that the blood itself is a sort of connective tissue and thus like a fluid fascia. There are three sorts of tissue you can find throughout the whole body, even in the smallest spaces: nerves, fascia, and blood vessels (Myers, 2009). All three are designed to inform and support all other cells by electrical, chemical, and mechanical signals and forces (Frucht, 1953).

The vascular system is able to inform other tissues via hormones and messenger peptides, but it has in addition a remarkable ability to take part in mechanical force transmission. Arteries of medium diameter especially can function as a tensional and bending-stiff structure because of their smooth muscles and the intravascular pressure (Bank & Kaiser, 1998; Faury, 2001; Han, 1995; Humphrey, 2009).

There is evidence too, that another sort of informative transfer could take place via the fluids themselves by using the tube content like a hollow conductor that works with the speed of sound in water (approximately 1500 m/s) (Riha, 2005). Taking all that into consideration, you can easily imagine the possibilities of vascular treatment for improving drainage and nutrition of tissues, and also the role of vessels in tissue mechanics and data transfer in the body.

Origins and history of vascular treatment

There are hints at manipulative treatment of blood vessels in early medical history, for example, in the ancient Indian medical system of Ayurveda (5000 BC) or ancient Egyptian and Chinese medicine (Bhishagratna, 2010). Ancient martial arts systems dealt with techniques of disturbing the blood supply of an enemy by striking or pressing special points of the body, like the system of *dim hsueh* in Chinese *win chun* or *kyoshu jutsu* in Japanese Kenpo Karate. The Egyptians learned from the Indians and the Greeks learned from the Egyptians. The Romans learned from the Greeks and whole of Europe learned from the Romans. The ideas of the Roman doctor Galen and his teachings of the four humors – blood, slime, yellow gall, and black gall – ruled medicine until medieval times. Times changed with the appearance of Andreas Vesalius, a Belgian doctor, who performed the first specimen section at the university of Ghent in 1485. During the Renaissance our knowledge of blood circulation and other physiological dependencies increased and experimental treatment of inner organs and blood vessels evolved mainly in France. Apart from the development of inner surgery in France, the Swedish doctor Lasse Brandt and Stapfer in Belgium were involved with the development of vessel treatment (Liem, 2013). In the last century the impetus for visceral treatment and vessel techniques arose in French osteopathy namely through Jean-Pierre Barral and Paul Mercier, and also by Jacques Weischenck, Paul Chauffour, and Eric Prat. A method inspired by the teachings of Rollin Becker was developed by Maxwell Fraval in Australia.

It has to be said that vascular treatment is far away from being an integrated part of the work of manual therapists worldwide. Even among osteopathic therapists, the idea of treating blood vessels as the targeted tissue is very new. A. T. Still himself, the founder of osteopathy, believed in the importance of an undisturbed blood supply to the body tissues, but even osteopathic therapists are used to treating the vessels more indirectly by treating the surrounding connective tissue and encouraging a better supply by decreasing the tissue tension of the fascia (Still, 1899).

Aims and objectives

As the founder of osteopathy, A. T. Still states in his autobiography that the objective of vascular treatment should be to irrigate the dry fields (Still, 1899). To achieve this aim, one has to look at the physiology of arteries and veins first and then evaluate their technical approximation to the tissue. One has to distinguish the empirical results of a treatment from the independent outcome of clinical research. The 'felt' result of a technique is often composed of the real reaction of the tissue, the reaction of the autonomic nervous system (ANS), the expectation of the client, the expectation of the therapist, short-term effects on the body, homeostasis, and so on (Vogt, 2008). How often do we just hope our treatment was successful as a result of our technique, but the way we spoke to our client, our touch, or maybe just the warmth of our hand might have had an even bigger effect (Venkatasubramanian, 2006). You can imagine that in order to reach the target of a better blood supply you would have to reassure yourself by use of sonography or thermography. To make an assessment in order to solve a dysfunction of a blood vessel that serves as a tensioner for structural elements, like the carotid artery as traction rein for the cervical spine, you have to control mobility or vitality of the spine before and after the treatment. And no matter how good our skills are, when we are dealing with vessels in treatment, we should not forget that the outcome or result of our treatment depends on many more things than just the technique used on the tissue (Barral & Croibier, 2011).

Indications and contraindications

Treatment of the vascular system is indicated in all forms of ischemia but could be performed for downregulating the sympathetic nervous system and treating vascular-dependent structural dysfunctions of the spine or other bony structures (Bevan et al., 1987). To be safe and in order not to do any harm to your client, you should know what to do and, even more essential, when to send your client to hospital or call the emergency doctor. There are some guidelines you should follow when treating the vascular system (contraindications):

1. Never treat a client with acute ischemia, for example, heart attack, stroke, mesenterial ischemia, subdural bleeding, or peripheral arterial lockdown. After your client is out of hospital, there would be no contraindication for indirect treatment.

2. You should not treat clients who are taking anticoagulant medicines like heparin or coumarin derivates because you may cause vessel rupture and bleeding.

3. It is a good idea when treating girls, very slim young women, or older people to measure the patient's blood pressure before treatment. When performing the treatment, you sometimes transport enormous amounts of blood from one place in the body to another. Visceral treatments especially allow a lot of blood to flow to the abdominal organs and that could cause dizziness or even fainting.

4. When treating patients with high blood pressure (more than 140/90), you have to make sure your treatment does not cause a hypertensive crisis (systolic pressure over 230 mm Hg).

5. The elasticity of blood vessels decreases in older people. To manage that disadvantage the vessels become longer and lie in curves or loops, so they can respond to increasing tension with loop elasticity instead of wall elasticity. However, the vessel wall becomes more vulnerable against shear stress and traction. So be especially gentle with older people.

6. You should handle clients with hyperactive immune systems with care. Sometimes they develop inflammation of blood vessels, for example, in Horton's disease, Takayasu's disease, or Kawasaki disease (in children). When the temporal artery or other vessels of the head are involved there is risk of severe headache.

Modalities of assessment

Your client should be calm and informed of your treatment, and he or she should be encouraged to observe the interoceptive signals of the body as far as possible. Like the nervous and the fascial system, the vascular system is represented even in the finest parts of any tissue of the body as capillary vessels (Myers, 2009). So the vascular system is only one possible window for looking at the client's system, or it can be the door by which you enter the system. But therapists can sometimes be cruel and overwhelming to their clients, even if they don't intend to be. When you enter an unfamiliar property, you would not jump over the fence, run to the door, smash it open, and enter the house, would you? But in treatment we are often a little aggressive toward our client. Even if he is paying for treatment, it isn't polite to let him strip down to his underwear and touch his or her body without being invited by the system to do so. So keep in mind that you should wait until you are allowed to enter the system, after checking nonverbal signals and the reaction of the body to your presence.

In addition, you have to be prepared for work by being calm yourself, with an attitude of benevolent awareness for the body under your hands. Beside the fascial and nervous listening there is always a type of fluidal listening that brings you to every place in the body as well: the vascular system. Here you can observe and find dysfunctions and deal with them one way or another.

Principles and methods of application

As mentioned earlier in this chapter, there are three main types of vascular treatment. But before we get to them, let's talk about diagnosis. It is a pity that there is so little training on vascular palpation in many osteopathic schools because such training is necessary for a proper approach. Not to mention the information that can be obtained from a proper clinical examination. In most cases pain results from ischemia or inflammation, one way or another. Blood vessels are involved in either case. By palpating an artery you can gather information about tension of the vessel wall itself, tension in the fascial track of the vessel, the heartbeat, the heart-rate variability (as a value for the

ANS), and pulse qualities – weak or strong, smooth or hard, and so on (Porges, 2010). By using inhibition, you can even detect dependencies of, for example, the cervical spine from a dysfunctional vertebral artery. The aforementioned methods of Barral and Chauffour involve working with stretching, meaning mechanical influence on the vessel or the fascial track of the vessel. Fraval's method is more indirect by inducing a point of balance in the vessel wall. Barral's technique is performed by using four different kinds of approach:

1. Slide–induction is a smooth, gliding movement along the arterial axis until it relaxes.

2. Stretch–induction is for muscular arteries to let them relax through longitudinal stretch.

3. Pressure–induction is for regions where you cannot palpate the course of the vessel but can use pressure on the assumed vessel until relaxation of the surrounding tissue occurs.

4. Combined stretch uses two points of a longer vessel, that are pressed, while the arm or leg is moved in all directions.

Barral suggests shortening the muscular parts by shoving them together, before stretching them (Barral & Croibier, 2011).

The Chauffour and Prat method is part of the concept of 'mechanical link' and works with a 'recoil' on the vessel. The vessel is stretched in the longitudinal axis and with amplification by breathing, then released at its highest tension (Chauffour & Prat, 2002). In addition, with my clients I am experimenting with balancing the blood flow itself, which is another story.

Possible physiological mechanisms

Speaking of physiology of the vascular system, you have to bear in mind that in rest our body has no need for a central regulation of blood flow. That means there is a local regulation of blood supply, regulated by the requirements of the tissues (Porges, 2010). Local blood supply and the diameter of the vessels depend either on tissue hormones like nitric oxide (NO) or local vasomotor nerves. When we are talking about the effects of osteopathic treatment on blood supply, we must consider several possible ways of creating vasodilation or vasoconstriction. The requirement for a change in blood supply can be metabolic (need for oxygen), myogenic (pressure or wall tension), endothelial (flow or shear forces), or neurogenic (epinephrine or similar) (Atienza et al., 2007; Bank & Kaiser, 1998; Burnstock & Ralevic, 1994; Gokina, 1998; Jaggar, 1998). When we are working on a local tissue, we will obviously get local effects first. That means, no effects from the ANS, neither sympathetic nor parasympathetic. Autonomous blood regulation will always be 'global' for the body, because the 'freeze' (parasympathetic) and 'flight or fight' (sympathetic) responses require vast amounts of blood that has to be transferred to, for example, big muscle groups and the lungs (Porges, 2010). Instead of that, local regulation will depend on the local needs of special tissues. First of all, we have therefore to be interested in tension receptors and other receptors that react on tension or on peptides produced by tension. The most well-known receptors are α- and β-receptors. These are adrenergic receptors, and are only of interest in the case of 'global' blood regulation (Watkins, 1980; Webb, 1981; Hermsmeyer, 1983). Beside these more or less well-known receptor types, there are others that take part in local vasomotor control. Here we find muscarinic receptors, histaminic receptors, adenosine receptors, to mention just a few (Voets, 2009; Zhang & Zhang, 2008; Webb, 1981; Smith, 1998; Scotland, 2000; Ren et al., 1993). To get vasoconstriction, L-type Ca^{2+} channels, have to be activated in vascular smooth muscle cells. This can be done by all kinds of receptors through depolarization of the muscle membrane. The activated receptor is building inositol trisphosphate IP3), which opens the intracellular Ca^{2+} channels and, together with cGMP (cyclic guanylate monophosphate), activates the myosin light chain kinase (MLCK). The myosin head can react with actin and we have a contraction. Obviously this is not the way our osteopathic treatment can work. We use another way to get vasodilation. Through mechanosensitive receptors our therapeutic touch activates unspecific endothelial outflow of nitric oxide (NO), which activates a form of cGMP by activating guanylate cyclase (Lu & Kassab, 2011). That modulates all Ca^{2+} transportation systems of the vascular muscle cell, Ca^{2+}-ATPase will be stimulated, IP3 will be inhibited, Ca^{2+} stays in the depots,

the potassium channels will be activated, and K^+ is streaming out of the membrane, which causes hyperpolarization and a shutdown of Ca^{2+} channels. We get a vascular dilation. At the present time there are discussions about the role of prostaglandin-2 (PGl2) and a suspected (but not yet found) endothelial-derived hyperpolarization factor (EDHF) (Jaggar, 1998; Jones, 1983; Schiffrin, 2001). So, when we talk about increasing the blood flow to a tissue to follow the ideas of our founder, A. T. Still, we can either improve the existing blood supply by reducing all obstacles in the form of fascial tension, muscular hypertonus, and possibly sympathetic influences, or we can try to induce vasodilation by changing the vascular tension itself. Bayliss (1902) delivered a description of a vasodilating effect by reducing the rectangular pressure against the wall by reducing the blood pressure behind a pressure point (Voets, 2009). It is a pity that our osteopathic approach can have both effects, dilation and also contraction, because we are often not specific enough in our approach.

Clinical integration and example

But, how to integrate vascular techniques into our everyday treatment? Let's imagine your client comes to you with left-sided headache. In the interview you get the usual stuff: too much work, too much stress, too little sports and fun. No relevant injuries or accidents, and clinical examination does not get you far. During fascial listening you get the impression of dural tension and myofascial restriction at the left side of the neck. But there is also tension at the right side, and when you bring the cervical spine in lateral flexion to the right with left-sided rotation it decreases the left-hand tension. Strange? Shouldn't that movement bring more tension to the left? Maybe you should examine the right vertebral artery, which is very often connected to headache of the opposite side, tinnitus, or partial deafness and, as a branch of the subclavian artery, is connected to the aortic arc and the heart. To treat the vertebral artery, you should approach the occipital bone near the right side of the foramen magnum and the anterior side of the transverse process of C6. Find the pulsation there and let the vessel unwind between occipital bone and C6. To use a fascial approach, you can stretch the anterior layer of the deep cervical fascia, which is connected with the vertebral artery, or you can stretch the cervical channel by using lateral flexion to the left with right-handed rotation. Headache or tension at the left side should be better after that. Another example could be as follows. Imagine a young woman with lumbosacral pain that's getting better with exercises or running, occasionally cold feet, and increasing heat waves and sweating during the night when she wants to sleep beside her husband. Hormonal laboratory tests have proved no disturbances of her monthly cycle. She also says that her knees sometimes feel weak during running. You find an outflare of the iliac bones at both sides, increased abdominal wall tension, and painful pubic bones. So, before spending a lot of time on other assessments to find out what on earth is wrong here, you should lift the aortic bifurcation, where it divides into the common iliac arteries, and you can increase her pain like that. This means that iliac artery dysfunction is her problem. So, by using the fascial 'railway' again you can relax the psoas muscles and stretch the pelvic fascia, not to mention the anteroposterior connective tissue, known as 'Delbet's fascia' in French-speaking countries. To summarize, you can integrate vascular treatment in your plans to achieve better drainage by softening the vein-guiding connective tissue. This will, in a way, increase the chances even more of getting better blood supply through the arteries, too. But blood itself is a kind of connective tissue with specialized abilities. So, as mentioned above, blood vessel walls can be manipulated to open or shut down the blood flow, not only because there is less tension in the guiding fascia, but by informing the vessel about a bigger demand via correct receptor arousal. And in spite of the fact that we have done so much research in many countries on blood pressure, receptors, fluid dynamics, and neurological influences on blood supply, vessel diameter, and endothelial factors, we have to admit, that our knowledge of the blood supply of the tissues is far from complete. With that in mind, I'm reminded of Rollin Becker DO's words: 'Often there were theories, killed by a gang of some simple, hard facts'.

References

Atienza J. M., Guinea G. V., Rojo F. J. et al. 2007. The influence of pressure and temperature on the behavior of the human aorta and carotid arteries. *Revista Española de Cardiología* [English Edition], 60, 259–267.

Bank A. J, Kaiser. D. R. 1998. Smooth muscle relaxation: effects on arterial compliance, distensibility, elastic modulus, and pulse wave velocity. *Hypertension*, 1998, 32, 356–359.

Barral J.-P., Croibier A. (eds) 2011. *Manipulation viszeraler Gefäße: Osteopathie in Theorie und Praxis*, München: Urban & Fischer/ Elsevier.

Bevan J. A., Duckworth J., Laher I. et al., 1987. Sympathetic control of cerebral arteries: specialization in receptor type, affinity, and distribution. *FASEB Journal*, 1(3), 193–198.

Bhishagratna K. L. (ed.) 2010. *An English Translation of the Sushruta Samhita, Based on Original Sanskrit Text* Charleston SC: Nabu Press.

Burnstock G. Ralevic V. 1994. New insights into the local regulation of blood flow by perivascular nerves and endothelium. *Brirish Journal of Plastic Surgery*, (1994) 47, 527–543.

Chauffour P., Prat E. (eds) 2002. *Mechanical Link – Fundamental Principles, Theory, and Practice Following an osteopathic approach*, Berkeley, CA: North Atlantic Books.

Duivenvoorden R., De Groot E., Elsen B. M. et al. 2009. In vivo quantification of carotid artery wall dimensions: 3.0-Tesla MRI versus B-mode ultrasound imaging. *Circ Cardiovasc Imaging*, 2, 235–42.

Faury G. 2001. Function–structure relationship of elastic arteries in evolution: from microfibrils to elastin and elastic fibres. *Pathol Biol*, 49, 310–325.

Frucht A. H. 1953. Die Schallgeschwindigkeit in menschlichen und tierischen Geweben. *Zeitschrift für die gesamte experimentelle Medizin*, Bd.120, 526–557.

Gokina N. I. 1998. Temperature and protein kinase C modulate myofilament Ca 2+ sensitivity in pressurized rat cerebral arteries. *Am J Physiol Heart Circ Physiol*, 274 (1998), H1920–H1927.

Han H. C.. 1995. Longitudinal strain of canine and porcine aortas. *J Biomechanics*, 28, No.5, 637–641.

Hermsmeyer K. 1983. Excitation of vascular muscle by norepinephrine. *Annals of Biomedical Engineering*, 1983, Vol.11, 567–577.

Humphrey J. D. 2009. Vascular Mechanics, Mechanobiology, and Remodeling. *J Mech Med Biol*, 9, 243-257.

Jaggar J. G. 1998. Ca2+ channels, ryanodine receptors and Ca2+-activated K+ channels: a functional unit for regulating arterial tone. *Acta physiol scand*, 1998, 64, 577–587.

Jones A. 1983. Membrane Transport in vascular smooth muscle and its relation to normal and altered excitation during hypertension. *Annals of Biomedical Engineering*, 11 (1983), 589–598.

Lu D. & Kassab, G. S. 2011. Role of shear stress and stretch in vascular mechanobiology. *J R Soc Interface*, 8, 1379–85.

Myers T. W. (ed.) 2009. *Anatomy Trains*, Edinburgh, London, New York: Chuchill-Livingstone Elsevier.

Porges S. (ed.) 2010. *Die Polyvagal-Theorie: Neurophysiologische Grundlagen der Therapie. Emotionen, Bindung, Kommunikation & ihre Entstehung*, Paderborn: Junfermann-Verlag.

Ren L. M., Nakane T., Chiba S. 1993. Muscarinic receptor subtypes mediating vasodilation and vasoconstriction in isolated, perfused simian coronary arteries. *J Cardiovasc Pharmacol.*, Dec.;22(6), 841–846.

Riha G. M. 2005. Roles of hemodynamic forces in vascular cell differentiation. *Annals of Biomedical Engineering*, 33, No.6, 772–779.

Schiffrin E. L., 2001. A critical review of the role of endothelial factors in the pathogenesis of hypertension. *Journal of Cardiovascular Pharmacology*, 38, Suppl.2, S3–S6.

Scotland R. S. 2000. Endogenous factors involved in regulation of tone of arterial vasa vasorum:

implications for conduit vessel physiology. *Cardiovascular Research*, 46 (2000), 403–411.

Smith P. H., 1998. A review of the actions and control of intracellular pH in vascular smooth muscle. *Cardiovascular Research*, 38, 316–331.

Still A. T. (ed.) 1899. *Philosophy of Osteopathy*, Kirksville: Truman State University Press.

LIEM, T., Dobler T. K., Puylaert M. (ed.) 2013. *Leitfaden Viscerale Osteopathie*, Munich: Urban & Fischer/Elsevier.

Venkatasubramanian R. T. 2006. Changes in arterial biomechanics following heat and cold treatments. *Journal of Biomechanics*, 2006, Vol.39, S380.

Voets T., 2009. TRPCs, GPCRs and the Bayliss effect. *EmboJ*, 28 (1), 4–5.

Vogt R. 2008. Über das mechanische Verhalten elastischer Arterien. *DO Deutsche Zeitschrift für Osteopathie*, 6(01), 6–7.

Watkins R. W., 1980. Contraction velocity analysis of norepinephrine and angiotensin-ii activation of vascular smooth muscle. *European Journal of Pharmacology*, 62 (1980), 177–189.

Webb R. C., 1981. Regulation of vascular tone, molecular mechanisms. *Progress in Cardiovascular Diseases,*, Vol.24, No.3, 213–243.

Zhang H. & Zhang L. 2008. Role of protein kinase C isozymes in the regulation of alpha1-adrenergic receptor-mediated contractions in ovine uterine arteries. *Biol Reprod*, 78, 35-42.

SKIN – THE KEY ELEMENT IN PALPATION OF FASCIA: FROM AN OSTEOSOPHICAL CONCEPTUALIZATION TO RESEARCH

Jean-Marie A. T. Beuckels

Introduction

Any osteopathic practitioner or physician (OPP) can imagine fascia, skin, and palpation, but what is an osteosophical conceptualization? Osteosophy© is a philosophical and conceptual theoretical thinking system that is based on observation of nature and humanity, in order to create and underpin synthesis and integration insights, and so to determine osteopathic strategies within nonsymptomatic or total osteopathic manual treatment. Osteosophy© forms one of the three pillars of the department of osteopathic medicine at Witten/Herdecke University, along with osteopathic manual medicine (OMM) and research. The conceptualizing aspect in Osteosophy© – as a term kept copyrighted to prevent nonosteopathic use of its content – precedes research questions in OMM. OMM is a medical system that is not determined by its techniques, but depends on understanding and insight, or even wakefulness and consciousness. Fundamental research questions in OMM should *not* consider whether an osteopathic technique provides a therapeutic effect (in a possible placebo or non-placebo way) because these therapeutic effects occur in most cases, as in every other type of therapeutic care. The fundamental questions to ask should be whether an OPP can respond adequately to what the body needs instead of reasoning just about possible effects of actions. Rollin Becker stated that only tissues know. Therefore, interactive and communicative testing of tissue according to ideas, insights, conceptualization, and translational research concepts could give the OPP a direction for knowing the tissues. Translational research supported by osteosophical conceptualization might address more effectively questions concerning adequate treatment of the body's needs – it should at least attempt to let the OPP 'know as the tissues know'.

The question and an idea

More than 25 years ago, while making my first steps in osteopathic education, I asked myself over and over again: how can my osteopathic teachers feel a deeper layer of tissue and analyze its movement? A lot of thoughts crossed my mind at that time: were they gifted people or maybe talented people? Or did they use a kind of 'energetic' secret technique? Or did they just use a physical concept, which has a logical explanation? Or maybe the secret technique just had a logical explanation? However, I remember the first observational insight I had at that time: my osteopathic teachers seemed to palpate and analyze different levels, but the only thing they touched was skin. So my questioning journey started off with this 'skin idea'.

My purpose now is to present to you 'an osteosophical idea' put together from different 'fascial-palpation' notions that have crossed my osteopathic path over the last 25 years. Some of these concepts were derived from conversations with many OMM teachers, students, colleagues, and retired OMM practitioners and physicians. Others just emerged from the conceptualization process itself.

The skin-matrix conceptualization

Different points of view

Most of my osteopathic teachers and retired OMM colleagues explained that this fascial touch or matrix touch of deeper layers was related to a specific feeling of touch of the skin. They discussed that there was a 'gel' involved and that the 'gel' would have a slow movement. It also would be voluminous and filled with up with 'life'. Anyhow, in the most diverse explanations of different lecturers, the skin always seemed to play a major role. Some of these aspects led me to think about the skin in different ways.

Maybe the 'fascia-movements' felt were just skin-on-skin movements. I observed that all my teachers and colleagues, who worked on a fascial level, were contacting with their own skin the skin of their patients. So movement between or on the skin of the OPP and the skin of the patient could give a specific sensation, which led the OPP or patient to believe they feel something like a fascial motion. It could just be some physical proprioceptive effect.

Maybe because the skin is thoroughly interlinked with the extracellular and intracellular matrix (ECM/ICM) complex, moving the skin could make sense to get an idea about the movement of matrix layers beyond the skin. Ingber (2008) suggested that pulling or pressing the skin communicates with deeper layers. Lee (2005) adds to this tensegrity and mechanotransduction other features that might play a role in the communicating skin–ECM/ICM complex, like light and electromagnetic interactions.

Maybe touching and testing deeper fascial layers was a bit 'metaphysical' anyway. The skin could be a kind of motion-transmitter, similar to the cell membrane that is transmitting the signals from the ICM to the ECM and vice versa. The skin would then be the body membrane, bringing the information of the content of the body and the information of the integrated and surrounding body field together. In evolutionary biology, this morphological field is discussed more and more and cannot be denied (Sheldrake, 2009). This field contains all the information to build the morphological expression of biological matter. It not only contains the living matter, but also surrounds it. In an analogy with the ICM/ECM complex, in which the cell membrane plays an interconnecting role, the skin might play a similar role in the physical/metaphysical complex. As the connective tissue matrix is the whole ICM/ECM complex, the morphological matrix would become the physical/metaphysical complex.

This last concept guided me from skin ideas to different considerations of matter and different ways of perceiving the ECM/ICM complex.

Considering matter or the ECM/ICM complex from a Newtonian perspective brings us straight into a biomechanical mode of observation. A fulcrum, an axis, and the physical description of motion (like amplitude, direction, force, velocity, and frequency) are used to describe its motion. But, considering the matter from the perspective of Max Planck (1922 [2013]), the concept of physical solid matter suddenly disappears:

'All matter originates and exists only by virtue of a force, which brings the particle of an atom to vibration and holds this most minute solar system of the atom together. We must assume behind this force the existence of a conscious and intelligent mind. This mind is the matrix of all matter.'

These insights show that a physical body, which is being surrounded by skin, is held together by the 'Planck intelligence' – also a morphological matrix, which finds an anchor in the core of the physical body, and expands in the form field through the skin outside this solid body.

But solid matter can be represented not only as small particles, but also as waves. Heisenberg's 'double slit' experimental data (1927) suggest that electrons (tiny bits of matter) react to observation: the double slit diffraction and interference pattern disappear under observation (Bach et. al., 2013). Heisenberg stated that the observer collapses the wave function into particles by simply observing the matter. The very act of observing (even in a palpatory way) lets the entire wave possibilities in superposition of each other collapse into an arrangement of particles (Wolf, 1989), which is expressed through morphology. This means that when we touch in OMM in a conscious observing way, we as observers let the matter express itself as a collapsed wave function through its morphological expression of the particles.

Focus or defocus

Therefore, different 'worlds of matter' might emerge under the hands of an OPP, depending on intentionalizing or attentionalizing the interaction with the matter or tissue and its transforming morphologic state. Here 'intention' implies a focus and a specific inward motion and 'attention' implies a defocusing and a global outward motion.

Some fascia instructors proposed visualization to palpate a specific layer. In the last few decades, it was one of the more popular ways to interact on the level of the morphological matrix. It could be called a mind–hand intention. Here, an imaginary information field seems to be projected in the morphological field and used as a template in order to construct form or movement. The problem here might be a possible stagnant imagination field, which could counteract the natural expression of the morphological matrix. Visualization in this case might be a form of 'particularization' (modification of the waves into particles) through which the tissue matrix can be observed through palpation and consequently morphologically influenced on a physical level.

Other fascia instructors advised keeping some intention while testing the matrix to be able to test the deformation possibilities of its morphological expression; still others advised keeping attention to let the morphological matrix express itself during the matrix testing. The individual decision to do one or the other in OMM testing and treatment might depend on what is needed: a natural expression of reality or an influenced or deformed expression in a trans-reality. Both ways, focusing or defocusing, might have a reason to be applied.

Consciousness

As the cell membrane interconnects and integrates qualities of both ICM and ECM, the skin might express in a similar way different qualities of the physical and metaphysical complex of the body matrix. The skin is first of all tissue and so also a form of matter. As matter can be observed from different perspectives, the way you observe matter can modify your ideas and your thinking pathways. These perspectives can then also alter the way you touch matter or touch skin. They can enable you to palpate 'differently'. If we in OMM want to test tissue layers without modifying the morphological matrix through visualization, then an open conceptualization is needed.

If the morphological matrix could be represented by the E-hologram or total energy-hologram then it includes the tissue matrix, which could be defined by the matter-hologram. This results in the following formula: E = {matter hologram}. 'E' as energy field, (McTaggart, 2008), energetic scaffolding of the physical body (Fulford, 2003), or energizer of matter (Gerber, 2001) is more than just a matter-hologram.

Something is added to the matter-hologram to transform it into a morphological matrix. If we observe Einstein's formula, then the transforming substance can only be c^2. The 'c' stands for a 'constant' with the value of 'light velocity'. But what on earth could conceptually have the velocity of light, transform a matter matrix into a morphological matrix, and be represented by the letter 'c'? The answer here could be consciousness. It takes a lot of consciousness to substantialize matter: $(consciousness)^2$.

Liquid substance

All matter that surrounds us is a result of a frequency. If you change the frequency, the structure of the matter will change. For example, it is known that oscillating a wine glass by playing sound at its resonance frequency will cause it to move, change and liquefy its structure, and eventually even break it.

This liquid state, in which matter is vibrating with its own resonance frequency, has a small expansive quality. A. T. Still (1910) emphasized this (liquid) 'Matter' behind the matter, which he called 'Substance'. The concept of 'substance' arose from the metaphysical philosophy of Aristotle (384–322 BC), in which Aristotle explained substance to be the building block of the universe, while defining it as a kind of consciousness (Aristotle & Bishop Jones, 2012). For some reason, science integrated the idea of having basic building blocks in the cosmos but replaced it with solid material or matter, which actually proves today to be mainly empty space. This 'substance-matter switch' also wiped out consciousness from the common cosmic vision of mankind and the world. In OMM, this cosmic vision of matter–motion–mind was well known in the beginning, but later replaced with the 'medicine fitting formula', body–mind–spirit. This provided a kind of scientific 'drive' to cut further metaphysical aspects out of palpation and treatment. However, in OMM the liquefied and expansive states of matter were still maintained in education. Different forms of listening to the tissue as in states of balanced ligamentous tension or cranial primary respiratory motion still include this palpatory liquid-expansive mode, which is felt by many OPPs and is accepted to be a reality in OMM. To be able to contact the liquid-expansive mode requires a certain wakefulness and consciousness.

Tissue could be a form of substance, maybe it might just contain substance, or it may behave as matter and/or as substance. All these tissue realities might be real, possibly depending on the kind of conditions that are integrated or perceived during the palpation in that moment. Although the OPP can consider tissue as a piece of matter, the OPP can modify the palpation conditions in such a way that matter presents itself as substance. Considering simple laws of physics, resonance can induce in the tissue a state of vibration. Under such conditions, tissue will then show its liquid, palpable state. To induce a resonating state, a specific frequency input is needed – the frequency of the kind of tissue itself.

To enable a palpatory substance transformation for a specific kind of tissue, the OPP needs in the first place to specify the kind of tissue that is to be liquefied under palpatory conditions. Anatomical and histological knowledge definitely supports this specification. However, the 'Descartes-hangover' keeps most OPPs imprisoned in their analyzing knowledge. A detailed, but sometimes 'unreal' knowledge about models of cells or dead anatomy merely offers one a glimpse of what nature actually presents. Anatomy, anatomy, and anatomy, or (Anatomy)[3], which is a world of 'changing' morphology, might provide the OPP with a more 'living' experience of a more real particularity of tissue. Experienced knowledge of tissue is one of the conditions to dock into the individualized frequency of the tissue in order to turn it into its liquid expansion. Certainly, other levels of consciousness might support similar liquefication processes of tissue palpatory information.

Once liquid expansive matter opens the water interface between the tissue matrix and the morphological matrix, it is opening its information capacity. The 'Emoto' characteristic of water – also well known as the water information capacity – defines water's ability to capture and stock information, but also to communicate its information (Emoto, 2011)

Intention – attention

In the teachings of fascial therapy, it was mentioned many times that one should develop an intention to ask the tissue about its movement. But to have an intention, one needs a plan, knowledge, self-knowledge, total experienced knowledge, or even consciousness ... In osteopathic practice, there exists an intentional interaction, which is called a mind–hand–intention–interaction.

Here an interpretation of reality is mentally composed as information in the thoughts of the OPP. The OPP then puts his/her hands on the body of the patient and intentionally projects this reality into the tissue in order to turn it into the desired tissue reality. The problem here is not the intention but the exclusion of the tissue reality. If the tissue reality loses its degrees of freedom, the 'injected' idea becomes fixated, an *idée fixe*. This turns the projected reality into a subreality or nonreality. The OPP is consequently fixated in his or her own information.

From an osteosophical perspective, there might also exist a hand–mind pathway. Here the information flow originates from the tissues underneath the hand of the OPP. The first tissue to be touched by the OPP's hand is skin tissue. If the total tissue matrix or the morphological matrix communicates some information to the OPP's hand, naturally it would be transmitted through the skin. The OPP needs attention to pick this information up. The common basic information communication between the OPP and the tissue occurs through movement, which itself can be generated by different forces – internal or external ones – in the form of a pull, a push, or even a frequency. This movement information can similarly be measured and decoded by physical laws.

Research starts

Skin motion

Later, after gathering these many different points of view on fascial-therapeutic touch, the possible mechanisms, and different perspectives on matter, I was able to do research at the department of osteopathic medicine at Witten/Herdecke University. There, I discovered that the skin carries different movement patterns depending on space–time conditions. The basic osteosophical consideration for this research was the interconnection between the skin and the rest of the total tissue matrix, in a totality of matter and motion.

Scientific literature in 2015 still considers (bio) mechanical testing of the skin more as skin or skin-fascial stretching. Different devices prove that the skin can stretch to a certain amplitude. This ability to stretch is mainly measured by holding two reference points and taking them apart.

The idea of 'dermatofascial motion testing'

The idea of 'dermatofascial motion testing' is not about the stretch capacity of the skin but about motion patterns of the skin. The idea came from measurements in sports motion analyses.

In sport science in the 1980s, experimental set-ups in biomechanical analysis of sport movements used to attach several adhesive markers as reference points on skin for two-dimensional (2D) positional and motion measurements. During these experiments, the researchers had to take into account a kind of measurement problem of the reference markers, which did not remain optimally in place; the markers actually moved according to the individual skin motion of the subjects. Up to the present day, the movement of the markers reveals soft tissue artefacts in the measurement of joint kinematics (Benoit et al., 2015) These biomechanical artefact analyses provided 2D data; correspondingly the individual skin motion data was also 2D.

This observation of 2D skin motion was applied in an osteosophical conceptualization. The complete individual skin has its own 2D movement possibility, which might be interconnected by the skin with the very tissue beyond or even with the total morphological matrix. The skin might have an imprint of movement patterns of the total matrix. In other words, dermatofascial motion testing might reflect the total movement pattern of the tissue matrix from a skin perspective. Considering the narrow interconnection with the fascial tissue or matrix tissue, it was plausible that the 2D skin motion or skin shift depends on the limiting motion of its underlying interconnected layers.

Shift motions

The objective of dermatofascial testing was to examine the shift motions of skin. Shifting the skin in different directions provides a skin motion pattern in ease (or in barrier). The skin motion cannot possibly have the same amplitude or 2D range of motion as its inferior layers, but as the skin is well interconnected, it might have the same or a similar motion pattern as the tissue layers beyond that are 'holding' the skin. Within the current osteosophical conceptualization, the location of interconnection of skin with deeper tissue layers was called a skin–fascial unit.

Shift motions are necessary minor motions to let three-dimensional (3D) major motions happen. Bois explains with sensory biomechanics that without shift motions, 3D motions cannot totally express in a harmonic way (Courraud-Bourhis, 2005). A simple but clear example of harmonic balancing of minor and major motions can be demonstrated by forward-bending while standing against a wall. If you bring your feet, knees, pelvis, and total spine against a wall, and you then try to bend forward, falling over becomes inevitable. The reason why this happens is that there is a lack of backward shifting of the pelvis region. This demonstrates the necessity of a backward shift motion of the pelvis during forward-bending. Bending forward is a circular motion around an axis. All circular motions need an opposite shift to balance the body or specific 3D matrix part. If there is no balance, there is no harmony in the proprioception. No adequate proprioception means no full-body consciousness. In a way, the shift movements are defining the body consciousness. They define possibilities to move. Less shift possibility indicates less total movement.

The 2D shift patterns that are present in the skin could contain information on shift possibilities in the 3D matrix. In other words, the outcome of the shift test of the skin could reveal the patterns that are related to circular motions such as flexion–extension, lateral flexion, and rotation in the matrix.

A testing device

An electromechanical 'dermatofascial motion test device' was developed at the department of osteopathic medicine at Witten/Herdecke University (Fig. 49.1). The aim of creating such a device was to discover whether dermatofascial patterns could be measured with a device in a valid and reliable way, without a metaphysical influence. During the first

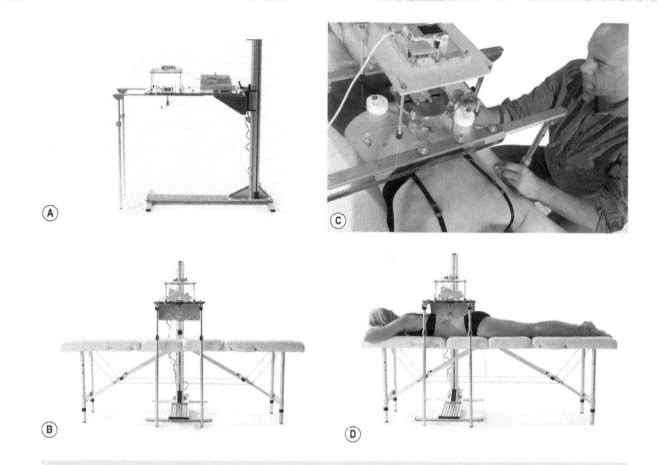

Figure 49.1

The skin motion analyzer. (A) Anterior view. (B) Side view in combination with a bench. (C) Preparing the patient's position for skin motion testing. (D) Side view of the patient in position for testing. Reproduced courtesy of Till Böcker

phase of the experimental setup, the device itself produced and demonstrated a valid and reliable outcome: different operators used the device to test dermatofascial patterns in the same skin and obtained the same results – a very good intra-rater reliability was reached.

However, the main idea of engineering such a device was to examine whether the device test and manual skin test could provide the same test results. Yet, the latest data showed that the test results are not the same, but the patterns sometimes seem to overlap. Compared to the device testing, which had a good intra-rater reliability, the manual testing achieved for the same skin–fascial unit a poor intra-rater

reliability. The main factor influencing this poor intra-rater reliability was a difference in OPPs' 'education'. OPPs with different educational backgrounds in dermatofascial testing seemed to produce different results during manual skin-pattern testing. Comparing the data of a manual tester subgroup that was educated in a specific way surprisingly demonstrated a much better intra-rater reliability.

Nevertheless, manual testing operators, even if educated in the same way, applied the proper idea of force and velocity during the manual testing. Their amplitudes differed but their pattern ranges overlapped. This also lead to the consequence that the data of the test device analysis did not provide the same amplitudes as the data of the manual dermatofascial motion analyses, but provided the same patterns of the skin–fascial unit. This means that overlapping of the pattern outcome between the device testing and manual testing only existed when the manual operators were specifically educated to perform the dermatofascial test in a similar way.

Thus, it could be concluded from this first experimental phase that it was possible to manually test shift patterns in the dermatofascial layer after a specific education, which corresponded with the patterns tested with a device.

Dysfunctional layers in the skin–fascial unit

In one of the following research phases, the dermatofascial shifts that were analyzed with the device were then compared with tissue motions of the related skin–fascial unit.

By the use of a pressure device, the deeper layers were investigated mechanically for dysfunctions. The results showed that the dysfunctions beyond the dermatofascial layer were spread out in more than just one anatomical or tissue layer. The dysfunction seemed to have a kind of amorphic feature or nonspecific morphology that interfered with the form motion of other adjacent layers. This interference or dysfunctional motion seemed to be projected in the dermatofascial layer in a 2D way. The shift motions at ease in the dermatofascial layer, which could be calculated as one vector, matched the 2D projection of the 3D vector (presenting amplitude, direction, and force) defining the major dysfunction in one of the layers beyond the skin.

Integrating depth as a third dimension constructs a volume

A later research idea questioned how the OPP could locate the major dysfunction beyond the skin layer in a specific skin–fascial unit. Interviews with colleagues and teachers in fascia therapy revealed that to test a location beyond the skin, logically the OPP needs to add depth as a third dimension to the palpatory information. Depth allows a perception of volume. The outcome of the interviews concluded

two extreme modes to integrate depth and pick up a volume.

Proprioceptive pressure volume

The first and easier way to pick up the sense of a volume could be achieved through proprioceptive information as a result of a colliding pressure interaction of the OPP's hand and a tissue resistance reaction in a deeper layer. This idea resembles the mechanism of the mechanical pressure device that was used to test the depth of the tissue resistance. The OPP should undergo specific educational steps to develop this kind of pressure palpation.

Proprioceptive sensorial volumes

A second, less obvious way to pick up the sense of a volume could be accomplished not via a physical pressure but via a 'sensorial set-up'. This sensorial volume is more a metaphysical volume or metavolume. It can be compared to a volume that is involved in the expression of the primary respiration mechanism (PRM). During the palpation of the PRM, the OPP has the impression that there is kind of volume involved, which feels like a soft electromagnetic charge that pushes one's hand off the skull or the skin. This sensorial volume manifests itself mainly from the inside outwards. But via a mind–hand–intention, a sensorial volume can be created and intentionally expanded inwards (in the tissue layers beyond the skin) and also moved inside the tissue matrix in various directions.

Using a metavolume, the OPP should be able to detect tissue layers beyond the skin that allow less inward expansion, less volume motion, and less specific expression of the possible features of the ECM/ICM complex. Precisely these tissue layers would contain the dysfunction.

A sensorial volume can also emerge from a hand–mind attention. Here attentionality creates the metavolume, which moves autonomously through the layers and scans them for resonating volume.

Both intentional and attentional metavolumes can be 'colored' by different palpatory features of the matrix like ECM/ICM tensegrity, light, and electromagnetic interactions. Even the 'Emoto' effect could play a role here. These 'colored' volumes can allow the OPP to interact on a different communication level with tissue layers of the matrix. To apply these sensorial volumes in order to analyze dysfunctions in deeper layers, a specific palpatory education is needed.

The sensorial method was studied in a research set-up and the latest research results demonstrate that testing the dysfunctional layers with a volume motion presents a motion pattern, which corresponds with the pattern of dermatofascial motion. The motion pattern of volume motion (manually tested) and the motion pattern of pressure motion (device tested) also seem to match. A preliminary 'correspondence of depth' analysis for OPP (with specific education in manual testing via sensorial volume and pressure volume) has been conducted. Early results seem to reveal a similarity of patterns, not of amplitudes.

Conclusion

The palpatory way to a deeper layer of tissue can be supported by the concept of mechanotransduction or other features in the communicating ECM/ICM complex like H_2O-plasticity, light and electromagnetic interactions, etc. As the OPP picks up different kinds of connecting tissue information through tactility, proprioception, or sensation in a focused or defocused way, tissue itself might be explored as a tissue matrix. This matrix is assumed to be integrated and embraced by a morphological field that contains all the information to build the morphological expression of biological matter. Supported by a Planckian view on matter and a Heisenbergian view on its observation, matter can be perceived during palpation as solid, gel, or as another state of aggregation, depending on the focus or defocus of the OPP. The non-solid palpatory observation demands a form of consciousness and resonance to interact with substantializing matter in its liquefication process.

Depending on a mind–hand–intention–interaction or a hand–mind pathway, the matter perceived as substance provides movement information, which can be measured and decoded by physical laws. The expression of this sensory information depends on the shifting properties of the skin. The skin shifts, measured by a testing device, seem to be an imprint of motion possibilities of the skin–fascial unit. A palpatory physical volume via a sol-pressure perception or

a palpatory metaphysical volume via a gel-substance perception can open the doors to deeper tissue layers.

For now, it can be concluded that the skin does play a major role in fascial or tissue matrix testing. The dermatofascial shift amplitudes in the test results are not supported by inter-rater reliability, but the patterns in the dermatofascial testing present a reliable (inter- and intra-rater) outcome.

References

Aristotle, Bishop Jones R., Ross W. D. *The Metaphysics*. CreateSpace Independent Publishing Platform, 2012.

Bach R., Pope D., Liou S-H., and Batelaan H. Controlled double-slit electron diffraction. *New J Physics*. 2013;15:033018

Benoit D. L., Damsgaard M., Andersen M. S. Surface marker cluster translation, rotation, scaling and deformation: their contribution to soft tissue artefact and impact on knee joint kinematics. *Journal of Biomechanics*. 2015;48(10):2124–2129.

Courraud-Bourhis H. Biomécanique sensorielle et biorythmie, Editions Point d'appui, 2005.

Emoto M., *The Miracle of Water*. Atria Books, reprint edition, 2011.

Fulford R., *Dr. Fulford's Touch of Life: The Healing Power of the Natural Life Force*. Gallery Books, 2003.

Gerber R. *Vibrational Medicine: The Handbook of Subtle-Energy Therapies*, 3rd edition. Bear & Company, 2001.

Ingber D. E. Tensegrity and mechanotransduction. *Journal of Bodywork and Movement Therapies*. 2008;12:198–200.

Lee R. P. *Interface: Mechanisms of Spirit*. Stillness Press LLC, 2005.

McTaggart L. *The Field: The Quest for the Secret Force of the Universe*. Harper Perennial. Updated edition, 2008.

Planck M. *The Origin and Development of the Quantum Theory Translated by Quantum Theory*. Classic Reprint Series. Forgotten Books, 1922 [2013].

Sheldrake R. *Morphic Resonance: The Nature of Formative Causation*. 4th edition. Revised and expanded edition of *A New Science of Life*. Park Street Press, 2009.

Still A. T. *Osteopathy: Research and Practice*. Kirksville, Mo: Andrew Taylor Still, 1910.

Wolf A. F. *Taking the Quantum Leap: The New Physics for Nonscientists*. Revised edition. Harper Perennial, 1989.

JARRICOT'S DERMALGIA APPLIED TO FASCIA

Michel Puylaert

Introduction

History

Reflex zones, or dermalgia zones, were first researched during the late nineteenth and early twentieth centuries:

- In 1841 Marshall Hall described a connection between points of focal tenderness and underlying visceral disease.

- A. Sherback introduced the concept of reflex zones between 1910–1936.

- In 1930, *connective tissue massage* was developed by W. Kohlrausch, H. Teirich-Leube and E. Dicke. The importance of their connective tissue zones was twofold: either during clinically active disease or as so-called 'clinically silent zones'.

- In 1955, O. Glaser and V. A. Dalicho further developed reflex-based techniques in relation to visceral and somatic dysfunction.

- After WWII a number of US scientists, including M. Beal, became interested in the relationship between skin and the viscera. This led to a further development of the so-called Chapman points.

These reflex zones were considered both diagnostic and therapeutic in nature.

Dr Jarricot (1903–1989) was a homeopath with additional training in Chinese acupuncture and ear acupuncture. Searching for objective signs of visceral dysfunction, he examined both thorax and abdomen and discovered superficial tissue changes in several distinct places. These were found to be specific skin changes originating from visceral disease. Jarricot compared these zones with findings from acupuncture-related research. He discovered that these zones, especially those of the anterior thorax, tend to disappear with the correct application of an acupuncture needle at specific locations distant from the zone of dermalgia, which often overlapped with acupuncture points. Conversely, treatment of these anterior zones of dermalgia normalized the respective Chinese pulse, an important diagnostic in acupuncture.

As early as 1932, Dr Jarricot described the relationship between skin and visceral organs, coining the term *'dermalgie réflexes'* or 'reflex dermalgias'. The construction of a reliable topographic map of these specific points took him almost half a century (Jarricot, 1975). Reflex points were included in the map only after numerous investigations, including laparoscopies, electrocardiograms, ultrasound, X-rays, etc. Additionally, these zones of skin were confirmed surgically. In general, these distinct tissue changes are found on the anterior aspect of the trunk and constitute projections of visceral organs and their supply. These zones serve both diagnosis and treatment. In his treatment of reflex dermalgias, Dr Jarricot often included acupuncture points.

Foundations

According to Dr Jarricot, reflex dermalgias are defined by a 'lipodystrophy' – a change of the dermis. Usually, the zone in which the reflex can be found is situated around the exit point of a cutaneous nerve. The size and shape of these zones differ depending on the viscera they relate to. Jarricot's reflex dermalgias are silent and do not cause pain spontaneously. Only during specific testing and in the case of underlying dysfunction can a tenderness, or sometimes even exquisite pain, be provoked. As external signs, the practitioner notes considerable skin thickening and is almost unable to lift the skin.

A hyperesthetic point can be found more or less centrally within the zone, usually corresponding with the point of exit of the perforating branch of a cutaneous nerve or with the crossing of a meridian.

A positive reflex dermalgia is an expression of the dysfunction of a visceral organ or its neurological, vascular, or lymphatic supply. It is a sign of a functional disturbance of the autonomic system of a visceral organ. The clinical relevance of reflex dermalgias has increased over the years and nowadays the concept of reflex dermalgias is taught in most osteopathic schools, often under the term 'viscerosomatic reflexes'.

Dr Jarricot undertook significant amounts of research in the fields of Chinese acupuncture and ear acupuncture. In his opinion, acupuncture points constitute 'mini reflex dermalgias'. Acupuncture points exist on a macroscopic level, usually comprising a nerve-vessel bundle enclosed by a thin sheet of loose connective tissue. The ground substance of the connective tissue can be submitted to mechanoelectrical transformations, thereby activating both autonomous nerves and sympathetic vasomotor plexuses of the vessels' adventitia, thus causing the cutaneous changes described.

Dermatomes

Each reflex dermalgia is located within a dermatome. A dermatome is considered the area of skin supplied by a single spinal nerve. Each dermatome is made up of three parts: a ventral, dorsal, and lateral aspect. These are innervated by ventral, dorsal, and lateral branches of a spinal nerve.

The diagnosis of a dermatome is an easy and efficient indication for the early detection of pathological processes within a segment. In internal disease, changes within a dermatome chronologically precede signs detectable by more technical means of diagnosis. It can thus be considered a form of early warning system. The 'reading' of a dermatome is a way for the practitioner to gain insight into the inside of the unharmed body. The deeper layers, for example, muscle, bone, and visceral organs, 'express' themselves by means of the epidermis, dermis, and subcutis.

In the literature, a distinction is made between subcutaneous dermatomes and dermatomes of the epidermis. Subcutaneous dermatomes are mapped out through anatomical preparation of the spinal nerve all the way to the subcutis. These are the dermatomes used by Dr Jarricot.

Dermatomes of the epidermis, on the other hand, are mapped out clinically through sensibility testing of the skin and observations from cases of herpes zoster infection. The well-known zones of Head are epidermal dermatomes. As they are not congruent with subcutaneous dermatomes, they will not be considered in more detail here.

Subcutaneous dermatomes, as opposed to dermatomes of the epidermis, are always subjectively verifiable demarcations.

Research

Dr Jarricot was mainly influenced by the work of three scientists: H. Head, J. Mackenzie, and, most crucially, J. Dejerine (1849–1917), a French neurologist investigating metamerization and dermatomes. He was mainly concerned with sensory dermatomes as opposed to autonomic or motor zones. Only dermatomes with visceral projections on the skin were examined and mapped out. Within each dermatome there exist several projections of visceral organs. Innervation of these organs is derived from the same spinal segment as the nerve fibers relating to the dermatome. Dr Jarricot adapted the dermatomal patterns from Dejerine.

The anterolateral aspect of the trunk between clavicle and pubic symphysis is covered by only 12 thoracic dermatomes, which are significantly easier to discern and anatomically more consistent than the posterior zones. On the ventral body surface, individual zones can be mapped out precisely. Additionally, there exist reflex zones at the head, back, and extremities. However, as they have not been considered by Dr Jarricot, they will not be discussed here.

With his work on the examination of dermatomes Sir H. Head (1861–1940), an English neurologist, clarified the existence of important viscerocutaneous connections. Head himself was inspired by the work of V. Ross (1880). Head noted that hypersensitive zones can develop in each dermatome and investigated the connection between a particular visceral complaint and the development of such hyperesthetic zones. Visceral dysfunction can manifest itself as a painful sensation at a distant area of the body surface. He called this phenomenon 'referred' or 'projected' pain. This transferred pain is specific in terms of the body's side and segment. Dr Jarricot emphasized the fact that early acupuncturists, almost 2000 years ago, already recognized such a topographic connection between cutaneous and visceral disease.

The English cardiologist Sir J. Mackenzie (1853–1925) examined the myotomal response and the tightening up of specific muscles during visceral dysfunction, thus developing the concept of a visceromuscular reflex (1923).

Despite all the evidence, there is as yet no clear explanation of the thickening of skin in positive reflex dermalgias. Generally, all cutaneous reflex zones are thought to have their origin in the embryological development of dermatomes, myotomes, and viscerotomes. A reflex arch was postulated but could not be scientifically validated.

Dr Jarricot, like other authors, suspected the skin changes to be mediated partly by the spinal nerve and mainly through sympathetic changes. The spinal nerve mainly influences the location of the changes observed, whereas the sympathetic fibers determine the nature and extent of such changes.

Reflex dermalgias

Overview

Prior to Dr Jarricot's investigations in the 1930s, the relationship between viscera and skin was mainly thought to be of a nociceptive nature. Dr Jarricot, however, postulated functional disturbances to be of much more significance. Positive reflex dermalgias are silent in the absence of an external stimulus, but already indicate the existence of an underlying dysfunction. The latter may be latent and often accompanies additional dysfunctions. In hypertension, for example, one can often find positive reflex dermalgias for the pancreas.

The appropriate treatment of a reflex dermalgia causes the diminution of the lipodystrophy and the hyperesthetic point to disappear. Occasionally, a reddening and increase in temperature can be observed at the level of the reflex dermalgia. Dr Jarricot noted this increase in temperature to amount to up to 1°C.

With some organs, a decrease in volume and a relaxation of the fascial surroundings of the organ is noted. Dr Jarricot also used ear acupuncture to complement his treatments.

These are a few examples from Dr Jarricot's practice:

The liver: The organ protrudes between two to four fingers' breadth from underneath the costal margin. A change in volume can occur immediately or with a delayed onset of a few minutes. In dysfunctions of the liver–gall bladder complex, quite regularly a positive reflex dermalgia for the pancreas can be detected.

Hemorrhoids: The swelling decreases immediately, unless there exists a thrombus within a vein. Thus, the treatment of the related reflex dermalgia can be considered a differential diagnostic tool to distinguish simple swelling and thrombosis.

Uterus: In case of congestion, the volume decreases and the uterus appears to relax and move cranially.

Ovaries: Congestion of the ovaries tends to normalize itself with treatment. There is, however, no response if the underlying cause is a cyst. The treatment of the reflex dermalgia is thus considered a way of differentiation between congestion and cyst.

Prostate: The prostate gland demonstrates an immediate relaxation in case of congestion. There is no response in case of underlying hypertrophy. Again, the treatment of the reflex zone is a useful diagnostic tool.

Examination

The position of the reflex dermalgia (i.e., the area of skin changes and tenderness) is consistently the same within the respective dermatome. For the unpaired organs, it is always situated ipsilaterally or in the midline, and symmetrically left or right for the paired organs.

Dr Jarricot proposed a protocol called the '*palper-rouler de Wetterwald*'. This examination protocol is the same for *all* reflex dermalgias.   AQ1

Positioning: The patient is in a supine or prone position. The practitioner is standing at pelvis level on the patient's right or left.

Technique: The practitioner takes up a fold of skin with both hands, lifting it slightly with the fingertips of his thumb and fingers. The thumbs are placed on one side, the fingers on the other side of the skin fold. Thumbs and index fingers are mainly palpating.

Whilst lifting up the skin it is gently rolled between the fingers. The practitioner tries to lift up as thin a skin fold as possible. The rolling movement is usually initiated from a more lateral position, away from the reflex dermalgia, where the skin is elastic and not thickened. The direction of movement is rectangular to the reflex dermalgia under examination.

Interpretation: If the reflex dermalgia is positive or active, this examination will provide both an objective and a subjective sign.

The objective measure is a clearly measurable thickening of the skin fold. The subdermal layers feel sticky and the palpatory quality is altered. It is hard to lift or roll the skin fold.

Subjectively, the patient reports pain. The closer the rolling of the skin gets to the reflex dermalgia, the more painful the examination is for the patient. A hyperesthetic point exists where the dermal adhesions are strongest.

The precise location of the hyperesthetic point can be determined not only using the '*palper-rouler*' test, but also using any current means of examining cutaneous sensibility, for example, electricity, needling, etc. According to Dr Jarricot, however, the technique described is easier, quicker, and just as precise as any classical method. Also, in most of these alternative examination techniques, an objective indication of dysfunction is missing.

Each individual reflex dermalgia is of a clearly defined shape, for example, oval for bile ducts and pancreas, or round for the gall bladder itself.

There is no visceral pain without a corresponding reflex dermalgia. Each functional or reactive disturbance of a viscerum causes a positive reflex dermalgia.

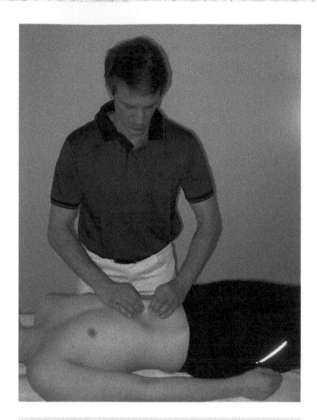

Figure 50.1
Anterior reflex dermalgia of the stomach

Any change of these zones is an indication of either an improvement or a deterioration of the underlying dysfunction.

Exceptions

It may happen that reflex dermalgias are found to be larger in size than the zones described by Dr Jarricot, or they may not be included in Dr Jarricot's maps at all (for example, in the 11th and 12th dermatomes). In these cases, often the reflex zones relate to musculoskeletal dysfunctions of, for example, the spine, rather than the viscera. The same may be the case when two symmetrical reflex dermalgias are detected.

Specific reflex dermalgias

Cardiac plexus and superficial fascia

This reflex dermalgia zone is situated at the 3rd and 4th left intercostal spaces (ICS), just parasternally.

This zone is found to be positive in functional disturbances of the heart. The dysfunction is a minor one if the hyperesthetic point is located only within the 4th ICS. When the 3rd and 5th ICSs are involved, the case requires significantly more attention.

If the painful zone extends further than the 3rd ICS, the pathology may be more serious, even more so if the pain extends all the way to the axilla.

The examination of the heart's reflex zones is not dangerous.

Treatment:

Positioning: The patient is in a prone position. The practitioner is standing at pelvis level on the patient's right or left.

Phase 1: Lift the painful and thickened fold of skin and wait until the pain and tension have decreased.

Phase 2: Stretching the superficial fascia between the ribs.

With the finger of one hand, fix the anterolateral sternum at the level of the 3rd ICS. From here, the middle finger of the other hand is used to apply a lateral tension along the ICS toward the medioclavicular line. The tension is held for several seconds.

Phase 3: Longitudinal stretch of the pectoral fascia at the sternal attachment.

The fingertips of one hand fix the sternum at the level of the 2nd ribs. The middle finger of the other hand is used to apply a caudal tension toward the 5th costal cartilage. The tension is held for several seconds.

Phase 4: Transverse stretch of the pectoral fascia.

The thumb of one hand fixes the anterolateral border of the sternum at the level of the 2nd rib, while the middle finger of the other hand applies a transversal drag toward the same side along the fibers of the pectoralis major. The technique is repeated at the level of the 3rd, 4th, and 5th ribs and can be used bilaterally.

'Zone of fear'

Reflex dermalgia: Dr Jarricot described a zone that is situated within the left 5th ICS and that he found to relate to the emotion of fear. This is the only reflex dermalgia that can cause pain spontaneously and can be found at the center of a line drawn between the sternum and the left nipple.

Treatment:

The treatment is the same as for the cardiac plexus, but is, however, focused more on the 5th ICS. The 'zone of fear' is often found with a positive celiac plexus reflex dermalgia.

Celiac plexus

The celiac plexus is made up of both sympathetic and parasympathetic fibers. It is formed by the semilunar ganglia, the superior mesenteric ganglion, and the aorticorenal ganglion. Any stimulation of this area spreads throughout the entire visceral system.

In Dr Jarricot's opinion, this plexus constitutes 60 per cent of the autonomous nervous system and is the key to any autonomic dystonia. The relating reflex dermalgia is positive, irrespective of which organ is dysfunctional. Both an anterior and posterior zone have been described, with the anterior zone being of more significance clinically.

Anterior: the reflex dermalgia is situated within the dermatome of T7, inferior to the xiphoid process and within the upper third of a line between the process and the umbilicus. Often, this zone is found to be mildly thickened.

Posterior: Within the dermatome of T7, close and bilateral to the transverse processes of the vertebra.

Treatment of anterior reflex dermalgia

Positioning: The patient is in a prone position with the knees slightly flexed. The practitioner is standing on the right-hand side of the patient.

Phase 1:

Positioning: The practitioner places his hands anterolaterally on the thorax with the thumbs resting inferiorly to the right and left costal margins.

Technique: A sliding and pushing movement is applied along the costal margins until a recess is formed underneath the hands.

Phase 2:

Positioning: The left costal margin, diaphragm, and stomach are fixed with the distal hand, which is pointing toward the sternum. The fingers are placed laterally on the ribs and the thumb is resting just distal to the left costal margin.

The practitioner places the fingers of the proximal hand over the thumb of the distal hand.

Technique: The fingers of the proximal hand apply a sliding and pushing movement towards the linea alba whilst the thumb of the distal hand holds on to the fasciae of diaphragm and stomach. The fingers slide along the fascia with a medium pressure.

Phase 3:

Positioning: The right costal margin is fixed using the proximal hand, the thumb being placed just distal to the costal margin. The fingers of the distal hand are resting on the thumb of the proximal hand.

Technique: The fingers of the proximal hand apply a sliding and pushing movement toward the linea alba. The fingers are sliding along the fascia with a medium pressure.

Phase 4:

Positioning: The practitioner's fingers are lying vertically on the linea alba.

Technique: Apply a straight posterior pressure until a release is felt.

Treatment of posterior reflex dermalgias

Positioning: The patient is in a supine position. The practitioner is standing next to the patient at pelvis level.

Technique:

Phase 1: Lift the tender and thickened skin and hold until the tension is felt to release. The pain decreases significantly and the thickness of the skin fold seems to go down.

Phase 2: Apply a focal pressure with the thumb over the zone's most sensitive point. Small stretching and rotating movements are performed. Slowly increase the pressure and feel for a change in the fasciae. The pressure is held for a few seconds, then removed and repeatedly applied again until the zone feels soft and elastic.

Phase 3:

Positioning: The patient is in a supine position. The practitioner is standing next to the patient at pelvis level.

Technique: With a medium amount of pressure, slide the thumbs along the skin just lateral to the spinous processes of T7, T8, and T9. The zone of tenderness is removed using stretching and rotational movements. Change the direction of the movements as appropriate.

The removal of the reflex dermalgias relating to the celiac plexus causes an immediate relaxation, mainly of the upper abdomen. The duration of this relaxed state depends on the underlying pathology.

Greater splanchnic nerve

This nerve contributes to the celiac plexus and originates at a thoracic chain ganglion at the level of T7, T8, and T9. The reflex dermalgias are located superficial to the 8th ribs, at a point where, a small indentation can often be found in the curvature of the rib. This point is tender to the touch.

Right side: Amongst other roles, the greater splanchnic nerve controls the functional organization of the biliary system. It executes a decisive control over the sphincter of Oddi.

Left side: This reflex dermalgia influences the pancreas, also regulating the autonomic balance of the abdominal region. Dr Jarricot recognized a remote effect on the thoracic diaphragm, the 'zone of fear' in the 5th ICS and the cardiac plexus.

Treatment:

Positioning: The patient is in a supine position. The practitioner is standing next to the patient at pelvis level.

Phase 1: Lift the fold of thickened skin and hold without pressure until a relaxation is felt.

Phase 2: The tender area is treated using gentle kneading and squeezing movements. The thumb applies a focal pressure with an element of multidirectional rotation until relaxation is achieved.

Topography of anterior reflex dermalgias (Fig. 50.2)

Ovaries and testes: Bilaterally within L1 and L2 dermatomes. The reflex zone is round in shape and measures about 4 cm in diameter. It is found halfway between the anterior superior iliac spine (ASIS) and the pubic tubercle.

Kidneys: Bilaterally within the dermatomes of T12. This zone is round and 1.5 cm in diameter, located medial and slightly proximal of the ASIS. In cases of renal colic, the laterality of the reflex zone will confirm the side of the kidney involved.

Urinary bladder: Located in the dermatome of T12, this zone measures 3 cm in diameter and can be found in the midline about a finger's breadth proximal to the pubic symphysis. Treatment of this reflex dermalgia can positively influence the symptoms of cystitis.

Uterus: An oval zone found in the dermatome of T11, halfway between the pubic symphysis and umbilicus and thus about three fingers' breadth cranial to the reflex dermalgia relating to the urinary bladder. It is found to be positive at the beginning of menstruation and in early pregnancy.

Prostate: The reflex dermalgia of the prostate is the same zone as for the uterus.

Ascending colon: Within the right T10 dermatome, this zone is located around the umbilicus and shaped like a quarter circle. The reflex dermalgia of the appendix is also found within this zone but has not been specified more precisely. A chronic inflammation of the appendix may cause a failure of the colon-reflex to respond to treatment.

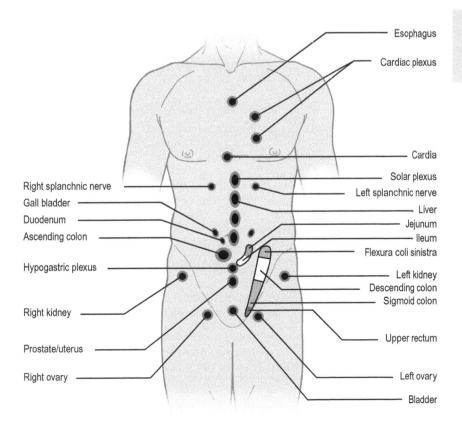

Figure 50.2
Topography of anterior reflex dermalgias

Esophagus
Cardiac plexus
Cardia
Solar plexus
Left splanchnic nerve
Liver
Jejunum
Ileum
Flexura coli sinistra
Left kidney
Descending colon
Sigmoid colon
Upper rectum
Left ovary
Bladder

Right splanchnic nerve
Gall bladder
Duodenum
Ascending colon
Hypogastric plexus
Right kidney
Prostate/uterus
Right ovary

Furthermore, the ascending colon often causes dysfunction of the ileum, with removal of the reflex dermalgia of the ascending colon having a positive effect on the ileum.

Descending colon: This band-shaped reflex zone is found in the left-sided dermatomes of T10–L1. Measuring about a finger's breadth in width, the zone extends from superolateral to inferomedial. The dermatome of T11 contains the reflex areas for the sigmoid colon, whereas the zone relating to the rectum can be found in L1. Frequently, the entire reflex occurs in union with the reflex of the left greater splanchnic nerve.

Ileum: In the left T10 dermatome, closely surrounding the umbilicus and about 1 cm wide. The zone is often found together with the reflex zone of the ascending colon.

Jejunum: Within left T9 dermatome, just lateral to the umbilicus and with 2 cm slightly wider, this zone forms an extension of the ileum zone. This reflex seems to be connected to the reflex dermalgias of both liver and pancreas and, when found positive, may contribute to generalized and unspecific digestive problems.

Duodenum: This zone is located directly superior to the reflex of the ascending colon, in the distal third of the right T9 dermatome and three fingers' breadth lateral to the umbilicus. In duodenal ulcers, this zone is always found to be positive. Treatment often causes the ulcer to stagnate or even to disappear. Additionally, the duodenal zone is always positive in dysfunction of the ascending colon.

Stomach: In the midline within the T9 dermatomes, this zone is located in the lower third of a line drawn between xyphoid process and the umbilicus. The zone relating to the pylorus is situated just proximal to the navel.

Pancreas: Left T9 dermatome. This zone extends cranially from the umbilicus toward the costal margin and forms a 45° angle with an imagined horizontal line through the umbilicus. Any patient suffering from diabetes will have positive reflex dermalgias in this area. Dysfunctions of the pancreas are often connected to other visceral dysfunctions.

Gall bladder: Right T9 dermatome. This zone is ovally shaped and located at 5–7 cm distance from the linea alba and 6–7 cm from the umbilicus. It extends diagonally to the costal margin. After a cholecystectomy, the reflex dermalgia often remains positive and indicates a dysfunctional supply of the gall bladder.

Liver: Found within the T8 dermatome, this zone lies centrally on a line between the xyphoid process and the umbilicus. It is about one finger's breadth. Whether the liver is in dysfunction or not, the organ is often not tender on palpation. Also, a dysfunction of the liver may often be clinically silent and asymptomatic. Examining the reflex dermalgia, on the other hand, may provide very useful information regarding the organ's functional state.

Esophagus: Located in the dermatomes of T2 and T5, two zones are differentiated – an inferior zone just lateral to the right of the sternum within the 5th ICS, and a superior zone on the sternal surface extending from the suprasternal notch to the right 2nd ICS.

Hypogastric plexus: T11 dermatome. In acupuncture literature, this reflex dermalgia is described as an expression of the parasympathetic state within the pelvis.

Treatment of anterior reflex dermalgias

General

Periphery

Positioning: The patient is lying prone, knees slightly flexed.

Technique: A slide–push technique is employed, where thumbs or fingers are used to trace lines on the patient's skin, which have been described as follows:

1. Starting on the left, trace an imaginary line from the tip of the 11th rib to the pubic symphysis.

2. Again on the left-hand side, trace a line from the xyphoid process to the tip of the 11th rib, parallel to the costal margin.

3. Moving to the right side of the abdomen, trace a line from the tip of the 11th rib to the xyphoid process, parallel to the costal margin.

4. Now, trace a line from the pubic symphysis to the tip of the 11th rib on the right.

Lower abdomen, abdominal fascia

1. The zone to be treated is located between the umbilicus and the pubic symphysis, extending laterally up to the outer margin of the rectus abdominis. To begin with, the practitioner's thumbs and fingertips meet at a rather proximal point over the linea alba. From this point, the fingers apply a stretch on the fascia and move toward the lateral borders of the rectus abdominis. The pressure is moderate. When both hands have reached the lateral borders of the zone, the movement is repeated further distally along the linea alba until the entire zone has been treated.

2. The distal zone (urinary bladder) is treated individually. The practitioner's fingertips trace short lines towards the pubic symphysis, both from left to right and from cranial to caudal. This, again, is a slide–push technique working mainly on the fascia.

3. Two techniques are performed on the lateral margins of the right and left rectus abdominis. First, the practitioner traces a line with his fingers from the pelvis to the costal margin. Secondly, short, parallel movements are made over the lateral margin of the muscle, both in lateromedial and caudocranial directions.

Periumbilical area

The practitioner traces several lines with his fingers, always starting from lateral position and moving medially toward the umbilicus. The proximal hand fixes a point about 3-4 cm from the umbilicus. The distal hand glides with moderate pressure across the skin toward the umbilicus. In this way, the entire area surrounding the umbilicus can be stimulated.

Specific

Reflex dermalgias caudal to the umbilicus

Positioning: The patient is in a supine position with the practitioner standing at hip level, the dorsal aspects of his hands pushed together and placed vertically against the patient's abdomen.

Technique: The abdominal fasciae are put under tension by applying a posterior pressure with the fingertips. Index fingers remain in contact and form the axis of rotation while the hands move away from each other in a motion resembling the opening of a fan. Hold until the tissue begins to relax.

Midline reflex dermalgias (linea alba)

Positioning: The patient is supine with the knees slightly flexed. The practitioner is at pelvis level next to the patient. Both hands take hold of a broad fold of skin between the pubic symphysis and the umbilicus.

Technique: The skin fold is lifted and held without squeezing. When a relaxation has been noted, the skin is pulled cranially and again held until another distinct release occurs.

Reflex dermalgias cranial to the umbilicus

Positioning: The patient is side-lying with the practitioner standing behind the patient at the level of the pelvis. The practitioner's hands are placed on the patient's side at the level of the upper abdomen. The proximal hand fixes the skin of the patient's flank, while the distal hand points toward the umbilicus.

Technique: The fingertips of the distal hand apply moderate pressure to the skin and glide toward the linea alba. The technique is repeated until the entire area above the umbilicus has been treated.

Topography of posterior reflex dermalgias (Fig. 50.3)

Esophagus (proximal part): right T2 dermatome. An oval zone located between the transverse processes of T2–T3.

Heart: Within the left T4 dermatome, at the tip of the T4 transverse process, this zone is known as 'sympathetic hyperesthesia of the heart'.

Cardiac sphincter and distal part of the esophagus: At the angle of the 6th rib on the right.

Liver: T8 dermatome on the right, at the level of the T10 transverse process.

Spleen: Left T8 dermatome, near the T10 transverse process.

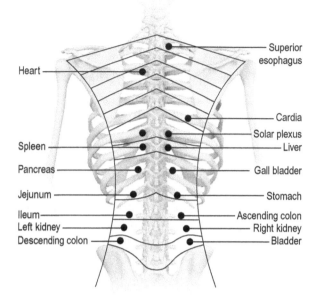

Figure 50.3
Topography of posterior reflex dermalgias

Stomach: This zone can be found at the angle of the right 12th rib, within the right T9 dermatome.

Gall bladder: Right T9 dermatome, superior border of the 11th rib near its angle.

Pancreas: Left T9 dermatome, superior border of the 11th rib near its angle.

Jejunum: Left T9 dermatome, at the level of the costal angle of the 12th rib.

Ileum: T10 dermatome, left side. This zone is located slightly lateral to the transverse processes of L1 and L2.

Ascending colon: In the T10 dermatome on the right, this zone is located slightly lateral to the transverse processes of L1 and L2.

Kidneys: Both left and right side of the T11 dermatome, this zone is found just lateral to the tips of the L3 transverse processes.

Urinary bladder: T12 dermatome on the right, lateral to the transverse process of L3.

Descending colon and rectum: T12 dermatome on the left, lateral to the transverse process of L3.

Treatment of posterior reflex dermalgias

General

Positioning: The patient is sitting on the edge of the treatment plinth, both feet on the floor. Standing behind the patient, the practitioner places the fingertips of his hands bilateral to the spinous process of L4, just proximal to the iliac crest.

Technique:

Phase 1: The patient bends forward and supports himself with his hands on his knees.

Phase 2: The practitioner pushes anterocranially with his fingertips.

Phase 3: The patient slowly sits back up as the practitioner continues to move his fingertips cranially towards T1.

Specific

Lumbosacral region

Positioning: The patient is in a prone position. The practitioner is standing next to the patient, with his hands placed on the bulk of the lumbar erector spinae muscles, parallel to the spine, and fingers pointing caudally.

Technique: The practitioner applies an inward pressure and fine-tunes his forces to find a position of ease: cranially, caudally, lateral right and left, rotation clockwise or counterclockwise. This position is held until a fascial relaxation (release) is attained.

Thoracolumbar region

Positioning: The patient is lying prone and the practitioner is standing at his side. The practitioner places both hands next to each other, transversely over the thoracolumbar junction.

Technique: The practitioner applies an inward pressure and fine-tunes his forces to find a position of ease: cranially, caudally, lateral right and left, rotation clockwise or counterclockwise. This position is held until a fascial relaxation (release) is attained.

Thoracic region

Positioning: The patient is in a prone position. The practitioner is standing next to the patient, with his hands lying on the costal angles left and right of the spine.

Technique: The practitioner applies an inward pressure and fine-tunes his forces to find a position of ease: cranially, caudally, lateral right and left, rotation clockwise or counterclockwise. This position is held until a fascial relaxation (release) is attained.

References and further reading

Dicke E. Schliack H., Wolff A. (1981). *Therapie manuelle des zones réflexes du tissu conjonctif.* Paris: Maloine.

Jarricot H. (1971). De certaines relations viscero-cutanées métamériques en acupuncture.. *Meridiens* 15–16:87–126.

Jarricot H. (1985). Plexus solaire et acupuncture, *Méridiens* 71–72:119–138.

Netter Frank H. (2003). *Atlas der Anatomie des Menschen.* Stuttgart, New York: Thieme.

UNDERSTANDING AND APPROACH TO TREATMENT OF SCARS AND ADHESIONS

Susan L. Chapelle

Introduction

The modern education system for manual therapy, including massage therapy, physiotherapy, osteopathy, and chiropractic works on the acceptance that manipulation of tissues for scars and adhesions is of therapeutic value. Manual therapy in its various forms is now being introduced in a growing number of integrated health clinics, and is accepted by many to be a valuable addition to allopathic care. Much of the manual therapy literature is innately conceptual, sometimes for lack of data, often using outdated concepts that may have been dispelled by modern science's ability to accurately measure and observe cellular-level mechanisms. Manual therapy education splits systems and practices into various camps, including central versus peripheral nervous system, visceral work, and connective tissue/fascia manipulation. There are various conjectures as to how mechanical forces affect these different systems of anatomy, despite almost no directly relevant science. The manipulation of fascia as a technique is relatively recent in manual therapy history, and has been separated out by various schools of thought. Patients seem to receive benefit from the treatments they receive. Interest in the mechanisms at the cellular level that govern wound healing and an understanding of the mechanisms of pain are critical to the practice and diagnostic reasoning of tissue manipulation for scars and adhesions.

Fascia is generally defined as connective tissue composed of irregularly arranged collagen fibers, in contrast to the regularly arranged collagen fibers seen in tendons, ligaments, or aponeurotic sheets. The irregular arrangement of collagen fibers allows fascia to fulfill a role as packing tissue and resist tensional forces universally (Willard et al., 2012). Conversely, tendons, ligaments, and aponeuroses have a pronounced regular arrangement of collagen fibers equipping them to resist maximal force in a limited number of planes, while rendering them vulnerable to tensional or shear forces in other directions.

In 1939, an article appeared in the *Journal of the American Medical Association* written by Mennell called 'The science and art of joint manipulation' (Mennell, 1939). The author states: 'It is not an easy task to present a subject as controversial as is the question of manipulative surgery to the circle of a critical profession'. His critics later comment on Mennell's ability to apply his hypothesis on manipulations by stating that in view of the 'careful restraint with which he handles physiologic and anatomic facts as a background for his indications, there is no tendency to admit any fantastic or forced theories into his field of reasoning' (JAMA, 1951).

These comments are relevant to an understanding of the science in manual therapy. Manual therapy and its effect on tissues has been weakly understood. There is a growing skepticism amongst allopathic practitioners due to claims made outside of evidence, and anatomic facts that are not held to reason. This chapter will follow biological mechanisms of healing, and present the up-to-date scientific knowledge that may be relevant to the formation of adhesions and scar tissue and the potential role of manual therapy.

Scars and adhesions

The formation of scars and adhesions is a ubiquitous and naturally occurring process that, most often, is not pathological. As a profession, manual therapists have long held the belief that local restrictions in tissue movements can result in a more global dysfunction. There is little support for this concept. There are few data available that would suggest the validity of applying manual treatment to existing scar tissue. In addition, the innervation of fascia is poorly understood, with obvious clinical implications for local pain and presumed pathology.

In this chapter, we will explore the healing mechanism as it relates to different types of tissue, and the best treatment protocols and outcomes based on current published evidence for tissue manipulation and manual therapy.

Scarring is a multifactorial process with different clinical presentations that affects over 40 million people worldwide (Bloemen et al., 2009). Scars can be categorized either as pathological or nonpathological. Understanding the difference between a scar and an adhesion is essential to the diagnostic reasoning necessary to designing a manual therapy treatment protocol and assessing possible outcomes. Treatment of scars or fibrotic thickening of tissue after a wound presenting as a consistent pathology may not be supported by peer-reviewed literature. The availability of information online has made this important distinction more difficult, with case reports on scar reduction flourishing in the manual therapy education system. Understanding the difference between pathological adhesion formations, innervated versus noninnervated structures, and how and where adhesions are formed compared to the formation of a scar is critical to devising an evidence-based approach to treatments.

An adhesion is an attachment of tissues at unusual nonanatomic sites, which can be flimsy or dense, vascular or avascular, innervated or not innervated (Epstein et al., 2006). A scar is a mark left on the skin or within body tissues where a wound, burn, or sore has not healed completely by primary intention, and fibrous connective tissue has developed. There is still poor understanding of the complex mechanisms surrounding scarring and wound contraction (Gauglitz et al., 2011). Sensory nerve fibers have been found in adhesive tissue samples (Sulaiman et al., 2001a), although the relationship to pain or pathology is yet to be established.

The literature suggesting that massage following burns leads to reduced scarring seems promising (Roques, 2002; Roh et al., 2007; Hallam et al., 2009;

Cho et al., 2014) but is largely anecdotal. More experiments are required in order to make sound recommendations (Shin & Bordeaux, 2012). Elucidating the contribution of inflammatory pathways and hypoxia may lead to a deeper understanding of the effect that manual therapy can have in affecting scars and adhesions.

Wound healing

Humans desire wound healing through complete regeneration of damaged tissue. However, the reality is that after tissue maturation, humans do not heal by regeneration, but via wound healing or repair, which leaves scars or forms adhesions. Healing involves a complicated process that takes place in the extracellular matrix. Healing proceeds through four overlapping stages; hemostasis, inflammation, proliferation, and remodeling (Olczyk et al., 2014). All soft tissue injuries require wound healing. This involves, in part, the coagulation and fibrinolytic pathways. The extracellular matrix orchestrates molecular interactions, and is where wound healing takes place. Morphogenic changes such as angiogenesis, fibrinolysis, and neural sprouting (Tonnesen et al., 2000) contribute to the appropriateness of any wound repair, and are the factors that determine whether cellular differentiation of a less specialized cell type into a more specialized cell type takes place. The most relevant molecules to wound healing and repair may be the fibroblast growth factors. Studies suggest a basic antiscarring effect of fibroblast growth factors during wound healing, the mechanisms of which are still poorly understood (Shi et al., 2013).

Mesenchymal stem cells reside within the extracellular matrix. These cells are pluripotent in their respective tissues, and have similar sensitivities and functions. Fibroblasts, chondrocytes, osteocytes, and adipocytes are derived from these cells. The contents of the extracellular matrix mediate the inflammatory response, as well as growth factors that control proliferation, differentiation, and metabolism of cells involved in the healing process.

Fibroblasts and fibrocytes create and maintain the extracellular matrix (Bellini & Mattoli, 2007). These cells show some response to mechanical strain. Manual therapists apply mechanical stress to tissues. This is the common denominator in all professions that use tissue manipulation to achieve the goal of affecting sensitivity or pain perception. There is little scientific evidence to support the hypothesis that fibroblasts communicate with each other. A differentiation must be made between meaningful communications such as transmission of information between cells via protein receptors, versus having an effect on cellular neighbors via neural connections. There is no evidence that such communication occurs between fibrocytes.

The changes of a fibrocyte to a fibroblast, and from a fibroblast to a myofibroblast are called differenti-ation. There are various factors that play a role in this process, such as physiological changes in the extracellular matrix, changes in gene expression, and upregulation of genes, which lead to cell differentiation in the extracellular matrix (Parker et al., 2014).

In humans, wound healing is complete with the formation of a permanent scar consisting of collagen fibers, fibroblasts, and small blood vessels. During granulation tissue formation, fibroblasts undergo extensive changes. Some fibroblasts start to express smooth muscle cell markers such as smooth muscle actin, resulting in a phenotype referred to as myofibroblasts (Shephard et al., 2004). Myofibroblasts acquire morphological and biochemical features of contractile cells. They are responsible for contraction of granulation tissue to assist wound closure (Desmouliere et al., 1995). Although the contractile nature of myofibroblasts shows many similarities to smooth muscle cells, they fail to express the full repertoire of smooth muscle cell markers (Darby et al., 2014). Smooth muscle cells are organized to perform a contractile function under the influence of (primarily) neural control, whereas myofibroblasts are not under similar control. The difference is fundamental; the cells are not linked or coordinated. The relevance of differentiation of fibroblasts into myofibroblasts is not understood when it comes to manual therapy for wound healing and scar formation. It is unclear as to whether stimulation or mechanical strain may lead to further differentiation due to an increase in inflammatory response dependent on dose and timing of intervention. It is believed that differentiation into myofibroblasts happens within the extracellular matrix, with gene expression causing differentiation from fibroblasts into myofibroblasts

that deposit fibrin (Sassoli et al., 2012; Parker et al., 2014). There is little understanding of the precursor cells and the interrelationships between phenotypes when it comes to the myofibroblast/fibroblast relationship. Once a wound is repaired, most myofibroblasts and cells that cause fibrosis disappear. Fibroblasts are viewed as being in a resting state in normal skin, but become active during tissue repair. They proliferate during wound repair, and synthesize new connective tissue. What has been established through in vitro studies is that mechanical forces do affect fibrocytes (Pietramaggiori et al., 2007). What we can glean from the literature on fibroblasts that may be relevant to manual therapy is that there has been a measurable response to mechanical stimuli (Klotzsch et al., 2015), and that fibroblasts respond to stretch (Abbott et al., 2013). This response has been observed in vitro, but not measured in humans. Other interesting responses that have been examined are the tissue growth factors such as transforming growth factor-β1 (TGFβ-1) for scarring and TGFβ-3 for regeneration (Campbell et al., 2004). Mechanical stimulation effects COX-2, MMP-1, and PGE-2, which are important markers for the modulation of the inflammatory response.

TGFβ is central to many of the mechanisms of pathological scarring and fibrosis. Platelets are a major source of TGFβ-1 and, in a wound event, cause coagulation and enable wound repair. In the early stages of a wound, TGFβ-1 is deposited but not activated. TGFβ may cause chemotaxis with inflammation, but is not in itself chemotactic. This cellular response to a stimulus may only be in response to inflammation (Sato et al., 2000), which is important in understanding its role in the immune response to injury. Research shows that fibroblasts in both dense connective tissue and stiff cross-linked gels did not exhibit cytoskeletal remodeling in response to tissue stretch (Abbott et al., 2013). However, a loosely arranged compliant collagen matrix, characteristic of areolar connective tissue, promoted fibroblast cytoskeletal remodeling in response to stretch regardless of the fibroblast's tissue of origin. This finding by Abbott et al. shows that, with pathological healing processes such as fibrosis that increase cross-linkage of collagen, the fibroblast loses its responsiveness in connective tissue.

TGFβ-1 is a potent regulator of extracellular matrix production, wound healing, differentiation, and immune response, and is implicated in the progression of fibrotic diseases (Venkatraman et al., 2012). Platelets are a major source of TGFβ-1 and in wound events cause coagulation and enable wound repair. The platelets deposit TGFβ in the extracellular matrix, which may act as a reservoir to store growth factor necessary in later stages of wound repair (Blakytny et al., 2004). In the early stages of a wound, TGFβ-1 is deposited but not activated.

It has been shown that, when there is tissue pathology from impaired wound healing states (such as venous or diabetic ulcers), TGFβ-1 expression is reduced. When administered topically, TGFβ-1 can assist healing through stimulation of wound contraction and increasing wound strength (Brunner & Blakytny, 2004). Embryonic wounds that heal without a scar have low levels of TGFβ-1 and TGFβ-2, low levels of platelet-derived growth factor, and high levels of TGFβ-3 (Ferguson & O'Kane, 2004). The functional and evolutionary differences between TGFβ-1, TGFβ-2, and TGFβ-3 have been demonstrated in experiments where topical treatments were applied. TGFβ-1 and TGFβ-2, showed more extracellular matrix deposition but no difference between wound treatments at long-term outcomes. The addition of the TGFα-3 peptide leads to reductions in monocyte and macrophage profile, fibronectin, collagen I, and collagen III deposition in the early stages of wound healing plus marked improvement of the architecture of the neodermis and reduced scarring (Shah et al., 1995).

It is important to keep in mind that our understanding of the effects of mechanical stimulation on the behavior of cells has come from studies performed in vitro. Case studies on outcomes of treatments are prolific, but they fail to address the specific effects of the various interventions. There is much work to be done in better developing clinical experiments. In manual therapy science, there is little understanding of what cells are affected, or what pathways are forged, broken or encouraged. There are no long-term, controlled outcomes of treatment to scars or adhesions in humans. Much literature is based on case studies, with little attention paid to dose, timing, techniques, or mechanisms.

At the cellular level, responses to trauma can be simple or complex (Fig. 51.1). Manual therapy entails use of external shearing or other forces on palpable tissue. The most relevant response to wound repair may be the treatment of interfaces, and the effect these forces have on the wound-healing cascade and extracellular matrix while healing is taking place.

Skin wounds heal by first intention, or by granulation. If a skin injury is a laceration without any tissue, loss, then first intention healing takes place. If there is a loss of tissue, such as in burns, ulcers, or with infections, the tissue will heal by granulation, in which case a scar will be formed.

Experiments have shown that with a subcutaneous injury, adding short stretch decreases the fibrotic response, which causes less collagen deposition and

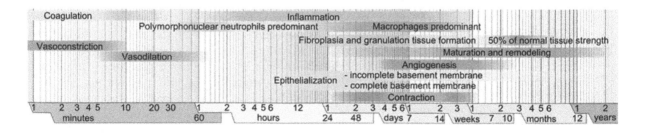

Figure 51.1
Subcutaneous tissue injury. Reproduced with permission from Mikael Häggström (2014)

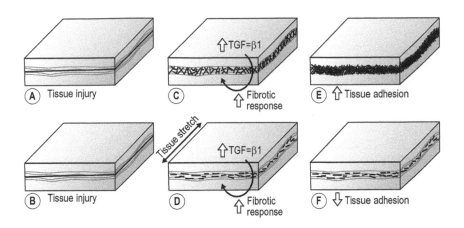

Figure 51.2

Proposed model for healing of connective tissue injury in the absence (A, C, E) and presence (B, D, F) of tissue stretch. In this model, brief stretching of tissue beyond the habitual range of motion reduces soluble TGF-β1 levels (D), causing a decrease in the fibrotic response, less collagen deposition, and reduced tissue adhesion (F) compared with no stretch (E). Black lines represent newly formed collagen. From Bouffard et al. (2008) Tissue stretch decreases soluble TGF-beta1 and type-1 procollagen in mouse subcutaneous connective tissue: evidence from ex vivo and in vivo models. J Cell Physiol 214:389–395. Reproduced with permission from John Wiley and Sons Publishing

reduced tissue adhesions (Bouffard et al., 2008). Tissue stretch to skin after injury reduced the amount of TGFß-1 inflammation and reduced macrophage expression in subcutaneous tissue (Corey et al., 2012). Fibroblasts in both dense connective tissue and stiff cross-linked gels did not exhibit cytoskeletal remodeling in response to tissue stretch. However, a loosely arranged compliant collagen matrix, characteristic of areolar connective tissue, promoted fibroblast cytoskeletal remodeling in response to stretch regardless of the fibroblast's tissue of origin. Mouse tissue loaded in a dish showed increased TGFβ-1, but with stretch added, the levels were reduced. Fibroblasts in connective tissue have shown extensive changes in response to stretch (Langevin et al., 2013). As in all wound healing, the control of inflammation may be the key to reduced fibrotic tissue deposition (Fig. 51.2).

Angiogenesis

Angiogenesis is a response of blood vessels to both pathological and normal physiology. Examples of normal angiogenesis can be seen in the female reproductive system during ovulation, menstruation, and formation of the placenta. Examples of pathological blood vessel formation can be seen in rheumatoid arthritis, tumor growth, and diabetes. Angiogenesis restores blood circulation where damage has occurred, and prevents the development of ischemic necrosis while stimulating the tissue repair process (Olczyk et al., 2014). Angiogenesis is stimulated by local environment such as low pH or high lactic acid concentrations (Gurtner et al., 2008). Inflammation and pathologies such as tumorigenesis typically lead to angiogenesis. During angiogenesis, endothelial cells migrate to the wound matrix, where they create a network of tubular structures (Schultz et al., 2011). When persistent inflammation or injury to tissue occurs, one of the hallmarks is vascular permeability. The inflammatory response increases capillary permeability and induces endothelial activation, which, when persistent, results in capillary sprouting (Arroyo & Iruela-Arispe, 2010). In the presence of

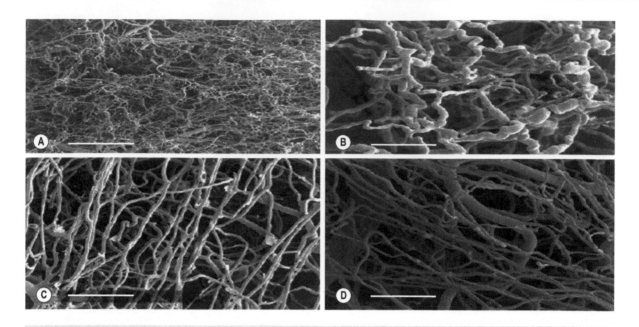

Figure 51.3

Scanning electron micrographs of casted microvascular networks of murine skin after stretching. (A) and (B) give some typical examples of stretched skin vasculature, showing tortuous elongation of dilated vessel bundles that build a transition zone of multidirectional vessel growth. (C) and (D) demonstrate densely packed, thin vessels assuring optimal blood flow towards an angiogenic transition zone. The bar on each image is equal to 100 μm. From Erba et al. (2011) A morphometric study of mechanotransductively induced dermal neovascularization. Plast Reconstr Surg 128:288e–299e. Reproduced with permission from Wolters Kluwer Health

newly formed blood vessels, fibroblasts proliferate and synthesize extracellular matrix components. This contributes to 'closing' wound surfaces.

The parallels between angiogenesis and other types of tissue development are numerous. In normal and pathological tissue development, angiogenesis is integral and has been suggested as an organizing principle underlying wound healing, tumor formation, and selected other conditions (Schultz et al., 2011). The presence of vascular endothelial growth factor (VEGF) can increase the efficiency of skeletal muscle repair by increasing angiogenesis and, at the same time, reducing the accumulation of fibrosis (Figs 51.3 and 51.4).

Several studies have shown that vascular endothelial growth factor increases angiogenesis in tissues that have been exposed to mechanical strain (Pietramaggiori et al., 2007). When cyclic stretch was applied to bladder tissue in vitro, the capillary bed showed increased density in formation of blood vessels (Yang et al., 2008). This finding, that under cyclical or stretch conditions angiogenesis is increased, shows that inflammation can lead to more vascularization. In the reverse situation, it may be that increased tension causes more inflammation, and therefore more permeability of the capillaries, perhaps prolonging an inflammatory state. There has been no relationship attributed directly to manual therapy.

Nerves

Any event that may compromise or disrupt the gliding movement of a nerve may result in epineurial and interfascicular fibrosis and scar formation. Reduction of intraneural blood flow from such scarring surrounding intraneural vessels causes ischemic

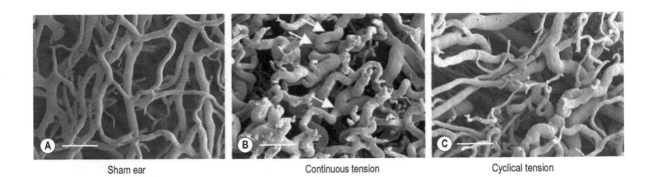

A — Sham ear   B — Continuous tension   C — Cyclical tension

Figure 51.4

Heterogeneity in caliber of the vessels and increased curvature are early signs of vascular remodeling. These peculiar changes are characteristic of the casts collected after the application of continuous force, and cyclical stretch regimens were also able to induce similar initial signs of vascular remodeling. The bar on each image is equal to 100 μm. From Pietramaggiori et al. (2007) Tensile forces stimulate vascular remodeling and epidermal cell proliferation in living skin. Ann Surg 246:896–902. Reproduced with permission from Wolters Kluwer Health

changes in intrafascicular tissue. In turn, these degenerative changes render nerves less elastic and more vulnerable to compression (Abe et al., 2005).

Muscles

Muscle fibrosis may be irrelevant to the application of manual therapy, due to the delicate balance between strength and healing (Jarvinen et al., 2007). The treatment outcome following an injury to skeletal muscle without tendon involvement has mostly focused on reduction of inflammation. In sports medicine studies this has led to suboptimal outcomes in comparison with natural healing times (Jarvinen & Lehto, 1993). Most timelines for the application of manual therapy to a muscle tissue repair have not been studied. Manual therapy has been assessed on the outcome of muscle recovery times from post-exercise stress and showed some benefit within the same day, but had no effect after multiple days (Crawford et al., 2014). The treatment approach that has been alluded to is that the reduction in the development of a fibrous scar may be beneficial to the increase of muscle fiber regeneration, and reducing the inflammatory response of a trauma or laceration. Muscle injury may also cause denervation of the distal

segments that will result in atrophy (Lim et al., 2006). The deposition of scar tissue in a muscle describes the extent to which a repair is functional, or leads to dystrophy. If the fibrotic tissue could be repaired and the dystrophic muscle redirected toward regeneration, thereby preserving muscle integrity, the health of the muscle tissue could be considerably improved (Mann et al., 2011). Nerve regrowth into muscle fibers does not seem to be inhibited by scarring; axon sprouts are able to penetrate scar tissue and are able to form new, functional neuromuscular junctions (Fig. 51.5) (Kaariainen et al., 2000).

Mechanical stimulation promotes growth, and this seems relevant to the healing of muscle fibers (Jarvinen et al., 2005). Gentle mobilization was shown to better align the developing fibers after a short period of immobilization allowed a firm scar to develop (Jarvinen & Lehto, 1993). The research showed that, with mobility, the scaffolding of the repairing tissue loses strength. Muscle tissue requires a firm scar in order to maintain its strength and not tear with contraction. Tissue that had been mobilized early was much more prone to reinjury, where the new trauma most often occurred in surrounding tissue, not in the initial wound repair (Jarvinen et al., 2000). One

Figure 51.5

Muscle injury and healing timeline with potential therapeutic opportunities. Courtesy of Dr Geoffrey Bove

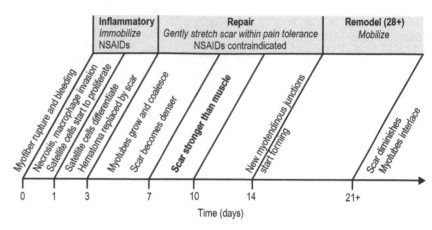

study performed muscle biopsy after manual therapy and did not observe any alterations in muscle glycogen levels or in muscle lactate, suggesting that the acute effects of massage occur independent of glucose uptake, or lactate clearance (Crane et al., 2012). The ameliorative effects may be that, when administered to skeletal muscle that has been acutely damaged through exercise, there appears to be a reduction in inflammation, and alterations in metabolites associated with mitochondrial biogenesis (Urakawa et al., 2015; Crane et al., 2012). This new literature supports the reduction of inflammation after exercise by manual therapy. The available data may not support utility of direct manual therapy to damaged or healing muscles until after the repair. Reduction in inflammatory mediators may inhibit muscle healing.

Ligaments and tendons

Ligaments and tendons are designed to transmit force. Although healing occurs to varying degrees, in general healing of repaired tendons follows the typical wound-healing course, including an early inflammatory phase, followed by proliferative and remodeling phases. Oxygen consumption by tendons and ligaments is 7.5 times lower than skeletal muscles (Sharma &

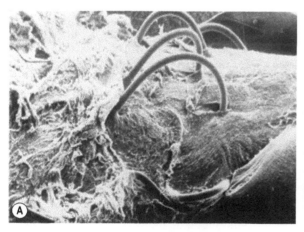

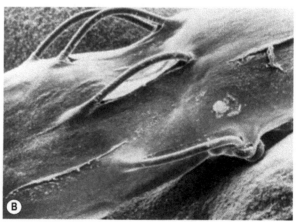

Figure 51.6

No mobilization (A) versus mobilization (B) on tendon. From Gelberman et al. (1983) Flexor tendon healing and restoration of the gliding surface: an ultrastructural study in dogs. J Bone Joint Surg Am 65:70–80. Reproduced with permission

Maffulli, 2006), which has advantages and disadvantages. Given that they have a low metabolic rate and well-developed anaerobic energy generation capacity, tendons are able to carry loads and maintain tension for long periods, while avoiding the risk of ischemia and subsequent necrosis. However, the low metabolic rate results in slow healing after injury. There has been considerably more literature on the effect of mechanical strain applied to tendons and ligaments after injury (Loghmani & Warden, 2009). The response of healing tendons to mechanical load or movement varies depending on anatomic location. Flexor tendons require motion to prevent adhesion formation between the sheath and the tendon surface. Excessive force results in gap formation and weakening of the repair (Killian et al., 2012). When damage occurs, cells from the intrasynovial sheath infiltrate to the repair site, leading to adhesions between the sheath and the tendon surface, which impairs tendon gliding, leading to a decrease in range of motion (Fig. 51.6).

Mobilization may decrease the amount of proinflammatory cytokines through movement of the extracellular matrix. Although an inflammatory response is essential for healing of a tendon to occur, high levels of inflammatory cytokines may result in collateral tissue damage and impaired tendon healing (Manning et al., 2014). In flexor tendon to bone repair, muscle loading across the repair site led to improved functional and biomechanical properties and was beneficial to healing. Complete removal of load by proximal transection resulted in tendon-to-bone repairs with less range of motion and lower biomechanical properties (Thomopoulos et al., 2008). In a systematic review of rotator cuff repair by (Shen et al., 2014) it was shown that long-term outcomes for mobilization versus immobilization showed no significant difference in repairs at one year. In general, data supports that some controlled loading is essential for development, homeostasis, and repair. However, excessive loading will result in a negative effect and reduced healing (Fig. 51.7) (Killian et al., 2012) .

Peritoneal cavity

Peritoneal adhesions are almost ubiquitous after surgery and can cause a number of complications. Peritoneal adhesions can lead to intestinal obstruction, infertility, and chronic pain (Herrick et al., 2000a). As many as 97% of women who undergo surgery for gynecologic indications have been shown to develop postoperative adhesions (Yelian et al., 2010). Peritoneal adhesions are fibrous bands of tissue that have connected viscera together, or attached organs to the abdominal wall. Adhesions have been found to be highly vascular, innervated, and cellular (Epstein et al., 2006). They are most often as a result of surgery, but can be formed from any defect that causes inflammatory exudate (Arung et al., 2011). Many approaches have been taken to resolve adhesion formation in the abdomen, but none offer reliable results (Alpay et al., 2008). Most often, patients are readmitted to hospital and require laparoscopic lysing of the fibrous bands that are causing pain, obstruction, or infertility. Surgery to lyse adhesions often results in reformation of adhesions (Bolnick et al., 2014). It is important to note that adhesions cannot be imaged accurately (Ghonge & Ghonge, 2014) and can only be accurately diagnosed upon reoperation by laparoscopy, which often leads to a reformation of adhesions (Mais, 2014).

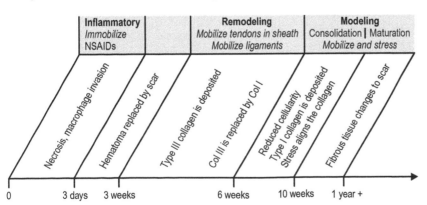

Figure 51.7

Tendon and ligament injury and healing time with potential therapeutic opportunities. Courtesy of Dr Geoffrey Bove

Despite claims by modern practitioners of visceral massage to have 'invented' techniques, the practice of visceral massage has been documented since the 1800s. Procedures used to reduce the burden of adhesions in clinical practice have not shown clinical effectiveness, and have lacked scientific validity. A few clinically relevant case studies have been published by one group (Wurn et al., 2008) but no mechanism, control group, or standardization was used.

Visceral massage has been documented since 1887, but the first text on the subject may be from Fielder (1955), who wrote *The Science and Art of Manipulative Surgery*. In his 1919 book *The Peritoneum*, Hertzler described management of permanent adhesions: 'Permanent adhesions require attention only when they limit the movement of a mobile organ or contract the lumen of a hollow one'. His observation on the application of manual therapy in his clinic showed little effect: 'Massage, particularly of the pelvic organs, once was in vogue but the results obtained were negligible'.

To date, there is little scientific evidence to confirm that there is any beneficial effect from the manipulation of viscera in relationship to pathological process.

In 1887 Symons Eccles, a surgeon, published his observations about his experience with atonic dyspepsia in the *British Medical Journal*. He noted that it occurred: 'where the abdominal organs partake of the generally anaemic, feeble, pathetic condition which appears to pervade the whole system and personality of the patient to such an extent that the disorder of digestion is overshadowed by the nervous system'. He noted: 'I have found it useless to practice massage too frequently at first' then, after bed rest, general corporeal massage including rapid effleurage to the limbs and trunk, then abdominal massage, the walls being vigorously rubbed and rolled between the hands, after which deeper kneading of the liver, stomach and intestines is carried out finishing with somewhat firm friction along the course of the colon. His prescription for massage was following treatment of two patients, and he noted that any increase from twice daily would retard recovery as opposed to advancing it (Eccles, 1887). Negative effects from the treatment were recorded, which are lacking in current literature.

These include acute painful sensations during or after massage, skin modification, parietal hematomas, and functional digestive symptoms.

There is inconsistent evidence in the literature that manual stimulation of the abdomen can impact neurogenic bowel dysfunction. The mechanistic hypothesis is that manual stimulation of the digestive pathway may enhance propulsive peristalsis and has been shown in spinal cord patients (Ayas et al., 2006). In the Ayas et al. study, the group discusses the same limitations that confound much manual therapy literature: lack of a control group, a small sample size, and a poor study design. Despite these considerable flaws, they recommend that manual therapy be included in any spinal cord injury bowel program.

Much work has been done in order to understand the formation of adhesions in the abdomen. They are a result of an inflammatory process, often caused by infections, endometriosis, and most often by surgical trauma (Saed & Diamond, 2004). Injury to the peritoneal cavity causes a loss of mesothelial cells and decreased plasminogen activator activity (PAA), then, underlying fibroblasts are exposed and adhesions result between two adjacent surfaces (Braun & Diamond, 2014). Many studies suggest that the reduction in peritoneal fibrinolysis during an abdominal surgery is a local response to trauma, and is a cause of adhesion formation (Holmdahl & Eriksson, 1998). It has been recently recognized that tissue hypoxia from surgery or an inflammatory event leads to a coordinated series of molecular actions that promote an inflammatory response leading to enhanced tissue fibrosis. These events are: reduced plasminogen activator activity (PAA), extracellular matrix deposition, increased cytokine production, increased angiogenesis, and reduced apoptosis (programmed cell death) (Saed & Diamond, 2004).

The intrinsic protective fibrinolytic activity of fibroblasts is essential to the normal healing mechanism of the peritoneal cavity. The tPA/PAI-1 ratio has been shown to be 80% higher in normal peritoneal fibroblasts than in adhesion fibroblasts. Under hypoxic conditions, this ratio significantly decreases in normal fibroblasts (90%), with an even more exaggerated decrease observed in adhesion fibroblasts (98%)

(Alpay et al., 2008). Collagen deposition and angiogenesis further result from conditions of hypoxia, and are key components of the infrastructure for postoperative adhesion formation (Awonuga et al., 2014; Bolnick et al., 2014).

Mechanical stimulation or massage to the abdomen aiming to affect bowel dysfunction has been documented (Le Blanc-Louvry et al., 2002). There appears to be some effect in reduction of symptoms, however the mechanisms remain unclear. Reduction in intraperitoneal inflammation and inhibition of macrophage function has also been postulated as a possible key in reduction of intraperitoneal adhesion formation (Bauer, 2008; Wehner et al., 2007).

Intraperitoneal protein concentration and the number of inflammatory cells were reduced by visceral massage, indicating a dilution of the inflammatory milieu (Chapelle & Bove, 2013) in postsurgical animals, however both protein and leukocyte numbers increased in normal animals with visceral treatment, indicating a proinflammatory response in the absence of pathology. In a rat model, visceral massage immediately following surgery interfered with the formation of postoperative adhesions (Bove & Chapelle, 2012) but failed to significantly reduce already formed adhesions after one week.

It may be possible that manual therapy performed on the abdomen may prevent or reduce the formation of adhesions when performed immediately after abdominal surgery. Postoperative soft adhesions form as early as from 72 hours to two weeks. Twenty per cent of these adhesions form within one month, while 40% form within one year (Menzies, 1992). Once formed, adhesions are difficult or impossible to disrupt (Bove & Chapelle, 2012). Pain may be caused by nerve infiltration into the adhesions (Sulaiman et al., 2001a), however, the presence of sensory nerves can be found in all peritoneal adhesion formations and size is not indicative of perception of pain (Almeida & Val-Gallas, 1997). A possible hypothesis to be explored with manual therapy is prevention of adhesions through reduction of hypoxia, and to understand introduction of macrophage and TGFβ cells. Yet another path to explore is the interruption of the fibrinolytic cascade, and the deposition of fibrin, or the conversion of plasmin to plasminogen at an early stage to encourage lysing of fibrin (Heydrick et al., 2007).

The dose and timing of postoperative prevention of adhesions with manual therapy is in need of significantly more scientific literature and exploration. The effect of manual therapy on the fibrinolytic cascade – in particular, plasminogen and the lysing of fibrin before forming fibrous bands, the timing of interventions, the possibility of effecting hypoxia, and vagal nerve involvement – are all in need of basic science.

The role of innervation in scars and adhesions

For the most part, people seek care from manual therapists for pain relief. When a link is made between a treatment and pathology such as a scar or an adhesion, it may be presumed that there is also some connection between the pathology and the symptoms, and thus, neurology. Every injury also involves nerves of some caliber. Mastectomy surgery involves cutting many intercostal nerve branches, and even a small cut in the skin damages a few axons. These damaged axons remain alive, and immediately start to regenerate. For the most part, nerves regrow appropriately, but in many cases they do not, and can lead to persistent pain.

It has been shown that scars and adhesions become innervated with nerve fibers that have properties consistent with nociceptors (Herrick et al., 2000b; Sulaiman et al., 2000; Sulaiman et al., 2001b; Liang et al., 2004). Endometrioma, the lesions that occur from endometriosis, also can become innervated with similar fibers (Berkley et al., 2005). Intraoperative mechanical stimulation of adhesions has led to reports of pain (Almeida & Val-Gallas, 1997; Almeida, 2002), supporting the idea that the innervation of adhesions is a functional response. While there may be anecdotal evidence that manual therapies reduce pain associated with scars and adhesions, we are unaware of any study that shows any effect on the sensory supply to either.

A direction research may wish to explore is the possible effects on inflammation. There is some evidence that manual therapy may reduce some inflammatory mediators (Corey et al., 2012; Crane et al., 2012; Haas et al., 2013). If this is found to be true, the effects on pain may be surmised based on known axonal biology. Nerves pass through many structures, and may be exposed to inflammation or become mechanically compromised by compression or adhesion (Araki & Milbrandt, 1996). For instance, the median nerve passes between the flexor muscles in the forearm, and the visceral nerves pass within a thin mesentery to reach the intestines. Inflammation in these areas, independent of any condition at their end-organ, will induce changes in the nociceptor axons seen as ongoing activity (which may be perceived as spontaneous pain) and mechanical sensitivity (which would be perceived as pain coming from the end-organ) (Bove et al., 2003; Dilley & Bove, 2008a). These changes are not permanent (Dilley & Bove, 2008b), resolving sometime after the stimulus is removed. If manual therapy reduces inflammation, it may also facilitate this recovery. These experiments have yet to be performed.

Discussion

While most of these examples of mechanical strain capture important aspects of tissue degeneration and the impact of injury, it is important to keep in mind that none captures the complete etiology of the injuries seen in human patients. Therefore, care must be taken in the choice and interpretation of the study model used to assess the impact of manual therapy on scars and adhesions. Further work is needed to validate the generalizability and translatability of basic science studies of healing mechanisms and the effect of mechanical strain in these models. Case studies and observation are important. Understanding basic cellular level function and response to mechanical strain are critical to the progression of manual therapy education and integration into the model of allopathic medicine.

It is important to recognize that regulated inflammation is largely beneficial to tissue repair, whereas excessive or persistent inflammation can be damaging. One consistent observation in all models and studies that include mechanical strain is that there is some effect on cell biology.

Whereas inflammatory cytokines attract fibroblasts to the repair site, excessive inflammation may lead to poor clinical outcome and an increase in fibrosis. Macrophages play essential roles in both promoting and resolving inflammation and in facilitating and moderating tissue repair. That a single cell type can serve opposing functions may seem counterintuitive, but dramatic phenotypic changes occur when macrophages respond to local stimuli. It has been shown that manual therapy evokes an immunomodulatory response to tissue, including an increase in macrophage activity (Crane et al., 2012; Waters-Banker et al., 2014a). By altering signaling pathways involved with the inflammatory process, manual therapy may decrease secondary injury, nerve sensitization, and collateral sprouting, resulting in more rapid recovery from damage and reduction or prevention of pain (Waters-Banker et al., 2014b).

The important role of the extracellular matrix in the formation of scars and adhesions cannot be overstated in this chapter. The interfaces between the following are important:

- skin to fascia
- epimysium to epimysium
- visceral peritoneum to visceral or parietal peritoneum
- nerve sheath to fascia
- tendon to tendon sheath or fascia.

Interfaces may prove relevant and possible to attenuate with manual therapy. There have been studies examining the relationship of lumbar fascia to lumbar pain (Schilder et al., 2014) but the differentiation of tissues may be irrelevant to the application of the techniques of manual therapy, since most tissues have been found to contain axons that are nociceptive. Clinical relevance may be the attenuation of inflammation to tissue healing cascades. Understanding the dose effect of pressure, techniques, and applications to acute or chronic tissue injuries is work that still needs to be done.

References

Abbott R. D., Koptiuch .C, Iatridis J. C. et al. (2013) Stress and matrix-responsive cytoskeletal remodeling in fibroblasts. *J Cell Physiol* 228:50–57.

Abe Y., Doi K., Kawai S. (2005) An experimental model of peripheral nerve adhesion in rabbits. *Br J Plast Surg* 58:533–540.

Almeida O. D., Jr. (2002) Microlaparoscopic conscious pain mapping in the evaluation of chronic pelvic pain: a case report. *JSLS* 6:81–83.

Almeida O. D., Jr., Val-Gallas J. M. (1997) Conscious pain mapping. *Am Assoc Gynecol Laparosc* 4:587–590.

Alpay Z., Saed G. M., Diamond M. P. (2008) Postoperative adhesions: from formation to prevention. *Semin Reprod Med* 26:313–321.

Araki T., Milbrandt J. (1996) Ninjurin, a novel adhesion molecule, is induced by nerve injury and promotes axonal growth. *Neuron* 17:353–361.

Arroyo A. G., Iruela-Arispe M. L. (2010) Extracellular matrix, inflammation, and the angiogenic response. *Cardiovasc Res* 86:226–235.

Arung W., Meurisse M., Detry O. (2011) Pathophysiology and prevention of postoperative peritoneal adhesions. *World J Gastroenterol* 17:4545–4553.

Awonuga A. O., Belotte J., Abuanzeh S., et al. (2014) Advances in the pathogenesis of adhesion development: the role of oxidative stress. *Reprod Sci* 21:823–836.

Ayas S., Leblebici B., Sozay S., Bayramoglu M., Niron E. A. (2006) The effect of abdominal massage on bowel function in patients with spinal cord injury. *Am J Phys Med Rehabil* 85:951–955.

Bauer A. J. (2008). Mentation on the immunological modulation of gastrointestinal motility. *Neurogastroenterol Motil* 20(Suppl 1):81–90.

Bellini A., Mattoli S. (2007) The role of the fibrocyte, a bone marrow-derived mesenchymal progenitor, in reactive and reparative fibroses. *Lab Invest* 87:858–870.

Berkley K. J., Rapkin A. J., Papka R. E. (2005) The pains of endometriosis. *Science* 308:1587–1589.

Blakytny R., Ludlow A., Martin G. E. et al. (2004) Latent TGF-beta1 activation by platelets. *J Cell Physiol* 199:67–76.

Bloemen M.C., van der Veer W. M., Ulrich M. M. et al. (2009) Prevention and curative management of hypertrophic scar formation. *Burns* 35:463–475.

Bolnick A., Bolnick J., Diamond M. P. (2014) Postoperative adhesions as a consequence of pelvic surgery. *J Minim Invasive Gynecol* 22:549–563.

Bouffard N. A., Cutroneo K. R., Badger G. J. et al. (2008) Tissue stretch decreases soluble TGF-beta1 and type-1 procollagen in mouse subcutaneous connective tissue: evidence from ex vivo and in vivo models. *J Cell Physiol* 214:389–395.

Bove G. M., Chapelle S. L. (2012) Visceral mobilization can lyse and prevent peritoneal adhesions in a rat model. *J Bodywork Mov Ther* 16:76–82.

Bove G. M., Ransil B. J., Lin H. C., Leem J. G. (2003) Inflammation induces ectopic mechanical sensitivity in axons of nociceptors innervating deep tissues. *J Neurophysiol* 90:1949–1955.

Braun K. M., Diamond M. P. (2014) The biology of adhesion formation in the peritoneal cavity. *Semin Pediatr Surg* 23:336–343.

Brunner G., Blakytny R. (2004) Extracellular regulation of TGF-β activity in wound repair: growth factor latency as a sensor mechanism for injury. *Thromb Haemost* 92:253–261.

Campbell B. H., Agarwal C., Wang J. H. (2004) TGF-beta1, TGF-beta3, and PGE(2) regulate contraction of human patellar tendon fibroblasts. *Biomech Model Mechanobiol* 2:239–245.

Chapelle S. L., Bove G .M. (2013) Visceral massage reduces postoperative ileus in a rat model. *J Bodywork Mov Ther* 17:83–88.

Cho Y. S., Jeon J. H., Hong A., et al. (2014) The effect of burn rehabilitation massage therapy on hypertrophic scar after burn: a randomized controlled trial. *Burns* 40:1513–1520.

Corey S. M., Vizzard M. A., Bouffard N. A. et al. (2012) Stretching of the back improves gait, mechanical sensitivity and connective tissue inflammation in a rodent model. *PLoS One* 7:e29831.

Crane J.D., Ogborn D.I., Cupido C. et al.(2012) Massage therapy attenuates inflammatory signaling after exercise-induced muscle damage. *Sci Transl Med* 4:119ra113.

Crawford S. K., Haas C., Butterfield T. A. et al. (2014) Effects of immediate vs. delayed massage-like loading on skeletal muscle viscoelastic properties following eccentric exercise. *Clin Biomech* 29:671–678.

Darby I. A., Laverdet B., Bonte F., Desmouliere A. (2014) Fibroblasts and myofibroblasts in wound healing. *Clin Cosmet Investi Dermatolo* 7:301–311.

Desmouliere A., Redard M., Darby I., Gabbiani G. (1995) Apoptosis mediates the decrease in cellularity during the transition between granulation tissue and scar. *Am J Pathol* 146:56–66.

Dilley A., Bove G. M. (2008a) Disruption of axoplasmic transport induces mechanical sensitivity in intact rat C-fibre nociceptor axons. *J Physiol* 586:593–604.

Dilley A., Bove G. M. (2008b) Resolution of inflammation induced axonal mechanical sensitivity and conduction slowing in C-fiber nociceptors. *J Pain* 9:185–192.

Eccles S. (1887) Massage as a means of treatment in chronic dyspepsia and sleeplessness. *Med J*

Epstein J. C., Wilson M. S., Wilkosz S. et al. (2006) Human peritoneal adhesions show evidence of tissue remodeling and markers of angiogenesis. *Dis Colon Rectum* 49:1885–1892.

Erba P., Miele L .F., Adini A. et al. (2011) A morphometric study of mechanotransductively induced dermal neovascularization. *Plast Reconstr Surg* 128:288e–299e.

Ferguson M. W., O'Kane S. (2004) Scar-free healing: from embryonic mechanisms to adult therapeutic intervention. *Philos Trans R Soc Lond B Biol Sci* 359:839–850.

Fielder S. L. (1955) *The Science and Art of Manipulative Surgery.* 2nd edition. American Institute of Manipulative Surgery.

Gauglitz G. G., Korting H. C., Pavicic T. et al. (2011) Hypertrophic scarring and keloids: pathomechanisms and current and emerging treatment strategies. *Mol Med* 17:113–125.

Gelberman R. H., Vande Berg J. S., Lundborg G. N., Akeson W. H. (1983) Flexor tendon healing and restoration of the gliding surface: an ultrastructural study in dogs. *J Bone Joint Surg Am* 65:70–80.

Ghonge N. P., Ghonge S. D. (2014) Computed tomography and magnetic resonance imaging in the evaluation of pelvic peritoneal adhesions: what radiologists need to know? *Indian J Radiol Imaging* 24:149–155.

Gurtner G. C., Werner S., Barrandon Y., Longaker M. T. (2008) Wound repair and regeneration. *Nature* 453:314–321.

Haas C., Butterfield T. A., Abshire S. et al. (2013) Massage timing affects postexercise muscle recovery and inflammation in a rabbit model. *Med Sci Sports Exerc* 45:1105–1112.

Hallam M. J., Shirley R., Dheansa B., Coker O. (2009) Scar massage therapy: a new technique. *J Wound Care* 18:258.

Herrick S. E., Mutsaers S. E., Ozua P. et al. (2000a) Human peritoneal adhesions are highly cellular, innervated, and vascularized. *The Journal of Pathology* 192:67–72.

Herrick S. E., Mutsaers S. E., Ozua P., et al. (2000b) Human peritoneal adhesions are highly cellular, innervated, and vascularized. *J Pathol* 192:67–72.

Heydrick S. J., Reed K. L., Cohen P.A. et al. (2007) Intraperitoneal administration of methylene blue attenuates oxidative stress, increases peritoneal fibrinolysis, and inhibits intraabdominal adhesion formation. *J Surg Res* 143:311–319.

Holmdahl L., Eriksson E. (1998) Depression of peritoneal fibrinolysis during operation is a local response to trauma. *Surgery* 123:539–544.

JAMA (1951) Manual Therapy. *JAMA* 147:1089.

Jarvinen M. J., Lehto M. U. (1993) The effects of early mobilisation and immobilisation on the healing process following muscle injuries. *Sports Med* 15:78–89.

Jarvinen T. A., Jarvinen T. L., Kaariainen M. et al. (2007) Muscle injuries: optimising recovery. *Best Pract Res Clin Rheumatol* 21:317–331.

Jarvinen T. A., Jarvinen T. L., Kaariainen M. et al. (2005) Muscle injuries: biology and treatment. *Am J Sports Med* 33:745–764.

Jarvinen T. A., Kaariainen M., Jarvinen M., Kalimo H. (2000) Muscle strain injuries. *Curr Opin Rheumatol* 12:155–161.

Kaariainen M., Jarvinen T., Jarvinen M., et al. (2000) Relation between myofibers and connective tissue during muscle injury repair. *Scand J Med Sci Sports* 10:332–337.

Killian M. L., Cavinatto L., Galatz L. M., Thomopoulos S. (2012) The role of mechanobiology in tendon healing. *J Shoulder Elbow Surg* 21:228–237.

Klotzsch E., Stiegler J., Ben-Ishay E., Gaus K. (2015) Do mechanical forces contribute to nanoscale membrane organisation in T cells? *Biochim Biophys Acta* 1853:822–829.

Langevin H. M., Fujita T., Bouffard N. A. et al. (2013) Fibroblast cytoskeletal remodeling induced by tissue stretch involves ATP signaling. *J Cell Physiol* 228:1922–1926.

Le Blanc-Louvry I., Costaglioli B., Boulon C et al. (2002) Does mechanical massage of the abdominal wall after colectomy reduce postoperative pain and shorten the duration of ileus? Results of a randomized study. *J Gastrointest Surg* 6:43–49.

Liang Z., Engrav L. H., Muangman P. et al. (2004) Nerve quantification in female red Duroc pig (FRDP) scar compared to human hypertrophic scar. *Burns* 30:57–64.

Lim A. Y., Lahiri A., Pereira B. P. et al. (2006) The role of intramuscular nerve repair in the recovery of lacerated skeletal muscles. *Muscle Nerve* 33:377–383.

Loghmani M. T., Warden S. J. (2009) Instrument-assisted cross-fiber massage accelerates knee ligament healing. *J Orthop Sports Phys Ther* 39:506–514.

Mais V. (2014) Peritoneal adhesions after laparoscopic gastrointestinal surgery. *World J Gastroenterol* 20:4917–4925.

Mann C. J., Perdiguero E., Kharraz Y. et al. (2011) Aberrant repair and fibrosis development in skeletal muscle. *Skelet Muscle* 1:21–21.

Manning C. N., Havlioglu N., Knutsen E. et al. (2014) The early inflammatory response after flexor tendon healing: a gene expression and histological analysis. *J Orthop Res* 32:645–652.

Mennell J. B. (1939) *The Science and Art of Joint Manipulation.* Philadelphia: P. Blakiston's Son & Co., Inc.

Menzies D. (1992) Peritoneal adhesions: incidence, cause, and prevention. *Surg Ann* 24:27–45.

Olczyk P., Mencner, Ł., Komosinska-Vassev K. (2014) The role of the extracellular matrix components in cutaneous wound healing. *BioMed Res Int* 2014:747584.

Parker M. W., Rossi D., Peterson M. et al. (2014) Fibrotic extracellular matrix activates a profibrotic positive feedback loop. *J Clin Invest* 124:1622–1635.

Pietramaggiori G., Liu P., Scherer S. S. et al. (2007) Tensile forces stimulate vascular remodeling and epidermal cell proliferation in living skin. *Ann Surg* 246:896–902.

Roh Y. S., Cho H., Oh J .O., Yoon C. J. (2007) Effects of skin rehabilitation massage therapy on pruritus, skin status, and depression in burn survivors. *Taehan Kanho Hakhoe Chi* 37.221–226.

Roques C. (2002) Massage applied to scars. *Wound Repair Regen* 10:126–128.

Saed G. M., Diamond M. P. (2004) Molecular characterization of postoperative adhesions: the adhesion phenotype. *J Am Assoc Gynecol Laparosc* 11:307–314.

Sassoli C., Formigli L. Chellini F., Pini A. et al. (2012) Fibroblast-myofibroblast transition and extracellular matrix remodeling in vitro: implication for Notch-1 pathway in muscle tissue repair/regeneration. *Ital J Anat Embryo* 117:172.

Sato K., Kawasaki H., Nagayama H. et al. (2000) TGF- 1 Reciprocally controls chemotaxis of human peripheral blood monocyte-derived dendritic cells via chemokine receptors. *J Immunol* 164:2285–2295.

Schilder A., Hoheisel U., Magerl W. et al. (2014) Sensory findings after stimulation of the thoracolumbar fascia with hypertonic saline suggest its contribution to low back pain. *Pain* 155:222–231.

Schultz G. S., Davidson J. M., Kirsner R. S. et al. (2011) Dynamic reciprocity in the wound microenvironment. *Wound Repair Regen* 19:134–148.

Shah, M., Foreman, D. M. and Ferguson, M. W. J. (1995) Neutralisation of TGF-β1 and TGF-β2 or exogenous addition of TGF-β3 to cutaneous rat wounds reduces scarring. *J Cell Sci* 108:985–1002.

Sharma P., Maffulli N. (2006) Biology of tendon injury: healing, modeling and remodeling. *J Musculoskelet Neuronal Interact* 6:181–190.

Shen C., Tang Z. H., Hu J. Z. et al. (2014) Does immobilization after arthroscopic rotator cuff repair increase tendon healing? A systematic review and meta-analysis. *Arch Orthop Trauma Surg* 134:1279–1285.

Shephard P., Martin G., Smola-Hess S., et al. (2004) Myofibroblast differentiation is induced in keratinocyte-fibroblast co-cultures and is antagonistically regulated by endogenous transforming growth factor-β and interleukin-1. *The Am J Pathol* 164:2055–2066.

Shi H. X., Lin C., Lin B .B. et al. (2013) The anti-scar effects of basic fibroblast growth factor on the wound repair in vitro and in vivo. *PLoS One* 8:e59966.

Shin T. M., Bordeaux J. S. (2012) The role of massage in scar management: a literature review. *Dermatol Surg* 38:414–423.

Sulaiman H., Gabella G., Davis C. et al. (2000) Growth of nerve fibres into murine peritoneal adhesions. *J Pathol* 192:396–403.

Sulaiman H., Gabella G., Davis M. C. et al. (2001a) Presence and distribution of sensory nerve fibers in human peritoneal adhesions. *Ann Surg* 234:256–261.

Sulaiman H., Gabella G., Davis M. C. et al. (2001b) Presence and distribution of sensory nerve fibers in human peritoneal adhesions. *Ann Surg* 234:256–261.

Thomopoulos S., Zampiakis E., Das R., Silva M. J., Gelberman R. H. (2008) The effect of muscle loading on flexor tendon-to-bone healing in a canine model. *J Orthop Res* 26:1611–1617.

Tonnesen M. G., Feng X., Clark R. A. (2000) Angiogenesis in wound healing. *J Investig Dermatol Symp Proc* 5:40–46.

Urakawa S., Takamoto K., Nakamura T. et al. (2015) Manual therapy ameliorates delayed-onset muscle soreness and alters muscle metabolites in rats. *Physiol Rep* 3:e12279.

Venkatraman L., Chia S. M., Narmada B. C. et al. (2012) Plasmin triggers a switch-like decrease in thrombospondin-dependent activation of TGF-beta1. *Biophys J* 103:1060–1068.

Waters-Banker C., Butterfield T. A., Dupont-Versteegden E. E. (2014a) Immunomodulatory effects of massage on nonperturbed skeletal muscle in rats. *J Appl Physiol* 116:164–175.

Waters-Banker C., Dupont-Versteegden E. E., Kitzman P. H., Butterfield T. A. (2014b) Investigating the mechanisms of massage efficacy: the role of mechanical immunomodulation. *J Athl Train* 49:266– 273.

Wehner S., Behrendt F. F., Lyutenski B. N. et al. (2007) Inhibition of macrophage function prevents intestinal inflammation and postoperative ileus in rodents. *Gut* 56:176–185.

Willard F. H., Vleeming A., Schuenke M. D., Danneels L., Schleip R. (2012) The thoracolumbar fascia: anatomy, function and clinical considerations. *J Anat* 221:507–536.

Wurn B. F., Wurn L. J., King C. R. et al. (2008) Treating fallopian tube occlusion with a manual pelvic physical therapy. *Altern Ther Health Med* 14:18–23.

Yang R., Amir J., Liu H., Chaqour B. (2008) Mechanical strain activates a program of genes functionally involved in paracrine signaling of angiogenesis. *Physiol Genomics* 36:1–14.

Yelian F. D., Shavell V. I., Diamond M. P. (2010) Early demonstration of postoperative adhesions in a rodent model. *Fertil Steril* 93:2734–2737.

FASCIAL TAPING

Kenzo Kase

During his early years practicing as a chiropractor, Dr Kenzo Kase experienced good results with the effects of his treatments but he was concerned that the effects were not long-lasting. It seemed that patients would walk out of the office feeling relief but in a short time begin to experience the same pain and symptoms that had led them to seek treatment in the first place. Dr Kase began looking for a technique or modality that could help his patients experience the same relief for longer periods of time. He experimented with rigid taping and strapping methods but was dissatisfied with the effects of the tape on patient skin. Many people had adverse reactions to the tape or it did not achieve the effect Dr Kase hoped it would have. The tape was often too rigid to allow normal movement patterns and quickly became uncomfortable. As he studied the structure of human skin, he began to think about the qualities a therapeutic tape would need to affect the fascia and muscle dysfunctions causing problems for his patients. At the same time, Dr Kase needed a tape that would be able to stay on the skin for longer periods of time without impacting the patient's comfort. He began developing and testing an elastic therapeutic tape that would have approximately the same weight and thickness as human skin, and be able to stretch and move with the patient rather than restricting the body's range of motion. Always as he was developing the tape he envisioned how it would work with the taping therapies he was creating. Thus the tape and the therapy work in harmony, because Dr Kase designed the tape specifically with the therapy in mind. Years of research and testing led to the production of Kinesio® Tex Tape. Having an elastic tape that moves with the skin allows the tape applications to provide continuous stimulation to the body through a normal range of motion.

Kinesio Taping® therapies affect five physiological systems of the body: skin, fascia, muscle, joint, and circulatory/lymphatic. The underlying concept can be expressed as *Ku Do Rei* – space–movement–cooling. Pain and dysfunction occur in the body when normal tissue movement and mobility is compromised by an injury or an abnormal movement or position pattern. Tissues become compressed and the function of underlying structures is hampered. Fascia is especially affected by injury or an compression of the tissues. Normal movements of the fascia are impaired and adhesions may develop. Fluid (lymph and blood) circulation is slowed and congestion occurs, causing body temperature in the affected area to become elevated. Above-normal tissue temperature

can affect cellular function. Kinesio Taping® therapies are designed to microscopically lift the epidermis and dermis to create more space in the underlying tissue layers (Fig. 52.1). As space is increased the movement of fluid (blood and lymph) through the tissues increases as constriction of the fluid vessels decreases. Less fluid congestion in the tissues leads to decompression of pain receptors, a restoration of normal tissue function, and cooling of tissue to normal temperatures.

When space–movement–cooling in the tissues is achieved, normal muscle function can be restored, joint biomechanics and alignment are improved, and fascial remodeling is assisted.

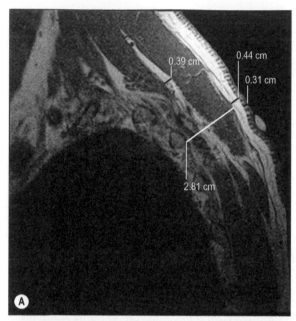

0.39 cm
0.44 cm
0.31 cm
2.81 cm

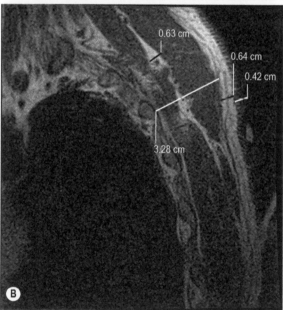

0.63 cm
0.64 cm
0.42 cm
3.28 cm

Figure 52.1

MRI slides showing increase in epidermis, dermis, and subcutaneous tissue compartments after application of Kinesio® Tex Tape. Courtesy of Dr Vivien C. Wong. Presented at the 2013 Kinesio Taping Association International Research Symposium held in Stanford, CA

Kinesio Taping® is designed to provide stimulus to the epidermis, the largest sensory and immune organ in the body. We know that the epidermis, the brain, and the central and peripheral nervous systems all develop from the same embryological tissue layer, the ectoderm. Traditionally, sensory perception in the skin was thought to be restricted to specific receptors found in the dermal layer. However, new research has shown that the epidermis itself can now be considered a sensory tissue where epidermal cells can participate in skin surface perception and interact with nerve fibers (Boulais & Misery, 2008). Epidermal stimulation seems to be able to transmit information to the nervous system much more than we had previously thought. We also have more evidence now of the extensive interconnections of the skin, fascia, and muscle. The idea that the layers of the skin were separate from the layers of the fascia, and that fascia was distinct from muscle, has been shown to be a misconception. The video images taken by Dr Jean-Claude Guimberteau in the DVD *Strolling Under the Skin* (2005) have shown the intricate blending of epidermis, dermis, and subcutaneous tissue with the fascial layers of the epimysium and perimysium. No clear separation can be seen between the different tissue layers, illustrating my belief that stimulation of the skin will affect deeper tissue layers in the body.

Another important foundation of the Kinesio Taping® Method is the concept of biotensegrity as conceptualized by Stephen Levine and based on the 'tension integrity' concept advanced by Fuller and Snelson. Biotensegrity models theorize that every part of the body is interconnected and that the body's tissues are continuously under tension. Balance must be maintained within the structure to ensure normal healthy functioning. Tension on one part of the system affects all other parts of the system and compensations are made when tension is applied to the body. Fascial systems react to injuries or imbalance by pulling toward the imbalance. Wang & Li (2010) have demonstrated that mechanical forces elicit chemical changes in the cells and that mechanical loads are essential for cellular repair of damaged tissue. The mechanism that changes physical forces to chemical signals in the body is known as mechanotransduction. Epidermal keratinocytes have been found to be instrumental in translating mechanical stimulation to chemical signals that can then excite the peripheral nervous system (Denda et al., 2007). Applying Kinesio® tape to the epidermis provides the mechanical stimulus.

Kinesio® Tex Tape is an elastic tape that stretches longitudinally, allowing the practitioner to vary tension in the tape to achieve the desired results. Tape applications are applied to the skin with varying tensions, shapes, and directions to stimulate changes in targeted tissues. Target tissue is the area of the body we are trying to affect – this is the area where tape will be applied. Stretching the target tissue before tape application increases the amount of stimulus to the tissues by increasing contact with skin receptors and sending more sensory messages to the nervous system. Less tension in the tape provides gentle stimulus and is less likely to irritate sensitive skin or thinner tissues. Pediatric and geriatric populations should always be treated with tape applications utilizing less tension. Less tension on the tape also has a greater effect on surface tissues such as the epidermis, and is more suitable for use on thinner tissues such as the face. More tension is used to hold tissues

in position and provide more support, and is used to target deeper tissues. Practitioners must be careful to use the appropriate amounts of tension on the tape. Applying too much tension on the tape can pull the skin, causing microtrauma or edema. Taping with too much tension can also cause pain by over-stimulating skin receptors. The shape of the tape applied to the body affects the way in which tension in the target tissue is dispersed. There are six basic shapes or cuts of tape used in Kinesio Taping® therapies: the Y-strip, the X Cut, the Fan Cut, the Donut Hole, the I-strip, and the Web Cut (Fig. 52.2). The cut of the tape often mirrors the shape of the tissue being taped. For example, the I-strip would be used over a long, narrow muscle, while a Y-strip is used on muscles with wide origins and narrow insertions. I-strip applications focus the tension directly over the target tissue. A back application targeted on the erector muscles would utilize the I-strip. Y-strips disperse the tension between the two tails over the target tissue. A muscle application focusing on the gastrocnemius muscle would utilize the Y-strip. X Cuts focus the tension directly over target tissue and disperse it through the tails at each end. X Cuts work

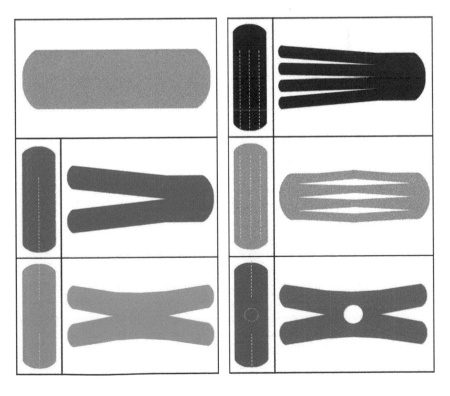

Figure 52.2

The six basic shapes or cuts of tape used in Kinesio Taping® therapies: the I-strip, the Y-strip, the X Cut, the Fan Cut, the Web Cut, and the Donut Hole

well with muscles having broad or multiple attachments, such as the rhomboids. Fan Cuts disperse tension through multiple tails applied over the target tissue, and are used for muscles having multiple tendons originating from one muscle belly. This cut works well on the plantar surface of the foot. The Web Cut is used primarily for applications designed to treat pain and dysfunction in a large, diffuse area. This cut is very effective for creating space in the tissues by reducing swelling and softening indurated tissues. The Donut Hole is used to decrease pressure over a small area of target tissue that is defined by the Donut Hole.

The original use of the Kinesio Taping® Method was muscle inhibition and muscle facilitation. Muscle function can be either inhibited or facilitated depending on the direction of the tape application. The start of the taping application is known as the anchor. The anchor is always laid down on the skin with no tension. As tape is stretched away from the anchor over the tissue it recoils back toward the start of the application, pulling the tissue along with it. The direction of recoil is actually considered to be the therapeutic direction of the tape action. Taping a muscle from insertion to origin (distal to proximal) recoils the tissue toward the insertion, which provides a stimulus to inhibit the overcontracted muscle, and provide rest for the overused muscle (Fig. 52.3).

Determining the appropriate Kinesio Taping® therapy to use begins with a patient assessment. Patients are first interviewed to determine the nature and duration of the dysfunction. Reports from the patient of pain and limitations in movement will inform the clinician's choice of further assessment techniques. Observation of the patient's skin color and temperature, palpation of the affected area for swelling or pain with direct pressure, and range-of-motion testing will give valuable information. In addition, the Kinesio Taping® Method uses unique screening assessments that incorporate standard orthopedic screenings but also require the clinician to look at movement patterns in a different way. Tissue movement is observed when certain motions are performed by the patient either actively or passively with the help of the clinician. Muscle,

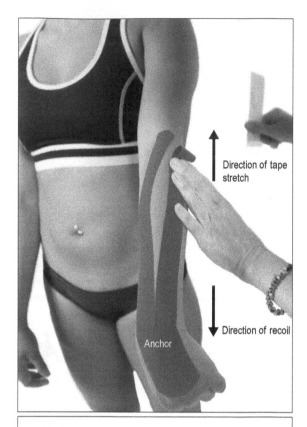

Direction of tape stretch

Direction of recoil

Anchor

- Tape is applied from distal attachment to proximal attachment (insertion to origin)

- Tension in the tape is 15% to 25%

- Tape recoils toward anchor to inhibit the muscle

Figure 52.3

Kinesio Taping® Method inhibition concept. Applying tape over the muscle from the insertion to origin (distal to proximal) direction inhibits muscle functioning by relaxing muscle contraction

joint, skin, and fascia restrictions are observed while the clinician also looks for necessary movement compensations. The clinician then determines an appropriate taping application to treat the patient's dysfunction. After the taping application is administered, reassessment is needed to determine if the application achieves the desired results and to ensure that it does not cause any patient discomfort or loss of range of motion. Taping applications applied directly over compromised tissue are not suitable for patients with irritated or fragile skin, sunburn, open wounds, or skin infections. Taping patients with serious health issues such as diabetes, kidney disease, congestive heart failure, and so forth may require consultation with the patient's physician prior to application. Any patient reports of itching, irritation, or pain should result in immediate removal of the tape.

Kinesio Taping® corrective techniques can be targeted specifically to muscle; tendons and ligaments; and fascia. Taping applications to different tissues use different shapes, directions of application, and tape tension. Corrective techniques are defined by the tissue to be taped and by the goal of the taping application. Corrective techniques can be combined and different techniques can be used at each stage of the rehabilitation process. In each stage the clinician needs to assess the needs of the patient and choose the application most appropriate for their needs at that point.

There are six types of corrective techniques. The first five techniques are listed below, followed by the sixth – fascial correction – technique.

1. Mechanical corrections provide a positional hold for stability and improved proprioceptive stimulus. This technique is typically used on muscle, fascia, or joints to inhibit pathological movement and maintain functional range of motion. Tension in different areas of the tape provides varying levels of stimulus to the target tissue to achieve different levels of hold. Downward, inward pressure is applied with the tape to hold tissues in the desired position without inhibiting circulation or range of motion.

2. Ligament/tendon corrective techniques are used to decrease stress on ligaments and tendons. Stimulation is provided to the mechanoreceptors to provide a perception of support and sense of normal movement patterns. High tape tension is used to provide support to the injured tissue at the joint. Since most ligament injuries are caused by overstretch of the tissue, taping applications on ligaments are not applied to stretched target tissue. However, tendon applications are applied to stretched tissue but with less tension than is applied on the ligament. Tendon applications stimulate the Golgi tendon receptors to assist in protection of the joint.

3. Functional corrective techniques are designed to provide sensory stimulation to either assist or limit a motion. This application uses movement of the joint to create tape tension, and is intended to prevent joint hypermobility and reinjury. Restoring functional movement patterns is the goal of this technique. Tape is anchored on either side of the joint and then the joint is moved into the desired functional position.

4. Lymphatic/circulatory corrective techniques are used for acute conditions, often involving bruising or lymphatic congestion due to surgical removal of lymph nodes. Tape is applied with a directional pull that channels lymphatic fluids toward less congested areas or a healthy lymph duct. Numerous thin cuts of tape are applied with zero to minimal tension to lift the skin and decrease pressure in injured tissues. Lymphatic corrections are often used in the treatment of hematomas and sprained joints. Areas peripheral to the injury need to be treated also to create space for fluids moving away from the injury.

5. Space corrections are applied in order to create space by lifting the skin in a specific location. Target tissue is generally an area of pain and inflammation. By creating lift over the area of pain, pressure is decreased on skin receptors and circulation is improved. I-strips can be used on tissues that are not very sensitive and are very effective on conditions such as bursitis or sacroiliac dysfunction. The space correction reflects the original idea of the Kinesio Taping® Method – lifting tissues to create space for balancing fluid flow, decreasing pressure on pain receptors, and normalizing tissue function.

Fascial correction techniques

The aim of the fascial correction is to create, unwind, or direct movement of fascia, and it is often used to treat chronic conditions. Superficial or deep fascia can be targeted by varying the amount of tension on the tape. Super-light (0–5%) and light (5–10%) tensions provide more superficial stimulation and gentle treatment of the fascia. More tension (11–50%) is used for deeper and stronger treatment of fascia. Oscillating or vibrating the Kinesio® Tex Tape as it is applied to the skin adds a micromassaging effect to the tissues. Oscillating the tape from side to side (horizontal to the start of the application) creates a light stimulus with a smooth recoil toward the start of the application. This provides a gentle stimulus for movement in the superficial fascia. Oscillating the tape in a long and short direction (perpendicular to the start of the application) creates more moderate stimulation to the deeper fascia. As the tape is applied it is lengthened, then shortened, creating zones of higher and lower tension.

Fascial corrective techniques are often used with a Y-shaped piece of Kinesio® Tex Tape to allow targeted treatment of specific areas of fascial limitation. Adding tension in the base of the application treats a smaller, more localized area of fascial limitation. Tension in the tails treats a larger area of tension and allows for more dispersal of tension between the tails. Adding differing amounts of tension to the base or to the tails varies the amount of stimulus added to the target tissue. The fascial correction illustrated here (Fig. 52.4) shows a treatment for the condition of lateral epicondylitis, also known as tennis elbow.

Tennis elbow is caused by repetitive overuse of the wrist extensor muscles. Evaluation and assessment is performed first to determine an appropriate taping application. In Figure 52.4, a muscle inhibition application is combined with a fascial correction to treat both the muscle group and the fascial connections involved. The muscle inhibition application (the Y-strip) is applied first to treat the overcontracted wrist extensor muscles contributing to the patient's pain. The inhibition application is applied in a distal to proximal direction to recoil the target tissues toward the muscle insertion. This relaxes the overcontracted extensor muscles. The Y-strip is used to release tension between the tails and is used because of the specific area of pain reported by the patient. The Y-strip tails can be used to bracket the localized area of pain. The Y-strip fascial correction is then applied over the elbow retinaculum with tension in the tails to apply a low level of stimulation to a larger area of tissue. Oscillation is applied to the tails as they are stretched over

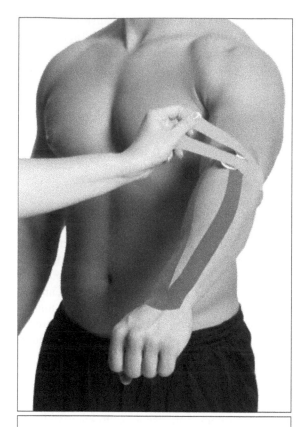

- Measure and cut Kinesio Tex Y Strip

- Position: elbow extension, forearm pronation and wrist flexion

- Anchor below or behind the target tissue with no tension

- 10% to 50% tension through tails with oscillation

Figure 52.4

Fascia correction elbow retinaculum application. A muscle inhibition application is combined with a fascial correction to treat both the muscle group and the fascial connections involved

the fascia. Applying manual stretch with the hand to the tissue before applying the taping application helps add movement to the tissue. This manual glide technique is helpful for loosening tissue too compromised to move in a normal fashion. It can also be used to treat deeper levels of fascia. After application the patient's range of motion is checked to make sure it is not compromised, and the patient is asked to report any sensations of discomfort.

Results of research into the Kinesio Taping® Method have been mixed. Too many research studies have focused on proving that the Kinesio Taping® Method improves strength and performance. This has never been the goal of the Kinesio Taping® Method. Instead, the aim has always been to restore normal functioning and balance in the body. For the past 35 years the Kinesio Taping® philosophy of how to do this has continued to evolve. In its original conception, the Kinesio Taping® Method was focused on affecting the muscle and fascia function. Further research and clinical practice have shown that the body responds best when its own healing process is facilitated. We live in a very stimulating, fast-paced world that has caused many people to live in a state of hyperarousal. Applying tape that uses too much tension or applies too much stimulation to the skin can be counterproductive. The conclusions of current research that epidermal cells can actually be involved in the sensory process and interact closely with the nervous system has enhanced my theory that lighter tape applications to the epidermis can actually be perceived very well by the body and can begin to make change faster than a traditional muscle tape application. This is not to say that the traditional muscle applications have no place anymore. Rather they must be used in conjunction with the epidermal applications to best serve the patient. Our goal as healthcare practitioners is to reduce pain and improve the normal body function of our patients. To do this we must continue to expand our methods of treatment and search for new and better ways to help our patients. Research continues to test new ways to use Kinesio® Tex Tape for the benefit of all who have found it useful.

Acknowledgements

This chapter was written with the assistance of Kinesio Taping Association International staff member Linda Delker BA, MS, LMT, RMTI, CKTP.

References

Boulais N., Misery L. The epidermis: a sensory tissue. *Eur J Dermatol* 2008;18:119–127.

Denda M., Nakatani M, Ikeyama K., Tsutsumi M., Denda S. Epidermal keratinocytes as the forefront of the sensory system. *Exp Dermatol* 2007;16:157–161.

Guimberteau J.-C. Strolling Under the Skin. DVD, 2005.

Wang J., Li B. Mechanics rules cell biology. *Sports Med Arthrosc Rehabil Ther Technol* 2010;2:16.

OSTEOPATHIC TREATMENT OF THE DURA

Torsten Liem

General treatment advice

The following are useful tips relating to the treatment techniques described in this chapter.

- It is generally useful to support the patient at the beginning of the treatment, to downregulate the sympathetic tone and reach the best possible autonomic balance. 'Slowing down' techniques should be at the forefront here.

- It is important for all the techniques that the practitioner does not concentrate himself into the structure, but rather lets the structure come forward to him.

- This is aided by using not only the palpating hand but the proprioceptive feedback from the whole body of the practitioner to sense patterns of tissue-tension, follow them, and possibly reinforce them.

- If the tissue dynamics repeat themselves, they are suppressed and we then 'wait' for the appearance of a new tissue dynamic with a relaxed presence.

- When carrying out a technique the attention should not just be focused on the treated tissue relationship. The awareness should also and always be on regional surroundings of the structure that is to be treated, the whole organism, and the field around the body. At the same time the attention expands to rest in the far distance, reaching out to the horizon and beyond. It is like relaxing your gaze and looking into the far distance.

- Dynamic developmental patterns or emotional reciprocities that aren't included in this chapter can be integrated depending on the case (Liem, 2013, pp. 87, 98, 106, 116, 223, 235, 249, 286, 362, 407, 416).

- It is generally useful to use integrative techniques (e.g., treatment of the three midlines by Van Den Heede [Liem, 2013]) at the end of the special treatment of the particular structure or structures.

Cranial dura mater (CDM)

The elastic collagen fibers of the dural membrane are interwoven. They are organized according to the tensile forces within the dura and run parallel to those forces.

The bony attachment points of the dural membrane to the skull, the sacrum, the coccyx, and irregularly within the vertebral canal, can be used as levers to examine and treat tensile patterns. In order to understand and correctly apply the techniques it is useful to know the insertion points.

The resolution of abnormal hypertonic dural tension will be displayed as a combination of direct and indirect techniques.

Approaches for examining the CDM

The intracranial tension of the falx and tentorium is examined passively and then actively using the following hand-holds: frontal bone lift, parietal bone lift, decompression of the sphenobasilar synchondrosis/synostosis, internal rotation of the temporal bone, and the 'ear-pulling' technique.

Treatment techniques for the CDM

General approach:

- Initially the practitioner synchronizes himself with the inherent tissue dynamics of the respective dura-osseous complex.

- With the spread technique (indirect) we follow the dural tension. Through this an initial temporary technique, compensatory release of the tension occurs.

- If a 'gasp of relief' and relaxation of the tissue can be sensed, we seamlessly transition into the lift technique (direct).

- With the lift technique the tissue is raised gently. It is not necessary to challenge the restriction, but enough just to raise the tissue until the dural membrane starts unfolding.

- A slight pull on the double folds of the dura (falx and tentorium) allows for expression of present patterns of tension and their unfolding. It also allows the release of excessive energy to the outer world, which in turn allows release from those binding forces and patterns of tension and results in a deconditioning.

- Not the practitioner but the forces of the inherent tissue dynamic accompany the tissue to a point of balance. This equilibrium can also embrace the whole patient.

- At this point of balance, the practitioner stays alert to all changes that occur. The attention of the practitioner opens itself toward all fluid, fascial, and electromagnetic interactions.

It is not the primary goal to accompany a specific tissue toward a point of greatest relaxation and best possible equilibrium. We try to support the whole homeostasis of the organism, no matter which processes, ways, or dynamics are needed to achieve this.

Frontal bone spread-and-lift technique

Positioning of hands

- The ring fingers hook around the zygomatic processes of the frontal bone and use them as an anchor.

- The little fingers support the ring fingers.

- The middle and index fingers lie laterally to the midline of the frontal bone.

- The thumbs touch or cross over each other posteriorly.

- The index fingers induce a slight pressure posteriorly at the midline of the frontal bone so that the

anteroposterior diameter of the falx reduces and the membranous tension reduces (spread).

- In order to lift, this is followed by a gentle, medially directed pressure to the zygomatic processes of the frontal bone, applied by the ring fingers. This allows gentle release from the sphenoid and parietal bones.

- An anterior pull is induced subsequently by putting weight through the elbows.

Parietal bone spread-and-lift technique

Positioning of hands

- The index, middle, ring and little fingers lie laterally on the parietal and temporal bones. The little fingers lie anteriorly to the asterion and the lambdoid suture.

- The thumbs are crossed over each other and lie on the contralateral side of the parietal bone.

- The membranous tension of the falx in the craniocaudal plane gets reduced by exerting a gentle caudal pressure with the thumb pads onto the parietal bone so that the sagittal suture depresses.

- In order to lift all fingers, move cranially and stop just above the squamous suture of the parietal bone. The thumb pads don't contact the bone anymore but touch each other above the sagittal suture.

- The index, middle, ring, and little fingers exert a gentle, medially directed pressure at the lower border of the parietal bones. This allows the release of the parietal bones from the temporal bones and is followed by the exertion of a cranial pull.

Sphenobasilar synchondrosis compression and decompression

- The thumbs lie on the large wings of the sphenoid posteriorly to the lateral edge of the eyes.

- The ring finger and little finger touch the lateral aspects of the occiput.

- The thumbs exert an initially posteriorly and then anteriorly directed pull.

Internal rotation of the temporal bone

- The thenar eminences lie bilaterally on the mastoid part of the temporal bones.

- The thumbs lie bilaterally on the anterior points of the mastoid processes.

- The thenar eminences exert a posteromedial pressure bilaterally.

'Ear-pulling' technique

- The thumbs lie in the external acoustic meatus.

- The index and middle fingers lie just posteriorly to the earlobe as close as possible to the temporal bones.

- The thumbs and fingers reach around the antitragus and the earlobes.

- A posterolaterally and cranially directed pull is exerted in the approximate plane of the petrous part of the temporal bone without challenging any restrictions.

Spinal dura mater (SDM)

After fetal development atlantodural and sacral ligaments are normally present and fix the dural sac (Munkácsi, 1990). The SDM separates from the vertebra in the area of the foramen magnum, creating an epidural space within the spinal canal that doesn't exist within the cranium. This space allows a gliding movement between the dura and the vertebral column (shearing).

The inner layer of the CDM is continuous with the SDM and the outer layer blends with the periosteum of the vertebrae. The epidural space is filled with connective and adipose tissue, and contains the internal vertebral venous plexus. The spinal epidural adipose tissue in the upper cervical area is only poorly developed (Breig, 1960).

Approaches for examining the SDM

General examination of the SDM

Both hands are in the area of the occiput. The head is slightly extended to take the superficial muscles off stretch. Initial passive palpation allows the practitioner to sense any tension within the SDM and the adjacent tissues. After this an active cranial pull is exerted to establish if there are any regions of resistance within the SDM and the surrounding tissues.

This is used in a similar manner at the sacrum.

We try to distinguish if these areas of tension come from any of the following structures:

- spinal dura mater

- spinal cord (and denticulate ligaments)

- ligamentum nuchae

- ligamentum flava

- dural sheath of the spinal nerves

- suboccipital muscles

- fascia of the muscles of the back

- posterior longitudinal ligament and deep posterior sacrococcygeal ligament

- anterior longitudinal ligament and anterior sacrococcygeal ligament

- prevertebral fascia (running from close to the pharyngeal tubercle and the occipitomastoid suture along the anterior parts of the vertebral fascia to the sacrum).

Treatment techniques for the SDM

Ligamentum craniale durae matris spinalis (lig. CDMS)

Positioning of hands for the upper level (Fig. 53.1)

- The index finger and middle finger of one hand are placed medially at the lower border of the occiput.

- The middle finger of the other hand is placed directly under the occiput in the region between the occiput and the atlas or, should this not be possible, on the atlas.

Positioning of hands for the middle level

- The middle finger of one hand is placed on the axis and the middle finger of the other hand is placed on the atlas (Fig. 53.2).

- The middle finger of one hand is placed on the axis, and the middle and index fingers of the other hand are positioned laterally at the lower border of the squama of the occipital bone (Fig. 53.3).

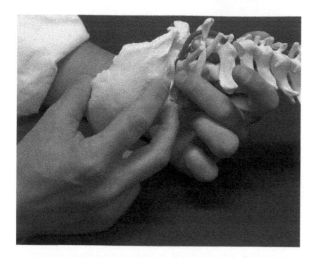

Figure 53.1
Hand-hold during treatment of lig. CDMS.
Positioning of hands for the upper level

- The middle finger of one hand is on the axis, and the middle and index fingers of the other hand are positioned laterally on the atlanto-occipital joint (Fig. 53.4).

Positioning of hands for the lower level

- The index, middle, and ring fingers are placed on the spinal processes of C3–C5.

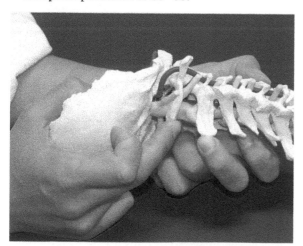

Figure 53.2
Hand-hold during treatment of lig. CDMS.
Positioning of hands for the middle level (step 1)

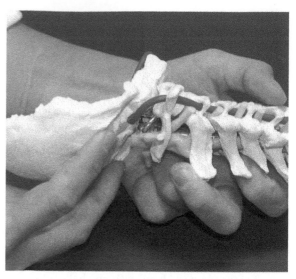

Figure 53.3
Hand-hold during treatment of lig. CDMS.
Positioning of hands for the middle level (step 2)

- The index and middle fingers of the other hand are on the atlanto-axial joint (Fig. 53.5).

Performance of the technique

- The head is brought into slight extension to relax the superficial musculature of the neck. A gentle divergent pull is built up between the two hands until the tissue starts responding (usually this is under the perception of a restriction).

- Follow the tissue dynamics to a release.

SDM and suboccipital muscles

Indications

- Cervical headaches, especially in combination with increased tone of suboccipital muscles and the SDM, or when the suboccipitals and the myodural bridge have a reduced tone that leads to subdural compression.

- The rectus capitis posterior minor (RCPmi), rectus capitis posterior major (RCPma), and the obliquus capitis inferior (OCin) muscles have myodural links to the dura and can be treated using the example of RCPmi.

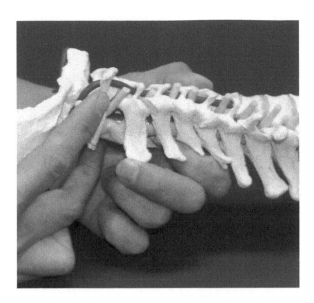

Figure 53.4
Hand-hold during treatment of lig. CDMS. Positioning of hands for the middle level (step 3)

Examination

The index, middle, and ring fingers are placed tightly and bilaterally at the palpable inferior edge of the

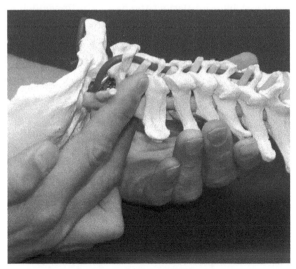

Figure 53.5
Hand-hold during treatment of lig. CDMS. Positioning of hands for the middle lower level

occiput to palpate the muscle tone of the suboccipitals, medially the RCPmi, next to it the rectus capitis posterior major, and laterally between C1 and C2 the obliquus capitis inferior muscles. Introduce a contralateral sidebend to test the link between RCPmi and SDM.

Introduce a contralateral sidebend and contralateral rotation to test the link between RCPma or OCin and SDM.

Treatment approach (for the RCPmi)

Positioning of hands

- The index finger of one hand lies paramedially directly under the lower palpable edge of the occiput.

- If possible, the middle finger of the other hand lies paramedially on the atlas on the side that is to be treated (Fig. 53.6 and 53.7).

Performance of the technique

- The head is brought into slight extension to relax the strong superficial cervical musculature.

- Introduce a contralateral sidebend at this level to engage the relationship between RCPmi and SDM.

- We then try to palpate the respective muscle between the atlas and the occiput. The dysfunctional myofascial patterns of tension are allowed to express themselves within a field of expansion in resonance to the myofascial tension. Sometimes a

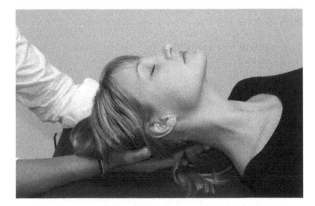

Figure 53.6
Treatment of the RCPmi

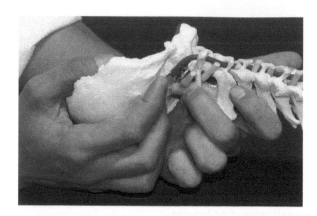

Figure 53.7
Treatment of the RCPmi

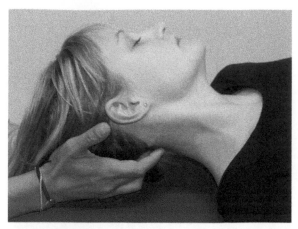

Figure 53.8
Treatment of the lig. nuchae

field of compression is needed as well. This is done until a balance between the forces is reached and a release occurs.

Note: for the treatment of the myodural links of the RCPma and the OCin with the SDM, the practitioner introduces contralateral sidebending and contralateral rotation.

Links between the SDM and the ligamentum nuchae at the level of C1–C2

Indications

Used for upper cervical rotatory dysfunction of the head in the sagittal and transverse planes.

Patient position

The patient lies supine and the practitioner is at the head end of the plinth.

Positioning of hands

- The middle fingers of both hands are placed laterally to the ligamentum nuchae at the level of C1–C2.

- The ring fingers of both hands lie superiorly to the middle fingers.

Performance of the technique

- To examine the ligament, gently push it from side to side.

- The restriction is treated by gently mobilizing the ligament toward the restriction. Doing this, the head is slightly rotated to the contralateral side (i.e., if the fingers lie on the right side of the ligament and gently mobilize to the left, the patient rotates his head toward the left) (Fig. 53.8).

Bilateral tenderness on palpation of the insertion of the ligamentum nuchae inferior from inion (protuberantia occipitalis inferior) and along the linea nuchae mediana at the occiput can be a sign of ligamentous tendinosis (or vertebral restrictions, which can be treated in this manner).

Note: The relationship to the rhomboid major, splenius capitis and cervicis, trapezius, and other cervical muscles, as well as superficial and deep cervical fascia, should be considered during the treatment.

Links between the SDM and the interspinal ligaments of the dura mater

Indications

Used for dysfunctional rotatory movements of the cervical spine (CSp).

Positioning of hands

- The index, middle, ring, and small fingers of both hands lie ipsilateral and as close as possible to the

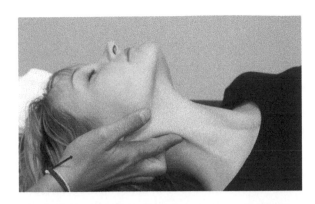

Figure 53.9
Treatment of the interspinal ligaments of the
dura mater

intervertebral foramina between the occiput and
C6 (Fig. 53.9).

Performance of the technique

- Sense the tension within the area of the interspinal
ligaments of the dura mater during rotation of the
CSp and by comparison of side-bending.

- It is possible to use a combination of direct and indirect techniques if there is tension in the area of the
interspinal ligaments of the dura mater (i.e., if there is
a dysfunctional ipsilateral, cranially directed increase
of tension within the right-hand side fibers during
side-bending to the left, we side-bend to the left to
come into resonance with the field of tension of interspinal ligaments of the dura mater on the right). Fine-
tuning using rotation is carried out at the same time
(possibly combined with slight flexion of the atlanto-
occipital joint and traction of the rest of the CSp*).

- Follow the tissue dynamics within this field of
tension, for example, by using a dynamic balanced-
ligamentous-tension technique (minimally reinforcing dysfunctional dynamics during inspiration, only
following them during expiration until there is a clear,
naturally occurring disengagement of the region).

---

*Note: the dorsal and intersegmental strings of the ligament
should be put under tension on the side of rotation and should
not be under tension on the contralateral side. During side-
bending the contralateral fibers should be pulled cranially.
Ipsilateral fibers in the area of the curve should be pulled
transversally, and fibers lying caudally to those cranially.

Links between the SDM and the ligamenta flava

Indications

- Used for upper cervical dysfunctions that sometimes show signs associated with a myelopathy
when held in flexion. Signs can include slight loss
of motor and sensory function in the upper and/or
lower extremities, and dissociated sensory symptoms.

- Note: It is important to include further differential
diagnosis for other causes of myelopathy.

- Narrowing of the spinal canal in the lumbar region
can cause neurogenic symptoms in the lower
extremities.

Positioning of hands

- The index fingers are placed bilaterally between
the atlas and the axis and the middle fingers are
placed between C2–C3. We try to palpate through
the muscular layers. It is also possible to encompass
the vertebrae C1–C2, and also C2–C3 (Fig. 53.10).

This description can also be used as a guide for the
ligamenta flava in the lower cervical and lumbar
region.

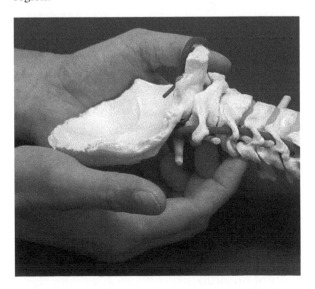

Figure 53.10
Treatment of the lig. flava

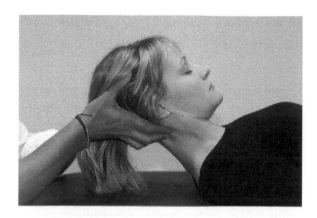

Figure 53.11
Treatment of the denticulate ligament

Performance of the technique

In all three cases we try to establish balanced ligamentous tension.

Posterior longitudinal ligament (PLL) and meningovertebral ligaments

Cranial examination

Patient position

The patient lies supine and the practitioner is at the head end of the plinth.

Positioning of hands

• The hands hold the occiput bilaterally.

Performance of the technique

• The head is brought into slight extension to relax the cervical musculature.

• A gentle cranial pull is exerted on the occiput whilst maintaining the extension.

• Parameters of tension between the dura and the PLL at the upper cervical region are registered.

Caudal examination

Patient position

The patient lies supine and the practitioner is next to the pelvis.

Positioning of hands

• One hand is on the sacrum.

Performance of the technique

• A gentle caudal pull is exerted to examine the patient.

• To treat, we place one hand above and one below the level of restriction.

• We then exert a divergent pull in order to contact the parameters of tension of the meningovertebral ligaments so they can disentangle themselves. We exert as little as or as much pull on the tissues as needed. Flexion, extension, and side-bending of the back can be used to aid the process.

Links between the SDM and the denticulate ligaments

Indications

• Dysfunctional stabilization of the spinal cord and the medulla during flexion of the upper cervical complex.

• The uppermost denticulate ligament is directed cranially (Rossitti, 1993). All other ligaments in the cervical and thoracic regions are almost horizontal. In the lumbar area they are directed caudally (Klein, 1986). Flexion of the head exerts a mechanical stress on the denticulate ligaments, moving their pyramidal attachment points on the dura further away from one another.

Treatment of cervical ligaments

Patient position

The patient lies supine and the practitioner is at the head end of the plinth.

Positioning of hands

• The fingers of both hands lie ipsilaterally and as close as possible to the vertebral column in the upper cervical area and on the occiput (Fig. 53.11).

Performance of the technique

• Head and CSp are brought into gentle flexion. This exerts a mechanical stress on the denticulate ligament so its pyramidal attachments move further away from each other (extension leads to a relaxation of the ligament).

- We try to sense asymmetric patterns of tension within the denticulate ligament.

- A balance is allowed to develop between the spinal cord, the denticulate ligament, the pia, and the dura mater.

Treatment of lumbar ligaments

For ligaments in the lumbar area we bring the lumbar spine into flexion by flexing the hips and the knees.

Patient position

The patient is side-lying with flexed hips and knees. The practitioner stands in front of the patient at the level of L5/S1.

Positioning of hands

- The cranial hand lies on the lumbar spine while the caudal hand lies on the sacrum.

- The knees of the patient lie between the thighs of the practitioner.

Performance of the technique

- The hand on the sacrum palpates at the level at which it meets resistance while exerting a caudally directed pull.

- The cranial hand is placed above this resistance, the caudal hand below.

- The hips of the patient can be flexed through the knees so that the tension is focused on the affected denticulate ligaments.

- This can be additionally supported with the hands by gently pulling caudally with the distal hand in order to release patterns of tension of the denticulate ligaments.

Dural sheaths of the spinal nerves

Indications

Radicular symptoms like paresthesia, paralysis, or changed reflexes in the area supplied by the affected spinal nerves.

Treatment using the example of the upper cervical region

Patient position

The patient lies supine and the practitioner is at the head end of the plinth.

Positioning of hands (Figs 53.12 and 53.13)

- The ring fingers lie bilaterally between C0 and C1, the middle fingers between C1 and C2.

- The index fingers lie between C2 and C3 and are as close as possible to the intervertebral foramina and the spinal nerves.

Performance of the technique

- The CSp is flexed and extended rhythmically. During flexion the spinal cord and the nerve root fold together. An unfolding occurs during extension.

- We try to sense tension within the area of the spinal nerves and reduce it with a combination of direct and indirect techniques.

- In order to do this we bring areas of increased tension into extension to stabilize the spinal

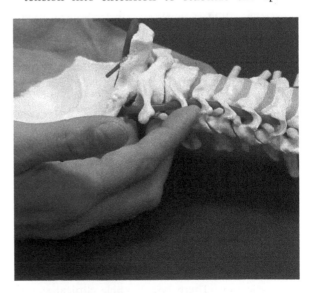

Figure 53.12
Treatment of the dural sheaths

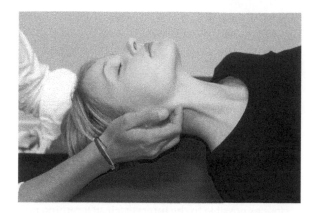

Figure 53.13
Treatment of the dural sheaths

nerve. Any patterns of tension are treated as described above.

The treatment of the dural sheaths includes treatment of the opercula of Forestier and the transforaminal ligaments. The opercula of Forestier lie at the height of each intervertebral foramina. They connect the dural sheath of the exiting spinal nerve with the periosteum of the corresponding vertebra (Forestier, 1922; Lazorthes, 1981; Trolard, 1890) and enclose the intervertebral foramina from the inside and the outside. The spinal nerve protrudes through the opercula of Forestier with the recurrent meningeal ramus. These structures may play a role in venolymphatic pumping (Van Dun & Giradin, 2006).

The transforaminal ligaments cover the intervertebral foramen along the exterior aspect and are described as incomplete opercula, part of the opercula of Forestier, or as 'false ligaments' (Giradin, 1996).

Treatment of the blood supply

According to Hu et al. (1995) a vascular irritation of the meninges can lead to persistent and reversible activation of the cervical muscles and muscles of mastication. There is a possible clinical significance of muscular tension and pain in relation to certain types of headaches. A vascular spasm can be caused by a mechanic, neurogenic, or chemical stimulus, and can last for minutes, days, or longer.

Usually there is a combination of stimuli involved, for instance, in an increased sympathetic tone that will lead to vasoconstriction by contraction of the smooth muscles. A vascular spasm of the vertebral artery can spread intracranially to the basilar artery and other intracranial arteries.

Osteopathic treatment of the vertebral artery or venous drainage is being taught (Barral, 2011). According to J. P. Barral it is possible to treat the vertebral artery directly.

Patient position

The patient lies supine and the practitioner is at the head end of the plinth.

Positioning of hands (Fig. 53.14)

- The tip of the thumb of the caudal hand fixes the subclavian artery posteriorly to the clavicle and laterally to the sternoclavicular joint
- The tip of the middle finger of the cranial hand lies at the lower edge of the transverse process of the atlas.
- The palm of the cranial hand lies gently at the lateral aspect of the head.

Performance of the technique

- A gentle increase of pressure is achieved by moving the transverse process of C1 cranially.

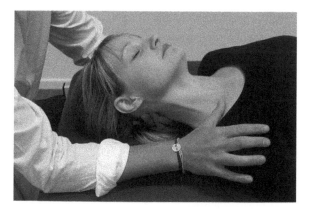

Figure 53.14
Treatment of the vertebral artery according to J. P. Barral

- This is aided by a gentle side-bend of the head to the contralateral side.

- We follow the dynamics of tension until the surrounding tissues become soft and reach an inherent relaxation.

- The joints of C0–C1 and C1–C2 can be manipulated additionally, and a direct release of tension can also be applied to the upper cervical dura.

- Venous drainage occurs through the vertebral plexus. It forms an anastomosis with the venous system of the brain and the venous sinuses of the cranium.

- Drainage through the venous plexus occurs externally to the vertebral column and the segmental veins.

Venous drainage can be treated with a modified J. P. Barral technique. For this the patient is side-lying. The osteopath palpates deeply between the anterior and middle scalene muscles close to the foramen spinosum whilst side-bending the CSp to the ipsilateral side (Fig. 53.15). The author usually exerts gentle and draining impulses (Barral, 2011).

Treatment of the innervation of the SDM

There is a controversial debate on the pathogenesis of pain in relation to the SDM. According to Kumar et al. (1996) the SDM functions mainly as a protec-

tive membrane as it encloses the spinal cord and the cerebrospinal fluid, and plays a smaller role in the pathogenesis of pain than the CDM.

Conversely Johnson (2004), Bogduk (2001), and Grgić (2007) say that the SDM is partly involved in the creation of radiating pain and cervical headaches because of these same anatomical features.

One source of cervical headaches apparently lies within the structures (upper cervical synovial joints and muscles, intervertebral discs C2 and C3, vertebral and internal carotid arteries, and the dura mater of the upper cervical region and the posterior cranial fossa) that are innervated by the spinal nerves of C1–C3 (Bogduk, 2001; Grgić, 2007). According to Grgić (2007) and Gasik (2008) the convergence of the nociceptive afferents of the spinal nerves C1–C3 with the spinal nucleus of the trigeminal nerve plays a significant role. According to Groen et al. (1988) the clear multisegmental innervation in the ventral region provides an anatomical basis for the explanation of the extrasegmental radiation of pain. Treatment can occur through the spinal nerves, for example.

The dura mater has a large amount of slowly adapting stretch receptors, the Ruffini corpuscles (SAII-sensors). They are activated by long-lasting tangential forces or lateral stretching. Therefore, the dura can be treated nicely with slow techniques. It is not uncommon for these techniques to also have a general relaxing effect. One explanation could be the inhibition of the sympathetic nervous system by the activation of Ruffini corpuscles.

Conclusion

The anatomical relationships of the spinal dura mater in the upper cervical region are complex. An osteopathic treatment should integrate these special anatomical relationships and acknowledge the articulate, ligamentous, fascial, muscular, arterial, venolymphatic and neural relations.

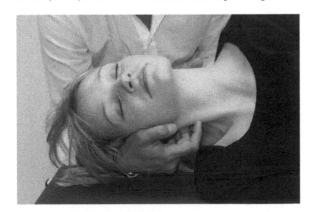

Figure 53.15
Venous drainage after J. P. Barral, modified

References

Barral J. P. (2011) *Kursmitschrift: Neue artikuläre Ansätze.* OSD Hamburg.

Bogduk N. (2001) Cervicogenic headache: anatomic basis and pathophysiologic mechanisms. *Curr Pain Headache Rep* 5:382–386.

Breig A. (1960) *Biomechanics of the Central Nervous System: Some Basic Normal and Pathologic Phenomena.* Almqvist and Wiksell.

Forestier J. (1922) *Le trou de conjugaison vertebral et l'espace epidural.* These de Paris.

Gasik R. (2008) Cervicogenic headache. *Pol Merkur Lekarski* 24:549–551.

Giradin M. (1996) Die caudale durale Insertion und das Ligamentum sacrodurale anterius (Trolard). *Naturheilpraxis* 4:528–535.

Grgić V. (2007) Cervicogenic headache: etiopathogenesis, characteristics, diagnosis, differential diagnosis and therapy. [in Croatian] *Lijec Vjesn* 129:230–236.

Groen G. J., Baljet B., Drukker J. (1988) The innervation of the spinal dura mater: anatomy and clinical implications. *Acta Neurochir* 92:39–46.

Hu J. W., Vernon H., Tatourian I. (1995) Changes in neck electromyography associated with meningeal noxious stimulation. *J Manipul Physiol Ther* 18: 577–581.

Johnson G. M. (2004) The sensory and sympathetic nerve supply within the cervical spine: review of recent observations. *Man Ther* 9:71–76.

Klein P. (1986) *Contribution à l'étude biomechanique de la moelle épinière et de ses envelop-pes.* Brussels: Mémoire.

Kumar R., Berger R. J., Dunkser S. B., Keller J. T. (1996) Innervation of the spinal dura: myth or reality? *Spine* 21:18–25.

Lazorthes G. (1981) *Le systeme nerveux peripherique.* Masson.

Liem T. (2013) *Morphodynamik in der Osteopathie.* Haug.

Munkácsi I. (1990) The epidural ligaments during fetal development. *Acta Morphol Hung* 38:1 89–197.

Rossitti S. (1993) Biomechanics of the pons-cord tract and its enveloping structures: an overview. *Acta Neurochir* 124:144–152.

Trolard P. (1890) De quelques particularités de la dure-mère. *Journal de l'Anatomie* 407–418.

Van Dun P. I. S., Giradin M. R. G. (2006) Embryological study of the spinal dura and its attachment into the vertebral canal. *Internat J Ost Med* 9:85–93.

THE PLEXUSES

Serge Paoletti

The plexuses comprise a concentration of different nerve fibers of the sympathetic and parasympathetic nervous systems, which interweave or anastomose in a complex fashion at specific points in the body. They enable organs to regulate the various functions of the body in an autonomous way, but can also be the origin of numerous dysfunctions. There are seven plexuses, which can be superimposed on the seven chakras of the Hindu tradition (Fig. 54.1). From bottom to top, these are:

- coccygeal plexus
- hypogastric plexus
- epigastric plexus
- cardiopulmonary plexus
- thyroid plexus.

The sixth and seventh plexuses of the Hindu tradition can be equated to the hypothalamic–pituitary axis, to which we add the amygdalae and the hippocampus. The pineal gland is considered to be the seventh plexus.

Even though they function autonomously, the plexuses are often sites of dysfunction, which we can qualify in simplified terms as, for example, hyperactivity or hypoactivity. By adapting osteopathic techniques, it is possible to treat these dysfunctions and restore normal physiology. As a result, we can influence the various autonomic functions that govern our daily lives.

Autonomic nervous system: sympathetic and parasympathetic nervous systems

These are two antagonistic systems that play a continuous role in the adaptation of all bodily functions to both the external and internal environments. Their

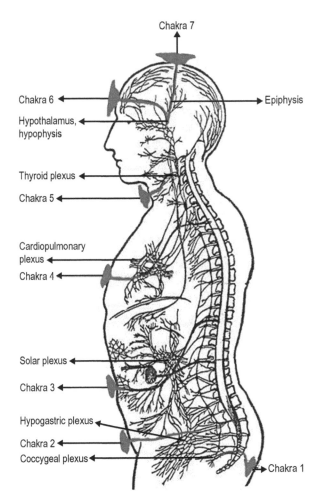

Figure 54.1
The seven plexuses superimposed on the seven chakras of the Hindu tradition

antagonistic effect acts especially on the following organs:

- heart
- respiratory system
- digestive system.

In an emergency the sympathetic system increases the heart rate and respiratory frequency and inhibits digestion and elimination. When a state of equilibrium is reached, the parasympathetic system intervenes to decrease the heart rate and respiratory frequency, to increase nutrition of cells, and to eliminate waste.

Vegetative centers

The vegetative centers have their own specific activity. They are located in the brainstem and in the spinal cord. They also establish the common final pathway toward the hypothalamic vegetative centers.

- The sympathetic centers are situated in the dorso-lumbar and cervical areas of the spinal cord.
- The parasympathetic centers are grouped together at both extremities of the spinal cord: on the 'floor' of the fourth ventricle and in the sacral part of the cord. The parasympathetic centers are subject to the activity of the higher centers.

These two systems receive information from baro-receptors in the blood vessels and chemoreceptors situated in the organs.

Sympathetic nervous system

The sympathetic nervous system consists of a succession of ganglia situated on either side of the vertebral column to form the lateral chain of sympathetic ganglia known as the paravertebral ganglia. All these ganglia are interconnected and extend upward via the three pairs of cervical sympathetic ganglia. The chains extend down to the coccyx where the two sympathetic trunks converge and terminate in a single ganglion, the ganglion impar. Sympathetic ganglions are the pathway through which sympathetic fibers must pass on their way to the viscera and glands in the head, neck, thorax, abdomen, and pelvis, as do the sympathetic fibers that supply the peripheral somatic areas.

Physiology

Globally, the sympathetic nervous system plays an antagonistic role to that of the parasympathetic nervous system. Generally speaking, it accelerates the metabolism and 'switches on' in situations of danger or fear to prepare the individual for escape (flight). When stimulated, it exerts an influence on the cardiovascular system: it increases the heart rate and induces peripheral vasoconstriction, which results in an increase in blood pressure. At the digestive level, it slows down contraction of the smooth muscles in the intestines, but promotes the liberation of glucose by the liver. It also has a bronchodilatory effect, inducing an augmentation of the diameter of the bronchi. It exerts its effects on cells and target organs mainly via neurotransmitters called catecholamines (noradrenaline and, to a lesser extent, adrenaline). Disturbance of the system leads either to hypertonia or hypotonia.

Parasympathetic nervous system

The parasympathetic nervous system consists of a cranial part comprising the following:

- oculomotor nerve (III)
- facial nerves (VII)
- glossopharyngeal nerves (IX)
- vagus nerves (X).

Sacral nerve fibers

Sacral nerve fibers originate from sacral segments S2–S4. Also called the vagal system, the parasympathetic nervous system is an integral part of the autonomic nervous system. It plays a major role in the involuntary actions of the organs, blood vessels, and glands. The parasympathetic nervous system is also involved in certain pathological events such as fainting, also known as vasovagal syncope.

Physiology

The role of the parasympathetic nervous system is multiple, and often antagonistic to that of the sympathetic nervous system. It intervenes mainly in situations of peace and rest. In general, it slows body functions in order to conserve energy. It lowers the heart rate and blood pressure through vasodilation or causes bronchoconstriction. It also facilitates digestion by increasing the secretion of saliva and also by increasing gastric and intestinal secretions. It also stimulates sexual appetite. Its actions are mediated by cholinergic neurotransmitters. The receptors are located in the walls of the organs. They provide information about the functional status or the composition of the internal environment of these organs. The parasympathetic tone prevents acceleration of the heart rate and maintains normal digestive and urinary function. In the case of disturbance, we see either hypertonia or hypotonia.

The seven plexuses

Coccygeal plexus (plexus no. 1)

The coccygeal plexus has rarely been studied by anatomists.[1] It is made up of sacrococcygeal sympathetic and parasympathetic nerve branches. The parasympathetic branch consists of the ventral rami originating from S4 (in part), S5, and the first coccygeal ramus.

The anococcygeal nerves that arise from this plexus pass through the coccygeal ligament and the sacrotuberous ligament, and supply a small area of skin between the tip of the coccyx and the anus. The anococcygeal nerve provides sensory innervation of the ischiococcygeal area as well as perianal sensitivity; it probably contributes to the innervation of the coccygeus muscle, the sacrospinous ligament, the ligaments of the coccyx, and the adjacent periosteum. There are also visceral branches, forming part of the erector nerves that anastomose with the hypogastric plexus.

The coccygeal plexus seems to be particularly implicated in coccydynia. One factor could be that some nerve branches from the coccygeal plexus perforate the sacrococcygeal ligament.[2] This region is also innervated by the sympathetic system via the ganglion impar. It has been established that these two systems exchange anastomotic fibers. Irritation of the ganglion impar also seems to be a factor in the aetiology of coccydynia.[3]

Hypogastric plexus (plexus no. 2)

The fibers of the hypogastric plexus supply the pelvic viscera and the perineum. This is the only paired plexus and consists of two quadrilateral sheaths located in the pelvis on either side of the viscera. The fibers that constitute the hypogastric plexus arise from the sympathetic system, from T1 to L2, and also from the sacral parasympathetic system, from S2 to S4. These latter fibers constitute the erector nerves.[4] The nerve fibers follow the trajectory of the vascular system as they make their way to the organs.[5] This system is much more complex than previously thought. Recent research has revealed the coexistence of cholinergic and adrenergic fibers in the sympathetic and parasympathetic systems.[6]

Epigastric plexus (plexus no. 3)

The epigastric plexus is also called the solar plexus because of its radiating nerve fibers. It is made up of branches of the vagus, splanchnic nerves, and the right phrenic nerve.[7] The sympathetic branches come from the splanchnic nerves, which arise from T5 to T12.[8]

The epigastric plexus is located on each side of the celiac artery (also known as the celiac trunk), close to the origin of the superior mesenteric artery and the renal arteries. The afferent fibers travel to different abdominal organs alongside the periarterial plexuses and the retroportal nerves.

The epigastric plexus consists of different ganglia linked together by multiple webs of nerves. It is also called the 'abdominal brain' because it comprises the greatest concentration of sympathetic fibers in the body. The largest and the most recognizable ganglia are the semilunar ganglia. The epigastric plexus is richly vascularized by branches from the aorta and its collateral arteries: the celiac artery, the superior mesenteric artery, the capsular artery, and the renal arteries. Its role is to control and regulate the digestive functions concerned with the absorption and assimilation of food. The epigastric plexus is also involved in the innervation of the bronchi and the pulmonary vessels.[9]

Research has also highlighted nerve connections between the hepatic plexus and the left atrium via branches (on the left-hand side) that travel along the hepatic artery, the hepatic portal vein, the hepatic vein, and the inferior vena cava.[10]

Popular expressions describe symptoms associated with the hypogastric plexus as a ball in the stomach, a feeling of a weight on the stomach, nausea, or a knot in the stomach. These expressions are not entirely meaningless and can be taken into account when expressed by the patient because they describe signs of dysfunction with no obvious clinical signs, which often indicate a state of stress or anxiety, suggesting the involvement of the autonomic nervous system.

Cardiopulmonary plexus (plexus no. 4)

The cardiopulmonary plexus controls and regulates circulatory and respiratory functions. It is formed by the anastomosis of fibers from the cervical sympathetic ganglia and superior thoracic ganglia with fibers of the hypogastric nerve. There are three types of fibers:

- *Cardioaccelerator fibers:* of sympathetic origin, centered in the lateral horn of the spinal cord (C4–D4).

- *Cardiomoderator fibers:* of vagal origin, centered in pneumogastric ganglion (below the 'floor' of the fourth ventricle).

- *Vasomotor fibers:* of mixed origin, they innervate the smooth muscle of the coronary blood vessels.

The nerves of the cardiac plexus extend by means of intracardiac fibers. These are controlled in part by the vagus nerve, in part by the stellate ganglion, and, in about 50% of cases, by the two ganglia. They control cardiac function and may be the cause of disease such as palpitations and cardiac arrhythmias.[11] It is accepted that stimulation of the vagus increases heart rate and contractility, while sympathetic stimulation improves variability and heart rate. Irritation of both the sympathetic and parasympathetic systems causes an increase in systemic blood pressure, as well as an increase in aortic pressure.[12] Stimulation of the vagus can improve heart failure, but side-effects may include bradycardia and hypotension. Stimulation of the sympathetic system can cause an imbalance due to sympathetic dominance. The stimulation of both systems increases myocardial contractility without increasing the frequency.[13,14] Hyperstimulation of the parasympathetic system is the cause of bradycardia, and can also cause apnea and cardiac arrest.[15] It is interesting to note that meditation has an effect on the regulation of the heart rate through its action on the cardiac plexus.[16]

Thyroid plexus (plexus no. 5)

The thyroid plexus, in correlation with the adrenal glands, interacts with the thyroid hormone (TH) at different levels, particularly in the stimulation of the thermogenic mechanisms that generate heat and maintain body temperature.[17] The nerves of the thyroid gland originate in the superior, middle, and lower cervical sympathetic ganglia. They reach the gland via the cardiac nerves and the superior and inferior periarterial thyroid plexuses that accompany the thyroid arteries. These are vasomotor, not secretomotor fibers. They provoke constriction of blood vessels. The endocrine secretion of the thyroid gland is controlled by hormones secreted by the pituitary gland.

Pituitary gland (plexus no. 6)

The pituitary gland is situated at the base of the brain in a bony cavity called the sella turcica. It is the size of a hazelnut and weighs about half a gram. It is connected to the hypothalamus by a stalk called the pituitary stalk. The average dimensions are 4.8 mm for the longitudinal axis and 2.4 mm for the transverse axis. The size of the pituitary decreases with age.[18] Note that raised intracranial pressure is often associated with widening of the sella turcica.[19]

The pituitary gland is divided into two lobes:

- anterior pituitary (or adenohypophysis)

- posterior pituitary (or neurohypophysis).

The pituitary gland is one of the organs with the richest blood supply and with the greatest number of nerve connections. Consequently, it is connected with all the organs in the body. Due to the nature of its hormonal secretion, the pituitary gland plays an essential role in metabolism, growth, and reproduction. It is closely linked to the hypothalamus.

Anterior pituitary

The hormones secreted by the anterior pituitary or adenohypophysis are essential for reproduction, growth, homeostasis, response to stress, and adaptation to environmental changes. Each hormonal secretion is controlled by the central nervous system through a complex interaction between hypothalamic neuroendocrine pathways and neural feedback from peripheral hormones and pituitary mechanisms.[20]

Anterior pituitary hormones

Anterior pituitary hormones are:

- Growth hormone (GH), which stimulates the tissues and energy metabolism and ensures harmonious growth.

- Adrenocorticotropic hormone (ACTH), which acts on the adrenal glands by stimulating the production of corticosteroids (which act on the metabolism).

- Thyroid-stimulating hormone (TSH), which acts on the thyroid gland (which regulates metabolic activity).

- Prolactin, which acts on the mammary glands by stimulating their production of milk.

- Follicle-stimulating hormone (FSH) and luteinizing hormone (LH), which act on the reproductive organs. They stimulate the production and secretion of sex hormones.

Posterior pituitary

The posterior pituitary is a sort of extension of the hypothalamus. It does not secrete hormones directly but provides a reservoir for two hormones secreted by the anterior pituitary.

Posterior pituitary hormones

Posterior pituitary hormones are:

- Vasopressin or antidiuretic hormone.

- Oxytocin, which stimulates contraction of the uterus and the secretion of milk by the mammary glands.

Trauma can modify the function of the pituitary gland with consequences for the functioning of certain organs depending on which hormonal system has been disturbed. Tiredness is often associated with pituitary dysfunction.[21] Pituitary physiology controls the function of almost all organs and it therefore affects in some way almost all of the plexuses. This characteristic must be taken into account when treating the plexuses.

The epiphysis cerebri (plexus no.7)

Also called the pineal gland, the epiphysis cerebri is part of the diencephalon and is situated at the front of the midbrain and the cerebellum. It is also situated between the two superior colliculi, which form a sort of gutter in which the pineal gland lies. It is held in place by expansions of the pia mater as well as a number of extensions that travel from its base to terminate in neighboring formations. The gland is oriented from the back to the front. It is the size of a pea, measuring 7–8 mm in length and 4–6 mm in width. It weighs 25 cg. It is suggested that some of the pineal cells migrate to form the suprachiasmatic nucleus, which, as their name suggests, are situated above the optic chiasm – the intersection of the optic nerves in front of the third ventricle. The pineal gland receives fibers from the superior cervical ganglion.[22] It is also called the third eye in the Hindu tradition.

We know that the pineal gland is not an endocrine gland in the classical sense, but it contributes to the synchronization of a number of rhythmic functions (diurnal and seasonal) responding to variations in physical factors and the environment.

The pineal gland was generally considered to be a photoreceptor sensory organ in lower vertebrates and an endocrine gland with a more or less well-defined antigonatotropic function in mammals.

Functions of the epiphysis cerebri

The epiphysis cerebri secretes melatonin (isolated in 1959 by the American researcher A. B. Lerner). Melatonin synthesis is controlled by the alternation of day and night. It is involved in the control of seasonal cycles (circadian and circannual). It can affect sexual development and reproductive function. It also reduces oxidative stress.[23] In 1969 W. B. Quay suggested that the pineal gland is mainly involved in the adaptation of animals to their environment. Light has a great influence on the function of the pineal gland. The secretion of the pineal is greater in adults than in children. There is also a gender difference, with a higher peak in women.[24] The pineal gland plays an important role in the regulation of the rhythmic functions of the endocrine system.

Tests for the plexuses

It is obvious that we cannot establish direct contact with the plexuses through palpation, so we should place our hands in such a way so as to project our palpatory awareness as precisely as possible toward the plexus in question. Since the plexuses are supported by fascia, the best way to reach them is via the fascia. In addition, these structures are too small for us to claim to be able to feel and palpate them directly.

However, as we have seen previously, the plexuses innervate all the internal structures of the body. Therefore, the effects of dysfunction of the plexuses will be felt all the way to the periphery due to disturbance of the tonus of the organs and the structures that support them, namely the fascia, which is itself also innervated by the plexuses. One of the important features of the fascia is to spread information about the state of the deeper tissues to the periphery, which for the practitioner is an important means of investigation that enables him to reach an accurate diagnosis of the functional state of the plexus and the structures that depend on it.

Dysfunction of the plexuses

As already pointed out, dysfunction of the plexuses occurs in two ways: hypertonia or hypotonia. However, it is necessary to know what normal tone is. This could be defined as moderate resistance to palpation. This resistance can vary from one person to another, but always within reasonable limits. This is above all a matter of experience and the repeated practice of palpation on many patients will enable the practitioner to 'record' what normal tone feels like. Let us not forget that our best tools are our hands, and that no instrument, no matter how sophisticated, can replace a well-trained hand.

Treatment of the plexuses requires a precise knowledge of the topographical anatomy of the areas concerned. The topography must be 'recorded' both in the brain and the hands. This will enable the practitioner to locate the area of dysfunction deep in the tissues with great precision. With diligent practice, this can be achieved quite easily and with maximum precision. Let us not forget that the accuracy of location (of tissue dysfunction) and the precision of the correction are essential factors in the success of osteopathic technique, irrespective of the technique being employed.

Hypertonia

In the case of hypertonia, the practitioner will feel a significant increase in tissue tonus during the diagnostic palpation. The palpating hand encounters significant resistance and it is difficult to depress the underlying structures. Tissue listening, or micro-movements of mobility, may be disturbed along a preferential axis. This indicates that the dysfunction of the plexus is specifically affecting an organ that is under its control, rather than acting in a global manner.

Hypotonia

Conversely, hypotonia manifests as a decrease in tissue tonus. The tissues are easily depressed. No resistance is encountered during palpation and the palpating hand seems to 'fall' into the body.

Test for the coccygeal plexus

The coccygeal plexus is located in the area of the central annulus of the perineum ('central tendinous point of the perineum' in *Gray's Anatomy*). This is midway between the anus and the scrotum and the lower part (posterior commissure) of the labia majora. Note that almost all the muscles and fascial structures of the perineum are attached to the annulus/central tendinous point. We can therefore consider this structure to be a faithful indicator of the status of perineal tonicity. The central annulus is normally the size of a hazelnut, easily palpable, and has a certain tonicity that means that it is easily identified.

- The thumb or middle finger is positioned on the central fibrous ring of the perineum.

- In a case of hypotonia, the finger can easily depress the tissues, the ring offers no resistance (and often cannot be distinguished from other fascias), and the finger penetrates deep into the perineum.

- Inversely, hypertonia manifests as abnormal tissue resistance with highly increased density. The fibrous ring is easily palpated.

- During the test the finger may be moved in any direction that allows the practitioner to determine whether or not the dysfunction is particularly concentrated in a specific area.

Test for the hypogastric plexus

The hypogastric plexus is located in the lower part of the abdomen at the level of the pubic symphysis.

- Sit at the side of the patient and place a flat hand on the abdomen, just above and parallel to the pubic symphysis. The pressure of the palpating hand must be less than the full weight of the hand.

- Hypertonia is characterized by increased tissue resistance. Hypotonia palpates as a soft abdomen, with the sensation of the hand sinking in with no resistance from the tissues, and coming into contact easily with the sacral promontory in some cases.

- In a case of hypertonia, the hand must be projected progressively deeper into the tissues in order to 'scan' all the different levels.

- If all the structures that depend on the plexus are dysfunctional, the resistance is uniform and it is difficult to penetrate deep into the tissues. This is not exceptional, but in many cases only a few structures dependent on or influenced by the plexus are dysfunctional, and in these cases the resistance encountered is not uniform.

- We can easily confirm these palpatory findings by testing the micromobility of the tissues. This is done by moving the palpating hand very slightly in all directions, which will confirm the site of the restriction.

Test for the epigastric plexus

The practitioner's hand is placed on the upper part of the abdomen, just below the ribs. It is placed transversely to provide a wide contact area because this plexus is very broad. Differential diagnosis of this plexus is particularly complex because of the large number of organs it controls. Very precise anatomical knowledge is required for accurate testing of the plexus, and the treatment that follows.

- Hypertonia manifests as significant tonus of the abdomen. In extreme cases it feels as if there is a stone beneath the palpating hand.

- In the presence of hypotonia the hand sinks into the abdomen with no resistance. Sometimes we get the impression that no organ interferes with the progression of the hand.

- In order to reach an accurate diagnosis, it is necessary for the hand to 'scan' the tissues, layer by layer, as it penetrates progressively deeper into the

tissues, down to the most posterior planes. In this way the practitioner can determine which structures should be treated preferentially.

- When performing this technique, it sometimes happens that when we exert light pressure, this acts as a sound box, and we feel beneath the hand an amplification of the heartbeat. This is also felt by the patient, who may express concern. If this happens, simply reassure the patient that this phenomenon does not indicate any serious pathology.

Test for the cardiopulmonary plexus

The cardiopulmonary plexus is located in the area beneath the middle of the sternum, spreading out laterally on both sides.

- Place a flat hand on the sternum, extending laterally to the ribs on both sides, as a rule slightly obliquely for enhanced perception ('a better feel'). The difficulty in palpating this area is due to the fact that a bony structure (the sternum) comes between the palpating hand and the plexus. This can interfere with deep palpation and therefore make diagnosis more difficult.

- Diligent practice combined with precise anatomical knowledge will allow us to make an accurate diagnosis in different planes.

- The palpatory feel is different compared to the other plexuses due to the anatomical particularity of this area.

- Hypotonia manifests as a hypodensity of the tissues of the chest, and of the bony resistance. This gives the feeling that the hand can easily sink into the rib cage.

- Conversely, hypertonia is felt as an increased resistance to pressure on the thorax, and as significantly increased density.

As we have already mentioned, the epigastric plexus and the cardiopulmonary plexus are (inter) connected, though the functions they control are different.

- The cardiopulmonary plexus plays a role in the circulation of fluids because it controls blood flow and oxygenation.

- The epigastric plexus plays a role in digestion and assimilation, providing energy and eliminating metabolic waste.

The diaphragm separates the two areas and influences both. It is therefore important to ensure that both plexuses function correctly in relation to each other, and that the flow of energy is unimpeded.

- Place one hand over the cardiopulmonary plexus and the other over the epigastric plexus to ensure that no outside interference comes between the two hands.

- If you feel a lack of synchronization, don't forget to test the diaphragm and normalize it if necessary, because the diaphragm is responsible for the synchronization of these two areas.

Once this has been accomplished, we can move on to the next plexus.

Test for the thyroid plexus

As we have seen previously, the thyroid plexus is located roughly at the level of the thyroid gland and therefore the thyroid cartilage.

- Certain preliminary precautions are necessary before performing this test. In some people this area is extremely sensitive to pressure, and a contact that is too firm often triggers an immediate defensive reaction, or even panic. Incidentally, this reaction should not be ignored as it may be indicative of trauma, which could have been caused by something tied round the neck or an attempt at strangulation.

- The practitioner is positioned on the patient's lateral side. The side of the thumb is in contact with the cartilage and the index and middle fingers are in contact with the opposite side of the cartilage, so as to move the cartilage to the right and to the left.

- To avoid any unpleasant reactions, place the thenar and hypothenar eminences on the sternal notch, with the rest of the hand making very light contact with the thyroid and cricoid cartilage.

- The practitioner's other hand is placed on the frontal bone to rotate the head opposite to the direction of traction on the cartilage.

- As with other areas, hypotonia manifests as tissue lacking in tone, which offers no resistance to mobilization.

- Conversely, hypertonia manifests as hypomobile, tense tissue.

- Pathology can manifest globally or unilaterally. This is easily confirmed by testing the micromobility of the tissues.

Test for the pituitary gland

Since it is located deep in the skull, it is obvious that the practitioner can only approach the pituitary gland by projection through all the cranial structures (Fig. 54.2). The pituitary gland is located in a well-defined bony landmark – the sella turcica. This will facilitate the method of palpation. Laterally, the pituitary gland is situated at the level of the wings of

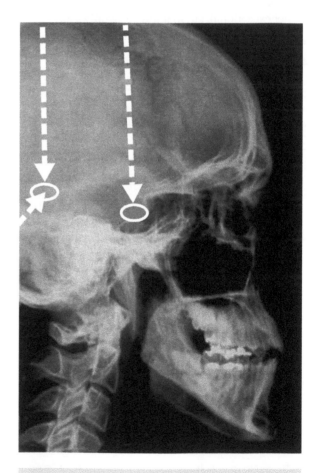

Figure 54.2
Location of the pituitary gland

the sphenoid. Vertically, it is situated roughly at the top of the cranial vault.

- The practitioner sits at the head of the subject.
- The technique is performed with two hands:
  - the two middle fingers make contact with the wings of the sphenoid
  - the thumbs make contact with the top of the skull.
- In this way we create two axes that allow us to approach the pituitary gland along different planes.
- The test consists of very light progressive pressure with the practitioner projecting his palpatory perception 'inside' the skull through the various structures, bringing it to focus in the area of the pituitary.

It seems illusory to want to 'feel' the pituitary gland in this way. However, with experience we can pick up disturbances in the sella turcica, especially by using fascial tension, and then go on to make effective corrections.

Palpatory findings often manifest as abnormal tension, usually unilateral, and as deviated axes that are not orthogonal.

Test for the epiphysis cerebri

The epiphysis cerebri is also located deep in the skull in the posterior part of the archicerebellum. Its landmarks are not easy to define. It is behind and above the pituitary gland.

- Starting from the same position as that of the previous test, the practitioner moves the middle fingers backward and upward, roughly the width of two fingers in each direction. The thumbs are placed over the lambda.
- The test is virtually the same as that for the pituitary. However, it must be noted that the palpatory sensations are much less obvious.

Treatment of the plexuses

This follows on directly from the tests.

Treatment of plexuses 1 to 5

As indicated, the practitioner will be faced with two possibilities: hypotonia or hypertonia.

Hypotonia

This causes the most problems in osteopathy, regardless of the area of dysfunction. This is because the tissues are lacking in tonicity and are hypomobile, which complicates the practitioner's osteopathic action. When dealing with a hypotonic plexus, the hand seems to sink into the body without any resistance. The technique consists of placing the hands flat over the area in question, and then seeking to tonify the tissues by imagining that you want to 'draw up' the underlying area with your hand. This takes place in conjunction with a tissue test to focus the work more precisely in a specific area if necessary. This is what happens in most cases and, curiously, it seems that the plexuses 'understand' what they need to do.

Hypertonia

This is easier to test and to treat by addressing areas of increased tissue tone that must be progressively released. The principle of treatment, in this case, is to lay the hand flat over the area and then gradually and gently penetrate deeper and deeper to the posterior structures where the plexuses are situated. Treatment is carried out at successive levels in order to normalize all the layers from superficial to deep. As we penetrate deeper into the tissues, we must also perform tests of micromobility so that we can treat the preferential axes of dysfunction (as and when we encounter them), which will enable us to progress more easily. The treatment is finished when the tissues beneath our hand are free in all dimensions and are 'able to float without restriction', and when, concomitantly, tissue tone has been 'normalized'. The basic principle of normalization applies to plexuses 1 to 5, with some local nuances depending on the underlying structures.

Treatment of plexuses 6 and 7

Here the treatment is slightly different. As we have already pointed out, it is much more difficult to identify hypotonia in these areas. We are dealing with hormonal function and the dysfunctions will instead be related hormonal hyperactivity or hypoactivity. However, this difference is still felt in the surrounding fascia and manifests as modified fascial tone.

- Starting with the hands in the same position as for the test for the pituitary gland, the practitioner tries, by using light pressure of the fingers, to project himself to the pituitary gland or the epiphysis, gradually normalizing tissue dysfunctions that he encounters (that interfere with this process). At the same time, he must also normalize the axes until they are orthogonal.

- The treatment is considered to be finished when no resistance is felt beneath the fingers, everything seems fluid, and it feels as if the fingers can penetrate the skull and follow an ebb and flow pulsation.

- When all the plexuses have been treated, an additional global test can be performed.

Additional global test

- The practitioner sits at the head of the subject with both hands together at the occiput using the same hold as for a compression of the fourth ventricle.

- Introduce light traction downwards and visualize at the same time a belt turning in an anticlockwise direction.

- Starting from the top, descend along the spine (the practitioner should project his attention downward along the spine) and then back up again along the anterior aspect of the spine, checking each plexus along the way to ensure that no restriction remains in any of the plexuses.

- This technique enables us to ensure the correct functioning of the plexuses, and therefore the proper flow of energy, while at the same carrying out a final verification of the treatment and, if necessary, making additional corrections to any plexus that still shows signs of dysfunction.

The tests and corrections have been described with a single hand placed on the front of the body. In most cases, this is sufficient to obtain satisfactory corrections. However, in some cases, it is clear that an anterior approach alone is insufficient and does not improve dysfunction. In these cases, it will be necessary to use both hands in order to improve the effectiveness of the technique, with the second hand positioned on the posterior aspect of the body opposite the anterior hand. This is especially true for plexuses 1 to 5. However, if you wish to start using both hands from the beginning, this poses no problem.

Chronology of treatment

Treatment always begins with plexus no. 1 and proceeds to plexus no. 7. We only pass on to the next plexus once we have normalized the plexus being treated, or have at least obtained an improvement. We end the treatment with the final global test and, if necessary, go back and treat any plexus that still shows signs of dysfunction. By proceeding in this way, treatment will be more effective, and we will obtain both a quicker response and improvement of the symptoms.

Value of treatment and mode of action

Value of treatment

The value of treating the plexuses is obvious when we consider their physiology. All autonomous body functions are under their control, including respiration, circulation, the secretion of hormones, assimilation, stress management, etc. It is thanks to them that physiological functions take place, and for this reason we can say that they are guarantors of good health.

Plexus dysfunction may have different origins: stress, vertebral dysfunction, fascial tensions, all types of irritation, lifestyle, etc. All these disturbances act directly or indirectly on the plexuses. They act directly by disturbing the function of one or several plexuses, by disturbing heart rate, or by disturbing digestion. Stress in the broadest sense directly affects the plexuses, resulting in a modification of physiological functions and tissue tone, especially of the fascia. Indirectly, such disturbances affect fascial tension. Remember that fascia provides support for the plexuses and therefore disturbance of the fascia will easily affect the function of the plexus. A feedback will be established so that dysfunction of one will result in dysfunction of the other and, if the body is unable to 'normalize' the resulting vicious cycle, this will (in the long term) lead to a pathological process.

Mode of action of treatment

It follows from what has been stated previously that osteopathic treatment of dysfunction of the plexuses enables the osteopath to normalize the status of the plexus, thus restoring normal physiological function of the body and thereby guaranteeing good health. Many diseases are the result of persistent dysfunction, having evolved over a long period of time, leading to chronicity and disease. By extrapolating this line of thought, we can say that the ultimate goal of all osteopathic treatment, by 'normalizing' the different structures, particularly the fascia, is to 'normalize' the tonicity of the sympathetic and parasympathetic systems and thus restore normal physiological function.

Response to treatment

Response to treatment of the plexuses, especially in the presence of dysfunction, is very rapid. It can manifest immediately during the treatment session, or within a few days after the intervention. In any case, there should be a rapid functional response. A lack of response is in most cases due to inadequate treatment.

Indications for treatment of the plexuses

Given the omnipresence of the plexuses, there can be no treatment without influencing these subtle structures, so therefore any treatment will affect the plexuses. However, we should keep in mind that treatment of all the plexuses is a lengthy process that requires a complete course of treatment that can only be carried out systematically.

Treatment of *all* the plexuses is generally successful:

- when the patient complains of prolonged fatigue and lack of energy

- in the case of mild seasonal depression.

In most cases the results are immediate, with complete disappearance of the symptoms. In all other cases we treat individual plexuses when necessary, based on the presenting dysfunction and the area to be treated:

- If we are dealing with a urogenital problem, the plexuses involved will usually be plexuses no. 1 and 2, as well as plexus no. 6 in some cases.

- Plexus no. 3 and sometimes plexus no. 2 are usually involved in digestive problems.

- In the case of cardiopulmonary problems, plexus no. 4 is primarily involved, without forgetting the inter-relationships with plexuses no. 5 and 3.

There are many other examples, but a sound knowledge of anatomy, physiology, and pathology will direct the practitioner toward the appropriate treatment.

Conclusion

The sympathetic and parasympathetic nervous systems, and by extension the plexuses, are still poorly understood systems in medicine. The subtleties of their functions and their actions on human physiology remain elusive due to a lack of comprehensive, in-depth studies. This system clearly intervenes continuously in all physiological functions of the body and is one of the main guarantors of good health. Its omnipresence means that all osteopathic treatment has an effect on this system. Working on the plexuses is therefore very helpful in the treatment of patients. It reinforces our osteopathic action, increases the efficiency of our treatment, and ensures more stable results. Further in-depth study of the fascia will undoubtedly enable us to improve our performance in the future.

References

1. Woon J. T, Stringer M. D. The anatomy of the sacrococcygeal cornual region and its clinical relevance. *Anat Sci Int* 2014;89:207–214.

2. Woon J. T, Stringer M. D. The anatomy of the sacrococcygeal cornual region and its clinical relevance. *Anat Sci Int* 2014;89:207–214.

3. Ellinas H., Sethna N. F. Ganglion impar block for management of chronic coccydynia in an adolescent. *Paediatr Anaesth* 2009;19: 1137–1138.

4. Alsaid B., Diallo D., Benoit G., Bessede T. Identification of the origin of adrenergic and cholinergic nerve fibers within the superior hypogastric plexus of the human fetus. *J Anat* 2013;223:14–21.

5. Baader B., Baader S. L, Herrmann M., Stenzl A. [Autonomic innervation of the female pelvis. Anatomic basis]. *Urologe A* 2004;43:133–140

6. Alsaid B., Bessede T., Karam I., Abd-Alsamad I., Uhl J. F, Benoît G., Droupy S., Delmas V.

Coexistence of adrenergic and cholinergic nerves in the inferior hypogastric plexus: anatomical and immunohistochemical study with 3D reconstruction in human male fetus. *J Anat* 2009;214:645–654.

7. Sişu A. M., Petrescu C. I, Cebzan C. C., Motoc A., Bolintineanu S., Vaida A. M., Niculescu M. C., Rusu M. C. The adult coeliac ganglion: a morphologic study. *Rom J Morphol Embryol* 2008;49:491–494.

8. Loukas M., Klaassen Z., Merbs W., Tubbs R. S., Gielecki J., Zurada A. A review of the thoracic splanchnic nerves and celiac ganglia. *Clin Anat* 2010;23:512–522.

9. Andriesh V. N. [The participation of the celiac plexus in the innervation of the bronchi and pulmonary vessels]. *Arkh Anat Gistol Embriol* 1981;81:51–57.

10. de Carvalho C. A., Rodrigues Júnior A. J., Chih C. L. [Innervation of the heart from an abdominal plexus in man]. *Arq Gastroenterol* 1985;22:7–11.

11. Beaumont E., Salavatian S., Southerland E. M., Vinet A., Jacquemet V., Armour J. A., Ardell J. L. Network interactions within the canine intrinsic cardiac nervous system: implications for reflex control of regional cardiac function. *J Physiol* 2013;591:4515–4533.

12. Kobayashi M., Sakurai S., Takaseya T., Shiose A., Kim H. I., Fujiki M., Karimov J. H., Dessoffy R., Massiello A., Borowski A. G., Van Wagoner D. R., Jung E., Fukamachi K. Effects of percutaneous stimulation of both sympathetic and parasympathetic cardiac autonomic nerves on cardiac function in dogs. *Innovations* 2012;7:282–289.

13. Kobayashi M., Massiello A., Karimov J. H., Van Wagoner D. R., Fukamachi K. Cardiac autonomic nerve stimulation in the treatment of heart failure. *Ann Thorac Surg* 2013;96:339–345.

14. Hotta H., Lazar J., Orman R., Koizumi K., Shiba K., Kamran H., Stewart M. Vagus nerve stimulation-induced bradyarrhythmias in rats. *Auton Neurosci* 2009;151:98–105.

15. Hotta H., Lazar J., Orman R., Koizumi K., Shiba K., Kamran H., Stewart M. Vagus nerve stimulation-induced bradyarrhythmias in rats. *Auton Neurosci* 2009;151:98–105.

16. Chang C. H., Lo P. C. Effects of long-term dharma-chan meditation on cardiorespiratory synchronization and heart rate variability behavior. *Rejuvenation Res* 2013;16:115–123.

17. Silva J. E., Bianco S. D. Thyroid-adrenergic interactions: physiological and clinical implications. *Thyroid* 2008:157–165.

18. Côté M., Salzman K. L., Sorour M., Couldwell W. T. Normal dimensions of the posterior pituitary bright spot on magnetic resonance imaging. *J Neurosurg* 2014;120:357–362.

19. Kyung S. E., Botelho J. V., Horton J. C. Enlargement of the sella turcica in pseudotumor cerebri. *J Neurosurg* 2014;120:538–542.

20. Samarasinghe S., Emanuele M. A., Mazhari A. Neurology of the pituitary. *J Clin Endocrinol Metab* 2014;99:1758–1766.

21. Kaltsas G., Vgontzas A., Chrousos G. Fatigue, endocrinopathies, and metabolic disorders. *PM R* 2010;2:393–398.

22. Csernus V., Mess B. Biorhythms and pineal gland. *Neuro Endocrinol Lett* 2003;24:404–411.

23. Shi L., Li N., Bo L., Xu Z. Melatonin and hypothalamic-pituitary-gonadal axis. *Curr Med Chem* 2013;20:2017–2031.

24. Pallotti S., Nordio M., Giuliano S. [Melatonin/circadian rhythm. Is there a feedback between epiphysis and hypophysis?]. *Minerva Endocrinol* 2002;27:73–77.

TECHNIQUES FOR BODY CAVITIES

Torsten Liem, Rüdiger C. Goldenstein, Patrick Van Den Heede

Summary

In this chapter, a brief introduction is given to the morphodynamic osteopathic approach. The functions of the fascial tissue will be briefly described, in relation to space formation during embryonic development. Following this, the practical treatment approach is outlined in general before relevant techniques are described in more detail.

Introduction

Although the term 'techniques' is used in the title of this chapter, we would like to point out that morphodynamic treatment is not so much about certain techniques; a better phrase would be 'ways to approach the tissue'. What is presented here are insights into the developmental processes of the body. Technique in the framework of morphodynamics means the intention to listen to the body, in line with the phrase: 'treatment occurs during treatment'. In this sense, there is no treatment technique, other than supporting the physiology of the body. This goes in line with the traditional view of 'looking for health and the unperturbed expression of the body'.

As with all written work, we also stress the fact that the following techniques can be described but never properly taught within the framework of a book. To study certain treatment approaches, appropriate practical courses are necessary with supervisory guidance and instructions. The palpatory perception of stress patterns is highly individual, so the studying practitioner can be guided to identify possible expressions of developmental patterns in the body of the patient. Moreover, as will be described at the beginning of the practical examples, as a practitioner it is important to know to what extent one's own patterns could influence the perception and interpretation of palpatory findings in patients.

Morphodynamic osteopathic therapy

As Patrick Van Den Heede says: 'I do not want to perform techniques. I am trying to approach the body of the patient with my own consciousness'. The mental image of body structures and knowledge of the developmental patterns serves as a way to achieve an approximation of the patient's tissues. The mesenchyme (in this context we can call it a fascia) has stored all information, and thus all encountered events that occurred during its development, in its tissues.

The morphodynamic osteopathic contact makes this information accessible to the body's awareness and helps to bring processes in which the body was 'stuck' and that have not been fully processed or completed to a conclusion. Osteopathy does not treat – osteopathy informs.

We should therefore allow the body to ask: what has compromised health and where is the compromised health expressed? Health in this context is understood as the highest achievable potential of vitality that can be reached through genetic and epigenetic factors. The body tries to perform its duties with minimum energy consumption, like a watercourse that always seeks the path of least resistance. If somewhere in the body obstacles are formed, this may lead to a correspondent increased force, which may be expressed in increased tensions at certain balance points. The osteopathic treatment, at whatever level it may occur, whether with more mechanical intention to improve movement around joints, muscles, or tendons, or more focused on a holistic energetic point of view, should always serve the body as a whole, to allow energy-efficient work and expression. The movements in the compartments and segments of the body as well as the tissues will be facilitated by the treatment. As a result, energy consumption can be reduced, and more energy and space (freedom) is available for further 'development' of the organism.

The role of body cavities

As already described in Chapter 000, the role of the fascia within the framework of development and from a morphodynamic standpoint consists of creation of space and connection between the various body compartments.

Figure 55.1 shows an example of the formation of body cavities through the fascia (mesenchymal wrappings/linings) in the embryo. The internal fascia borders the visceral structures (visceral fascia) and the meningeal structures (meningeal fascia). Both fascias provide spaces for movement and shifting, through which the developmental movements of the embryo become possible. Hence, at different time points, different space-time patterns occur. This leads to the formation of hinge joints: contact and turning points of movements. Ultimately, all these movement patterns

- Visceral fascia
- Meningeal fascia
- Cylinders surrounded by axial fascia
- *The fascial being looks like embryonic being missing arms and legs* (F. Willard)

1 Develop_ment of CNS
a Ascencus cerebri
b Mesencephalic flexure and pontine flexure
c First stage of telencephalisation
d Final telencephalisation
e Cerebellar development

2 Development of cardiac cavity
a Cardiac tube formation
b Outflow tract anlage
c Torque and cropping of the heart

3 Development of lungs
a Budding and sprouting of bronchi
b Segmentation of lung Anlagen

4. Development of liver/pancreas
a Liver bud / pancreas bud
b Development of liver
c Development of pancreas

5 Development of digestive tract
a Stomadeum
b Descensus viscerum
c Looping of digestive tract

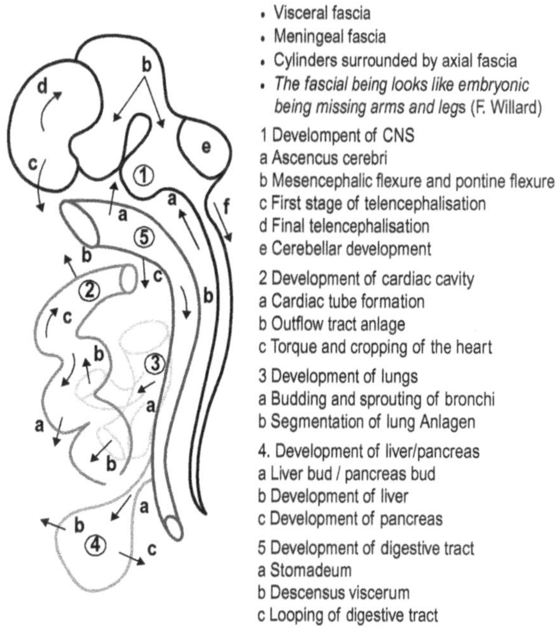

Figure 55.1

Formation of body cavities by the internal fascia.

serve the alignment of the various body structures but also the creation of physiological compounds. These space-time patterns are stored in the tissues (space-time units) and can be used at a later time as approximation points.

The specific roles/tasks of the body cavities are:

- compartmentalization, involving the formation of different spatial areas, both structurally and physiologically

- protection of organs

- organ mobility

- physiological integrity

- to provide guidance and freedom of arterial, venous, and lymphatic flow

- organization of fields.

Early in embryonic development the flow of directions is defined by spatial boundaries (Figure 55.2).

Note: The first space formations by mesenchymal cells can be traced back to very early embryonic development. This function is already evident in the development of the yolk sac and amniotic cavity. The developmental patterns repeat themselves. The mesenchyme or mesenchymal cells repeatedly form spaces during the entire development, segregate spaces from each other, and enable movement and contact between each other.

In the context of this chapter, techniques (or rather approximations) for body cavities and possible treatment approaches are described.

Treatment aims

We are not able to heal pathologies. However, we do believe that by osteopathic treatment we will be achieving an improvement of exchange between the tissues and better communication amongst the different body areas. If imbalancing influences and tensions are resolved, it may be possible that covert pathologies in the context of self-healing processes disappear. In this way, as already pointed out, the energy required for the maintenance of homeostasis will be reduced, which in turn promotes the health of the organism. This in turn means it can respond better to internal and external influences.

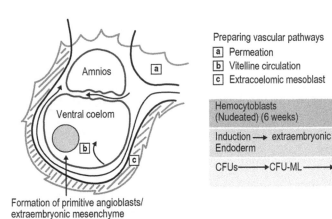

Preparing vascular pathways

- [a] Permeation
- [b] Vitelline circulation
- [c] Extracoelomic mesoblast

Hemocytoblasts (Nudeated) (6 weeks)	Pluripotent

Induction → extraembryonic Endoderm

CFUs——→CFU-ML——→ Lymphoid stem cells
Myeloid stem cells

Figure 55.2
Representation of the early flow patterns. CFUs = colony-forming units of spleen; CFU-ML = colony-forming units myelolymphoid)

Formation of primitive angioblasts/ extraembryonic mesenchyme

Treatment procedure

General preparation for techniques in view of morphodynamic treatment

For this type of palpation, it is important that the practitioner is continuously aware of his own position in the room; his own midlines; and his body, mood, and energy states. This serves to avoid interpretation of his own imbalanced patterns as being the pattern of the patient.

The practitioner centers himself before physically contacting the patient, in order to refine his perception and for him to be receptive. Once physical contact is made with the patient, the practitioner may recenter himself again.

Generally, as a practitioner, I should ask myself the following questions:

- Where in the body do I feel my greatest silence/ peace?

- How do I sit or stand most efficiently?

- In palpating, how do I feel best and most relaxed?

- What, for me, is the optimum height of the treatment couch?

Specific examples of techniques

Relationship between heart cavity and coelom cavity (visceropleura)

In its own development the heart has followed the development of all other organs and has stored this information in its own structure and orientation. It is almost pure mesenchymal tissue and, as such, it is in close contact with all developmental processes of the body. Therefore, the mesenchymal heart field can be included in the process of approximation of tissue memory.

The heart gets the first information through the splanchnopleura. Via currents and field effects, further developments of the body occur that go beyond the organ boundaries. Each organ is assigned a certain space in its development, and its boundaries are determined by other organ fields. Structurally, the mesenchymal tissue (fascia in the broadest sense) is always involved. Fascial tissue facilitates space formation, differentiation, and contact between different cavities.

Figure 55.3 shows the positional relationships between heart cavity and coelom cavity. Palpation is aimed at perception of motion patterns. Early fluctuations are caused by segmentations and axis-and-space formation.

Patient position

The patient is lying relaxed in supine position. Further relaxation of the patient can be achieved by placing pillows under the knees or by bending the knees and placing the feet flat on the treatment couch.

Position of practitioner and hand position

- The practitioner stands at the right side of the treatment couch. The right hand is in contact with the heart mesenchyme. The left hand is placed on the abdomen, in contact with the visceropleura.

Figure 55.3

Relationships between heart cavity and coelom cavity. (A) A Primitive coelomic cavity; (1) Cardiac coelom; (2) Centrum phrenicum; (3) Hepatic coelom; (4) Intestinal coelom; (5) Perineal coelom

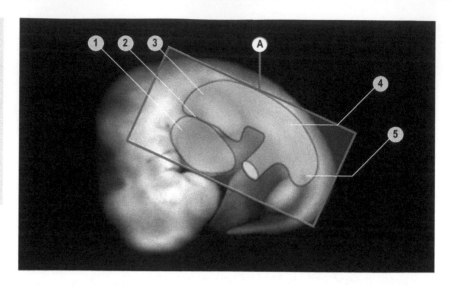

- Note: The practitioner needs to achieve a stable fulcrum. Frequently, the treatment couch is adjusted too high, hence the practitioner will loose his own fulcrum in the process of tissue approximation.

Implementation

After the information from these two areas is recorded, both areas will be brought into relationship with each other. Possible tension patterns will be detected and a balance between the two visualized cavities will be restored.

Heart mesenchyme and splanchnopleura (two practitioners)

This treatment approach aims to identify any points of tension during the development of these two regions and, if they are present, to achieve a balance point between them. The heart field is to be regarded as a mesenchymal developmental area or developmental field. There is a relationship to somitomeres 1–4 of the occiput as the ectodermal developmental field and the underlying following four somitomeres.

The sacrum as the counterpart of the cranium represents the final structure of the erection. It is also a densification of somitomeres and is formed of paraxial mesoderm. It provides the connections to the peritoneal field via the splanchnopleura.

Technique for two practitioners (Fig. 55.4)

The patient is lying relaxed in supine position at a sufficient distance from the head of the table. This allows the practitioner to easily (depending on hand positions at the head) place their forearms or elbows on the table, which serves to establish a corresponding fulcrum without introducing further tensions in the practitioner. Further relaxation of the patient can be achieved by placing pillows under the knees or by bending the knees and placing the feet flat on the treatment couch.

Practitioner 1: sitting and hand position

Practitioner 1 sits at the head end of the patient, who lies supine. The left hand is placed in contact with the occiput from the dorsal direction, the palm of the right hand lies ventrally over the sternum, in contact with the heart field.

Implementation

- An approximation of the heart mesenchyme is performed (i.e., the practitioner does not actively seek structural information but waits until a tissue information of a developmental field is perceived).

- The dorsal left hand under the occiput takes up the information of the development of the somitomeres. The ventral hand takes up information from the heart field. Between both hands the achievement of a balance point is encouraged.

Practitioner 2: sitting and hand positions

Practitioner 2 sits next to the patient on the right-hand side. The right hand is placed between the legs of the patient underneath the sacrum. The left hand rests flat, with the heel of the hand on the patient's pubis, fingers directed toward the head and placed on the abdomen.

Implementation

- After contact with the patient has been established as described above, the practitioner awaits information about individual developmental patterns, thus being able to perceive the different depths and developmental dynamics information from the caudal somitomeres, which built the sacrum. Information from the splanchnopleura of the abdomen will most likely also be perceived. Again, a balancing point between the two fields is anticipated.

- When both practitioners have reached the balance point within the fields that they are working on, both fields are balanced with each other. A so-called 'hinge' is created – a balance point at the level of the diaphragm.

- Note: This technique can also be performed by one practitioner in succession, for example, by contacting the heart field first, then both fields are placed in relation to each other by placing one hand ventrally onto the heart field and one hand onto the peritoneal field.

Technique in the peritoneal developmental area (Fig. 55.5)

Patient position

The patient is lying relaxed in supine position. Further relaxation of the patient can be achieved by placing pillows under the knees or by bending the knees and placing the feet flat on the treatment couch.

Practitioner sitting and hand positions

The practitioner stands laterally on the right-hand side of the lying patient at the level of the hips. Contact with the lateroconal fascia is made by placing the right hand in the region of the descending colon and the left hand in the region of the ascending colon.

Implementation

The deveopmental information of these regions will be compared according to the tension patterns and a balance encouraged.

Technique for balancing the meningeal space with the visceropleura (two practitioners) (Fig. 55.6)

Practitioners 1 and 2: sitting and hand positions

- Practitioner 1 establishes contact as described above (see the section on 'Technique in the peritoneal developmental area').

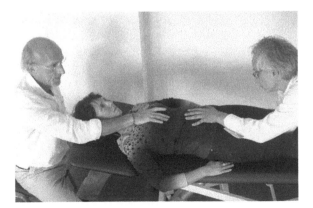

Figure 55.4
Technique for balancing heart mesenchyme – splanchnopleura

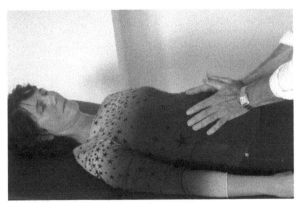

Figure 55.5
Technique in the peritoneal developmental area

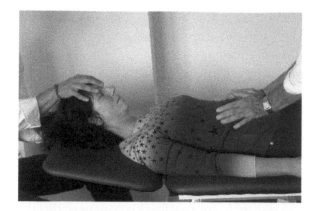

Figure 55.6
Technique for balancing the meningeal space with the visceropleura

- Practitioner 2 sits at the head end of the patient, the palm of the left hand lies flat under the occiput, the index and middle fingers of the right hand in contact with the glabella.

Implementation

- Practitioner 1: see the section on 'Technique in the peritoneal developmental area'.

- Practitioner 2 generates a balance via his two hands through the falx cerebri and the venous sinus.

- Following that, a balance between both therapeutic fields is anticipated.

Technique for balancing the pleural area (Fig. 55.7)

Patient position

The patient lies in supine position.

Practitioner: sitting and hand positions

The practitioner takes up a position at the head end of the patient, placing his hands under the shoulder blades of the patient.

Implementation

The practitioner establishes contact with the pleural cavity of the lungs. By imagining the appropriate cavities, tension patterns will be detected and brought to a balance.

Technique of pelvic compression – erection of the peritoneal sac against the retroperitoneal space and the diaphragma (Fig. 55.8)

Patient position

The patient lies on the left side, legs bent, head supported by a pillow.

Position of practitioner and hand position

The practitioner is standing behind the patient, well supported by the edge of the treatment table, at the level

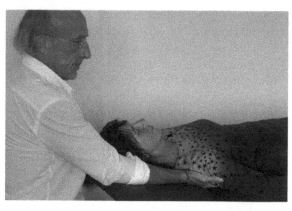

Figure 55.7
Technique for balancing the pleural area

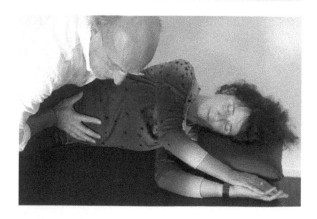

Figure 55.8
Technique for pelvic compression – erection of the peritoneal sac against the retroperitoneal space and the diaphragm

of the patient's pelvic area. The practitioner performs a compression of the patient's pelvis with his own body. He also establishes dorsal contact with the patient's body with his left hand at the level of T12. Ventrally, contact is established with the palm of the right hand, and a caudocranial compression to the peritoneal sac of the patient will be performed. At the same time, the rotational ability of the peritoneal sac is tested.

Implementation

The practitioner determines the peritoneal movement patterns, exerts a counter pressure on T12, and waits for a balance point. This allows freedom of the peritoneal erection movement against the retroperitoneal space and the diaphragm.

Technique for balancing the mediastinal cavity against T6 in sitting (Fig. 55.9)

Patient position

The patient sits on the treatment table in a stable position.

Practitioner: sitting and hand positions

The practitioner sits next to the patient on the right-hand side. He establishes dorsal contact with the patient's spine with his left hand at the level of T6, and ventrally he places the palm of his right hand on the sternum.

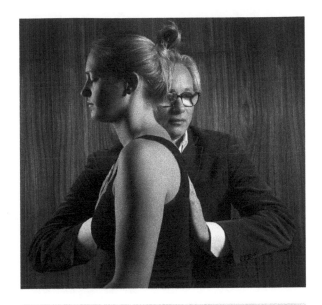

Figure 55.9
Technique for balancing the mediastinal cavity against T6 in seating

Implementation

The practitioner determines the developmental information and rotational movement of the mediastinal space, follows the occurring spiral movement to its base, and waits for a balance point.

Note: Page number followed by f and t indicate figure and table respectively.